Clinical Neurophysiology

Clinical Neurophysiology

Editor: Donald Chilton

AMERICAN
MEDICAL PUBLISHERS
www.americanmedicalpublishers.com

AMERICAN
MEDICAL PUBLISHERS
www.americanmedicalpublishers.com

Cataloging-in-Publication Data

Clinical neurophysiology / edited by Donald Chilton.
p. cm.
Includes bibliographical references and index.
ISBN 979-8-88740-000-6
1. Neurophysiology. 2. Neurobiology. 3. Physiology.
4. Clinical medicine. I. Chilton, Donald.
QP355.2 .C55 2023
612.8--dc23

American Medical Publishers,
41 Flatbush Avenue,
1st Floor, New York,
NY 11217, USA

ISBN 979-8-88740-000-6 (Hardback)

Contents

Preface

Neurophysiology is a branch of study that draws from two fields, namely, physiology and neurology. Physiology refers to the study of how human body works and neurology relates to the study of the nervous system. Therefore, the field of neurophysiology deals with the working of the nervous system and its components such as neurons and glia. The nervous system can be divided into two parts, namely, the central nervous system (CNS) and the peripheral nervous system (PNS). The CNS is made up of the brain and spinal cord, whereas the PNS comprises the nerves that extend from the CNS and branch out towards the muscles, glands, and sense organs. Clinical neurophysiology analyses the central and peripheral nervous systems by observing the spontaneous as well as induced electrical activity of neurons. It includes pathophysiology research and clinical strategies for diagnosing disorders affecting both the central and peripheral nervous systems. The significant treatment methods used in clinical neurophysiology include electromyography, nerve conduction studies (NCS), electroencephalography, and evoked potentials. This book elucidates the concepts and innovative models around prospective developments in clinical neurophysiology. It presents various researches and studies undertaken by experts across the globe. The readers would gain substantial knowledge that would broaden their perspective with respect to clinical neurophysiology.

This book is a result of research of several months to collate the most relevant data in the field.

When I was approached with the idea of this book and the proposal to edit it, I was overwhelmed. It gave me an opportunity to reach out to all those who share a common interest with me in this field. I had 3 main parameters for editing this text:

1. Accuracy - The data and information provided in this book should be up-to-date and valuable to the readers.

2. Structure - The data must be presented in a structured format for easy understanding and better grasping of the readers

3. Universal Approach - This book not only targets students but also experts and innovators in the field, thus my aim was to present topics which are of use to all

Thus, it took me a couple of months to finish the editing of this book.

I would like to make a special mention of my publisher who considered me worthy of this opportunity and also supported me throughout the editing process. I would also like to thank the editing team at the back-end who extended their help whenever required.

Editor

1

Inference of human affective states from psychophysiological measurements extracted under ecologically valid conditions

Alberto Betella[1†], Riccardo Zucca[1†], Ryszard Cetnarski[1], Alberto Greco[2,3], Antonio Lanatà[2,3], Daniele Mazzei[2], Alessandro Tognetti[2,3], Xerxes D. Arsiwalla[1], Pedro Omedas[1], Danilo De Rossi[2,3] and Paul F. M. J. Verschure[1,4]*

[1] *Synthetic, Perceptive, Emotive and Cognitive Systems group (SPECS), Universitat Pompeu Fabra, Barcelona, Spain*
[2] *Research Centre "E. Piaggio", University of Pisa, Pisa, Italy*
[3] *Information Engineering Department, University of Pisa, Pisa, Italy*
[4] *ICREA, Institució Catalana de Recerca i Estudis Avançats, Barcelona, Spain*

***Correspondence:**
Paul F. M. J. Verschure, Synthetic, Perceptive, Emotive and Cognitive Systems group (SPECS), Universitat Pompeu Fabra, C/Roc Boronat 138, Barcelona 08018, Spain
e-mail: paul.verschure@upf.edu

† These authors have contributed equally to this work.

Compared to standard laboratory protocols, the measurement of psychophysiological signals in real world experiments poses technical and methodological challenges due to external factors that cannot be directly controlled. To address this problem, we propose a hybrid approach based on an immersive and human accessible space called the eXperience Induction Machine (XIM), that incorporates the advantages of a laboratory within a life-like setting. The XIM integrates unobtrusive wearable sensors for the acquisition of psychophysiological signals suitable for ambulatory emotion research. In this paper, we present results from two different studies conducted to validate the XIM as a general-purpose sensing infrastructure for the study of human affective states under ecologically valid conditions. In the first investigation, we recorded and classified signals from subjects exposed to pictorial stimuli corresponding to a range of arousal levels, while they were free to walk and gesticulate. In the second study, we designed an experiment that follows the classical conditioning paradigm, a well-known procedure in the behavioral sciences, with the additional feature that participants were free to move in the physical space, as opposed to similar studies measuring physiological signals in constrained laboratory settings. Our results indicate that, by using our sensing infrastructure, it is indeed possible to infer human event-elicited affective states through measurements of psychophysiological signals under ecological conditions.

Keywords: affect, conditioning, ecological validity, EDR, ECG, emotions, VR, wearable devices

1. INTRODUCTION

Decades of psychophysiological studies have demonstrated the role of the Autonomic Nervous System (ANS) in modulating human physiological responses (Andreassi, 2006; Cacioppo et al., 2007; Boucsein, 2012). This has facilitated an important channel for the inference of human affective states. In particular, two important physiological measurements of autonomic responses, namely, the electrodermal response (EDR) and electrocardiogram (ECG), have been widely used as indicators of psychological internal states and processes, due to their relative non-invasiveness, easy quantification and reliability (see Berntson et al., 2007; Dawson et al., 2007 for a review). ECG and EDR allow the extraction of heart-rate variability (HRV) and skin conductance (SC), respectively. HRV constitutes an objective index of sympatho-vagal balance (Stein et al., 1994; Acharya et al., 2006), while SC is a direct measure of eccrine sweat glands activity and reflects activity within the sympathetic axis of the ANS (Fowles et al., 1981; Valenza et al., 2010; Boucsein, 2012). EDR is acquired by measuring the electrical conductance on the skin of the hand palm (normally on the fingertips), where the concentration of eccrine glands is higher. The recorded signal consists of a superposition of two main components: a tonic level of skin conductance (SCL), representing the baseline of the signal, and a series of superimposed phasic increases in conductance. Each of these phasic elements represents a unitary skin conductance response (SCR), which reflects the response of eccrine sweat gland activity to an external stimulus (Boucsein, 2012). Heart rate is controlled by both the sympathetic and the parasympathetic branches of the ANS (Berntson et al., 2007). Among features that characterize cardiac response, one of the most reliable and robust measures with regard to ANS dynamics is HRV, which reflects the fluctuations of the cardiac beat-to-beat time distance (Acharya et al., 2006) and previous research has already shown that several HRV spectral measures are strictly related to sympatho-vagal balance variations (Stein et al., 1994; Valenza et al., 2013b). A broad consensus now exists among researchers that variations in electrical properties of the skin and cardiac activity are physiological markers of specific internal states associated to cognition and emotion

(Ekman et al., 1983; Lang et al., 1993; Lang, 1995; Healey and Picard, 2005; Greco et al., 2012; Lanatà et al., 2012; Valenza et al., 2014).

Nonetheless, these physiological measures are prone to contamination by noise and artifacts that dramatically reduce their quality and reliability (Boucsein, 2012) and often occur on the same bandwidth as the signal, thus affecting its precision and informative utility. As a matter of fact, both ECG and EDR can be severely affected by such artifacts if not properly treated. External sources, such as the common power line noise (hum), can be detected from the spectrogram of the recorded signal and successfully reduced employing online or offline filters (or a combination of both). Other artifacts are due to physiological factors and are more difficult to treat. For instance, deep or irregular breathing, as well as speech, often induce an increase of non-specific EDR components (Hygge and Hugdahl, 1985; Schneider et al., 2003). In addition, physical activity itself can covary with the recorded physiological signals (Picard and Healey, 1997). The latter becomes a crucial issue in wearable systems, when acquisition is performed under real life conditions. For this reason, most research is often conducted under strictly controlled laboratory settings or artificial clinical environments, where the subject is usually wired to a fixed equipment and asked to avoid gross body movements in order to ensure optimal conditions in the acquisition of high quality signals. Strict laboratory settings, however, introduce other limitations. For instance, physiological responses, which are normally recorded for short segments of time (mainly due to the discomfort produced by long term use of the equipment) may not reflect the entire spectrum of emotional experiences that occur under everyday situations (Picard, 2000; Healey and Picard, 2005; Healey et al., 2010). These shortcomings spurred an increased interest in the development and application of wearable technologies to different fields of research from clinical and rehabilitation to behavioral studies (Valenza et al., 2008; Lanatà et al., 2010a; Pantelopoulos and Bourbakis, 2010; Poh et al., 2010; Lanatà et al., 2011; Boucsein, 2012; Patel et al., 2012). In addition, a good amount of ambulatory physiological research has recently been directed toward the development of devices that are both accurate and robust to motion artifacts, while, at the same time, comfortable to wear, easy to use (Picard and Healey, 1997; Ebner-Priemer and Kubiak, 2007) and reliable for investigating physiological correlates of emotions in natural settings. Despite these advances, experiments involving psychophysiological measures of affective states in the natural world still present a number of technical drawbacks such as loss of connectivity during signal acquisition, fitting problems with the wearable devices, difficulty in accurately labeling data (which often relies exclusively on subjects' self-assessment) and other external factors, such as social interactions, that cannot be fully controlled by the experimenter.

In this context, laboratory settings and life-like conditions do not have to be seen as mutually exclusive paradigms, but can rather be viewed as complementary to each other (Fahrenberg et al., 2007). For instance, the use of Virtual Reality (VR) offers an excellent compromise between the laboratory and natural world. Through VR it is possible to create life-like environments where users can act through natural movements and gestures, while, at the same time, accounting for a systematic control of the stimuli and the variables that are studied. For this reason, we have built the eXperience Induction Machine (XIM), an immersive space we previously used to study human behavior in ecologically valid conditions (Eng et al., 2005; Bernardet et al., 2007, 2010). More recently, we used the XIM to investigate the salience of social stimuli by measuring participants' physiological responses induced by spatial interaction with humans and avatars using a commercial data acquisition system (g.MobiLab, g.Tec, Austria). We showed that the salience of a social stimulus is directly mapped onto the physiological correlates of arousal (Inderbitzin et al., 2013). With the aim of conducting ambulatory emotion research, we expanded the XIM's capabilities with the integration of new wearable sensors for the acquisition of psychophysiological signals (Omedas et al., 2014). These devices are capable of real-time measurements of body posture, arm orientation, hand position, fingers movements, as well as psychophysiological signals such as ECG and EDR. These signals were specifically selected because of their reliability in inferring affective states and the possibility to integrate dedicated textile-based sensors on small-scale wearable devices (Paradiso and Caldani, 2010; Carbonaro et al., 2012).

In this paper we present results from two different studies conducted to validate the XIM as a general-purpose sensing infrastructure for investigating human affective states in life-like conditions. In the first investigation, we aimed to validate the quality of the signals acquired through our new pool of wearable sensors. To do so, we exposed subjects to pictorial stimuli, covering the full range of arousal levels, while walking and performing hand gestures in the XIM environment. By interpreting the participants' ECG and EDR signals we were able to correctly classify and predict the presented stimuli in terms of arousal classes (a short version of the results was presented in Betella et al., 2014).

In the second study, we investigated whether we can correctly infer the features of conditioning from the signals recorded in a subject freely acting in a physical space while trained with a classical conditioning protocol. Classical conditioning has for long been a well-grounded paradigm in cognitive and clinical neuroscience. In particular, conditioning has been widely investigated using EDR (see Boucsein, 2012 for a comprehensive review) and applied to different clinical treatments for anxiety, phobias and other behavioral disorders (Field, 2006). Our results not only demonstrate behavioral features of conditioning in an ecological setting, but also show how psychophysiological signatures of conditioning can be effectively extracted from the acquired signals.

In both our studies, the main goal was to use our sensing infrastructure (i.e., the XIM and the wearable sensors) to tackle the well-known challenge of measuring psychophysiological signals in the presence of movements and gestures, thus advancing beyond standard laboratory protocols. The obtained results confirm the validity of our approach for the inference of human event-elicited affective states in life-like conditions. We show that using our custom-made technology, it is indeed possible to infer participants' emotional states (i.e., arousal) from acquired psychophysiological signals.

2. MATERIALS AND METHODS

2.1. THE SENSING INFRASTRUCTURE

2.1.1. The eXperience Induction Machine (XIM)

The XIM (see an illustration in **Figure 1**) covers an area of about 25 m^2 and is equipped with a number of effectors that include 8 projectors, 4 projection screens, a luminous interactive floor (Delbruck et al., 2007) and a sonification system (Le Groux et al., 2007). Along with the effectors, the XIM features a pool of sensors to measure users' explicit behavior and implicit states, including a marker-free multi-modal tracking system (Mathews et al., 2012), microphones and floor-based pressure sensors.

2.1.2. Wearable sensing systems

The wearable devices used in this study were integrated into two main interfaces: a sensing glove for the simultaneous acquisition of hand gestures and EDR, and a sensing shirt for the acquisition of ECG and respiration. The choice of textile integrated sensors was primarily dictated by the advantages in terms of portability and usability for long-term monitoring and because they provide minimal constraints in terms of natural gestures and movements.

2.1.2.1. Sensing glove. The sensing glove (**Figure 2**) was specifically designed for the XIM space and it was conceived to measure both explicit (gestural information through forearm orientation and finger positions) and implicit (psychophysiological inference through EDR) signals. Two textile electrodes interwoven in the index and middle fingertips are used to measure EDR. In a previous work, electrical characteristics of interwoven textile electrodes were investigated in comparison with standard Ag/AgCl electrodes through simultaneous acquisition of the same EDR signals (Lanatà et al., 2012), where the impedance of textile electrodes in the EDR bandwidth was evaluated using a standard reference electrolytic cell and a high precision impedance meter. This study demonstrated that textile electrodes are equivalent to standard Ag/AgCl electrodes, thus allowing the acquisition of high quality signals. Grounded on previous results obtained with conductive elastomer sensors (Tognetti et al., 2006; Vanello et al., 2008), finger motion tracking is obtained through five

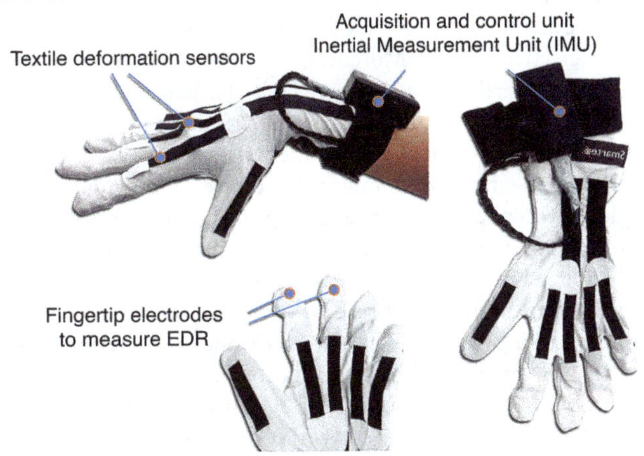

FIGURE 2 | The sensing glove and its main components. We refer the reader to the main text (Section 2.1.2.1) for a detailed explanation of the features.

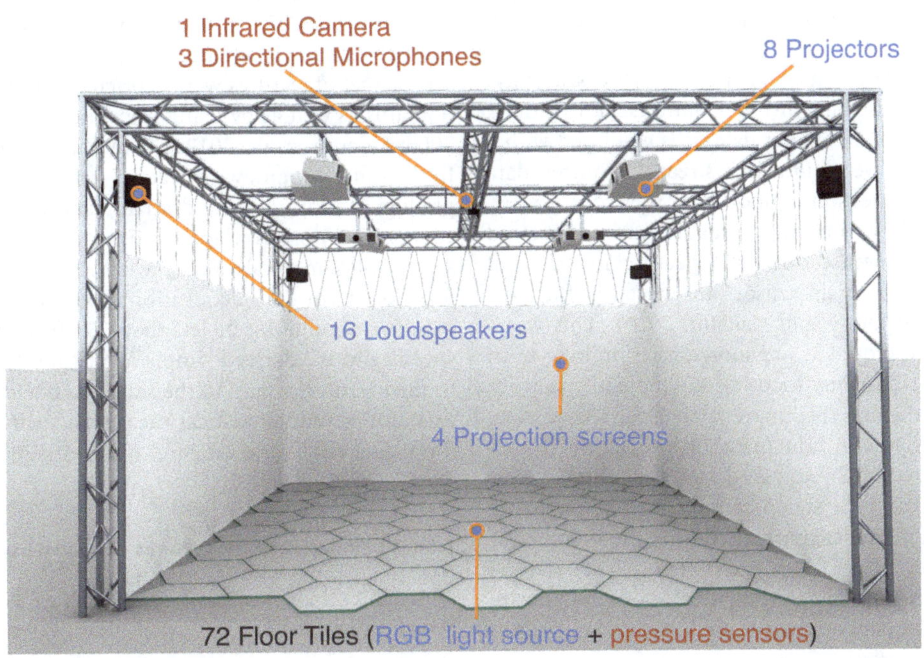

FIGURE 1 | Schematic illustration of the eXperience Induction Machine (XIM). XIM is a 5 × 5 × 4 m infrastructure equipped with a number of effectors (8 projectors, 4 projection screens, a luminous interactive floor and a sonification system) and sensors (marker-free multi-modal tracking system, microphones and floor-based pressure sensors). In addition, a custom-built sensing glove is used for the acquisition of hand gestures and electrodermal response (EDR), while a sensing shirt is used for the acquisition of electrocardiogram (ECG) signals and respiration (BR).

textile deformation sensors integrated on the glove metacarpophalangeal hand joints. Sensors are made of knitted piezoresistive fabric (KPF) material, previously demonstrated to be a valid choice for biomechanical and cardiopulmonary data acquisition (Taccini et al., 2008; Pacelli et al., 2013). Finger movements produce local deformations in the fabric that modify the electrical resistance of the sensors, which is highly correlated with the single finger degree of flexion. A customized algorithm for hand gestures recognition was developed (Carbonaro et al., 2012) to deal with the slow baseline drift of the sensor signal which is due to intrinsic characteristics of the textile substrate. Both EDR and deformation signals are acquired in real-time through a dedicated wearable and wireless electronic unit. Moreover, forearm orientation is measured by an Inertial Measurement Unit (HMC6343, Honeywell, MN, USA) embedded in the glove's electronics and worn on the dorsal area of the forearm close to the wrist.

Compared with other similar devices (e.g., the Aladin sensor glove Ritter, 2009), our sensing glove is not limited to the measurement of EDR, yet it integrates a broader pool of sensors while maintaining a high level of comfort and usability. Acquisition of fingers position and forearm orientation through wearable sensing systems allows to track fine user's actions more precisely and enable multi-user scenarios (i.e., avoiding the common problem of camera occlusion). In immersive environments, such as XIM, the use of low cost video-based systems like Kinect and LeapMotion does not guarantee an optimal resolution to track finger angles and hand/forearm orientation, especially when the users are not correctly positioned with respect to cameras. In addition, professional infrared (IR) sensors and magnetic or radio based tracking systems are usually prone to interference in cave-like environments due to the simultaneous presence of light projection systems, metal scaffolding and wireless devices.

2.1.2.2. Sensing shirt. The sensing shirt (Smartex srl, Italy) (Paradiso et al., 2005) is used in XIM to acquire ECG, Breathing Rate (BR) and tri-axial accelerometer data. It is equipped with a tiny electronic battery-powered unit that streams acquired data through a Bluetooth connection contained in the front pocket. ECG is acquired through two interwoven textile electrodes placed inside the shirt near the lower section of the pectoral muscles. BR is acquired through a KPF strain sensor interwoven in the shirt (Lanatà et al., 2010b; Paradiso and Caldani, 2010). This wearable system has been employed in previous studies on long-term monitoring of chronic patients, focusing on the early prevention of cardiovascular diseases (Scilingo et al., 2005). This sensing shirt has also been adopted in human-robot interaction studies aimed to investigate psychophysiological states of autistic children (Mazzei et al., 2012). The states were inferred by analysing signals acquired through the sensing shirt during the therapeutic protocol (Mazzei et al., 2010, 2011; Lazzeri et al., 2014) and the obtained results empirically validated the device's capabilities in the acquisition of high quality signals suitable for the analysis of psychophysiological measures.

2.1.3. Data recording

The data coming from the wearable devices is conveyed to the XIM sensing platform that captures and processes in real-time raw sensors data (Wagner et al., 2013a). This platform is implemented using the Social Signal Interpretation (SSI) framework (Wagner et al., 2013b), a set of tools for the recording, analysis and recognition of human behavior in real-time. The data stream of each sensor is transmitted through dedicated separate channels and preprocessed. The sensing platform then synchronizes the incoming streams by establishing a stable connection with all the sensors and by buffering data streams. Single buffers are compared upon regular time intervals according to an internal timestamp and synchronized, if necessary. Following the synchronization, each signal is processed separately to isolate noise and artifacts from relevant information.

2.2. ELECTROCARDIOGRAM

From the data recorded via the sensing shirt we computed the HRV signal as the variability of the distance between consecutive R-peaks over time. Currently, R-wave peaks were taken as the reference point. It is worthwhile noting that R-peak is the most reliable ECG-measure against noise-artifact that can be made with respect to other possible points of the QRS complex. Before extracting the R-peaks, the ECG signal was filtered using a Moving Average Filter (MAF) to extract and subtract the baseline since it is commonly affected by low frequency disturbances (e.g., respiration activity). The Heart Rate (HR) was defined as HR$= 60/t_{R-R}$, where t_{R-R} is the time interval between two successive R-peaks. In order to detect QRS complexes, we treated the ECG signal using the automatic QRS detection algorithm proposed by Pan and Tompkins (Pan and Tompkins, 1985) and after this procedure R-peaks could be extracted. The obtained HR resulted in a time series of non-uniform RR intervals, hence it was interpolated and re-sampled in accordance to the recommendations of Berger et al. (2007). In this study, we solely focused on the intervals between normal (sinus) beats (NN-intervals). Given RR time series, a set of features were extracted in both time and frequency domains as well as by using non-linear methods (Acharya et al., 2006; Valenza et al., 2012a), which are summarized in **Table 1**. In the time domain, we extracted statistical parameters and morphological indices. Time-domain features were computed within consecutive non-overlapping time windows of 30 s in which a series of RR intervals were present. It is worthwhile noting that, for short-term ECG acquisitions (i.e., lower than several hours), windows should not be less than 20 s (Camm et al., 1996). More specifically, we derived simple MNN and SDNN, corresponding to the mean value and to the standard deviation of the NN intervals, and several statistical measures, such as standard error of the mean, root mean square, mean of squares, sum of squares,

Table 1 | Summary of the features extracted from HRV/HR and SC signals.

Features extracted	Signal
MNN, SDNN, RMSSD, pNN50, VLF, LF, HF, LF/HF, SD1, SD2, E	HRV/HR
Lat, nSCR, Mean.SCR, Var.SCR, Max.SCR AmpSum, AUC.SCR, Mean.Tonic, Var.Tonic, NSR	SC

skewness, kurtosis' excess coefficient, mean absolute deviation, root mean square of successive differences of intervals (RMSSD), as well as several central moments. We also computed the number of consecutive differences of intervals, which differ by more than 50 ms (NN50) and the same features normalized with respect to the total number of intervals (pNN50).

In addition to the above statistical measures, a series of geometric measures were calculated from the RR intervals histogram. The HRV triangular index was obtained as the integral of the histogram (i.e., total number of RR intervals) divided by the height of the histogram, which was dependent on the selected bin width. Finally we extracted the TINN which corresponds to the baseline width of the RR histogram evaluated through triangular interpolation (see Camm et al., 1996 for details).

In the HRV frequency domain analysis, three main spectral components were distinguished in a spectrum calculated from short term recordings: Very Low Frequency (VLF) [0.003–0.04 Hz], Low Frequency (LF) [0.04–0.15 Hz], and High Frequency (HF) [0.15–0.4 Hz]. Short term recordings were intended as the time duration of HRV signal segments. In this work, HRV segments were in agreement with the picture presentation time. It is well known from the literature that the distribution of the spectral power gives an indication of modulations in the Autonomic Nervous System (ANS). Current HRV research in the frequency domain suggests that even though the frequency band division represents a unique non-invasive tool to achieve an assessment of autonomic function, the use of HF and LF components does not allow to precisely assess the state of sympathetic activation. Therefore, along with the estimation of the Power Spectral Density in the VLF, LF and HF band, we also calculated the LF/HF PSD Ratio which provides information about the Sympatho-Vagal balance (Camm et al., 1996).

In regards to non-linear analysis of HRV, it is reasonable to assume that non-linear mechanisms are involved in the genesis of HRV. In the latest decade, several non-linear measures have been used to investigate HRV behavior that do not fully comply with standard measures, neither in the time domain nor in the frequency domain. Further details on HRV non-linear methods can be found in Fusheng et al. (2000); Zbilut and Webber (2006); Chua et al. (2008); Valenza et al. (2012a,b, 2013a). In this work, we used the Poincaré plot (a graphical representation of the correlation between successive RR intervals) and entropy. More specifically, from the Poincaré plot we used the short and long term variability (i.e., SD1 and SD2). Moreover, non-linear measures often suffer from the curse of dimensionality, i.e., they cannot reliably be estimated because of the lack of a sufficient number of points in the time series. For this reason, we estimated system complexity which allows to quantitatively characterize the dynamics even with short time series (Kurths et al., 1995; Wessel et al., 2000). Entropy was also employed since it has already been adopted in HRV analysis with encouraging results (Pincus and Goldberger, 1994).

2.3. ELECTRODERMAL RESPONSE

EDR was obtained as the ratio between an imposed continuous voltage of 0.5 V applied to the index and middle fingers and the flowing current. In order to analytically split the EDR signal into its tonic (SCL) and phasic (SCR) components we adopted a convolution model (Benedek and Kaernbach, 2010a) where the Sudo-Motor Nerve Activity (SMNA) can be seen as the input of the model whose output is the EDR. The Impulse Response Function (IRF) is represented by a biexponential function (called the Bateman function) (Garrett, 1994), which is defined as follows:

$$IRF(t) = (e^{-\frac{t}{\tau_1}} - e^{-\frac{t}{\tau_2}}) \cdot u(t) \tag{1}$$

where $u(t)$ is the stepwise function. Consequently, the result of the deconvolution between the EDR signal and IRF can be defined as the *driver function*, describing the SMNA behavior. This processing method allows for the identification of intrinsically overlapped inter-stimulus phasic responses, which are due to a sequence of stimuli in time. Further details on the EDR deconvolution method can be found in Benedek and Kaernbach (2010a).

Skin conductance decomposition to its components was performed using Ledalab software package in MATLAB (Benedek and Kaernbach, 2010b). The signal was filtered by means of a low pass zero-phase forward and reverse digital filter (Mitra and Kuo, 2006) with a cutoff frequency of 2 Hz. The phasic features were calculated within a time window (response window) up to 5 s length following the stimulus onset. We extracted the number of SCRs within the response window (nSCR), the latency of the first SCR (Lat), the Amplitude-Sum of SCRs reconvolved from phasic driver-peaks (AmpSum), the average phasic driver activity (Mean.SCR) as the time integral over response window by size of response window, the variance of the phasic driver signal (Var.SCR), the Phasic driver area under curve (AUC.SCR) and the maximum phasic driver amplitude (Max.SCR).

From the tonic driver signal, we obtained the following features: average level of (decomposed) tonic component (Mean.Tonic), variance of the tonic driver signal (Var.Tonic) and number of the non-specific response (i.e., the spontaneous skin conductance response unrelated to a specific stimulus) (NSR). See **Table 1** for a summary of the features extracted.

2.4. MOVEMENT DETECTION AND ARTIFACTS

Along with the acquired ECG and EDR signals, acceleration, finger flexion and forearm orientation were also recorded using the tri-axial accelerometer, textile deformation sensors and the Inertial Measurement Unit embedded in the sensing shirt and glove (see Section 2.1.2 for more details). Moreover, in the first study all the subjects were video recorded for the entire duration of the experiment, and a precise annotation of the type of movements performed by the subjects was obtained. These sources of information were then used to isolate body movements (e.g., in our scenario the subject walks in XIM, grabs virtual objects and/or points with the hand toward different parts of the virtual scene), and subsequently identify those parts of the physiological signals that were potentially affected by motion artifacts.

In general, we expect portions of the acquired signals to be affected by artifacts, that are alternated with unaffected "clean" segments. The amount of affected signal increases depending on the intensity of the physical activity and frequency of movement. In this context, we hypothesize that, at least in the case of mild physical activity related to interaction in virtual reality, the segments of clean signals that can be extracted are sufficient to allow for a reliable identification of event-elicited affective states. Motion artifacts mostly affected the EDR signal due to the gesture of grabbing that induces a physical movement of the EDR electrodes. ECG signal measured on the subject's chest, instead, is normally not affected by hand or arms gestures. For this reason ECG recording was preprocessed as reported in Section 2.2 and the entire time window related to the stimuli presentation was used to further analyze the ECG signal.

An example of EDR signals acquired from the sensing glove in a representative subject, with and without the motion artifact induced by a series of grabbing gestures, is provided in **Figure 3A.** To do so, we acquired simultaneously EDR using two gloves, on the left and on the right hand, respectively. We instructed the subject to relax as much as possible (to avoid changes in affective states) and to use only the right hand to perform a series of grabbing gestures. Given the high impact of this gesture on the acquired EDR measure, the signal affected by this artifact cannot be used for affective states classification. These artifacts are due to skin stretch and/or compression and are particularly evident during the grabbing events, when the electrodes mounted on the glove fingertips physically touch the hand palm. **Figure 3B** illustrates the glove finger signals in correspondence to the EDR red trace in **Figure 3A** and clearly shows that fingers motion and EDR signal affected by the gesture are highly correlated. This qualitative observation is further confirmed by a Fourier analysis performed on fingers flexion and EDR during slow hand grabbing

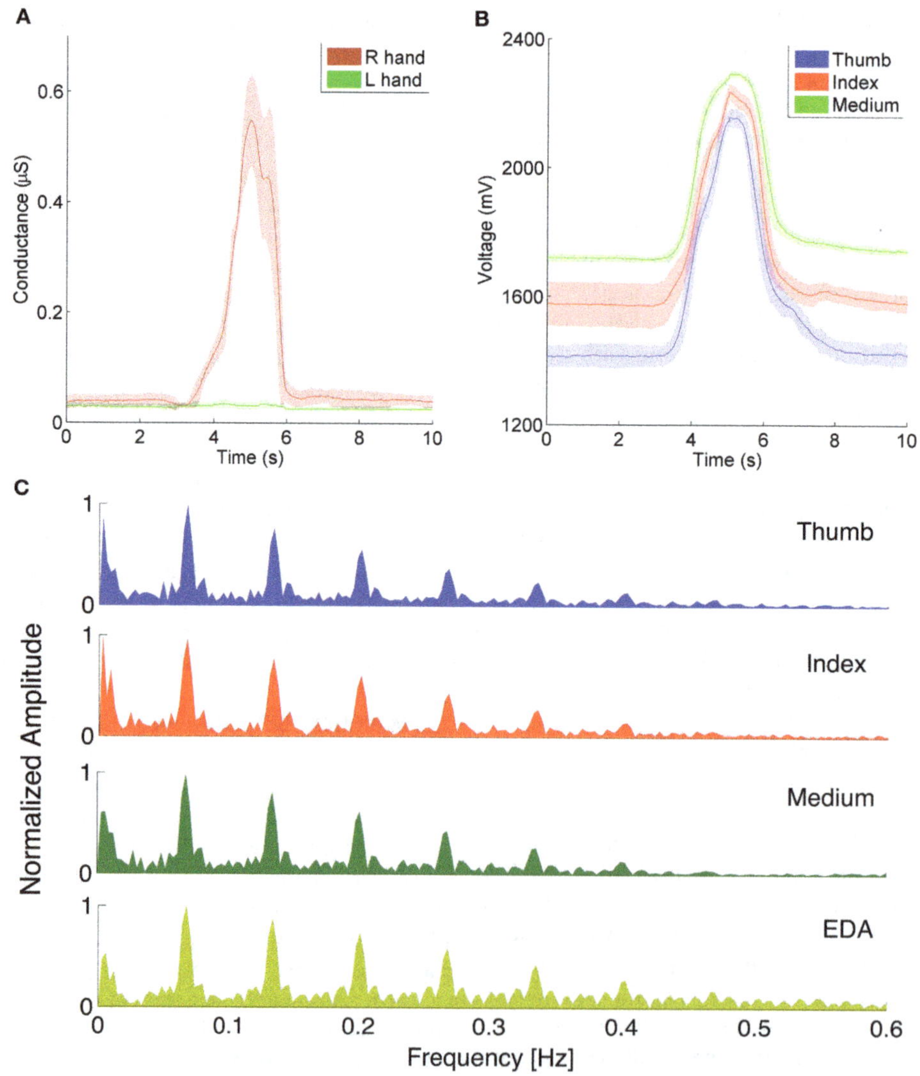

FIGURE 3 | (A) Averaged EDR signals of a subject while performing a grabbing gesture with the right hand (red trace) whereas the left hand is in rest conditions (green trace). **(B)** Right hand fingers flexion signals acquired in correspondence of the EDR recordings of **(A)**. The peaks of the flexion occur at the same time of the peaks observed in the EDR. Each trace in **(A,B)** is the average of three sweeps ± standard deviation. **(C)** Comparison of EDR and finger flexion spectral contents. The Y axis shows the normalized amplitude of the Fourier transform.

tasks (**Figure 3C**) showing a strong correlation in frequency content of EDR and motion signals.

The portions of the signals that were strongly affected by artifacts (e.g., grabbing gestures) were excluded from the analysis with the aim of demonstrating that the remaining physiological signals associated to the induced stimuli were sufficient to accurately classify users' affective states. **Figure 4** shows a 90-s segment of annotated recording of one participant in our first study (Section 3), where the motion events captured through the sensors and the EDR signal are labeled according to the natural movements of the subject extracted from the analysis of the video recorded during the experimental trial. With the exception of the right hand grab event occurring after 12 s of recording (and thus excluded from the analysis), the impact of the body movements on the remaining portion of the EDR signal did not produce strong artifacts and allowed for the extraction of the features used to classify the subject's affective state. Motion events, such as hand grabbing, generate synchronous spikes on the EDR signal, as shown in **Figure 3**. The grabbing event can be easily extracted from the finger sensors through adaptive threshold based algorithms such as the one described in Carbonaro et al. (2012), that were implemented directly in our sensing platform SSI (see Section 2.1.3). In the specific context of ambulatory research of event-elicited emotion using our sensing infrastructure (i.e., the

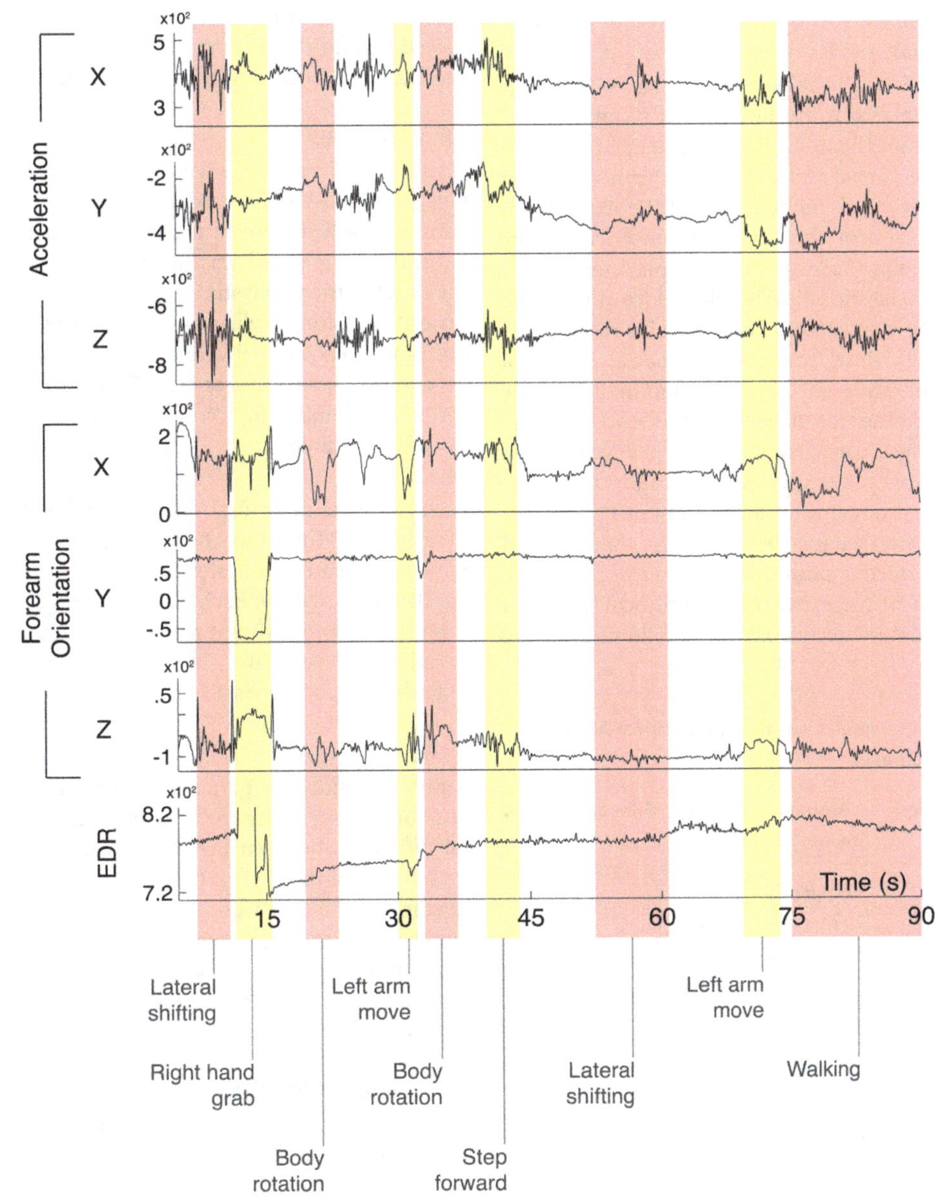

FIGURE 4 | 90-s recording from a subject while conducting the experiment described in study 1. The signals were acquired from the accelerometer (sensing shirt), the IMU and the EDR sensors (sensing glove). The annotated body movements events were extracted from the recorded video and synchronized with the signals. Y axis of the EDR signal is truncated to allow a better visualization of the signal.

work here presented), strong artifacts produced by movements accounted only for a small portion of the data collected (corresponding to the grabbing events) and were manually excluded from the analysis by means of post-processing techniques.

3. STUDY 1

The aim of the first study was to correctly discriminate stimulus–elicited subjective arousal levels from the ECG and EDR recorded signals. We expected to observe a significant increase in SC peaks and HR when the subjects were exposed to highly arousing pictures. Moreover, we expected to observe significant changes in the values of the features extracted from the psychophysiological signals, in accordance to the arousal of the stimuli.

3.1. SAMPLE AND PROTOCOL

A total of 7 voluntary subjects (4 females and 3 males, mean age $= 29.7$, $SD = \pm 3.9$) recruited from the University campus participated to this empirical validation. Before participating to the experiment, all the subjects read and signed an informed consent form declaring that they clearly understood all the experimental procedures and the aim of the study. The protocol of the experiment was approved by the local Ethical Committee.

Twelve different pictorial stimuli were selected from the IAPS pictures collection (Lang et al., 2008). Each stimulus represented a different rating value of arousal, thus covering the entire scale of arousal from a minimum rating of 1.72 to a maximum of 7.34 (see **Table 2** for a summary of the stimuli used for this study). Before being exposed to the images, participants were helped wearing the sensing shirt and the glove by the experimenter. A short test phase to verify the correct positioning and functioning of the sensors followed. Participants were then instructed to enter the XIM and stand at the designated starting point in the center of the room. A schematic illustration of the experimental protocol is shown in **Figure 5**. A 5-min baseline recording phase followed, during which a black screen was displayed while participants were asked to maintain a natural standing and relaxed posture. After baseline acquisition, participants were told that they were free to walk and to assume a natural posture during the entire duration of the experiment. Subsequently, the first image was displayed on the frontal screen of the XIM. The order of presentation of the stimuli was randomized for each experimental session and subject. Each stimulus was displayed for 20 s and it was followed by a "beep" sound to alert the user about the possibility to proceed with the following trial. To start the new trial, the participant was instructed to make a "grabbing" gesture with the hand that wore the sensing glove. This event was interpreted and recorded by the sensing platform to provide an accurate time annotation for each stimulus. A 20 s black screen was inserted between each trial. All the subjects were video recorded using a video camera placed behind them on the XIM floor and the information was used as an additional source for movements' annotation.

Table 2 | Selection of the 12 stimuli from the International Affective Picture System (IAPS) database.

ID	IAPS Catalog ID	Description	Arousal mean (SD)	Subset α	Subset β	Subset γ
1	7175	Lamp	1.72 (±1.26)	A_1	A_1	A_1
2	7020	Fan	2.17 (±1.71)	A_1	A_1	A_1
3	5030	Flower	2.74 (±2.13)	A_1	A_1	A_1
4	7547	Bridge	3.18 (±2.01)	A_1	–	A_1
5	7512	Chess	3.72 (±2.07)	A_1	–	A_2
6	9280	Smoke	4.26 (±2.44)	–	–	A_2
7	9171	Fisherman	4.72 (±2.17)	–	–	A_2
8	9582	Dental Exam	5.29 (±2.21)	A_2	–	A_2
9	9611	Plane Crash	5.75 (±2.44)	A_2	–	A_3
10	9622	Jet	6.26 (±1.98)	A_2	A_2	A_3
11	9412	Dead Man	6.72 (±2.07)	A_2	A_2	A_3
12	3000	Mutilation	7.34 (±2.27)	A_2	A_2	A_3

The arousal ratings are reported for each stimulus, along with the class assigned in the data subsets α, β, and γ.

3.2. DATA ANALYSIS

A number of fixed time windows were used to segment the signals (EDR, HRV) in accordance to the experimental protocol. To compute each feature of the skin conductance's phasic component, the EDR signal was segmented in 5 s windows aligned to the onset of the visual stimulus. To compute the HRV features we instead used longer windows of 20 s corresponding to the entire duration of each visual stimulus.

The extracted features (see **Table 1**) were divided into three subsets α, β and γ in accordance with the arousal ratings of the stimuli (see **Table 2**):

- α: A_1 refers to arousal ratings 1–3 (low), A_2 refers to arousal ratings 5–7 (high). Each class comprises 5 stimuli.
- β: A_1 refers to arousal ratings 1–2 (low), A_2 refers to arousal ratings 6–7 (high). Each class comprises 3 stimuli.
- γ: A_1 refers to arousal ratings 1–3 (low), A_2 refers to arousal ratings 3–5 (medium), A_3 refers to arousal ratings 5–7 (high). Each class comprises 4 stimuli.

A statistical inference analysis was conducted by means of both parametric and non-parametric tests, in accordance to the data distribution, to verify the null-hypothesis of having no statistical difference between the classes for both the 2-class (datasets α and β) and the 3-class (dataset γ) problems. The significance level for all the tests was set to 0.05. A pattern recognition phase followed the statistical analysis to investigate whether the arousal content of the stimuli could be discriminated in 2 and 3 classes of α, β and γ respectively, considering the aforementioned subset of features.

3.3. PATTERN RECOGNITION

An inter-subject analysis was performed for all subjects and all extracted features. The subsets α and β represent a 2-class problem, while subset γ represents a 3-class problem. Taking into account the entire dataset of features, the dimensionality of the features space was reduced through the application of Principal Component Analysis (PCA), considering the number of PCs that would be sufficient to explain 90% of the total variance.

We performed a classification phase to classify each sample of the dataset according to the set of classes. Among different classifiers, the Linear Discriminant Classifier (LDC) (Härdle and Simar, 2007), was the one that performed better in terms of accuracy and consistency in arousal discrimination. The performance of the classification process was examined through the confusion matrix, which expresses the capacity of the algorithm to recognize each sample as belonging to one of the predefined classes (a more diagonal confusion matrix corresponds to a higher degree of classification). The validity of the classification model was evaluated through the cross-validation method. For each validation step, the classifier was trained on the 80% of features randomly extracted from the whole dataset (training set) and tested on the remaining 20% (test set). More specifically, we performed 40-fold cross-validation steps in order to obtain unbiased results. The final results were expressed as the mean and the standard deviation of the 40 computed confusion matrices.

3.4. RESULTS

We assessed the non-Gaussianity of the features distribution using Kolmogorov–Smirnov tests with Lilliefors correction ($p < 0.05$). The α and the β datasets were submitted to a Mann–Whitney test to check for a difference between class A_1 (low arousal) and class A_2 (high arousal). The performed analysis on the α subset of features showed no statistical significance, whilst for the β subset LF resulted to be significantly higher in A_2 than A_1 ($p < 0.05$; Mdn A_1 1097; Mdn A_2 1684).

We conducted a Kruskal–Wallis (KW) test among the three classes A_1 (low arousal), A_2 (medium arousal) and A_3 (high arousal) of the γ dataset. The obtained results showed a significant effect ($p < 0.01$). Mann–Whitney tests were used to follow up these findings. A Bonferroni correction was applied to compensate for multiple comparisons. The pairwise comparisons showed a significantly higher value of RMSSD for A_3 as opposed to A_1 ($p < 0.05$; Mdn A_1 195.98; Mdn A_3 218.67) and a significantly higher value of HF for A_3 as opposed to A_1 ($p < 0.05$; Mdn A_1 528.22; Mdn A_3 727.46).

We assessed the parametric distribution of the mean HR values for each one of the three datasets by means of a Kolmogorov–Smirnov test with Lilliefors correction ($p > 0.05$). We submitted the mean HR in the α and the β datasets to an Independent Samples T-test. The results showed no statistical differences ($p > 0.05$) between the two classes in both the α dataset (mean $A_1 = 82.40$, $SD = \pm 16.5$; mean $A_2 = 80.31$, $SD = \pm 12.9$) and the β dataset (mean $A_1 = 82.17$, $SD = \pm 15.6$; mean $A_2 = 79.85$, $SD = \pm 13.4$). To test for differences in mean HR between the 3 classes of the γ dataset, we conducted an ANOVA. No significant effect was found (mean $A_1 = 82.88$, $SD = \pm 16.9$; mean $A_2 = 82.94$, $SD = \pm 15.4$; mean $A_3 = 79.93$, $SD = \pm 13.1$). Given all of the physiological features extracted from HRV and SC, we discriminated by a pattern recognition stage (Section 3.3) the two levels of arousal for the α and β datasets and the three levels of arousal for the dataset γ. As a result of the pattern recognition phase, the LDC classifier accounted for a high accuracy in the recognition of both the 2-class and the 3-class problems (**Tables 3, 4** respectively).

The multivariate analysis with LDC for the entire dataset accounted for an accuracy between 73.3% and 88.9% in the 3-class problem (low, medium and high arousal), and exceeding 87% in the 2-class problem (low and high arousal).

3.5. BODY MOVEMENTS AND SIGNALS ACQUISITION

To exclude the possibility that the overall accuracy of the classification could be biased by body movements systematically associated to the arousal of the stimuli presented, we quantified the subjects' motor activity for each class of stimuli. To do so, we calculated the sum of the standard deviation for the three axes for both acceleration and orientation data within time windows equal to (or greater than) 20 s, that correspond to the presentation

Table 3 | Confusion matrix of the LDC classifier for the 2-class problem for α and β datasets.

	Dataset α		Dataset β	
LDC	A_1	A_2	A_1	A_2
A_1	**87.27 ± 6.19**	7.72 ± 15.12	**95.36 ± 6.77**	0.00 ± 0.00
A_2	12.72 ± 6.19	**92.27 ± 15.12**	4.64 ± 6.77	**100.0 ± 0.00**

The results were obtained after 40 cross-fold validations.

Table 4 | Confusion matrix of the LDC classifier for the 3-class problem for γ dataset.

LDC	A_1	A_2	A_3
A_1	**88.89 ± 10.19**	2.78 ± 6.11	5.56 ± 10.44
A_2	7.72.56 ± 7.45	**85.56 ± 12.01**	21.11 ± 13.74
A_3	3.89 ± 5.43	11.67 ± 11.09	**73.33 ± 11.29**

The results were obtained after 40 cross-fold validations.

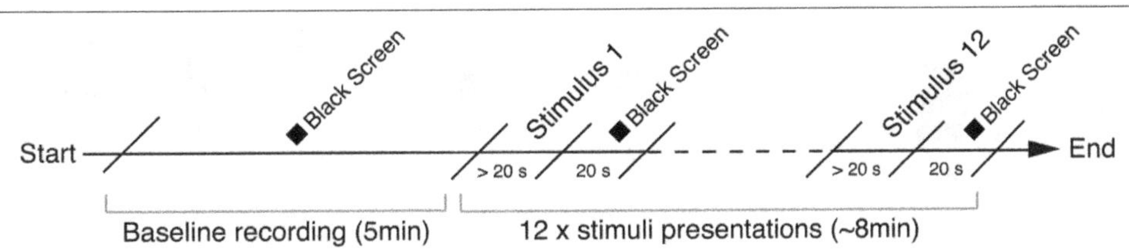

FIGURE 5 | Experimental protocol of Study 1. A black screen is presented during the first 5 min of the experimental session while the subject is maintaining a natural standing and relaxed posture. A sequence of 12 pictorial images extracted from the IAPS database and followed by a black screen is then presented and the physiological measures collected.

of the pictorial stimuli, thus obtaining two maximized activity indexes (Maximized Acceleration Index and Maximized Rotation Index). Using these indexes, we conducted an intra-subject analysis to compare the subjects' motor activity to the arousal classes identified in the 3 data subsets (see Section 3.3). We assessed the homogeneity of variance between the classes by conducting within-subject Levene tests. Our results did not show statistically significant differences across classes neither in the α and β subsets, nor in the γ subset ($p > 0.05$).

Additionally, we conducted an inter-subject analysis. We computed the standard deviation of acceleration and orientation for all the subjects within the time window that corresponds to the stimuli exposure and compared the obtained values to the classes of the 3 data subsets. Using the Levene test for both the activity indexes, we did not find statistically significant differences across classes neither in the α and β subsets ($p > 0.05$), nor in the γ subset ($p > 0.05$) (**Figure 6**).

The outcome of these two analyses indicates the homogeneity of variance in the activity indexes across the classes in the 3 data subsets, hence showing that the results obtained through the acquired psychophysiological signals were not due to artifacts produced by the subjects' motor activity.

4. STUDY 2

The second study was designed to empirically validate the XIM infrastructure and its wearable sensors using a classical conditioning (CC) task. Classical conditioning has been extensively used to study autonomic responses in humans and other species due to its non invasiveness and the relatively fast underlying learning processes (Fanselow and Poulos, 2005; Boucsein, 2012), allowing a direct comparison with results already present in literature. In the CC paradigm, subjects learn to predict the occurrence of an aversive event (unconditioned stimulus or US, i.e., a mild electrical shock or a loud noise) from contextual cues (conditioned stimulus or CS, i.e., a tone or a light), which, after several presentations of the CS–US pairings, results in the expression of an anticipatory conditioned response (CR) (Pavlov, 1927; Rescorla, 1966; Dickinson and Mackintosh, 1978; Clark and Squire, 1998; Maren, 2001; Inderbitzin et al., 2010). In summary, our primary objective was to verify whether we can reliably extract signatures of EDR and ECG conditioning from the recordings of freely moving subjects in a VR scenario using virtual objects and IAPS pictures as conditioned and unconditioned stimuli, respectively. We expected to observe significantly stronger skin conductance responses to the CS events that were followed by a high arousing US by the end of the acquisition protocol. We further expected to observe longer reaction latencies during the trials where the CSs were followed by an aversive US image. In regards to the HRV, we expected to find a significant variation in the vagal control of the heart going from the acquisition to the extinction phase, along with a reduction of the global activity.

4.1. SAMPLE

A total of 11 voluntary subjects (7 females and 4 males, mean age = 27, $SD = \pm 4.51$) recruited from the University campus participated in the study. All participants completed and signed an informed consent providing information about the motivation of the study, the procedures adopted and the storage policy of the data collected. Subjects were informed about the possibility to leave the experiment at any moment if they were not

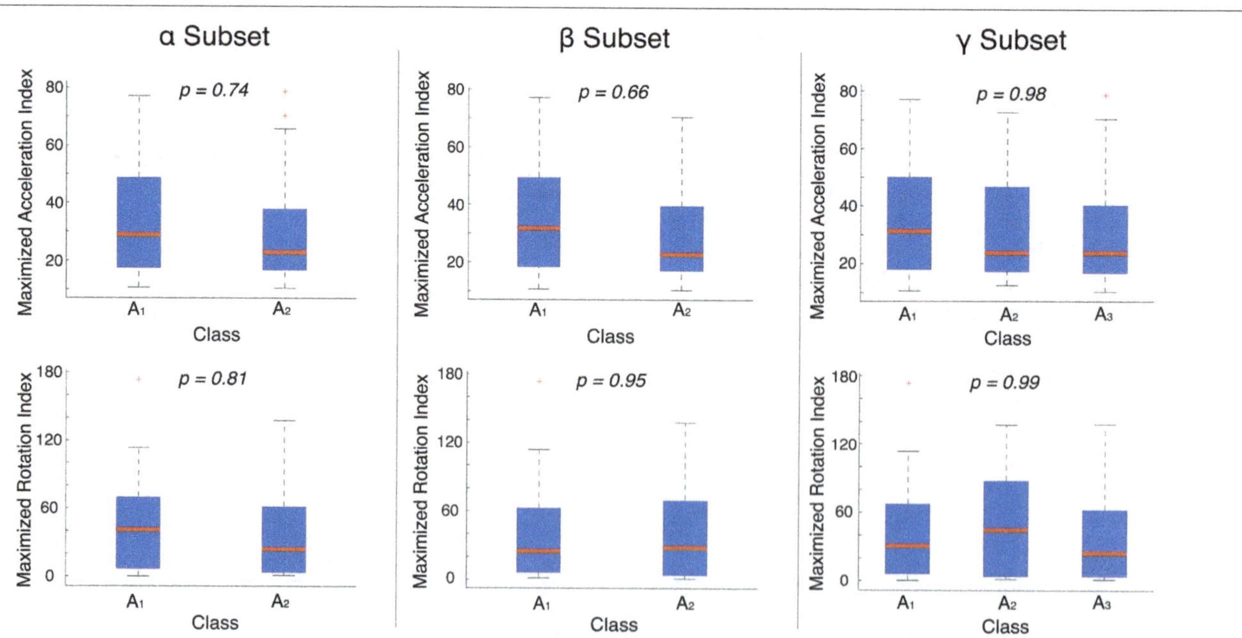

FIGURE 6 | Acceleration (top) and rotation (bottom) of all the subjects across the classes of arousal of the stimuli for the 3 data subsets. The Maximized Acceleration Index and the Maximized Rotation Index are calculated as the sum of the standard deviation of the 3 axes ($\sigma_X+\sigma_Y+\sigma_Z$) of the accelerometer and the IMU embedded in the sensing shirt and glove, respectively. The *p*-values reported in each plot indicate homogeneity of variance across the classes.

feeling comfortable with the experimental settings. The study was reviewed and approved by the local Ethical Committee.

4.2. CONDITIONING PROCEDURE AND EXPERIMENTAL DESIGN

Before starting the experimental session, participants were provided with task instructions and fitted with the sensors by the experimenter. Subjects were then left alone in the XIM for 5 min to relax and get acquainted with the sensors and the XIM environment. An interactive virtual scenario consisting of a realistic 3D model of an equipped living room designed with SketchUp (http://www.sketchup.com) and rendered using Unity3D (http://unity3d.com) was then projected on the frontal and the two lateral screens of the XIM (**Figure 7**).

The experimental protocol consisted of three different sessions in a within-subjects design: an acquisition and an extinction session that were followed by a self-assessment questionnaire to test for awareness of the contingencies between the stimuli presented. During each learning phase, participants were presented with a conditional visual stimulus (a photo camera, CS+, or a remote control, CS−, representing the reinforced and non-reinforced stimuli, respectively) that they had to collect from the virtual cabinet through a grabbing gesture. Once collected, a high or low arousal IAPS classified image (representing US+ and US− respectively), was displayed on the virtual TV screen. Based on the image segmentation obtained in the first study, we selected our stimuli from two subsets of images belonging to the negative (high arousal ratings) and neutral (low arousal ratings) categories of the IAPS database. In more detail, the acquisition phase consisted of 18 intermixed trials for each CS type presented in a random order (**Figure 8**). Each one of the 9 CS+ stimuli was followed by a high arousing image (US+, mean valence = 2.02, $SD = \pm 1.44$ and mean arousal = 6.95, $SD = \pm 2.04$), while the CS− stimuli were followed by a low arousing image (US−, mean valence = 5.06, $SD = \pm 1.13$ and mean arousal = 2.42, $SD = \pm 1.65$). Each trial followed a fixed guided sequence that drove the participant through the trial. USs were displayed for 15 s and during the acquisition phase they were followed by a black image for an interval of 17 ± 3 s. Following the acquisition phase, participants were left inside the room for 5 min to rest before starting the following session. The extinction phase consisted of 18 intermixed trials for each CS within the same context (**Figure 9**), always followed by a neutral image (US− trials only). At the end of the extinction phase the participants were asked to fill the self-assessment questionnaires, then they were assisted by the experimenter in the removal of the equipment and finally dismissed.

4.2.1. *Questionnaires*

To measure subjective affective reactions to the stimuli, we used both a computer interactive version of the Self-Assessment

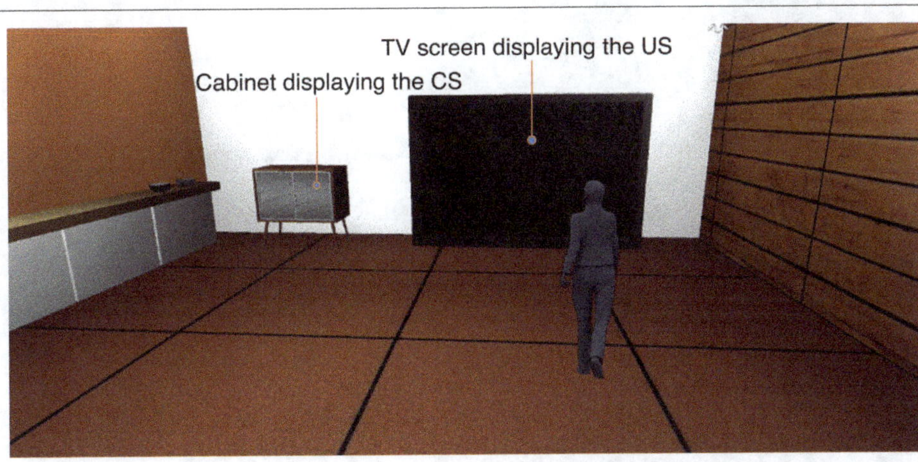

FIGURE 7 | Study 2: the VR scenario displayed in XIM with 180 degrees immersive projections. The participant (here represented as an avatar) starts at the center of the room. The cabinet on the left contains the CS (either a photo camera or a remote control), while the TV displays the US (images from IAPS database).

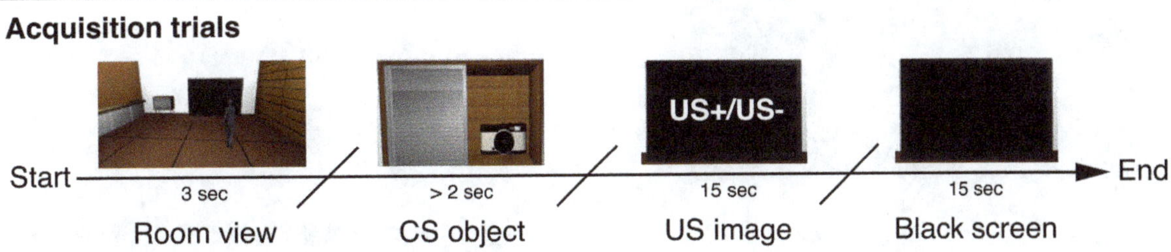

FIGURE 8 | Study 2: timeline of an acquisition phase trial. The CS is displayed in the cabinet as a virtual object (photo camera or remote control). As soon as the participant grabs the CS, the US is displayed for 15 s. A black screen follows for 15 s.

Manikin (SAM) (Bradley and Lang, 1994) and the Affective Slider. The latter is an alternative scale under development in our group that measures the same dimensions as the SAM questionnaire, but on a continuous scale (**Figure 10**). In addition, a second interactive questionnaire was delivered to each participant to asses the level of explicit awareness about the relation between the CSs and USs. Participants were shown a picture of the CS+ and asked to rate on a Likert scale ranging from −5 (strong disagreement) to

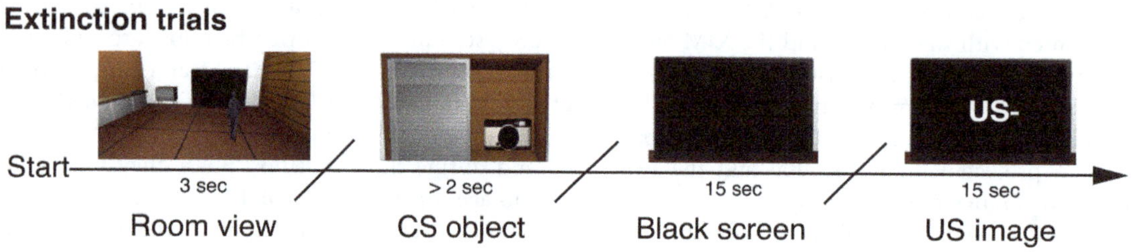

FIGURE 9 | Study 2: timeline of an extinction phase trial. The CS is displayed in the cabinet as a virtual object (photo camera or remote control). As soon as the participant grabs the CS, a black screen is displayed for 15 s. Subsequently US− is displayed.

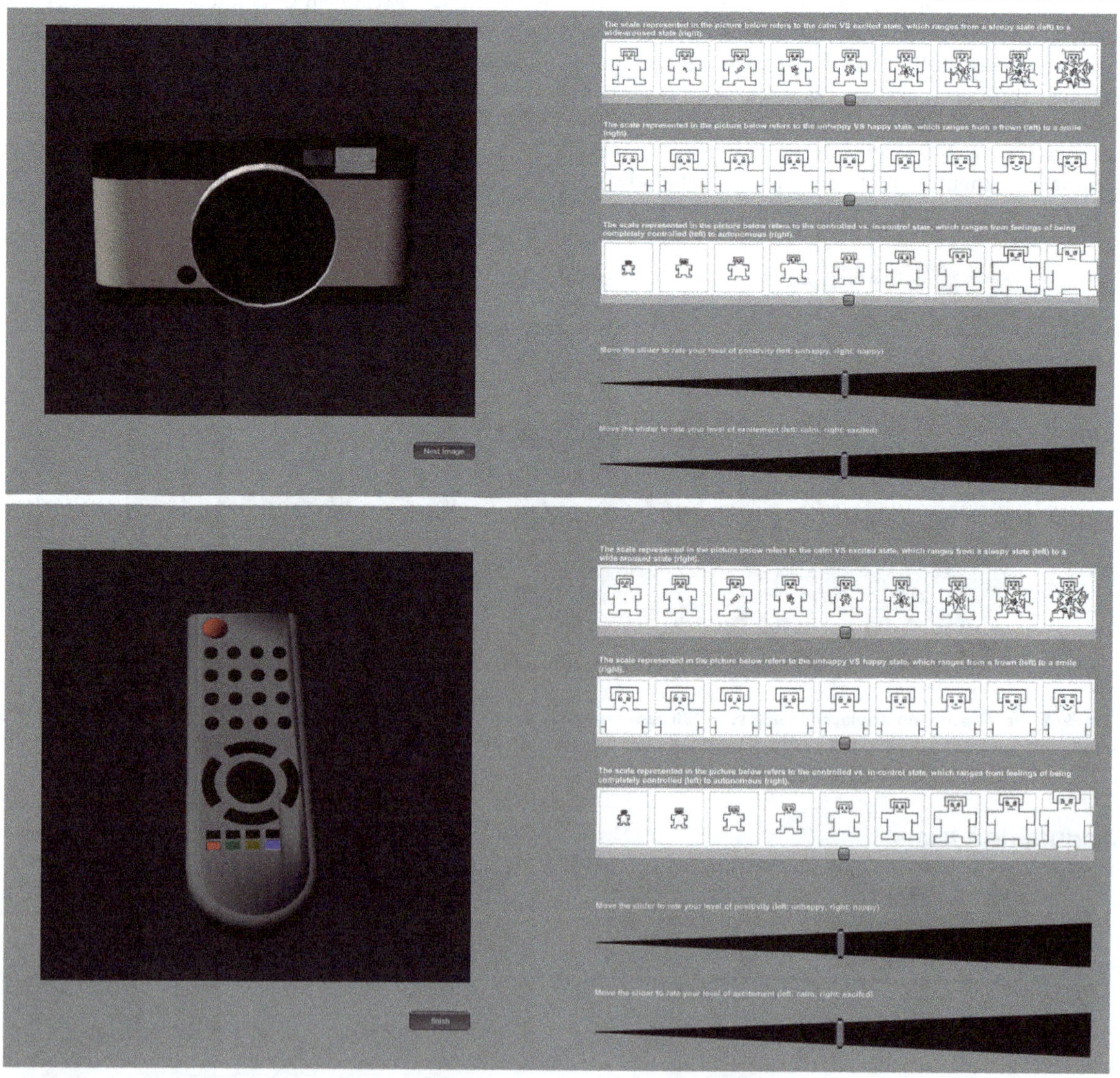

FIGURE 10 | Study 2: self-assessment questionnaire (based on SAM and Affective Slider) to test for awareness of CSs. CS+ (photo camera) and CS− (remote control) were presented separately and in random order.

5 (strong agreement) the level of self-awareness about any causal relationship between the CS and the following US.

4.3. PSYCHOPHYSIOLOGICAL MEASURES AND DATA ANALYSIS

Electrodermal responses were acquired through the sensing glove, sampled at 100 Hz and stored for off-line analysis, whilst the ECG signals were acquired through the sensing shirt with a sampling frequency of 250 Hz. As already detailed in the Section 2.2, ECG was used to extract HR and HRV related features.

The recorded EDR waveforms were visually inspected and the analysis of skin conductance components was performed using Ledalab (Benedek and Kaernbach, 2010b). Before being decomposed into its phasic and tonic components, the signal was low pass filtered with a cut-off frequency of 2 Hz. For the event-related analysis, a number of fixed time windows were used to segment the signal according to the conditioning protocol and a set of phasic component features were extracted (see Section 2.3). A segment of the signal time-locked to each CS onset was used to derive a dependent measure of the cued response (separately for the CS+ and the CS−). In accordance to the EDR literature, for the analysis of cued responses we considered only those responses starting one second after the stimulus presentation.

The EDR and latencies to the grabbing data for each CS type were analyzed both in aggregated form by dividing each session into early, middle and late blocks of three trials, and on a trial by trial basis. The Amplitude-Sum of SCRs in a time window of 3 s after the CS onset was considered (first interval response), and the values were normalized with respect to subject's own maximum value for between-subjects comparison. Statistical analysis was performed with non-parametric tests (Wilcoxon ranksum, Kruskal-Wallis and Friedman) given the non-Gaussianity of the distributions, as assessed by independent Kolmogorov–Smirnov tests with Lilliefors correction. When required, the statistics were corrected for multi-comparisons. The significance level α for all tests was set to 0.05.

HRV analysis was conducted in accordance to the recommendations of Task Force on HRV (Camm et al., 1996). While for the event-related analysis of EDR we defined short time windows starting after the CS onset, to analyze HRV we extracted features using time windows of 30 s corresponding to the US and the black screen together. We refer to these time windows in the text as "CS+ trials" and "CS− trials," in accordance to the nature of the preceding CS. Four participants were excluded from the HRV analysis due to technical problems (i.e., signal degradation due to low battery charge) that occurred during the acquisition phase of the ECG signal (hence resulting in $N = 7$). Statistical analysis of HRV included non-parametric Wilcoxon and Friedman rank-based tests, due to the non-Gaussianity of the distributions, as assessed by Kolmogorov–Smirnov tests with Lilliefors correction. The significance level α for all the tests was set to 0.05.

4.4. RESULTS

4.4.1. Time to grab

We looked for any significant difference in the latencies to the grabbing of the virtual object. Reaction times to the CS+ (mean = 3.7238 s, $SD = \pm 0.76$) were significantly longer than the latencies for CS− (mean = 3.3998 s, $SD = \pm 0.73$) during acquisition (paired Wilcoxon ranksum test, $p < 0.05$), while no significant differences were found for the extinction phase (mean CS+ = 3.5640 s, $SD = \pm 1.3$; mean CS− = 3.5696 s, $SD = \pm 1.1$). A significant difference was also found for CS+ reaction times between acquisition and extinction sessions (paired Wilcoxon ranksum test, $p < 0.05$), with longer reaction times during the acquisition session.

4.4.2. Self-assessment and awareness questionnaires

The self-assessment ratings of arousal collected through the questionnaire were tested for normality with a Kolmogorov–Smirnov test with Lilliefors correction ($p > 0.05$), and a paired-samples T-test between the arousal ratings for CS+ and CS− was then conducted. We found a significant difference between the two stimuli: CS+ was rated as more arousing than the CS− (mean CS− = 3.23, $SD = \pm 1.4$; mean CS+ = 4.62, $SD = \pm 2.7$, $p < 0.05$) showing that the subjects differentiated between the two stimuli by the end of the experiment, thus demonstrating a trace of conditioned response being maintained after extinction. In addition, 95% of the participants explicitly reported that they strongly agreed with the statement "In the first level I noticed a relationship between the object in the cabinet and the image displayed on the TV" (mean rating = 4, $SD = \pm 1.28$), hence suggesting a causal contingency between CS+ and US+.

4.4.3. EDR

A statistically significant difference was found for the CS+ amplitudes between the second three (middle block) and the last three (late block) trial during acquisition, with larger amplitudes during the late block (KW, $p = 0.047$, corrected for multi comparisons). A significant difference was also found for CS− amplitudes during extinction between the first three (early block) and the last three trials, with significantly smaller amplitudes in the last part of the extinction session (KW, $p = 0.024$, corrected for multicomparisons). A close to significance difference ($p = 0.06$) was found for the CS+ between acquisition and extinction trials. The other comparisons did not differ significantly, but overall the EDR showed characteristic trend patterns both in the acquisition and extinction phases (**Figure 11**).

4.4.4. HRV

To analyze HRV, we performed a series of inter-subject comparisons for each one of the extracted features (see **Table 1**). We conducted a Friedman test between all the stimuli presentations in both acquisition and extinction phases, which consisted of 4 groups of data (i.e., all the CS+ trials and CS− trials in the 2 sessions). The results of the test indicate a significant difference between acquisition and extinction in Mean ($p < 0.02$), Median ($p < 0.02$) and RRmean ($p = 0.01$). These 3 features show a significantly higher mean value for CS+ trials than CS− trials during the acquisition phase and a significantly higher mean value of CS− trials as opposed to CS+ trials in the extinction phase (see **Table 5**).

An inter-subject comparison between CS+ trials and CS− trials in both the acquisition and extinction sessions was then conducted through means of Wilcoxon tests. No statistically significant results were found in the acquisition session, with the

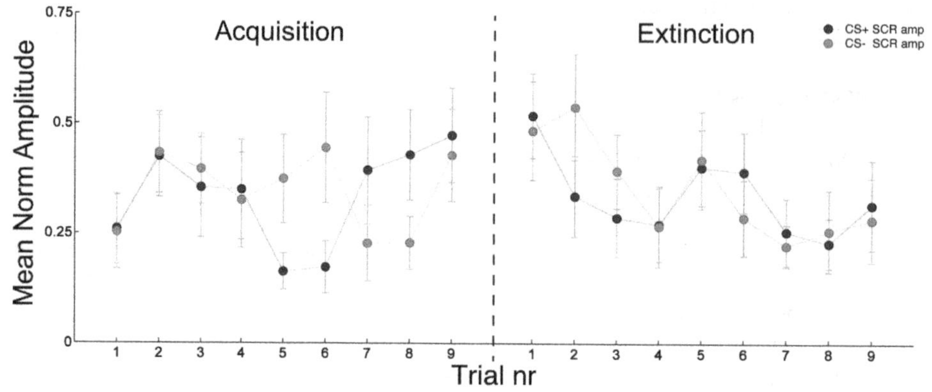

FIGURE 11 | Study 2: trial by trial evolution of the normalized sum of amplitudes of the significant SCRs averaged over all the subjects in a window of 1–4 s after the CS onset during acquisition and extinction session. Data are normalized for each subject's maximum. Bars indicate ± sem.

Table 5 | Mean values and SD of statistically significant features extracted from HRV (Mean, Median and RRmean) between CS+ trials and CS− trials.

HRV Feature	Acquisition			Extinction		
	Mean	Median	RRmean	Mean	Median	RRmean
CS+ trials mean (SD)	0.91 (±0.021)	0.86 (±0.017)	0.90 (±0.022)	0.92 (±0.033)	0.87 (±0.038)	0.91 (±0.032)
CS− trials mean (SD)	0.90 (±0.028)	0.85 (±0.022)	0.89 (±0.027)	0.93 (±0.025)	0.88 (±0.029)	0.92 (±0.024)

For all these features, CS+ trials show a higher mean than CS− trials during acquisition, while this trend is inverted during the extinction phase.

exception of a close to significance difference between CS+ trials and CS− trials for RR_tri ($p = 0.07$). In the extinction phase, we found statistically significant differences in the first 4 consecutive CS+ trials between acquisition and extinction for RRmean, Mean and Median ($p < 0.05$).

Finally, taken the first 4 consecutive CS+ trials in the extinction phase, a number of features showed significantly lower in values in the last occurrence, as opposed to the first: RMSSD, HF, SD1 ($p < 0.05$). **Figure 12** shows that RMSSD, HF and SD1 decreased their ranks value from the first to the fourth CS+ trial. These features are indeed representative of the vagal control of the hearth (Camm et al., 1996; Tulppo et al., 1996; Berntson et al., 2005), therefore their concurrent decrease during the extinction phase represents a significant variation in the parasympathetic heart activity.

5. DISCUSSION

The role played by psychophysiological correlates of human affective states has been investigated for more than a century, dating back to James-Lange's theory of emotions (Cannon, 1927) in the late 19th century. Until recently, most of the studies that measured psychophysiological signals, such as EDR and ECG, were conducted under strictly controlled laboratory settings. However, due to the improvements in hardware portability, the last decade has witnessed an increasing interest in the real world domain.

The bottleneck of conventional laboratory settings is created by the artificial conditions in which experiments are conducted, because they may or may not induce genuine emotions. When studying anxiety disorders, for instance, an unfamiliar laboratory environment can generate apprehension and stress in the participants, thus interfering with the natural emotional phenomena investigated. Similarly, the study of stress in a social context, such as family or workplace, necessarily requires investigation under naturalistic conditions (Wilhelm and Grossman, 2010). However, the discrepancy between the laboratory and the real world can be considerably minimized when investigating other topics, such as stress or mental workload detection during driving. Healey and Picard (2005), for instance, measured physiological data during a real-world driving task and classified the driver's stress using a recognition algorithm (Healey and Picard, 2005), while Stuiver et al. (2014) used cardiovascular measures to detect drivers' mental workload. The act of driving a real car (while wearing sensors with the awareness of being exposed to an experiment) or performing the same task in a laboratory using virtual reality would probably lead to similar results since the subjects' body motion is limited in both the approaches.

Moreover, in some cases, the laboratory can present a number of advantages when compared to life-like conditions. The latter, for instance, often present the problem of loss in connectivity between the sensors and the recording devices, while in controlled laboratory settings (even though there is a possibility of disconnection of devices) the probability of a data loss is extremely reduced. In addition, experiments that investigate affect recognition in life-like conditions are often aimed to measure long-term components of psychophysiological signals, such as tonic activity in EDR (see, as an example Healey et al., 2010), but can produce ambiguous results when investigating event-related states since the participants in the natural world

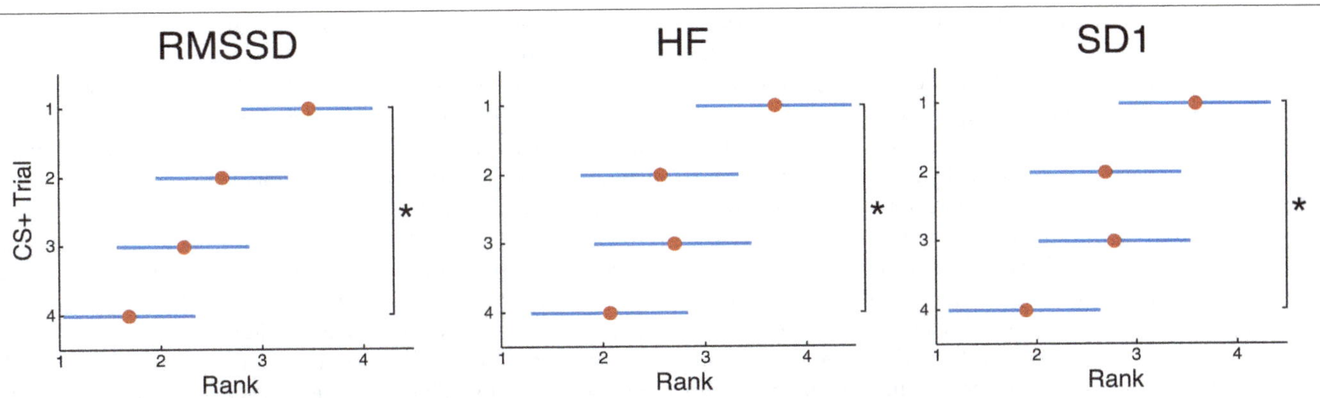

FIGURE 12 | Study 2: statistical comparison of the features RMSSD, HF and SD1 (extracted form HRV) among the first 4 CS+ trials (i.e., US + black screen that follow a CS+) in the extinction phase. Specifically, a statistically significant difference was found between the 1st CS+ trial and the 4th CS+ trial presented ($p < 0.02$), along with a clear decreasing trend in terms of ranks. The marker represents the median of the ranks, while the whiskers indicate the median absolute deviation (MAD).

perform other activities than merely experiencing emotions (e.g., reading, talking, etc.). Furthermore, in the laboratory it is possible to investigate reactivity to specific classes of emotion-eliciting stimuli, while in life-like conditions there can be avoidance of negative emotion-eliciting situations (Wilhelm and Grossman, 2010; Valenza et al., 2012c). Additionally, data labeling in life-like conditions relies almost exclusively on self-assessment. For an effective analysis, it is crucial to accurately annotate the data collected, since physical activity in ambulatory subjects can overwhelm the physiological effect of affective responses (Picard and Healey, 1997). A controlled laboratory environment, instead, provides all the means to easily annotate events along with the recorded signals with high accuracy and minimal delays, to determine a baseline for the acquired psychophysiological signals, and does not necessarily require the participants' self-assessment.

While we acknowledge the importance of achieving ecologically valid conditions in order to get genuine insights in the field of emotion research, we do believe that the definition of ecological validity in literature is often vague. Fahrenberg et al. (2007) support this viewpoint by presenting the laboratory and the field as alternatives that are not fundamentally opposed and by stressing the importance of removing this antithesis by developing new research strategies, that can be validated in the laboratory, while, at the same time, being close to daily life conditions (Fahrenberg et al., 2007). This is exactly why we built an immersive sensing infrastructure, the eXperience Induction Machine (XIM), which provides the unique opportunity to investigate human affective states in more ecologically valid environments than those offered by standard laboratory settings. By taking this hybrid approach, we are able to conduct ambulatory emotion research through the use of virtual reality and custom-made unobtrusive wearable technology suitable for the acquisition of psychophysiological signals without the constrains typical of standard laboratory settings, while, at the same time, ensuring that the subjects are timely exposed to systematically controlled stimuli according to the experimental design. This makes the XIM an ideal environment to conduct research on emotion-eliciting events and reactions, such as the two studies that we conducted to validate our infrastructure which are discussed in this work.

In the first study, we exposed participants to a set of visual stimuli that covered the full range of arousal levels while they were free to walk around in the space and gesticulate with the aim of observing different psychophysiological signatures related to the arousal of the stimuli. Using a classifier, we were successful in discriminating and predicting arousal classes of the stimuli presented by only measuring participants' ECG and EDR, with an accuracy between 73% and 88% in the 3-class problem, and exceeding 87% in the 2-class problem. Although we found clear classification results, the analysis of psychophysiological data did not show a full consistency between the signals and the classes of arousal. We found significant trends for some of the features extracted from HRV, however these trends were not visible in all the data subsets. The α subset, for instance, did not present any trend. This result could be due to the fact that it comprised 5 stimuli per class (thus including almost the entire pool of stimuli), while classes in β and γ comprised 3 and 4 stimuli, respectively, hence covering just more extreme arousal levels. In the frequency domain, the β subset showed a significantly higher value for LF, while the γ subset resulted in significantly higher values for HF when associated to the presentation of highly arousing pictures as opposed to neutral images. In the time domain, we found significantly higher values of RMSSD in the γ subset for the high arousal class, whereas, contrary to our expectations, the analysis of the HR did not show any statistically significant result. Similar studies that address the effect of arousal on HR present heterogeneous results, in some cases even showing a decrease in HR following highly arousing stimuli. One explanation for this mixed outcomes can be the dominance of other cognitive processes (e.g., attention) during the experimental task (Brouwer et al., 2013).

Following the first study, we designed a second experiment using VR that goes beyond the standard laboratory setup used in the well-known classical conditioning paradigm. Previous researchers have, in fact, investigated conditioning in VR using psychophysiological measures (Grillon et al., 2006; Huff et al., 2011; Greville et al., 2013), albeit with one caveat; in all those studies participants were constrained to a chair and used devices such as joysticks to move in the virtual space, while keeping the non-dominant hand (where the EDR electrodes were mounted) still for the entire duration of the experimental session in order to minimize signal artifacts. This is precisely what we wanted to avoid in our experiment: by providing an ecological form of interaction and using our wearable technology, we tackled the challenge of acquiring meaningful psychophysiological recordings related to emotion-eliciting events in an ambulatory context. Additionally, we used the recorded motion events (e.g., hand grabbing) not only to isolate motion-related artifacts, but also to further support the results obtained through physiological measures (i.e., grabbing latencies and reaction time). Consistent with our hypothesis, we found an anticipation of the US manifested as longer response times to the CS+. These results are in line with other studies on classical and context conditioning in VR. Dawson et al. (1982) observed longer reaction times to a stimulus during the CS−US interval only for the CS+ that they interpreted as the CS+ allocating more attentional resources. In other studies the presentation of CS+ led to behavioral avoidance of certain locations (Grillon et al., 2006) or resulted in a negative performance in an interactive task requiring precise motor control (Greville et al., 2013). The results of the HRV analysis suggest that learning took place and was detected through psychophysiological measures. The values in time of Mean, Median and RRmean for CS+ trials as opposed to CS− trials inverted their trend from the acquisition to the extinction phase. Additionally, our findings show statistical changes in the activity related to the vagal control of the heart for time-dependent features such as RMSSD, which is associated with short-term, rapid changes in heart rate, and is correlated with vagus mediated components of HRV (Malik et al., 1996). From the analysis of the EDR, we observed significantly stronger skin conductance responses following the presentation of CS+. The significant difference in CS+ during the acquisition phase between the middle and the late block confirms the expected outcome and is consistent with previous research on conditioning (Grings and Dawson, 1973; Öhman and Bohlin, 1973; Prokasy and Kumpfer, 1973). During the extinction phase, we also found a significant reduction in the amplitudes of the responses related to CS− toward the end of the session. This result can be explained by the fact that the acquisition protocol followed in previous studies, normally, did not include the presentation of any US following the CS−, while in our experimental design neutral IAPS images were used as US− in order to ensure the ecological setting we designed (i.e., the virtual living room where the TV screen always displays an image after the subject collects the CS from the cabinet). The close to significant difference found for CS+ between acquisition and extinction suggests that a complete extinction probably did not occur. This interpretation is supported by the results of the self-assessment questionnaire administered at the end of the experiment, where the subjects reported higher arousal levels associated to CS+. To be more effective, experiments on conditioning conventionally adopt strong USs, such as electrical shocks, loud sounds, bright lights and evolutionary fear-relevant images as CSs. In our data we did observe characteristic trial-by-trial trends in the amplitude of SCRs for both the acquisition and extinction phases, however, these trends were not statistically significant. A possible interpretation of this outcome relies in the nature of the stimuli used in our experimental design (i.e., IAPS pictures with negative arousal and common objects as conditional stimuli) for the sake of ecological validity, while the adoption of fearful images would have produced stronger emotional responses than negative images (Courtney et al., 2010).

The results reported here are in line with previous research. Nevertheless, some of these findings also reflect the complexity in obtaining a homogeneous interpretation of psychophysiological signals across studies. One example we observed, in contrast to our expectations, is the similarity of the mean values of HR obtained when the subjects were exposed to stimuli conveying different arousal content. As a matter of fact, the uniform inference of psychophysiological correlates of emotions in life-like settings still constitutes a challenge in the field. This is mainly due to the concurrence of multiple cognitive processes that modulate both sympathetic and parasympathetic activity, and that are difficult to isolate, especially under ecologically valid conditions (i.e., short time windows, artifacts, etc.). Along with future improvements in hardware technology, one further step to tackle this issue is the addition of more (direct and indirect) physiological measurements, such as an eye-tracker, that can be used to measure attention and estimate mental workload.

AUTHOR CONTRIBUTIONS

Alberto Betella, Ryszard Cetnarski, Riccardo Zucca, Paul F. M. J. Verschure: experimental design. Alberto Betella, Ryszard Cetnarski, Riccardo Zucca: data collection, data pre-processing. Alberto Betella, Riccardo Zucca: data analysis (accelerometers, IMU, video, questionnaires). Riccardo Zucca, Alberto Greco, Antonio Lanata: EDR analysis. Antonio Lanata: HRV analysis. Daniele Mazzei: Sensors and devices control software development and integration. Alessandro Tognetti: Design and development of wearable sensors and devices; algorithms for hand gesture tracking. Xerxes D. Arsiwalla: critical revision of the work. Pedro Omedas: integration of the sensors in XIM. Danilo De Rossi, Paul F. M. J. Verschure: supervision and final approval of the work. Alberto Betella, and Riccardo Zucca, contributed equally to this work. All the authors contributed to the draft and following revisions of the manuscript.

FUNDING

The research leading to these results has received funding from the European Community's Seventh Framework Programme (FP7-ICT-2009-5) under grant agreement n. 258749 [CEEDS]. The Generalitat de Catalunya (CUR, DIUE) and the European Social Fund are supporting this research.

ACKNOWLEDGMENTS

Thanks to Gaetano Valenza (Centro Piaggio, UNIPI) for helping with data pre-processing and to Ivan Herreros-Alonso (SPECS, UPF) for his critical comments on the manuscript.

REFERENCES

Acharya, U. R., Joseph, K. P., Kannathal, N., Lim, C. M., and Suri, J. S. (2006). Heart rate variability: a review. *Med. Biol. Eng. Comput.* 44, 1031–1051. doi: 10.1007/s11517-006-0119-0

Andreassi, J. (2006). *Psychophysiology: Human Behavior and Physiological Response*. New York, NY: Lawrence Erlbaum Assoc Inc.

Benedek, M., and Kaernbach, C. (2010a). A continuous measure of phasic electrodermal activity. *J. Neurosci. Methods* 190, 80–91. doi: 10.1016/j.jneumeth.2010.04.028

Benedek, M., and Kaernbach, C. (2010b). Decomposition of skin conductance data by means of nonnegative deconvolution. *Psychophysiology* 47, 647–658. doi: 10.1111/j.1469-8986.2009.00972.x

Berger, R., Akselrod, S., Gordon, D., and Cohen, R. (2007). An efficient algorithm for spectral analysis of heart rate variability. *Bio. Eng. IEEE Trans.* 33, 900–904.

Bernardet, U., Bermúdez i Badia, S., Duff, A., Inderbitzin, M., Le Groux, S., Manzolli, J., et al. (2010). "The eXperience induction machine: a new paradigm for mixed-reality interaction design and psychological experimentation," in *The Engineering of Mixed Reality Systems, Human-Computer Interaction Series*, eds E. Dubois, P. Gray, and L. Nigay (London, UK: Springer), 357–379.

Bernardet, U., Bermúdez i Badia, S., and Verschure, P. F. M. J. (2007). "The eXperience induction machine and its role in the research on presence," in *Proceedings of the 10th Annual International Workshop on Presence* (Barcelona: Xim), 1–7.

Berntson, G. G., Lozano, D. L., and Chen, Y.-J. (2005). Filter properties of root mean square successive difference (rmssd) for heart rate. *Psychophysiology* 42, 246–252. doi: 10.1111/j.1469-8986.2005.00277.x

Berntson, G. G., Quigley, K. S., and Lozano, D. L. (2007). Cardiovascular psychophysiology. *Handb. Psychophysiol.* 3, 182–210. doi: 10.1017/CBO9780511546396.008

Betella, A., Pacheco, D., Zucca, R., Arsiwalla, X. D., Omedas, P., Lanatà, A., et al. (2014). "Interpreting psychophysiological states using unobtrusive wearable sensors in virtual reality," in *ACHI2014: The Seventh International Conference on Advances in Computer-Human Interactions* (Barcelona), 331–336.

Boucsein, W. (2012). *Electrodermal Activity*. New York, NY: Springer Verlag. doi: 10.1007/978-1-4614-1126-0

Bradley, M., and Lang, P. J. (1994). Measuring emotion: the self-assessment manikin and the semantic differential. *J. Behav. Ther. Exp. Psychiat.* 25, 49–59. doi: 10.1016/0005-7916(94)90063-9

Brouwer, A.-M., van Wouwe, N., Mühl, C., van Erp, J., and Toet, A. (2013). Perceiving blocks of emotional pictures and sounds: effects on physiological variables. *Front. Hum. Neurosci.* 7:295. doi: 10.3389/fnhum.2013.00295

Cacioppo, J., Tassinary, L., and Berntson, G. (2007). *Handbook of Psychophysiology*. 3rd Edn. Cambridge, UK: Cambridge University Press. doi: 10.1017/CBO9780511546396

Camm, A., Malik, M., Bigger, J., Breithardt, G., Cerutti, S., Cohen, R., et al. (1996). Heart rate variability: standards of measurement, physiological interpretation, and clinical use. *Circulation* 93, 1043–1065. doi: 10.1161/01.CIR.93.5.1043

Cannon, W. B. (1927). The James-Lange theory of emotions: a critical examination and an alternative theory. *Am. J. Psychol.* 39, 106–124. doi: 10.2307/1415404

Carbonaro, N., Greco, A., Anania, G., Dalle Mura, G., Tognetti, A., Scilingo, E. P., et al. (2012). "Unobtrusive physiological and gesture wearable acquisition system: a preliminary study on behavioral and emotional correlations," in *Global Health 2012, The First International Conference on Global Health Challenges* (Venezia), 88–92.

Chua, K., Chandran, V., Acharya, U., and Lim, C. (2008). Cardiac state diagnosis using higher order spectra of heart rate variability. *J. Med. Eng. Technol.* 32, 145–155. doi: 10.1080/03091900601050862

Clark, R. E., and Squire, L. R. (1998). Classical conditioning and brain systems: the role of awareness. *Science* 280, 77–81. doi: 10.1126/science.280.5360.77

Courtney, C. G., Dawson, M. E., Schell, A. M., Iyer, A., and Parsons, T. D. (2010). Better than the real thing: eliciting fear with moving and static computer-generated stimuli. *Int. J. Psychophysiol.* 78, 107–114. doi: 10.1016/j.ijpsycho.2010.06.028

Dawson, M. E., Schell, A. M., Beers, J. R., and Kelly, A. (1982). Allocation of cognitive processing capacity during human autonomic classical conditioning. *J. Exp. Psychol.* 11, 272–295.

Dawson, M. E., Schell, A. M., and Filion, D. L. (2007). "The electrodermal system," in *Handbook of Psychophysiology, 3rd Edn.*, eds J. T. Cacioppo, L. G. Tassinary, and G. Berntson (New York, NY: Cambridge University Press), 157–181. doi: 10.1017/CBO9780511546396.007

Delbruck, T., Whatley, A., Douglas, R., Eng, K., Hepp, K., and Verschure, P. F. M. J. (2007). A tactile luminous floor for an interactive autonomous space. *Robot. Auton. Syst.* 55, 433–443. doi: 10.1016/j.robot.2007.01.006

Dickinson, A., and Mackintosh, N. J. (1978). Classical conditioning in animals. *Annu. Rev. Psychol.* 29, 587–612. doi: 10.1146/annurev.ps.29.020178.003103

Ebner-Priemer, U. W., and Kubiak, T. (2007). Psychological and psychophysiological ambulatory monitoring: a review of hardware and software solutions. *Eur. J. Psychol. Assess.* 23:214. doi: 10.1027/1015-5759.23.4.214

Ekman, P., Levenson, R. W., and Friesen, W. V. (1983). Autonomic nervous system activity distinguishes among emotions. *Science* 221, 1208–1210. doi: 10.1126/science.6612338

Eng, K., Douglas, R., and Verschure, P. F. M. J. (2005). An interactive space that learns to influence human behavior. *IEEE Trans. Syst. Man Cybern. A Syst. Hum.* 35, 66–77. doi: 10.1109/TSMCA.2004.838467

Fahrenberg, J., Myrtek, M., Pawlik, K., and Perrez, M. (2007). Ambulatory assessment - monitoring behavior in daily life settings. *Eur. J. Psychol. Assess.* 23, 206–213. doi: 10.1027/1015-5759.23.4.206

Fanselow, M. S., and Poulos, A. M. (2005). The neuroscience of mammalian associative learning. *Annu. Rev. Psychol.* 56, 207–234. doi: 10.1146/annurev.psych.56.091103.070213

Field, A. P. (2006). Is conditioning a useful framework for understanding the development and treatment of phobias? *Clin. Psychol. Rev.* 26, 857–875. doi: 10.1016/j.cpr.2005.05.010

Fowles, D., Christie, M., Edelberg, R., Grings, W., Lykken, D., and Venables, P. (1981). Publication recommendations for electrodermal measurements. *Psychophysiology* 18, 232–239. doi: 10.1111/j.1469-8986.1981.tb03024.x

Fusheng, Y., Bo, H., and Qingyu, T. (2000). Approximate Entropy and its application in biosignal analysis. *Nonlinear Biomed. Signal Process.* 2, 72–91. doi: 10.1002/9780470545379.ch3

Garrett, E. (1994). The Bateman function revisited: a critical reevaluation of the quantitative expressions to characterize concentrations in the one compartment body model as a function of time with first-order invasion and first-order elimination. *J. Pharmacokinet. Pharmacodyn.* 22, 103–128. doi: 10.1007/BF02353538

Greco, A., Lanatà, A., Valenza, G., Rota, G., Vanello, N., and Scilingo, E. (2012). "On the deconvolution analysis of electrodermal activity in bipolar patients," in *Engineering in Medicine and Biology Society (EMBC), 2012 Annual International Conference of the IEEE* (San Diego, CA: IEEE), 6691–6694.

Greville, W. J., Newton, P. M., Roche, B., and Dymond, S. (2013). Conditioned suppression in a virtual environment. *Comput. Hum. Behav.* 29, 552–558. doi: 10.1016/j.chb.2012.11.016

Grillon, C., Baas, J. M. P., Cornwell, B., and Johnson, L. (2006). Context conditioning and behavioral avoidance in a virtual reality environment: effect of predictability. *Biol. Psychiat.* 60, 752–759. doi: 10.1016/j.biopsych.2006.03.072

Grings, W. W., and Dawson, M. E. (1973). "Complex variables in conditioning," in *Electrodermal Activity in Psychological Research*, eds W. F. Prokasy and D. C. Raskin (New York, NY: Academic), 203–254.

Healey, J., Nachman, L., Subramanian, S., and Shahabdeen, J. (2010). "Out of the lab and into the fray: towards modeling emotion in everyday life," in *Lecture Notes in Computer Science*, 156–173. doi: 10.1007/978-3-642-12654-3_10

Healey, J. A., and Picard, R. W. (2005). Detecting stress during real-world driving tasks using physiological sensors. *Intell. Trans. Syst. IEEE Trans.* 6, 156–166. doi: 10.1109/TITS.2005.848368

Härdle, W., and Simar, L. (2007). *Applied Multivariate Statistical Analysis*. Berlin; Heidelberg: Springer.

Huff, N. C., Hernandez, J. A., Fecteau, M. E., Zielinski, D. J., Brady, R., and Labar, K. S. (2011). Revealing context-specific conditioned fear memories with full immersion virtual reality. *Front. Behav. Neurosci.* 5:75. doi: 10.3389/fnbeh.2011.00075

Hygge, S., and Hugdahl, K. (1985). Skin conductance recordings and the NaCl concentration of the electrolyte. *Psychophysiology* 22, 365–367. doi: 10.1111/j.1469-8986.1985.tb01616.x

Inderbitzin, M., Herreros-Alonso, I., and Verschure, P. F. M. J. (2010). "An integrated computational model of the two phase theory of classical conditioning," in *Neural Networks (IJCNN), The 2010 International Joint Conference on* (Barcelona: IEEE), 1–8. doi: 10.1109/IJCNN.2010.5596874

Inderbitzin, M. P., Betella, A., Lanatà, A., Scilingo, E. P., Bernardet, U., and Verschure, P. F. M. J. (2013). The social perceptual salience effect. *J. Exp. Psychol. Hum. Percept. Perform.* 39, 62–74. doi: 10.1037/a0028317

Kurths, J., Voss, A., Saparin, P., Witt, A., Kleiner, H., and Wessel, N. (1995). Quantitative analysis of heart rate variability. *Chaos* 5, 88–94. doi: 10.1063/1.166090

Lanatà, A., Scilingo, E. P., and De Rossi, D. (2010a). A multimodal transducer for cardiopulmonary activity monitoring in emergency. *Inf. Technol. Biomed. IEEE Trans.* 14, 817–825. doi: 10.1109/TITB.2009.2024414

Lanatà, A., Scilingo, E. P., Nardini, E., Loriga, G., Paradiso, R., and De-Rossi, D. (2010b). Comparative evaluation of susceptibility to motion artifact in different wearable systems for monitoring respiratory rate. *Inf. Technol. Biomed. IEEE Trans.* 14, 378–386. doi: 10.1109/TITB.2009.2037614

Lanatà, A., Valenza, G., Mancuso, C., and Scilingo, E. P. (2011). Robust multiple cardiac arrhythmia detection through bispectrum analysis. *Exp. Syst. Appl.* 38, 6798–6804. doi: 10.1016/j.eswa.2010.12.066

Lanatà, A., Valenza, G., and Scilingo, E. (2012). A novel EDA glove based on textile-integrated electrodes for affective computing. *Med. Biol. Eng. Comput.* 50, 1163–1172. doi: 10.1007/s11517-012-0921-9

Lang, P. (1995). The emotion probe. *Am. Psychol.* 50, 372–385. doi: 10.1037/0003-066X.50.5.372

Lang, P., Greenwald, M., Bradley, M., and Hamm, A. (1993). Looking at pictures: affective, facial, visceral, and behavioral reactions. *Psychophysiology* 30, 261–273. doi: 10.1111/j.1469-8986.1993.tb03352.x

Lang, P. J., Bradley, M. M., and Cuthbert, B. N. (2008). *International Affective Picture System (IAPS): Affective Ratings of Pictures and Instruction Manual.* Technical Report A-8, The Center for Research in Psychophysiology, Gainesville, FL: University of Florida.

Lazzeri, N., Mazzei, D., and De Rossi, D. (2014). Development and testing of a multimodal acquisition platform for human-robot interaction affective studies. *J. Hum. Robot Inter.* 3, 1–24. doi: 10.5898/JHRI.3.2.Lazzeri

Le Groux, S., Manzolli, J., and Verschure, P. F. M. J. (2007). "Interactive sonification of the spatial behavior of human and synthetic characters in a mixed-reality environment," in *Proceedings of the 10th Annual International Workshop on Presence* (Barcelona), 27–34.

Malik, M., Bigger, J. T., Camm, A. J., Kleiger, R. E., Malliani, A., Moss, A. J., et al. (1996). Heart rate variability standards of measurement, physiological interpretation, and clinical use. *Eur. Heart J.* 17, 354–381. doi: 10.1093/oxfordjournals.eurheartj.a014868

Maren, S. (2001). Neurobiology of Pavlovian fear conditioning. *Annu. Rev. Neurosci.* 24, 897–931. doi: 10.1146/annurev.neuro.24.1.897

Mathews, Z., Bermúdez i Badia, S., and Verschure, P. F. M. J. (2012). PASAR: An integrated model of prediction, anticipation, sensation, attention and response for artificial sensorimotor systems. *Inf. Sci.* 186, 1–19. doi: 10.1016/j.ins.2011.09.042

Mazzei, D., Billeci, L., Armato, A., Lazzeri, N., Cisternino, A., Pioggia, G., et al. (2010). "The face of autism," in *RO-MAN, 2010 IEEE* (Viareggio, LU: IEEE), 791–796.

Mazzei, D., Greco, A., Lazzeri, N., Zaraki, A., Lanatà, A., Igliozzi, R., et al. (2012). "Robotic social therapy on children with autism: preliminary evaluation through multi-parametric analysis," in *Privacy, Security, Risk and Trust (PASSAT), 2012 International Conference on and 2012 International Confernece on Social Computing (SocialCom)* (Amsterdam: IEEE), 955–960. doi: 10.1109/SocialCom-PASSAT.2012.99

Mazzei, D., Lazzeri, N., Billeci, L., Igliozzi, R., Mancini, A., Ahluwalia, A., et al. (2011). "Development and evaluation of a social robot platform for therapy in autism," in *Engineering in Medicine and Biology Society, EMBC, 2011 Annual International Conference of the IEEE* (Boston, MA: IEEE), 4515–4518. doi: 10.1109/IEMBS.2011.6091119

Mitra, S. K., and Kuo, Y. (2006). *Digital Signal Processing: A Computer-Based Approach, Vol. 2.* New York, NY: McGraw-Hill.

Öhman, A., and Bohlin, G. (1973). The relationship between spontaneous and stimulus-correlated electrodermal responses in simple and discriminative conditioning paradigms. *Psychophysiology* 10, 589–577. doi: 10.1111/j.1469-8986.1973.tb00809.x

Omedas, P., Betella, A., Zucca, R., Arsiwalla, X. D., Pacheco, D., Wagner, J., et al. (2014). "XIM-Engine: a software framework to support the development of interactive applications that uses conscious and unconscious reactions in immersive mixed reality," in *Virtual Reality International Conference (VRIC '14)* (Laval).

Pacelli, M., Caldani, L., and Paradiso, R. (2013). "Performances evaluation of piezoresistive fabric sensors as function of yarn structure," in *Engineering in Medicine and Biology Society (EMBC), 2013 35th Annual International Conference of the IEEE* (Osaka: IEEE), 6502–6505. doi: 10.1109/EMBC.2013.6611044

Pan, J., and Tompkins, W. (1985). A real-time QRS detection algorithm. *IEEE Trans. Biomed. Eng.* 32, 230–236. doi: 10.1109/TBME.1985.325532

Pantelopoulos, A., and Bourbakis, N. G. (2010). A survey on wearable sensor-based systems for health monitoring and prognosis. *Syst Man Cybern. C Appl. Rev. IEEE Trans.* 40, 1–12. doi: 10.1109/TSMCC.2009.2032660

Paradiso, R., and Caldani, L. (2010). Electronic textile platforms for monitoring in a natural environment. *Res. J. Text. Appar.* 14, 9.

Paradiso, R., Loriga, G., and Taccini, N. (2005). A wearable health care system based on knitted integrated sensors. *Inf. Technol. Biomed. IEEE Trans.* 9, 337–344. doi: 10.1109/TITB.2005.854512

Patel, S., Park, H., Bonato, P., Chan, L., and Rodgers, M. (2012). A review of wearable sensors and systems with application in rehabilitation. *J. Neuroeng. Rehabil.* 9:21. doi: 10.1186/1743-0003-9-21

Pavlov, I. (1927). *Conditioned Reflexes: An Investigation of the Physiological Activity of the Cerebral Cortex.* Oxford, UK: Oxford University Press.

Picard, R. (2000). *Affective Computing.* Boston, MA: The MIT Press.

Picard, R. W., and Healey, J. (1997). Affective wearables. *Pers. Technol.* 1, 231–240. doi: 10.1007/BF01682026

Pincus, S. M., and Goldberger, A. L. (1994). Physiological time-series analysis: what does regularity quantify? *Am. J. Physiol. Heart Circul. Physiol.* 266, H1643–H1656.

Poh, M.-Z., Swenson, N. C., and Picard, R. W. (2010). A wearable sensor for unobtrusive, long-term assessment of electrodermal activity. *Biomed. Eng. IEEE Trans.* 57, 1243–1252. doi: 10.1109/TBME.2009.2038487

Prokasy, W. F., and Kumpfer, K. (1973). "Classical conditioning," in *Electrodermal Activity in Psychological Research*, eds W. F. Prokasy and D. C. Raskin (New York, NY: Academic), 157–202.

Rescorla, R. A. (1966). Pavlovian conditioning. *Am. Psychol.* 43, 151–160. doi: 10.1037/0003-066X.43.3.151

Ritter, W. (2009). Measuring psychophysiological signals in every-day situations. *Univ. Access Hum. Comput. Inter.* 5615, 720–728. doi: 10.1007/978-3-642-02710-9_80

Schneider, R., Schmidt, S., Binder, M., Schafer, F., and Walach, H. (2003). Respiration-related artifacts in EDA recordings: introducing a standardized method to overcome multiple interpretations. *Psychol. Rep.* 93, 907–920. doi: 10.2466/pr0.2003.93.3.907

Scilingo, E., Gemignani, A., Paradiso, R., Taccini, N., Ghelarducci, B., and De Rossi, D. (2005). Performance evaluation of sensing fabrics for monitoring physiological and biomechanical variables. *Inf. Technol. Biomed. IEEE Trans.* 9, 345–352. doi: 10.1109/TITB.2005.854506

Stein, P., Bosner, M., Kleiger, R., and Conger, B. (1994). Heart rate variability: a measure of cardiac autonomic tone. *Am. Heart J.* 127, 1376–1381. doi: 10.1016/0002-8703(94)90059-0

Stuiver, A., Brookhuis, K. A., de Waard, D., and Mulder, B. (2014). Short-term cardiovascular measures for driver support: increasing sensitivity for detecting changes in mental workload. *Int. J. Psychophysiol.* 92, 35–41. doi: 10.1016/j.ijpsycho.2014.01.010

Taccini, N., Loriga, G., Pacelli, M., and Paradiso, R. (2008). "Wearable monitoring system for chronic cardio-respiratory diseases," in *Engineering in Medicine and Biology Society, 2008. EMBS 2008. 30th Annual International Conference of the IEEE* (Vancouver, BC: IEEE), 3690–3693.

Tognetti, A., Carbonaro, N., Zupone, G., and De Rossi, D. (2006). "Characterization of a novel data glove based on textile integrated sensors," in *Engineering in Medicine and Biology Society, 2006. EMBS'06. 28th Annual International Conference of the IEEE* (New York, NY: IEEE), 2510–2513.

Tulppo, M. P., Makikallio, T., Takala, T., Seppanen, T., and Huikuri, H. (1996). Quantitative beat-to-beat analysis of heart rate dynamics during exercise. *Am. J. Physiol. Heart Circul. Physiol.* 40:H244.

Valenza, G., Allegrini, P., Lanatà, A., and Scilingo, E. P. (2012a). Dominant Lyapunov exponent and approximate entropy in heart rate variability during emotional visual elicitation. *Front. Neuroeng.* 5:3. doi: 10.3389/fneng.2012.00003

Valenza, G., Citi, L., Lanatà, A., Scilingo, E. P., and Barbieri, R. (2013a). "A nonlinear heartbeat dynamics model approach for personalized emotion recognition," in *Engineering in Medicine and Biology Society (EMBC), 2013 35th Annual International Conference of the IEEE* (Osaka: IEEE), 2579–2582.

Valenza, G., Citi, L., Lanatá, A., Scilingo, E. P., and Barbieri, R. (2014). Revealing real-time emotional responses: a personalized assessment based on heartbeat dynamics. *Sci. Rep.* 4:4998. doi: 10.1038/srep04998

Valenza, G., Lanatà, A., Scilingo, E. P. (2012b). The role of nonlinear dynamics in affective valence and arousal recognition. *Affect. Comput. IEEE Trans.* 3, 237–249. doi: 10.1109/T-AFFC.2011.30

Valenza, G., Lanatá, A., Scilingo, E. P. (2013b). Improving emotion recognition systems by embedding cardiorespiratory coupling. *Physiol. Measure.* 34:449. doi: 10.1088/0967-3334/34/4/449

Valenza, G., Lanatà, A., Ferro, M., and Scilingo, E. P. (2008). "Real-time discrimination of multiple cardiac arrhythmias for wearable systems based on neural networks," in *Computers in Cardiology, 2008* (Bologna: IEEE), 1053–1056. doi: 10.1109/CIC.2008.4749226

Valenza, G., Lanatà, A., and Scilingo, E. P. (2012c). Oscillations of heart rate and respiration synchronize during affective visual stimulation. *Inf. Technol. Biomed. IEEE Trans.* 16, 683–690. doi: 10.1109/TITB.2012.2197632

Valenza, G., Lanatà, A., Scilingo, E. P., and De Rossi, D. (2010). "Towards a smart glove: arousal recognition based on textile electrodermal response," in *Engineering in Medicine and Biology Society (EMBC), International Conference of the IEEE* (Buenos Aires), 3598–3601.

Vanello, N., Hartwig, V., Tesconi, M., Ricciardi, E., Tognetti, A., Zupone, G., et al. (2008). Sensing glove for brain studies: design and assessment of its compatibility for fMRI with a robust test. *Mechatron. IEEE/ASME Trans.* 13, 345–354. doi: 10.1109/TMECH.2008.924115

Wagner, J., Lingenfelser, F., André, E., Mazzei, D., Tognetti, A., Lanatà, A., et al. (2013a). "A sensing architecture for empathetic data systems," in *Proceedings of the 4th Augmented Human International Conference*, AH '13 (New York, NY: ACM), 96–99.

Wagner, J., Lingenfelser, F., Baur, T., Damian, I., Kistler, F., and André, E. (2013b). "The social signal interpretation (SSI) framework: multimodal signal processing and recognition in real-time," in *Proceedings of the 21st ACM International Conference on Multimedia*, MM '13 (New York, NY: ACM), 831–834.

Wessel, N., Ziehmann, C., Kurths, J., Meyerfeldt, U., Schirdewan, A., and Voss, A. (2000). Short-term forecasting of life-threatening cardiac arrhythmias based on symbolic dynamics and finite-time growth rates. *Phys. Rev. E* 61:733. doi: 10.1103/PhysRevE.61.733

Wilhelm, F. H., and Grossman, P. (2010). Emotions beyond the laboratory: theoretical fundaments, study design, and analytic strategies for advanced ambulatory assessment. *Biol. Psychol.* 84, 552–569. doi: 10.1016/j.biopsycho.2010.01.017

Zbilut, J., and Webber, C. Jr. (2006). *Recurrence Quantification Analysis.* New York, NY: Wiley Online Library.

2

Combining and comparing EEG, peripheral physiology and eye-related measures for the assessment of mental workload

Maarten A. Hogervorst*, Anne-Marie Brouwer and Jan B. F. van Erp

TNO Human Factors, Netherlands Organisation for Applied Scientific Research, Soesterberg, Netherlands

Correspondence:
Maarten A. Hogervorst, TNO Human Factors, Netherlands Organisation for Applied Scientific Research, PO Box 23, 3769 ZG Soesterberg, Netherlands
e-mail: maarten.hogervorst@tno.nl

While studies exist that compare different physiological variables with respect to their association with mental workload, it is still largely unclear which variables supply the best information about momentary workload of an individual and what is the benefit of combining them. We investigated workload using the n-back task, controlling for body movements and visual input. We recorded EEG, skin conductance, respiration, ECG, pupil size and eye blinks of 14 subjects. Various variables were extracted from these recordings and used as features in individually tuned classification models. Online classification was simulated by using the first part of the data as training set and the last part of the data for testing the models. The results indicate that EEG performs best, followed by eye related measures and peripheral physiology. Combining variables from different sensors did not significantly improve workload assessment over the best performing sensor alone. Best classification accuracy, a little over 90%, was reached for distinguishing between high and low workload on the basis of 2 min segments of EEG and eye related variables. A similar and not significantly different performance of 86% was reached using only EEG from single electrode location Pz.

Keywords: EEG, physiology, eye, workload, classification, combination, ECG, skin conductance

INTRODUCTION

In the literature, mental workload has been associated with a range of physiological variables. These include heart rate (e.g., studies as reviewed by Vogt et al., 2006), different types of heart rate variability (reviewed by Hancock et al., 1985; Aasman et al., 1987), pupil size (reviewed by Beatty, 1982; May et al., 1990; Porter et al., 2007; Hampson et al., 2010), eye blink frequency and duration (Wilson and Fisher, 1991; Brookings et al., 1996; Veltman and Gaillard, 1996, 1998), electrodermal measures (Kohlisch and Schaefer, 1996; Reimer and Mehler, 2011), respiration frequency (Wientjes, 1992; Mehler et al., 2009; Karavidas et al., 2010) and various variables derived from EEG (most prominently power in the alpha and theta band—reviewed by Brouwer et al. (2012).

A question that arises when one aims to put this knowledge into practical use is which variable(s) one should measure in order to get the best workload assessment for a specific individual. It is not easy to answer this question based on the current literature because of several complications. Firstly, only a limited set of variables is recorded and analyzed in each study, precluding easy comparison of performance across variables. Secondly, variables are often analyzed and reported at a group level rather than used to assess workload in an individual. Associations between physiological variables and workload as found using a group level analysis may not generalize to the case of assessing workload in an individual since they may not be sufficiently strong to reliably assess workload at a certain moment in time for a single individual. On the other hand, physiological responses to workload may be consistent within and not between individuals, which would result in variables that are seemingly non-responsive to workload at a group level while they are actually valuable for assessing workload on an individual basis. Finally, many workload studies suffer from experimental flaws in which workload levels are confounded with for instance body movements (potentially affecting heart rate and related variables) or visual information processing (potentially affecting eye- and EEG based variables). We here aim to provide an overview of the workload assessment performance of a rather broad range of variables within the context of an experiment in which visual input and the amount of body movements are constant across workload levels. Classification analyses are used to get an impression of the quality of workload estimation within an individual. While analyses are performed offline, we simulate an online[1] situation, where our classification models are trained on data acquired at the start of the experiment and tested on data acquired at the end of the experiment, therewith avoiding inflation of classification accuracy due to time dependencies. The same data have been analyzed on a group level in Brouwer et al. (2014). That study gives an overview of the general magnitude and direction of effects of the different conditions on the studied variables.

[1] Note that here "online" and "real time" refer to using information as collected over the last half- or several minutes. Especially for certain non-EEG measures, it is not possible to retrieve reliable information from very short intervals.

Besides examining how well different variables can be used to estimate workload on their own, we examine to what extent combination of different variables improves performance. As discussed later, while some studies seem to suggest that assessment of mental state improves when combining physiological variables, reported improvements often are modest and not statistically significant or not statistically tested. We examine different ways of combining variables. Below we review the literature and formulate hypotheses as to what we expect to find.

SENSITIVITY OF SINGLE VARIABLES TO WORKLOAD

Studies on (neuro) physiological correlates of workload (or mental load) go back to at least the early sixties (Kalsbeek and Ettema, 1963). A range of variables has been examined over the years such as heart rate, different types of heart rate variability, pupil size, eye blink frequency and duration, saccade and fixation related measures, electrodermal measures, respiration, blood pressure, chemical measures, EMG and neurophysiological variables derived from EEG. To our knowledge, a substantial, recent review of physiological responses to workload is lacking. There does not seem to be an obvious "winning" variable that can effectively be used to determine workload. One review study (Hancock et al., 1985) suggested heart rate variability as the most reliable measure, whereas another (Vogt et al., 2006) reviewed 19 studies in which heart rate variability was not even recorded. In these studies, heart rate seemed to be relatively reliable. Most studies that examined EEG spectral variables next to physiological variables such as different eye and heart related measures, concluded or suggested EEG to be the most sensitive or promising indicator of workload (Brookings et al., 1996; Taylor et al., 2010; Christensen et al., 2012). The study by Christensen et al. (2012) showed that classification accuracy using only EEG data was only marginally lower compared to adding information about heart rate, blink rate, blink amplitude, blink duration and EOG. Berka et al. (2007) argue in their introduction that EEG is the only physiological signal that has been shown to accurately reflect subtle shifts in workload. However, in the three studies favoring EEG just mentioned, as well as in many other workload studies, workload was manipulated in the context of simulated realistic tasks involving potential confounds such as speech, body movement and visual information. In a recent study (Brouwer et al., 2014) we examined effects of workload and time using a task that controls for these kinds of confounds. Repeated measures ANOVA analyses did not mark EEG as the source of information that "best" indicated workload. Highly significant effects of workload were found for EEG in the alpha frequency band but also for mean and minimum skin conductance level, respiration frequency, heart rate, high frequency heart rate variability and pupil size. No significant effects were found for EEG in the theta frequency band, mid frequency heart rate variability, number of blinks and blink duration. Still, this study does not indicate which variables would be most useful for assessing workload based on a limited amount of physiological data of a single individual. This is especially the case since Brouwer et al. (2014) highlighted (strong) effects of time on most of the measured variables which could potentially complicate their use.

COMBINING VARIABLES - PROCESSES UNDERLYING THE ASSOCIATION BETWEEN WORKLOAD AND PHYSIOLOGICAL VARIABLES

Being interested in combining physiological variables in order to arrive at a better assessment of workload, it is of special importance to examine the background of the association between the variables and workload. This is because using a combination of variables reflecting workload is especially expected to improve workload assessment if these variables are not all associated with the same but rather with different aspects of workload. As described below, high workload likely goes hand in hand with increased cognitive processing, increased (emotional) arousal and increased energy demand; aspects of workload that are presumably reflected by different physiological variables that have all been associated with workload before.

COGNITIVE PROCESSING—EEG

EEG alpha activity (power in the 8–12 Hz band) has been linked to idling (Pfurtscheller et al., 1996), default mode brain activity (Laufs et al., 2003; Jann et al., 2009) and cortical inhibition (Foxe et al., 1998; van Dijk et al., 2008; Brouwer et al., 2009). This suggests that this measure would reflect different levels of workload, with high alpha for low levels of workload which indeed was reported in several workload studies (e.g., Fink et al., 2005; Brouwer et al., 2012). Another EEG frequency band that has been related to workload associated processes is theta (4–8 Hz). Evidence for an association between theta and working memory processes or mental effort has been summarized in several reviews by Klimesch (1996, 1997, 1999). Theta increases as task requirements increase (e.g., Miyata et al., 1990; Raghavachari et al., 2001; Jensen and Tesche, 2002; Esposito et al., 2009). A number of studies on workload reported both alpha and theta effects (e.g., Gundel and Wilson, 1992; Brookings et al., 1996; Gevins et al., 1998; Fournier et al., 1999).

Not only EEG spectral variables, also Event-Related-Potentials (ERPs) have been found to reflect different levels of workload. The P300 component of the ERP is a peak occurring 300 ms or somewhat later after an attended stimulus has been presented. It is thought to reflect attentional and working memory processes (Polich and Kok, 1995; Polich, 2007) and it is in particular this component that has been reported to decrease with increasing levels of memory or workload (Watter et al., 2001; Kida et al., 2004; Raabe et al., 2005; Allison and Polich, 2008; Evans et al., 2011; Pratt et al., 2011). Besides the P300, earlier ERP components like the N100 (Kramer et al., 1995; Ullsperger et al., 2001; Allison and Polich, 2008) the N200 (Kramer et al., 1995), the P1 (Pratt et al., 2011) and a positive-negative component between 140 and 280 ms (Missonnier et al., 2003, 2004) have been found to respond to task difficulty or workload. Finally, late positive or negative slow waves have been related to high memory load (Ruchkin et al., 1990) and amount of resource allocation (Rösler et al., 1997).

AROUSAL AND ENERGY DEMAND—PERIPHERAL PHYSIOLOGY

High mental workload is associated with high mental effort (Hockey, 1986; Gaillard and Wientjes, 1994). Mental workload or mental effort is associated with a decrease of the parasympathetic ("rest or digest") autonomous nervous system activity and an increase in sympathetic ("fight or flight") activity (Mulder and Mulder, 1987; Gawron et al., 1989). These changes in autonomous nervous system activity can be estimated through several peripheral physiological measures such as skin conductance (Roth, 1983), heart rate and heart rate variability (Berntson et al., 1997).

Electrical skin conductance varies with the moisture level of the skin. Since the sweat glands are controlled by the sympathetic part of the autonomous nervous system (Roth, 1983), electrodermal measures indicate the level of sympathetic activity or arousal. A large body of literature describes the positive effect of arousal on skin conductance (e.g., Winton et al., 1984; Greenwald et al., 1989; Boucsein, 1992, 1999; Brouwer et al., 2013). While increases in skin conductance may be viewed as reflecting sympathetic activity as a consequence of arousal due to mental effort, Reimer and Mehler (2011) and Kohlisch and Schaefer (1996) interpret their findings of heightened skin conductance with increased workload as reflecting emotional arousal.

Heart rate and its variability are affected by activation and suppression of both the sympathetic and parasympathetic nervous systems (Berntson et al., 1997). At normal breathing frequencies, fast changes in heart rate (0.15–0.50 Hz) reflect the adjustment of heart rate to breathing: breathing causes changes in blood pressure and by adapting heart rate, blood pressure is kept around a certain point (Mulder, 1980; Aasman et al., 1987). Also, the adaptation to breathing facilitates gas exchange between the lungs and the blood (Grossman and Taylor, 2007). High frequency heart rate variability reflects only the (fast) parasympathetic nervous system (Berntson et al., 1997). Mental effort has been reported to have the largest effect upon the mid-band (0.07–0.14 Hz; Mulder, 1980; Aasman et al., 1987). This band reflects not only parasympathetic but also sympathetic activity (Berntson et al., 1997; Veltman and Gaillard, 1998). For both bands, suppression of parasympathetic activity (associated with high workload) results in lower adaptation to changes in blood pressure and hence less heart rate variability.

Mental workload being associated with increased arousal and neural activity increases metabolic demand, which is probably the cause of observed increases in heart rate and respiration frequency with workload (Veltman and Gaillard, 1998).

EYE-RELATED MEASURES

Pupil dilation is not only caused by decreasing luminance but also by increasing workload (Beatty, 1982; May et al., 1990; Porter et al., 2007; Hampson et al., 2010). Consistent with this, the frontal cortex is involved in controlling pupil dilation (Hampson et al., 2010). The underlying function is unclear, but the fact that the effect has been observed in studies that varied task difficulty without varying the visual environment (Kahneman and Beatty, 1966; Kahneman et al., 1969) indicates that it does not primarily serve purposes related to visual perception. Reduction of blink frequency and duration with workload could be attributed to maximizing detection of visual information (Bauer et al., 1987; Fogarty and Stern, 1989). In this sense, the sensitivity of these parameters can often be explained by high workload being confounded by the presence of much visual information.

THREE SENSOR GROUPS

In sum, we can loosely divide physiological variables found to be associated with workload into three, what we call "sensor groups" that are assumed to reflect different aspects of workload. EEG measures are expected to mainly reflect cognitive processes. Peripheral physiological measures reflect arousal and energy demand. The third group of eye related measures have probably partly been found to covary with workload due to the often occurring confound of the amount of visual information, but for pupil dilation, the reason for its association with workload is unclear. Considering the idea that they reflect different aspects of workload, combination of these groups is expected to lead to better classification accuracy than either group alone, especially for the combination of EEG and peripheral physiology.

COMBINING VARIABLES—FUSION TECHNIQUES

In previous workload studies, EEG has been combined with other physiological signals for assessing workload. Coffey et al. (2012) found that classification of workload based on EEG was more accurate than when based on fNIRS (functional Near Infrared Spectroscopy), and that combining the two did not increase classification performance. Wilson and Russell (2003, 2007) combine respiration (Wilson and Russell, 2003), EEG, EOG and heart rate in their classification models to assess workload in simulated aviation-related tasks. However, they do not report on the relative contribution of these different signals to classification performance. Christensen et al. (2012) assessed workload in simulated remote piloting. Their classification models were based on EEG, EOG, heart rate, blink rate, blink amplitude, and blink duration. They did not extensively report on the relative contribution of these variables, but mention that when classification was performed on the basis of EEG only, classification accuracy hardly decreased (about 2%). Chanel et al. (2006) studied the relative contribution of EEG and peripheral physiological signals (skin conductance, heart rate, blood pressure, respiration and temperature) on classifying mental states as elicited by emotional pictures. They also did not find a strong advantage of fusion of EEG and physiology over EEG alone.

In all of these studies, combination of variables from different domains was achieved by simple concatenation of the input feature vectors. However, when combining EEG data with physiology, the large difference in length of the feature vectors forms a potential problem. While EEG spectral features are captured by power values in different frequency bands at different electrodes amounting to a large number of features, physiological or eye related features such as pupil size and heart rate are typically each represented by just one (average) value. This could lead to a priori small added value of these features. A possible solution is to use higher order combination of information by combing the assessments based on the various types of features. Such a method was used by Chanel et al. (2009) who studied classification of different emotions as elicited by emotional recall. Classification decisions were made by two different EEG based classifiers and one classifier based on physiology (skin conductance, heart rate, blood pressure and respiration) and these decisions were then combined. Adding the worst performing EEG set to the best performing one increased classification accuracy (that was generally between 70 and 80% for a two class problem) with about 2–4%, and adding physiology on top of that resulted in an additional increase of up to almost 3%. There was no direct comparison with the concatenation method (using all features as input to a single classifier) though the authors mention that this method did not lead to an increase in accuracy.

The improvements in classification accuracy as found by Chanel et al. (2009) are relatively small and are probably not statistically significant. However, the trend is positive and we think it is worthwhile to examine the case for workload where EEG and other types of signals are expected to complement each other. We will compare the discussed ways of combining information, i.e., fusion at the feature level or at the decision level. When combining decisions from different classifiers, a confidence measure of the decision is useful. Such a confidence measure is given by an elastic net model with logistic regression (Friedman et al., 2010). Therefore, besides using linear Support Vector Machine as the more standard classification model, we also use an elastic net model. This enables us to weigh information of the different sources before averaging (a similar method was used by Chanel et al., 2009). The potential advantage of fusion at a decision level is that smaller feature vectors reflecting physiology or eye related measures do not run the risk to be "flooded" by EEG—the disadvantage of fusion at the decision level is that interactions between different features or feature sets may be missed.

CURRENT STUDY: OVERVIEW AND HYPOTHESES

We study workload in an experiment in which we control for visual input and the amount of body movements by using an n-back task to vary workload. This task requires participants to indicate of each of successively presented letters whether it is a target or not. Workload is low when the target letter is an "x" (0-back), intermediate when the target letter is the same as the one before (1-back) and high when the target letter is the same as two letters before (2-back). In this task, visual input and number of button presses are the same across workload levels. This means that effects of workload can really be attributed to differences in mental processes and cannot be due to different amounts of hand or eye movements in the high workload condition compared to the low workload condition.

We determine the value of individual features and combinations for the assessment of individual workload level using individually trained classification models. We simulate an on-line situation in which a model is tuned to an individual using data from the first part of the experiment and in which the workload is predicted for the last part of the experiment. We record EEG, skin conductance, respiration, ECG, pupil size and eye blinks. Various variables are extracted from these measurements and used as features in classification models. Firstly, we examine how well classification models based on the various individual features perform. We expect EEG features to perform best given indications from earlier studies and given the fact that EEG is expected to reflect what can be considered to be the core of mental workload, namely cognitive processing. Next, we will look at combinations of features. We start by combining features originating from the same sensor (e.g., heart rate and heart rate variability that can both be determined from ECG). While these are not expected to strongly improve classification performance since they are probably largely reflecting the same underlying process, we think it is worth trying for the practical reason that these features are available without additional costs (i.e., without having to use an additional sensor). Subsequently, we combine features from different sensor groups "EEG," "Physiology," and "Eyes." Especially the combination of EEG with Physiology is expected to improve classification performance since these groups are assumed to reflect different general physiological processes associated with workload. For analyses at the sensor group level, we check whether taking time into account improves classification performance. An improvement of including information about time of measurement may be expected based on finding general effects of time on physiological variables (e.g., Fairclough et al., 2005; Brouwer et al., 2014). For analyses at the sensor group level, we also compare fusion at the feature level to fusion at the decision level. We use both SVM and elastic net classification models.

MATERIALS AND METHODS

PARTICIPANTS

Data of 14 participants are analyzed in this study. Participants were aged between 23 and 40 years (mean age 27.9), 8 female and 6 male. The experiment was performed in accordance with the local ethics guidelines and participants gave written informed consent[2].

MATERIALS

Stimuli (letters), subjective workload scales and announcements about the type of the n-back task to follow were presented on a Tobii T60 Eye Tracker monitor, at a distance of about 50 cm from the participants' eyes. Feedback about task performance was presented through Labtec LCS-1050 speakers in the form of beeps. Participants used a keyboard to indicate whether presented letters were targets or non-targets. Which of the keys (1 or 2 on the numerical pad) indicated "target" and which "non-target" was counterbalanced between participants. Participants used the mouse to rate subjective workload on a scale (RSME) between the stimulus blocks.

EEG (electro encephalogram) was recorded through a g.tec USBamp and g.tec Au electrodes placed at Fz, FCz, Pz, C3, C4, F3, and F4, referenced to linked mastoid electrodes. A ground electrode was placed at FPz. Impedance was kept below 5 kΩ. EEG data were filtered by a 0.1 Hz high pass- and a 100 Hz low pass filter and sampled with a frequency of 256 Hz (USB Biosignal Amplifier, g.tecmedical engineering GmbH).

ECG (electro cardiogram) and skin conductance were recorded using a MindWare BioNex 8-slot chassis with a 3-channel Bio-Potential and GSR amplifier. A 4-channel transducer amplifier was used to measure respiration. For ECG measurement, self-adhesive 1 1/2″ electrodes with 7% chloride wet gel

[2]A total of 35 participants took part in the original experiment (see also Brouwer et al., 2012, 2014). However, we here only considered participants with complete data sets. We also performed similar analyses for all participants for which a subset of data was available. The results from such partial analyses showed the same patterns as presented here.

were attached just below the right collarbone, just below the left lower rib and above the right hip. To record skin conductance, two self-adhesive 1 5/8″ electrodes with 1% chloride wet gel were attached to the palm of the left hand that was not used for pressing the keys—one below the thumb and one below the little finger. Respiration was recorded using an elastic band around the waist at the height of the lower side of the sternum. MindWare's BioLab software was used to acquire ECG, skin conductance and respiration. These signals were sampled with a frequency of 300 Hz. They were acquired with a gain setting of 1000, 10, and 500 and filtered with a 0.5, 1, and 5 Hz high-pass filters, respectively.

Pupil size, blink rate and blink duration were measured using a Tobii T60 Eye Tracker that was integrated into an 17″ monitor. Recording frequency was 60 Hz. All signals were synchronized using the TCAP signal from The Observer XT (Zimmerman et al., 2009).

We used the RSME scale (Rating Scale Mental Effort, Zijlstra, 1993) to measure subjectively experienced mental effort. This scale runs from 0 to 150 with higher values reflecting higher workload. It has nine descriptors along the axis, e.g., "not effortful" at value 2 and "rather effortful" at value 58. Verwey and Veltman (1996) concluded this simple one-dimensional scale to be more sensitive than the often-used NASA-TLX (Hart and Staveland, 1988).

TASK

Participants viewed letters, successively presented on a screen. For each letter, they pressed a button to indicate whether the letter was a target or a non-target. In the 0-back condition, the letter x is the target. In the 1-back condition, a letter is a target when it is the same as the one before. In the 2-back condition, a letter is a target when it is the same as two letters before. With this version of the n-back task, the level of workload is varied without varying visual input or frequency and type of motor output (button presses). A 3-back condition was not used, due to evidence that many participants find it too difficult and tend to give up (Ayaz et al., 2007; Izzetoglu et al., 2007).

Participants were informed after every button press whether it was a correct decision by a high (correct) or a low (incorrect) pitched tone. This was intended to help the participant, who in our experiment switched rather often between n-back conditions, and to increase the likelihood that participants would decide to invest effort since the participant knew the experiment leader would hear the sounds as well.

STIMULI

The letters used in the n-back task were black (font style: Matlab standard, approximately 3 cm high) and were presented on a light gray background. The letters were presented for 500 ms followed by a 2000-ms inter-stimulus interval during which the letter was replaced by a fixation cross. In all conditions, 33% of letters were targets. Except for the letter x in the 0-back task, letters were randomly selected from English consonants. Vowels were excluded to reduce the likeliness of participants developing chunking strategies which reduce mental effort, as suggested in Grimes et al. (2008).

DESIGN

The three conditions (0-back, 1-back, 2-back) were presented in 2-min blocks divided across four sessions. Each session consisted of two repetitions of each of the three blocks. Thus, for each of the three conditions participants performed 4 sessions *2 repetitions = 8 blocks. In each block, 48 letters were presented, 16 of which were targets. The blocks were presented in pseudorandom order, such that each condition was presented once in the first half of the session and once in the second half of the session, and that blocks of the same condition never occurred directly after each other. Before each session was a baseline block of 2 min in which the participant quietly fixated a cross on the screen. With 4 sessions *2 repetitions *3 conditions, plus 4 sessions *1 baseline block, the total duration of the n-back task was 56 min.

PROCEDURE

After entering the lab, participants read and were explained about the experimental procedure. They then signed an informed consent form. The physiological sensors were attached and the Tobii eye tracker was calibrated. The three conditions were practiced up to the point that the participant was familiar with the task. Regardless of this, all participants completed at least one block of the 2-back task in order to also practice the RSME rating that appeared at the end of the block. It was stressed that the 2-back task could be difficult, but that even when the participant thought it was too difficult he or she should keep trying to do as well as possible. Participants were asked to avoid movement as much as possible while performing the task and to use the breaks in between the blocks to make necessary movements. Before the start of each block, the participant was informed about the nature of the block (rest, 0-back, 1-back, or 2-back) via the monitor. After each block, the RSME scale was presented and the participant rated subjective mental effort by clicking the appropriate location on the scale using the mouse. The next block started after the participant indicated to be ready by pressing a button. Between sessions, participants had longer breaks, chatting with the experiment leader or having a drink.

DEFINITION OF FEATURES

EEG data were filtered by a 0.1 Hz high pass- and a 100 Hz low pass filter and sampled with a frequency of 256 Hz (USB Biosignal Amplifier, g.tecmedical engineering GmbH). Afterwards data was processed and analyzed using Matlab and the FieldTrip open source Matlab toolbox (Oostenveld et al., 2011). Epochs starting at 500 ms before stimulus onset and ending 2000 ms after were shifted such that the mean of the first 500 ms was zero. No eye blink artifacts were removed before classification which makes the implementation of online classification easier. Our previous analysis (Brouwer et al., 2012) showed that with EOG performance was not better or contribute to EEG-based workload classification, indicating that performance is only expected to get better when removing them. Over each block and each of the 7 EEG-channels (C3, F3, C4, F4, Fz, Pz, FCz) we calculated the average ERP over all trials after resampling the data to 100 Hz. The ($N =$ 101) samples between 0 to 1 s as ERP-features. Similarly, for each of the trials and channels the spectral power over complete trials (from −0.5 to +2.0 s) was calculated in ($N = 37$) bands ranging from 2 to 20 Hz (in steps of 0.5 Hz) following an FFT approach using a single Hanning taper. Next, the average spectral power was determined for each block and channel (by averaging over all trials within a block). Trials with extreme variance in the signal as defined by a standard deviation above 100 μV were discarded before calculating the average ERP and spectral power features (1% of the data). Apart from using the "raw" ERP and power spectra of the various EEG-channels we also used alpha power and theta power as feature input for classification. As a measure of alpha power we used the average over the natural log transformed power within the frequency band ranging from 8 to 13 Hz. As a measure of theta power we used the average over the natural log transformed power of frequencies between 4 and 8 Hz. Models that included alpha power and/or theta power as features did not also include the raw power values. Additionally, we examined alpha power of EEG as only recorded at Pz, theta power as only recorded at Fz and ERP as only recorded at Pz since it would be practical to attach only one electrode to the scalp, and those are the location-feature combinations that we a priori expect to produce the clearest results. Effects of workload on the alpha band are particularly expected around Pz (for effortful and attentive processing alpha reduction is observed at parietal regions—(Klimesch et al., 2000; Keil et al., 2006). Effects of workload on the theta band are particularly expected around frontal electrode locations such as Fz (e.g., Miyata et al., 1990; Raghavachari et al., 2001; Jensen and Tesche, 2002; Esposito et al., 2009). The P300 is expected to be most clearly visible at Pz (e.g., Ravden and Polich, 1999; Srinivasan, 2007). Since a priori Pz seems to be the most informative electrode, we also looked at EEG data in general coming only from this electrode.

Skin conductance level was determined by averaging skin conductance over each block. Inspection of the raw data showed that frequently, skin conductance peaks around the onset of a block (i.e., after rating subjective workload of the previous block) after which skin conductance rapidly decreases and remains around the same level. This led us to also use minimum skin conductance of each block as a feature.

As a measure of heart rate, we determined the mean RRI for each block. RRI is the interval between successive heart beats or more precisely, the interval between subsequent R-peaks in the ECG. Three measures of heart rate variability were computed. The root mean squared successive difference (RMSSD: Goedhart et al., 2007) between the RRIs reflects high frequency heart rate variability. High-frequency heart rate variability was also computed as the power in the high frequency range (0.15–0.5 Hz) of the RRI over time using Welch's method applied after spline interpolation; similarly, for mid-frequency heart rate variability the power in the frequency range of 0.07–0.15 Hz was used.

The respiration signal was filtered using a running Gaussian blurring window (with a kernel width of 0.39 s). Subsequently peaks and throughs were detected using the derivative of the signal. Breathing frequency was defined as the mean time interval between the peaks. Modulation depth was defined as the average difference between peak and through.

Pupil size as determined by the Tobii Eyetracker and the ClearView algorithms was averaged for each block. When the eyetracker did not detect the pupil for both eyes for minimally two successive frames (i.e., 33 ms) and maximally 25 successive frames (416 ms), this was considered to be a blink. For each blink, blink duration was determined. Blink rate is the average number of blinks per minute.

The feature "time" was operationalized as the mid-time of the corresponding data segment in seconds from the start of the experiment, discarding breaks and periods in between blocks in which the RSME was registered. For instance, the mid-time of the first 2-min workload block is 60 s and that of the second is 180 s.

Physiological features that were considered with respect to their capacity to estimate workload in this study are summarized in **Table 1**. This table also indicates the length of the corresponding feature vector ("Dimension"), as well as the single sensors and the sensor groups that the features belong to. For examining the usability of different variables for assessing workload, we follow the list of features as summed up in **Table 1**. Only for EEG, features can consist of multiple values (dimension larger than 1). The rationale behind this is that the mentioned features are the smallest possible pieces of information that are expected to reflect workload. For examining EEG sensors "all electrodes," "Pz," and "Fz," we only include features reflecting both ERP and spectral properties of the EEG signal as printed in italics. The EEG sensor group only includes ERP and spectral power features of "All electrodes."

CLASSIFICATION ANALYSIS

The first three sessions, each containing two blocks of each n-back condition, were used to train the model parameters to individual participants. The last session was used to evaluate the model's classification accuracy. This simulates estimating workload online, using model parameters that are adjusted to the individual participant in a training phase. As a default, the classification models were trained and applied to distinguish between 0- and 2-back blocks, each containing 2 min of data or 48 trials (letters). Average classification performance (fraction correct in the last session) over all participants was used as measure of model performance.

Feature vectors were constructed for each of the data segments. For instance, the feature vectors used for the model that includes all spectral power values over 120 s blocks of data contains 259 features (power at 37 frequencies × 7 channels, see **Table 1** second row) × 16 blocks (4 sessions × 4 blocks). The data from the first 3 sessions was used to train a classifier model for each individual participant. The features were standardized to have mean 0 and standard deviation 1 on the basis of data from the training set. The same standardization transformation was applied to the test data (the data of the 4th session). After training the model using the training data (12 blocks of 259 features in the example above), the classification was applied to the test data and the performance score of each of the individual models was determined. Finally, overall performance is calculated by taking the average score over all individual models.

Classification accuracy was determined for a range of models differing in the (types of) features that were included in the model, differing in the type of classifier and differing in the fusion rule that was used. Classification was performed using the Donders machine learning toolbox (DMLT) developed by

Table 1 | Examined (neuro)physiological features, sensors and sensor groups.

Sensor group	Sensor	Feature	Dimension
EEG	*All electrodes*	ERP (0–1 s from stimulus onset)	707
		Spectral power (2–20 Hz)	259
		Alpha power (8–13 Hz)	7
		Theta power (4–8 Hz)	7
		ERP + Spectral power features	966
	Pz (single electrode)	ERP (0–1 s from stimulus onset)	101
		Alpha power (8–13 Hz)	1
		ERP + Spectral power features	138
	Fz (single electrode)	Theta power (4–8 Hz)	1
Physiology	Skin conductance electrodes	Mean skin conductance level	1
		Minimum skin conductance level	1
	Respiration belt	Respiration frequency	1
		Respiration modulation depth	1
	ECG electrodes	HR (heart rate—RRI)	1
		RMSSD	1
		Mid frequency HRV	1
		High frequency HRV	1
Eye	Eye camera	Pupil size	1
		Blink rate	1
		Blink duration	1

For EEG, the sensors "All electrodes," "Pz" and "Fz" are examined using the features as defined by ERP and spectral power (printed in italics). The EEG sensor group only includes ERP and spectral power features of "All electrodes."

van Gerven et al. (2013). Two types of classifiers were used. We used a linear Support Vector Machine as representing a more standard model and, in order to obtain confidence measures that can be used to fuse information, we used an elastic net model with logistic regression (Friedman et al., 2010).

For combining information across sensor groups, both fusion at feature level and fusion at the decision level were investigated. In the first (default) case the concatenated feature vector containing all features was used as the input to a single model. In the latter case, the final decision was based on the average of the probability estimates supplied by the logistic regression from the different elastic net models, each based on the individual features (one model output for each feature). For instance, if estimated probabilities on high workload would be based on mean heart rate, mean skin conductance and blink rate with model output probabilities of $p1 = 0.2$, $p2 = 0.6$, $p3 = 0.5$, the average probability of the combination model is 0.43. Thus, these data would be assessed to reflect low workload.

STATISTICAL ANALYSIS

We used one-tailed binomial tests to determine whether classification accuracy was significantly higher than chance, which works as follows. In the default situation of classifying the 2-min high and low workload blocks (2- vs. 0-back), classification accuracy per participant could only take values of 0, 0.25, 0.50, 0.75, and 1 (correct classification of 0–4 blocks in the last session). To test whether on the whole, classification performance is above chance, we compute the averaged score over all 14 individual models as a measure of performance. This average score can take on values between 0/56, 1/56, 2/56,...1 (resolution of 1/56 where 56 is 4 possible scores higher than zero*14 participants). To determine whether this average score is significantly higher than chance we calculate the chance that a this score or higher is obtained when using a random classification model (i.e., with a probability of classifying a block as one or the other with a probability of 0.5). In this way, one can determine that the chance of obtaining a value of 0.61 or higher given a probability of 50% is equal to 0.05 (the level corresponding to $p = 0.05$ in e.g., **Figure 1**). We also calculated Bonferroni corrected levels per comparison/figure, and found that when the $p = 0.05$ significance level is corrected for multiple testing (using Bonferroni) this level goes up to the same level as the uncorrected $p = 0.01$ level. This means that the conditions that reach an uncorrected level of $p = 0.01$ maintain significance after Bonferroni correction (at $p = 0.05$).

Pairwise comparison tests were used to determine whether two accuracies were significantly different from each other. To indicate the level of significance chance and alpha levels are shown in the various figures. The figures also include estimates of the standard error in the fractions correct based on a binomial distribution. We did not correct for multiple testing which means that estimates of significance levels are on the low side.

Since the results suggested that EEG models might perform at ceiling level and that we could get a higher benefit of combining variables for a more difficult case where workload assessment did not reach ceiling, we also analyzed performance for classifying smaller workload differences (2- vs. 1-back and 1- vs. 0-back) and for classifying 30 rather than 120 s segments of data. In the latter case two of the participants' data were incomplete due to segments without blinks resulting in undefined blink duration and were discarded (leaving 12 participants). Using parts of blocks rather than complete blocks resulted in having 16 data sets (each 30 s long) per participant available to test the trained classification model rather than 4 (each 2 min long).

RESULTS

Task difficulty and subjective effort (workload) were successfully manipulated as indicated by the expected effects of n-back level on performance and subjective ratings (Brouwer et al., 2012). The different n-back levels resulted in the expected differences in performance for the 14 subjects with decreasing fraction correct (0.96, 0.94, and 0.90 for the 0-back, 1-back, and 2-back conditions) and increasing response times (560, 616, and 730 ms respectively). Perceived mental effort as measured by RSME increased with n-back level (31, 39, and 55 for the 0-back, 1-back, and 2-back conditions respectively).

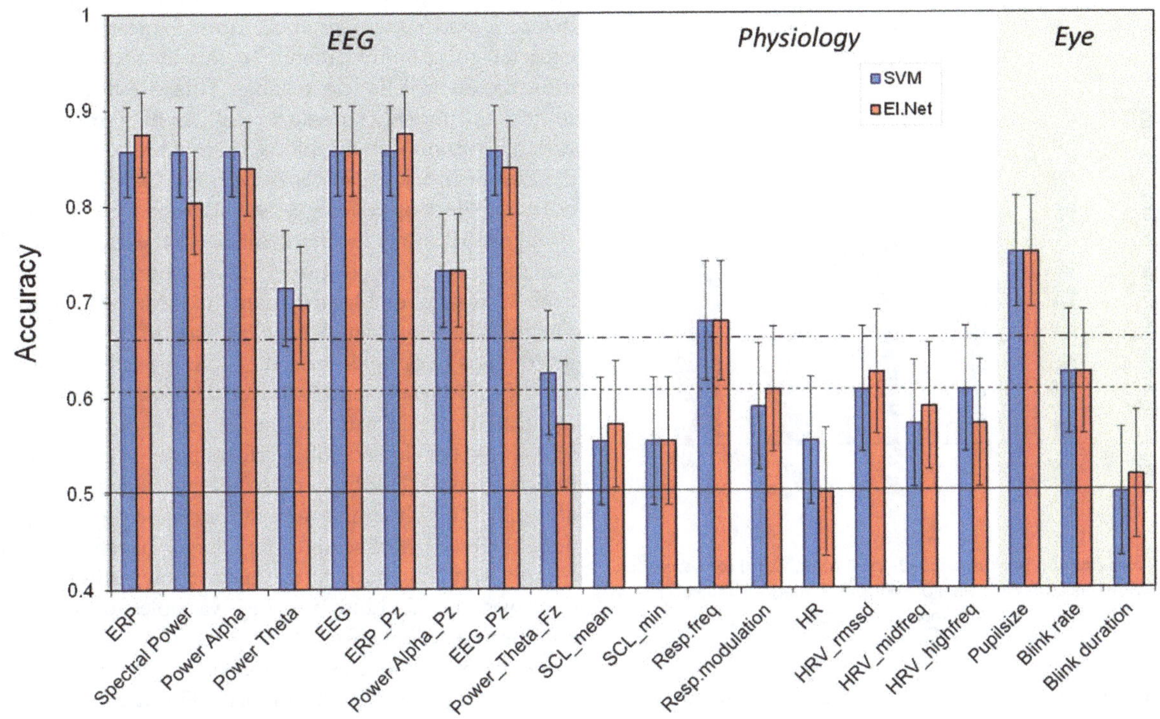

FIGURE 1 | Classification performance (2- vs. 0-back, 120 s) for separate features as resulting from SVM and elastic net classification models. The horizontal lines indicate chance level (**bottom**), 0.05 significance level (**middle**) and 0.01 significance level (**top**). Different shades in the background indicate the three different sensor groups EEG, Physiology and Eye. Error bars indicate estimates of the variance (s.e.m.s) based on the binomial distribution.

SINGLE VARIABLES

Figure 1 shows the performance of models that include a single variable or feature (as defined in the second column of **Table 1**), separately for the SVM and elastic net classification approaches (see below "Classification Approach"). The horizontal lines indicate chance level, and levels corresponding to a significant difference from chance, for $p = 0.05$ and $p = 0.01$. In general, performance of models based on EEG variables is much better than models based on the other (single) variables.

ERP and spectral power (when using SVM) lead to approximately the same high classification performance of over 0.85 as using all EEG features. Moreover, when reducing information from using EEG or ERP as recorded at all electrodes to only Pz classification performance remains at the same level. Also, when instead of using all frequency bands only alpha is used, performance does not deteriorate. Using only Pz for alpha alone does reduce performance relative to using all electrodes ($p < 0.05$). A model based on the theta band alone does not perform as well as using all frequencies ($p < 0.05$), indicating that the theta band is less informative in our case (in correspondence with our previous findings, see Brouwer et al., 2012).

Models based on the physiological variables perform relatively poorly with respiration frequency being the only feature that reaches the 0.01 significance level with an accuracy of 0.68. High frequency HRV (as defined by RMSSD and spectrally defined) is the only other physiological feature that, depending on the classification approach, just reaches significance ($p < 0.05$).

In comparison, models based on eye measures show relatively good performance with a classification accuracy of 0.75 for pupil size. Blink rate significantly performs above chance as well but blink duration does not.

SINGLE SENSORS

Figure 2 shows the performance of the "single sensor" models, i.e., the models that include all features belonging to a certain sensor. Also shown is the performance of the best performing single variable model for each sensor type (in which ERP and spectral power are regarded as the corresponding single features for EEG and EEG_Pz. Skin conductance reaches the significance level when features are combined using the elastic net model, while it remains below significance level for each individual feature. However, and as hypothesized, performance of models using combinations of features from a single sensor do not perform significantly better compared to using only the best performing single feature for any of the sensors. Again, the EEG model shows the best performance (with an accuracy of 0.86 for both classification approaches). Second best is the performance of the models based on eye measures (accuracy of 0.75 for SVM). Also the model based on respiration reaches a relatively high performance level (accuracy of 0.70 for both classification approaches). Models based on skin conductance (accuracy of 0.63 for elastic net) and ECG (accuracy of 0.61 for elastic net) show relatively poor performance, just reaching a level that is significantly higher than chance ($p < 0.05$). Pairwise comparison tests (using the SVM-data) show

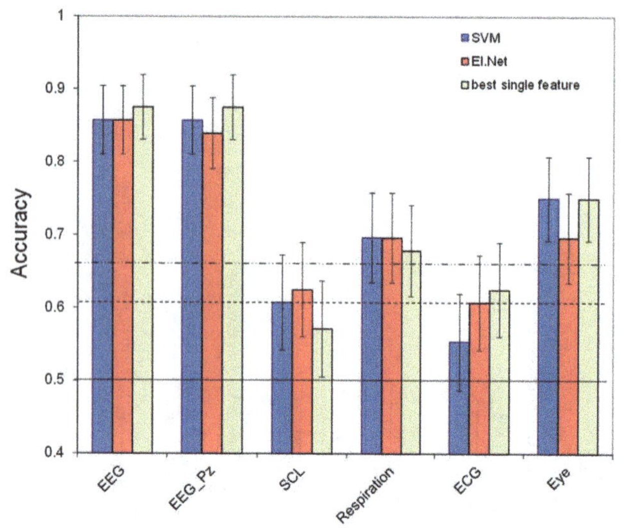

FIGURE 2 | Classification performance (2- vs. 0-back, 120 s) for separate sensors. Conventions as in **Figure 1**. For comparison, performance of the best performing feature for each of sensor is depicted.

that the EEG models are significantly different from the other models ($p < 0.01$), and that performance of the eye model is significantly better than that of the skin conductance and ECG models ($p < 0.05$).

COMBINATIONS ACROSS SENSOR GROUPS

Figure 3 shows the results for different (combinations of) sensor groups of SVM and elastic net, as well as the outcome of combining the outputs of different elastic net models ("decision level"). Shown are the results for the default case of classifying 2 vs. 0-back over 2 min. data segments (a) as well as for more difficult cases: using 30 s data segments (b), or classifying 2 vs. 1-back (c), or 1 vs. 0-back (d). Comparing performance in the default case (**Figure 3A**) with that of separate sensors (**Figure 2**) shows that for Physiology, combining the three sensors leads to a (non-significant) increase in performance (accuracy of 0.75 for SVM, compared to 0.70 for the best performing single physiological sensor respiration). Models that include EEG perform significantly better than physiology and eye models (SVM, pairwise comparisons, $p < 0.05$). Adding sensor groups to the already well performing EEG improves classification accuracy by 3–5% (for adding Physiology or Eye variables with elastic net). For SVM, the combination of physiology and eye measures tends to improve performance relative to either one alone by 7% as well. However, all of these improvements do not reach statistical significance. Using the assumption of a binomial distribution, significance ($p < 0.05$) is reached for differences of around 10%.

We may not observe a larger, statistically significant improvement of combining EEG with physiology (as we had hypothesized) because EEG alone is already performing very well. Therefore, we performed the same analyses on more challenging classification tasks, namely classification of shorter time segments (30 s rather than 120 s) and classification of more similar workload levels (2- vs. 1-back and 1-back vs. 0-back). In addition, this gives us an impression of how much lower classification performance is under these circumstances. Shorter time segments are expected to be more difficult to classify because the extraction information will be less reliable. This is especially obvious for some of the non-EEG measures (e.g., for high frequency heart rate variability minimum durations of 1 min are advised: Task Force of the European Society of Cardiology the North American Society of Pacing Electrophysiology, 1996; Berntson et al., 1997).

Figure 3B shows the performance of the models for classifying data segments of 30 s instead of 120 s. Note that this includes data from 12 instead of 14 participants (see Materials and Methods). The thresholds for significance decrease in this case since the test set contains 16 samples instead of 4. As expected, performance for classifying 30 s segments is lower than for classifying 120 s segments, with a performance that is (on average) 8% (SVM) and 5% (elastic net) lower. Still, performance for models that include EEG is around 0.8 or higher for the elastic net model. The pattern of results is highly similar to that for classifying 120 s segments—thus, there does not seem to be a larger benefit of sensor group combination than in the previous case, suggesting that the lack of improvement of adding non-EEG variables to the EEG model is not due to a ceiling effect.

Figure 3C shows classification performance for classifying 2-back vs. 1-back using 2-min blocks. **Figure 3D** shows 1-back vs. 0-back classification performance. As expected, performance for discriminating smaller differences in workload is lower than for discriminating 2-back vs. 0-back. Performance is on average 10% (SVM) and 6% (elastic net) lower for 2 vs. 1-back, with performance around 0.85 for elastic net models including EEG. It is 22% (SVM) and 18% (elastic net) lower for 1 vs. 0-back, with performance just below 0.70 for elastic net models including EEG. This suggests a larger increase in workload from 1-back to 2-back than from 0-back to 1-back in accordance with earlier findings (Brouwer et al., 2012, 2014). Again, models that include EEG variables show the best performance. Performance of classification models based on Physiology is not significantly different from chance for both small workload differences, and the Eye based model drops to chance level when distinguishing 1- from 0-back.

Also included in **Figure 3** is the performance of the "decision level" model that combines the output of different elastic net models (based on single features). We did not find any significant differences between performance of the elastic net models that use the two types of fusion; trends indicate an advantage of fusion at the feature level compared to fusion at the decision level.

Figure 4 shows the effect of adding the feature time (i.e., the time of measurement, since the start of the experiment) to the model input for the default case (2- vs. 1-back, 120 s of data). Adding time leads to an increase in performance of 9% (significant at $p < 0.05$) and 5% (not significant) for respectively physiological and eye sensor group models (SVM) when classifying 2- vs. 0-back using 120 s of data. For EEG and "All" the inclusion of time information does not improve performance. Further analysis of the data shows that when classification is more difficult due to shorter time intervals or smaller workload differences (see **Figures 3B–D**), the potentially beneficial effect of including time decreases.

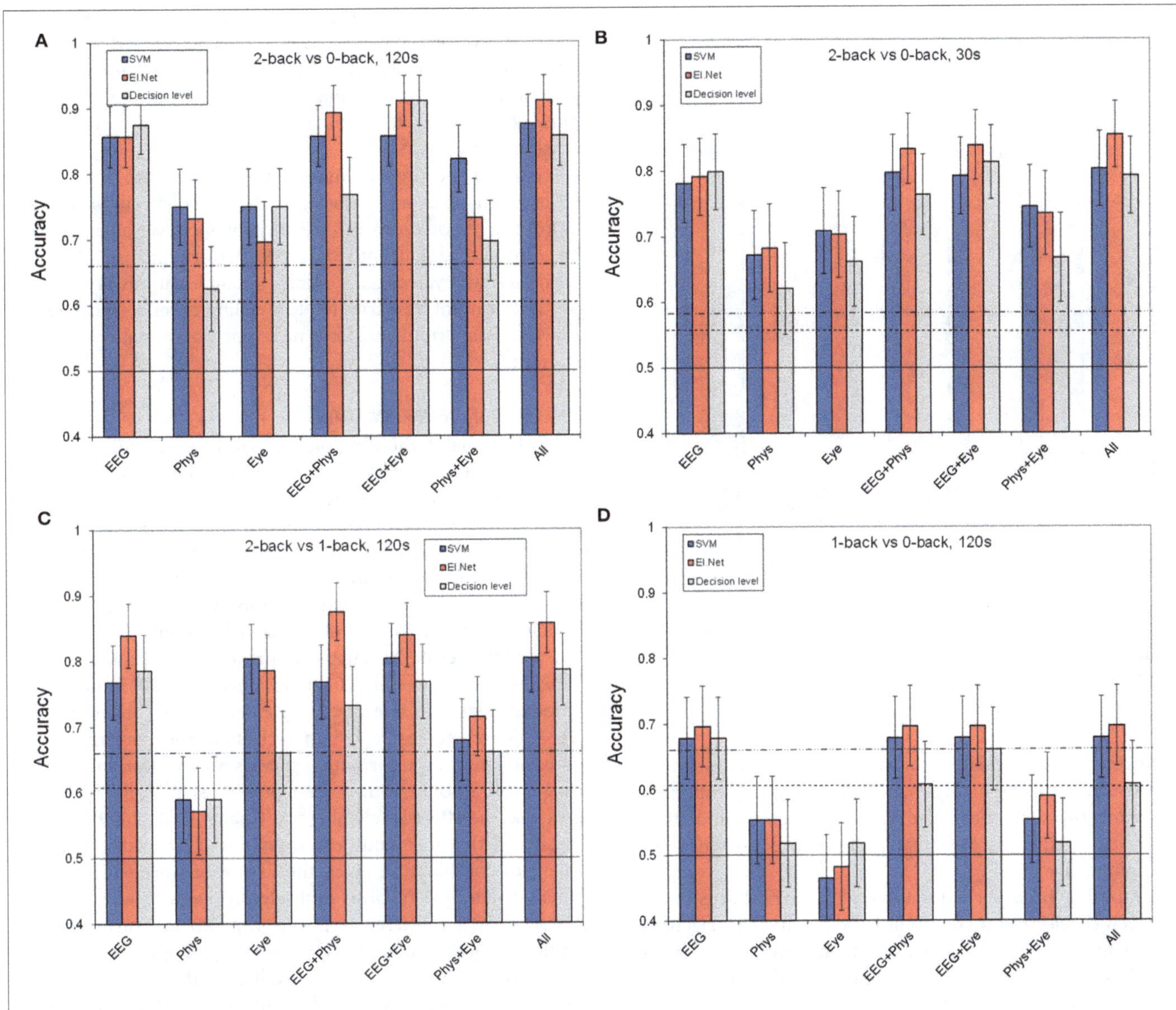

FIGURE 3 | Classification performance for separate and combined sensor groups for SVM, elastic net and a model that combines the outputs from different single feature models ("decision level"). (A) performance in the default condition (2- vs. 0-back, 120 s of data, **(B)** for comparing 2- vs. 0-back over 30 s of data, **(C)** for comparing 2- vs. 1-back (120 s of data), **(D)** for comparing 1- vs. 0-back (120 s of data).

CONCLUSION AND DISCUSSION

SUMMARY OF FINDINGS

In this study, we compared how well different physiological variables can be used to assess workload in (simulated) real time for a single individual, when the amount of body movement and visual information are controlled for. We also examined to what extent (different ways of) combining information leads to better classification performance, as well as whether taking time into account improves performance.

Classification models based on data from each of the three sensor groups perform above chance (distinguishing high from low workload) at a 0.01 significance level, where EEG reached around 86% classification accuracy and classification models based on peripheral physiology and eye-related variables reached between 70 and 75% accuracy. As hypothesized, the difference in classification accuracy between models based on EEG variables on the one hand, and models based on peripheral physiology and eye-related variables on the other hand was statistically significant. The best performing single variable was ERP at Pz with 88% accuracy (elastic net). All EEG variables (except power in the theta band measured at Fz) performed well above chance ($p < 0.01$). The only non-EEG variables exceeding the 0.01 chance level were respiration frequency (69% accuracy) and pupil size (75% accuracy).

As hypothesized, combining variables recorded using a single sensor (i.e., only the EEG electrodes, electrode Pz, skin conductance electrodes, respiration belt, ECG electrodes or eye camera) does not significantly improve performance over the best

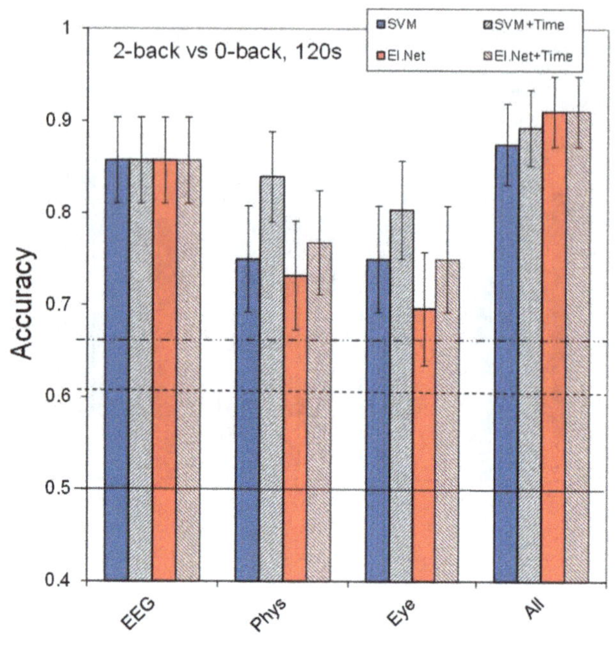

FIGURE 4 | Classification performance in the default condition (2- vs. 0-back, 120 s) for the different sensor types and using all available input. The striped bars show the effect of adding the time feature. Conventions as in **Figure 1**.

performing single variable from that sensor. Variables from the same sensor are likely highly correlated and, in our experiment, combining them has no added value. For four out of the six sensors the trend was even that performance worsened when combining data.

Combining variables of the three physiological sensors (skin conductance electrodes, respiration belt and ECG electrodes) resulted in a modest, non-significant improvement to around 75% classification accuracy with respect to the best performing single physiological sensor (respiration—around 70%). In contrast to what we expected, combining EEG with another sensor group (physiology and eyes) does not lead to a significant improvement in classification accuracy over EEG alone. Using elastic net, we only found non-significant trends of better performance for EEG combined with eye data (91% accuracy) and EEG combined with physiology (89%) than EEG alone (86% accuracy). Adding physiology to fused EEG and eye data does not further improve, or tend to improve, performance. Analysis of data from shorter time segments or smaller workload differences indicates that the fact that we did not get a stronger, significant improvement of adding physiological or eye data to EEG is not caused by a ceiling effect.

Fusion of variables by concatenating feature vectors could not be improved by fusing variables at the decision level. The latter approach results in a more balanced weighting of the different indicators compensating for the low number of features from physiological and eye-based variables relative to EEG, and could therefore have improved classification. As it turned out, the variables that may have profited of the decision level approach, i.e., physiological and eye data, performed lower than EEG variables. Giving more weight to variables with a lower performance is not necessarily beneficial. In addition, classification models based on concatenation may be making more optimal use of interactions between variables that are missed when fusion occurs at the decision level.

Including the time of measurement relative to the start of the experiment as a parameter leads to statistically significant improvements of up to 9% for physiological variables. Adding time did not significantly improve performance of classifiers based on EEG, eye-related variables or combinations of variables. The latter cannot be attributed to a ceiling effect, as indicated by analysis of data from shorter time segments or smaller workload differences.

COMBINATION OF INFORMATION

The notion that combining physiological variables that reflect a certain mental state will result in a more accurate assessment of this mental state compared to using these variables on their own seems very sensible and has frequently been suggested in the literature as a potential way to improve mental state assessment. However, we are not aware of studies that tried this and showed a statistically reliable and strong improvement. A few studies explicitly mention that combination of physiological information did not result in reliable improvement (e.g., Christensen et al., 2012; Coffey et al., 2012; Severens et al., 2013) or only to a modest degree in one of multiple conditions (Brouwer et al., 2012). Other studies report that classification performance of models combining information increases classification accuracy (by a small amount) but do not provide statistical evidence to show that the effect is reliable (e.g., Chanel et al., 2009). We had anticipated that our study could provide clear evidence for the benefit of combination given the nature of workload, which is a mental state that involves multiple processes that are presumably reflected by different types of physiological variables (e.g., cognitive processes by EEG and arousal by peripheral physiological measures). Also, while most studies combine information by fusion at the feature level, we thought that fusion of information at the decision level could have contributed to finding a strong reliable advantage of combining information. However, we did not find significant differences between the two methods, with the overall trend indicating worse rather than better performance for fusion at the decision. The fact that with this study, there is still no evidence of large benefits when combining physiological variables reflecting workload suggests that they are too highly related to gain a benefit of combination. It could be the case that meta-analyses or a study such as ours including more participants would turn non-significant trends of fusion benefits into statistically significant effects. However, if present at all, the effects of data fusion are at least small. Also, it may be the case that for other tasks (perhaps involving more strong emotional processing besides cognitive processes) benefits of feature fusion can be found more easily.

WORKLOAD ASSESSMENT PERFORMANCE

Classification accuracy for distinguishing 2-min segments of high vs. low workload for a single individual is relatively high (with an average over participants up to 91%), especially when considering the fact that the amount of movements and visual information was the same across workload levels, and that classification simulated a real time situation.

When the duration of to be classified data segments was decreased to 30 s, this resulted in a relatively small decrease in performance, of on average 5% (elastic net) to 8% (SVM). The results further show that discrimination between more subtle differences in workload is possible as well. These results are good news for potential use in applications. Another finding that is useful for practical applications is that performance based on a single Pz-channel was found to be comparable to that of a model using all EEG-channels. This means that in our case a single channel suffices to characterize the EEG.

As reported, we found EEG variables to be most informative when assessing workload. However, we also found pupil size and blink rate to reflect workload. This is interesting given the fact that lighting conditions and visual input were strictly controlled in our experiment. These results thus indicate that not only pupil size but also blink rate is affected by mental workload level apart from visual demands.

GROUP vs. INDIVIDUAL LEVEL

In the present study, we examine how well different variables can be used to assess workload in real time for a single individual by training classification models on different types of information and comparing performance. Sensitivity of physiological variables is often examined using group level analyses (e.g., using repeated measures ANOVAs). However, for various reasons (see Introduction) one cannot draw straightforward conclusions about assessing workload on an individual level from the results on a group level. For instance, in the current study we found that classification models based on heart rate performed badly, while, for basically the same set of data, this variable was found to be among the ones most strongly associated with workload in a repeated measures ANOVA (Brouwer et al., 2014). Brouwer et al. (2014) also found that heart rate strongly decreased over the time course of the experiment. Since we presented workload conditions in 2-min segments equally dispersed over time, even strong time effects are averaged out in repeated measure ANOVAs whereas they could overrule the comparatively small workload effects in classification type of analyses, especially when classification models are trained on data acquired at the start of the experiment and tested on data at the end. Thus, caution should be taken when generalizing results from studies using group level analysis to situations where momentary data of individuals is used.

NOISE AND CONFOUNDS IN REAL LIFE

In real-life, out-of-the-lab situations, the presence of factors like body movement and varying light conditions may act as noise, therewith diminishing the value of certain variables (e.g., pupil size). Also, levels of workload can be confounded with different levels of stimulus processing or motor actions. For example, workload in Air Traffic Control may be confounded by speech, where controllers talking more during high than during low workload situations. Such confounds may affect physiology (e.g., speech affects respiration), resulting in improved classification accuracy. One of the reasons for the fact that we only found a minor improvement in performance by fusing different workload measures may have been that the experiment controlled for many of such confounding factors, thus decreasing the additional benefit of recording various physiological measures. In this way we were better able to determine which factors directly reflect mental workload. However, in practical situations, physiological measures may supply information about the context and contribute to workload assessment in a more indirect way, i.e., via the confounds. In such a case one should determine whether physiological measures are the most convenient measures to supply workload information, or whether task or behavioral measures (such as the detection of speech through audio sensors with respect to our previous ATC example) are more suitable.

ACKNOWLEDGMENTS

We would like to thank Pjotr van Amerongen, Rob van de Pijpekamp, Tobias Heffelaar and Patrick Zimmerman (Noldus) for technical assistance, Marcel van Gerven and Jason Farquar for contributions to the multivariate analysis tools and the SVM method in the FieldTrip toolbox, Boris Reuderink and Robert Oostenveld for fruitful discussions. This research has been supported by the GATE project, funded by the Netherlands Organization for Scientific Research (NWO) and the Netherlands ICT Research and Innovation Authority (ICT Regie). Furthermore, the authors gratefully acknowledge the support of the BrainGain Smart Mix Programme of the Netherlands Ministry of Economic Affairs and the Netherlands Ministry of Education, Culture and Science.

REFERENCES

Aasman, J., Mulder, G., and Mulder, L. J. M. (1987). Operator effort and the measurement of heartrate variability. *Hum. Factors* 29, 161–170.

Allison, B. Z., and Polich, J. (2008). Workload assessment of computer gaming using a single-stimulus event-related potential paradigm. *Biol. Psychol.* 77, 277–283. doi: 10.1016/j.biopsycho.2007.10.014

Ayaz, H., Izzetoglu, M., Bunce, S., Heiman-Patterson, T., and Onaral, B. (2007). "Detecting cognitive activity related hemodynamic signal for brain computer interface using functional near infrared spectroscopy," in *3rd International IEEE/EMBS Conference on Neural Engineering* (Kohala Coast, HI), 342–345.

Bauer, L. O., Goldstein, R., and Stern, J. A. (1987). Effects of information-processing demands on physiological response patterns. *Hum. Factors* 29, 213–234.

Beatty, J. (1982). Task-evoked pupillary responses, processing load, and the structure of processing resources. *Psychol. Bull.* 91, 276–292. doi: 10.1037/0033-2909.91.2.276

Berka, C., Levendowski, D. J., Lumicao, M. N., Yau, A., Davis, G., Zivkovic, V. T., et al. (2007). EEG correlates of task engagement and mental workload in vigilance, learning, and memory tasks. *Aviat. Space Environ. Med.* 78(5 Suppl.), B231–B244.

Berntson, G. G., Bigger, J. T., Eckberg, D. L., Grossman, P., Kaufmann, P. G., Malik, M., et al. (1997). Heart rate variability: origins, methods, and interpretive caveats. *Psychophysiology* 34, 623–648. doi: 10.1111/j.1469-8986.1997.tb02140.x

Boucsein, W. (1992). *Electrodermal Activity*. New York, NY: Plenum Press.

Boucsein, W. (1999). Electrodermal activity as an indicator of emotional processes. *J. Sci. Emot. Sensib.* 2, 1–25.

Brookings, J. B., Wilson, G. F., and Swain, C. R. (1996). Psychophysiological responses to changes in workload during simulated air traffic control. *Biol. Psychol.* 42, 361–377. doi: 10.1016/0301-0511(95)05167-8

Brouwer, A.-M., Hogervorst, M. A., Herman, P., and Kooi, F. (2009). "Are you really looking? Finding the answer through fixation patterns and EEG. Lecture notes in artificial intelligence, Vol. 5638," in *Proceedings of the 5th International Conference on Foundations of Augmented Cognition* (Berlin; Heidelberg: Springer), 329–338.

Brouwer, A.-M., Hogervorst, M. A., Holewijn, M., and van Erp, J. B. F. (2014). Evidence for effects of task difficulty but not learning on neurophysiological variables associated with effort. *Int. J. Psychophysiol.* 93, 242–252. doi: 10.1016/j.ijpsycho.2014.05.004

Brouwer, A.-M., Hogervorst, M. A., van Erp, J. B. F., Heffelaar, T., Zimmerman, P. H., and Oostenveld, R. (2012). Estimating workload using EEG spectral power and ERPs in the n-back task. *J. Neural Eng.* 9:045008. doi: 10.1088/1741-2560/9/4/045008

Brouwer, A.-M., van Wouwe, N., Mühl, C., van Erp, J. B. F., and Toet, A. (2013). Perceiving blocks of emotional pictures and sounds: effects on physiological variables. *Front. Hum. Neurosci.* 7:295. doi: 10.3389/fnhum.2013.00295

Chanel, G., Kierkels, J. J. M., Soleymani, M., and Pun, T. (2009). Short-term emotion assessment in a recall paradigm. *Int. J. Hum. Comput. St.* 67, 607–627. doi: 10.1016/j.ijhcs.2009.03.005

Chanel, G., Kronegg, J., Grandjean, D., and Pun, T. (2006). "Emotion assessment: arousal evaluation using EEG's and peripheral physiological signals," in *Multimedia Content Representation Classification and Security. Springer Lecture Notes in Computer Sciences*, Vol. 4105, eds B. Gunsel, A. M. Tekalp, A. K. Jain, and B. Sankur (Berlin; Heidelberg: Springer), 530–537. doi: 10.1007/11848035_70

Christensen, J. C., Estepp, J. R., Wilson, G. F., and Russell, C. A. (2012). The effects of day-to-day variability of physiological data on operator state classification. *Neuroimage* 59, 57–63. doi: 10.1016/j.neuroimage.2011.07.091

Coffey, E. B. J., Brouwer, A. M., and van Erp, J. B. F. (2012). Measuring workload using a combination of electroencephalography and near infrared spectroscopy. *Proc. Hum. Factors Ergon. Soc. Annu. Meet.* 56, 1822–1826. doi: 10.1177/1071181312561367

Esposito, F., Aragri, A., Piccoli, T., Tedeschi, G., Goebel, R., and Di Salle, F. (2009). Distributed analysis of simultaneous EEG-fMRI time-series: modeling and interpretation issues. *Magn. Reson. Imaging* 27, 1120–1130. doi: 10.1016/j.mri.2009.01.007

Evans, J. L., Selinger, C., and Pollak, S. D. (2011). P300 as a measure of processing capacity in auditory and visual domains in specific language impairment. *Brain Res.* 1389, 93–102. doi: 10.1016/j.brainres.2011.02.010

Fairclough, S. H., Venables, L., and Tattersall, A. (2005). The influence of task demand and learning on the psychophysiological response. *Int. J. Psychophysiol.* 56, 171–184. doi: 10.1016/j.ijpsycho.2004.11.003

Fink, A., Grabner, R. H., Neuper, C., and Neubauer, A. C. (2005). EEG alpha band dissociation with increasing task demands. *Cogn. Brain Res.* 24, 252–259. doi: 10.1016/j.cogbrainres.2005.02.002

Fogarty, C., and Stern, J. A. (1989). Eye movements and blinks: their relationship to higher cognitive processes. *Int. J. Psychophysiol.* 8, 35–42. doi: 10.1016/0167-8760(89)90017-2

Fournier, L. R., Wilson, G. F., and Swain, C. R. (1999). Electrophysiological, behavioral, and subjective indexes of workload when performing multiple tasks: manipulations of task difficulty and training. *Int. J. Psychophysiol.* 31, 129–145. doi: 10.1016/S0167-8760(98)00049-X

Foxe, J. J., Simpson, G. V., and Ahlfors, S. P. (1998). Parieto-occipital ~10 Hz activity reflects anticipatory state of visual attention mechanisms. *Neuroreport* 9, 3929–3933. doi: 10.1097/00001756-199812010-00030

Friedman, J., Hastie, T., and Tibshirani, R. (2010). Regularization paths for generalized linear models via coordinate descent. *J. Stat. Softw.* 33, 1–22.

Gaillard, A. W. K., and Wientjes, C. J. E. (1994). Mental load and work stress as two types of energy mobilization. *Work Stress* 8, 141–152. doi: 10.1080/02678379408259986

Gawron, V. J., Schiflett, S. G., and Miller, J. C. (1989). "Measures of in-flight workload," in *Aviafion Psychology*, ed R. S. Jensen (Aldershot: Brookfield), 240–287.

Gevins, A., Smith, M. E., Leong, H., McEvoy, L., Whitfield, S., Du, R., et al. (1998). Monitoring working memory load during computer-based tasks with EEG pattern recognition methods. *Hum. Factors* 40, 79–91. doi: 10.1518/001872098779480578

Goedhart, A. D., van der Sluis, S., Houtveen, J. H., Willemsen, G., and de Geus, E. J. (2007). Comparison of time and frequency domain measures of RSA in ambulatory recordings. *Psychophysiology* 44, 203–215. doi: 10.1111/j.1469-8986.2006.00490.x

Greenwald, M. K., Cook, E. W., and Lang, P. J. (1989). Affective judgment and psychophysiological response: dimensional covariation in the evaluation of pictorial stimuli. *J. Psychophysiol.* 3, 51–64.

Grimes, D., Tan, D. S., Hudson, S. E., Shenoy, P., and Rao, R. P. (2008). "Feasibility and pragmatics of classifying working memory load with an electroencephalograph," in *Proceeding of the Twenty-Sixth Annual SIGCHI Conference on Human Factors in Computing Systems* (Florence: ACM), 835–844.

Grossman, P., and Taylor, E. W. (2007). Toward understanding respiratory sinus arrhythmia: relations to cardiac vagal tone, evolution and biobehavioral functions. *Biol. Psychol.* 74, 263–285. doi: 10.1016/j.biopsycho.2005.11.014

Gundel, A., and Wilson, G. F. (1992). Topographical changes in the ongoing EEG related to the difficulty of mental task. *Brain Topogr.* 5, 17–25. doi: 10.1007/BF01129966

Hampson, R. E., Opris, I., and Deadwyler, S. A. (2010). Neural correlates of fast pupil dilation in nonhuman primates: relation to behavioral performance and cognitive workload. *Behav. Brain Res.* 212, 1–11. doi: 10.1016/j.bbr.2010.03.011

Hancock, P. A., Meshkati, N., and Robertson, M. M. (1985). Physiological reflections of mental workload. *Aviat. Space Environ. Med.* 56, 1110–1114.

Hart, S. G., and Staveland, L. E. (1988). "Development of a multi-dimensional workload rating scale: results of empirical and theoretical research," in *Human Mental Workload*, eds P. A. Hancock and N. Meshkati (Amsterdam: Elsevier), 139–183.

Hockey, G. R. J. (1986). "Changes in operator efficiency as a function of environmental stress, fatigue, and circadian rhythms," in *Handbook of Perception and Human Performance*, Vol. 2, eds K. R. Boff, L. Kaufman, and J. P. Thomas (New York, NY: John Wiley), 44.1–44.49.

Izzetoglu, M., Bunce, S. C., Izzetoglu, K., Onaral, B., and Pourrezaei, A. K. (2007). Functional brain imaging using near-infrared technology. *IEEE Eng. Med. Biol. Mag.* 26, 38–46. doi: 10.1109/MEMB.2007.384094

Jann, K., Dierks, T., Boesch, C., Kottlow, M., Strik, W., and Koenig, T. (2009). BOLD correlates of EEG alpha phase-locking and the fMRI default mode network. *Neuroimage* 45, 903–916. doi: 10.1016/j.neuroimage.2009.01.001

Jensen, O., and Tesche, C. D. (2002). Frontal theta activity in humans increases with memory load in a working memory task. *Eur. J. Neurosci.* 15, 1395–1399. doi: 10.1046/j.1460-9568.2002.01975.x

Kahneman, D., and Beatty, J. (1966). Pupil diameter and load on memory. *Science* 154, 1583–1585. doi: 10.1126/science.154.3756.1583

Kahneman, D., Tursky, B., Shapiro, D., and Crider, A. (1969). Pupillary, heart rate, and skin resistance changes during a mental task. *J. Exp. Psychol.* 79, 164–167. doi: 10.1037/h0026952

Kalsbeek, J. W. H., and Ettema, J. (1963). Scored regularity of the heart rate pattern and the measurement of perceptual or mental load. *Ergonomics* 6:306.

Karavidas, M. K., Lehrer, P. M., Lu, S.-E., Vaschillo, E., Vaschillo, B., and Cheng, A. (2010). The effects of workload on respiratory variables in simulated flight: a preliminary study. *Biol. Psychol.* 84, 157–160. doi: 10.1016/j.biopsycho.2009.12.009

Keil, A., Mussweiler, T., and Epstude, K. (2006). Alpha-band activity reflects reduction of mental effort in a comparison task: a source space analysis. *Brain Res.* 1121, 117–127. doi: 10.1016/j.brainres.2006.08.118

Kida, T., Nishihira, Y., Hatta, A., Wasaka, T., Tazoe, T., Sakajiri, Y., et al. (2004). Resource allocation and somatosensory P300 amplitude during dual task: effects of tracking speed and predictability of tracking direction. *Clin. Neurophysiol.* 115, 2616–2628. doi: 10.1016/j.clinph.2004.06.013

Klimesch, W., Doppelmayr, M., Röhm, D., Pöllhuber, D., and Stadler, W. (2000). Simultaneous desynchronization and synchronization of different alpha responses in the human electroencephalograph: a neglected paradox? *Neurosci. Lett.* 284, 97–100. doi: 10.1016/S0304-3940(00)00985-X

Klimesch, W. (1996). Memory processes, brain oscillations and EEG synchronization. *Int. J. Psychophysiol.* 24, 61–100. doi: 10.1016/S0167-8760(96)00057-8

Klimesch, W. (1997). EEG-alpha rhythms and memory processes. *Int. J. Psychophysiol.* 26, 319–340. doi: 10.1016/S0167-8760(97)00773-3

Klimesch, W. (1999). EEG alpha and theta oscillations reflect cognitive and memory performance: a review and analysis. *Brain Res. Brain Res. Rev.* 29, 169–195. doi: 10.1016/S0165-0173(98)00056-3

Kohlisch, O., and Schaefer, F. (1996). Physiological changes during computer tasks: responses to mental load or to motor demands? *Ergonomics* 39, 213–224. doi: 10.1080/00140139608964452

Kramer, A. F., Trejo, L. J., and Humphrey, D. (1995). Assessment of mental workload with task-irrelevant auditory probes. *Biol. Psychol.* 40, 83–100. doi: 10.1016/0301-0511(95)05108-2

Laufs, H., Krakow, K., Sterzer, P., Eger, E., Beyerle, A., Salek-Haddadi, A., et al. (2003). Electroencephalographic signatures of attentional and cognitive default modes in spontaneous brain activity fluctuations at rest. *Proc. Natl. Acad. Sci. U.S.A.* 100, 11053–11058. doi: 10.1073/pnas.1831638100

May, J. G., Kennedy, R. S., Williams, M. C., Dunlap, W. P., and Brannan, J. R. (1990). Eye movement indices of mental workload. *Acta Psychol.* 75, 75–89. doi: 10.1016/0001-6918(90)90067-P

Mehler, B., Reimer, B., Coughlin, J. F., and Dusek, J. A. (2009). Impact of incremental increases in cognitive workload on physiological arousal and performance in young adult drivers. *Transport. Res. Rec.* 2138, 6–12. doi: 10.3141/2138-02

Missonnier, P., Gold, G., Leonards, U., Costa-Fazio, L., Michel, J.-P., Ibáñez, V., et al. (2004). Aging and working memory: early deficits in EEG activation of posterior cortical areas. *J. Neural Transm.* 111, 1141–1154. doi: 10.1007/s00702-004-0159-2

Missonnier, P., Leonards, U., Gold, G., Palix, J., Ibáñez, V., and Giannakopoulos, P. (2003). A new electrophysiological index for working memory load in humans. *Neuroreport* 14, 1451–1455. doi: 10.1097/00001756-200308060-00009

Miyata, Y., Tanaka, Y., and Hono, T. (1990). Long term observation on Fm-theta during mental effort. *Neuroscience* 16, 145–148.

Mulder, G. (1980). *The Heart of Mental Effort.* Thesis, University of Groningen, Groningen.

Mulder, L. J. M., and Mulder, G. (1987). "Cardiovascular reactivity and mental workload," in *The Beat-by-Beat Investigation of Cardiovascular Function*, eds R. I. Kitney and O. Rompelman (Oxford: Clarendon Press), 216–253.

Oostenveld, R., Fries, P., Maris, E., and Schoffelen, J. M. (2011). FieldTrip: open source software for advanced analysis of MEG, EEG, and invasive electrophysiological data. *Comput. Intell. Neurosci.* 2011:156869. doi: 10.1155/2011/156869

Pfurtscheller, G., Stancak, A. Jr., and Neuper, C. (1996). Event-related synchronization (ERS) in the alpha band: an electrophysiological correlate of cortical idling [review]. *Int. J. Psychophysiol.* 24, 39–46. doi: 10.1016/S0167-8760(96)00066-9

Polich, J., and Kok, A. (1995). Cognitive and biological determinants of P300: an integrative review. *Biol. Psychol.* 41, 103–146. doi: 10.1016/0301-0511(95)05130-9

Polich, J. (2007). Updating P300: an integrative theory of P3a and P3b. *Clin. Neurophysiol.* 118, 2128–2148. doi: 10.1016/j.clinph.2007.04.019

Porter, G., Troscianko, T., and Gilchrist, I. D. (2007). Effort during visual search and counting: insights from pupillometry. *Q. J. Exp. Psychol.* 60, 211–229. doi: 10.1080/17470210600673818

Pratt, N., Willoughby, A., and Swick, D. (2011). Effects of working memory load on visual selective attention: behavioral and electrophysiological evidence. *Front. Hum. Neurosci.* 5:57. doi: 10.3389/fnhum.2011.00057

Raabe, M., Rutschmann, R. M., Schrauf, M., and Greenlee, M. W. (2005). "Neural correlates of simulated driving: auditory oddball responses dependent on workload," in *Foundations of Augmented Cognition*, ed D. D. Schmorrow (Mahwah, NJ: Lawrence Erlbaum Associates, Inc.), 1067–1076.

Raghavachari, S., Kahana, M. J., Rizzuto, D. S., Caplan, J. B., Kirschen, M. P., Bourgeois, B., et al. (2001). Gating of human theta oscillations by a working memory task. *J. Neurosci.* 21, 3175–3183.

Ravden, D., and Polich, J. (1999). On P300 measurement stability: habituation, intra-trial block variation, and ultradian rhythms. *Biol. Psychol.* 51, 59–76. doi: 10.1016/S0301-0511(99)00015-0

Reimer, B., and Mehler, B. (2011). The impact of cognitive workload on physiological arousal in young adult drivers: a field study and simulation validation. *Ergonomics* 54, 932–942. doi: 10.1080/00140139.2011.604431

Rösler, F., Heil, M., and Röder, B. (1997). Slow negative brain potentials as reflections of specific modular resources of cognition. *Biol. Psychol.* 45, 109–141. doi: 10.1016/S0301-0511(96)05225-8

Roth, W. T. (1983). "A comparison of P300 and the skin conductance response," in *Tutorials in ERP Research—Endogenous Components*, eds A. W. K. Gaillard and W. Ritter (Amsterdam: North-Holland), 177–199.

Ruchkin, D. S., Johnson, R. Jr., Canoune, H., and Ritter, W. (1990). Short-term memory storage and retention: an event-related brain potential study. *Electroencephalogr. Clin. Neurophysiol.* 76, 419–439. doi: 10.1016/0013-4694(90)90096-3

Severens, M., Farquhar, J., Duysens, J., and Desain, P. (2013). A multi-signature brain-computer interface: use of transient and steady-state responses. *J. Neural. Eng.* 10:026005. doi: 10.1088/1741-2560/10/2/026005

Srinivasan, N. (2007). Cognitive neuroscience of creativity: EEG based approaches. *Methods* 42, 109–116. doi: 10.1016/j.ymeth.2006.12.008

Task Force of the European Society of Cardiology the North American Society of Pacing Electrophysiology. (1996). Heart rate variability: standards of measurement, physiological interpretation and clinical use. *Circulation* 93, 1043–1065. doi: 10.1161/01.CIR.93.5.1043

Taylor, G., Reinerman-Jones, L. E., Cosenzo, K., and Nicholson, D. (2010). "Comparison of multiple physiological sensors to classify operator state in adaptive automation systems," in *Proceedings of the Human Factors and Ergonomics Society Annual Meeting September 2010.* Vol. 54 (San Francisco, CA: Human Factors and Ergonomics Society), 195–199.

Ullsperger, P., Freude, G., and Erdmann, U. (2001). Auditory probe sensitivity to mental workload changes - an event-related potential study. *Int. J. Psychophysiol.* 40, 201–209. doi: 10.1016/S0167-8760(00)00188-4

van Dijk, H., Schoffelen, J. M., Oostenveld, R., and Jensen, O. (2008). Prestimulus oscillatory activity in the alpha band predicts visual discrimination ability. *J. Neurosci.* 28, 1816–1823. doi: 10.1523/JNEUROSCI.1853-07.2008

van Gerven, M., Bahramisharif, A., Farquhar, J., and Heskes, T. (2013). *Donders Machine Learning Toolbox (DMLT) for Matlab Version 26/06/2013.* Available online at: https://github.com/distrep/DMLT.

Veltman, J. A., and Gaillard, A. W. K. (1996). Physiological indices of workload in a simulated flight task. *Biol. Psychol.* 42, 323–342. doi: 10.1016/0301-0511(95)05165-1

Veltman, J. A., and Gaillard, A. W. K. (1998). Physiological workload reactions to increasing levels of task difficulty. *Ergonomics* 41, 656–669. doi: 10.1080/001401398186829

Verwey, W. B., and Veltman, H. A. (1996). Detecting Short Periods of Elevated Workload: a comparison of nine workload assesment techniques. *J. Exp. Psychol.* 2, 270–285.

Vogt, J., Hagemann, T., and Kastner, M. (2006). The impact of workload on heart rate and blood pressure in en-route and tower air traffic control. *J. Psychophysiol.* 20, 297–314. doi: 10.1027/0269-8803.20.4.297

Watter, S., Geffen, G. M., and Geffen, L. B. (2001). The n-back as a dual-task: P300 morphology under divided attention. *Psychophysiology* 38, 998–1003. doi: 10.1111/1469-8986.3860998

Wientjes, C. J. E. (1992). Respiration in psychophysiology: methods and applications. *Biol. Psychol.* 34, 179–204. doi: 10.1016/0301-0511(92)90015-M

Wilson, G. F., and Fisher, F. (1991). The use of cardiac and eye blink measures to determine flight segment in F4 crews. *Aviat. Space Environ. Med.* 62, 959–961.

Wilson, G. F., and Russell, C. A. (2003). Operator functional state classification using multiple psychophysiological features in an air traffic control task. *Hum. Factors* 45, 381–389. doi: 10.1518/hfes.45.3.381.27252

Wilson, G. F., and Russell, C. A. (2007). Performance enhancement in a UAV task using psychophysiological determined adaptive aiding. *Hum. Factors* 49, 1005–1019. doi: 10.1518/001872007X249875

Winton, W. M., Putnam, L. E., and Krauss, R. M. (1984). Facial and autonomic manifestations of the dimensional structure of emotion. *J. Exp. Soc. Psychol.* 20, 195–216. doi: 10.1016/0022-1031(84)90047-7

Zijlstra, F. R. H. (1993). *Efficiency in Work Behaviour. A Design Approach for Modern Tools.* Ph.D. thesis, Delft University of Technology, Delft University Press, Delft.

Zimmerman, P. H., Bolhuis, J. E., Willemsen, A., Meyer, E. S., and Noldus, L. P. (2009). The Observer XT: a tool for the integrations and synchronization of multimodal signals. *Behav. Res. Methods* 41, 731–735. doi: 10.3758/BRM.41.3.731

3

Errare machinale est: the use of error-related potentials in brain-machine interfaces

Ricardo Chavarriaga *, Aleksander Sobolewski and José del R. Millán

Defitech Chair in Non-Invasive Brain-Machine Interface, Center for Neuroprosthetics, School of Engineering, Ecole Polytechnique Fédérale de Lausanne, Lausanne, Switzerland

***Correspondence:**
Ricardo Chavarriaga, Defitech Chair in Non-Invasive Brain-Machine Interface, Ecole Polytechnique Fédérale de Lausanne, EPFL-STI-CNBI, Station 11, Lausanne 1015, Switzerland
e-mail: ricardo.chavarriaga@epfl.ch

The ability to recognize errors is crucial for efficient behavior. Numerous studies have identified electrophysiological correlates of error recognition in the human brain (error-related potentials, ErrPs). Consequently, it has been proposed to use these signals to improve human-computer interaction (HCI) or brain-machine interfacing (BMI). Here, we present a review of over a decade of developments toward this goal. This body of work provides consistent evidence that ErrPs can be successfully detected on a single-trial basis, and that they can be effectively used in both HCI and BMI applications. We first describe the ErrP phenomenon and follow up with an analysis of different strategies to increase the robustness of a system by incorporating single-trial ErrP recognition, either by correcting the machine's actions or by providing means for its error-based adaptation. These approaches can be applied both when the user employs traditional HCI input devices or in combination with another BMI channel. Finally, we discuss the current challenges that have to be overcome in order to fully integrate ErrPs into practical applications. This includes, in particular, the characterization of such signals during real(istic) applications, as well as the possibility of extracting richer information from them, going beyond the time-locked decoding that dominates current approaches.

Keywords: brain-machine interface, error-related potentials, reinforcement learning, EEG, neuroprosthesis, hybrid BCI

1. INTRODUCTION

Errare humanum est, perseverare autem diabolicum
–Seneca the younger

The ability of human and non -human animals to learn and adapt their behavior is largely based on their capacity of identifying erroneous actions (Rabbitt, 1966). Several studies have reported that such events elicit distinct neural responses, which can be observed using different neuroimaging techniques including fMRI, scalp and intracranial electroencephalography (EEG), and magnetoencephalography (MEG). In particular, it has been demonstrated that the electrophysiological signatures of this error processing—i.e., error-related potentials, ErrPs– can be reliably decoded on a single-trial basis, thus allowing their use through brain-machine interface (BMI) systems as a means to improve the machine's performance, similarly to animals. For instance, typically BMIs aim at decoding user's intentions from the neural activity (e.g., as recorded by EEG). Misclassification of these intentions results in an erroneous command. The user's subsequent perception of such error can elicit an ErrP and the successful decoding of this response would allow the system to take corrective actions, e.g., by preventing the erroneous command from being fully executed or reverting its outcome (Schalk et al., 2000; Ferrez and Millán, 2008a; Dal Seno et al., 2010). Alternatively, ErrPs can be used to reduce the possibility of the error reappearing in the future through re-calibration of the system, allowing it to "learn from its mistakes" (Artusi et al., 2011; Llera et al., 2011). These approaches are illustrated in **Figure 1**. They combine the decoding of one brain signal (e.g., correlates of motor imagery or stimulus recognition) for controlling the device and the ErrP as a corrective mechanism, thus corresponding to hybrid BMI systems (Pfurtscheller et al., 2010). Notably, the same principles can also be applied to human-computer interaction (HCI) systems when input devices other than BMI are employed (Parra et al., 2003; Chavarriaga and Millán, 2010; Wang et al., 2011; Zander and Kothe, 2011; Zander and Jatzev, 2012). Interestingly, these ErrPs are naturally elicited during human interaction with the machine. This means that information about the user's cognitive assessment of such interaction can be obtained implicitly, without a need for training or asking the users to actively generate them. Systems that decode this information are sometimes referred to as *passive* BMIs; as opposed to the so-called *active* BMIs where the brain signals are consciously modulated by the user to control a given device or application (Zander and Kothe, 2011). However, caution should be taken not to interpret this as if the user played an entirely passive role during the interaction. In fact, ErrPs have been shown to be modulated by the user's level of engagement in the task (Hajcak et al., 2005).

In the last decade, researchers have provided ample evidence of the feasibility of such approaches. Here we review this work, starting with a short description of different error-related electrophysiological patterns (section 2). For more detailed account of the neural basis of these signals, readers can refer to reviews by Taylor et al. (2007); Hoffmann and Falkenstein (2012); Wessel

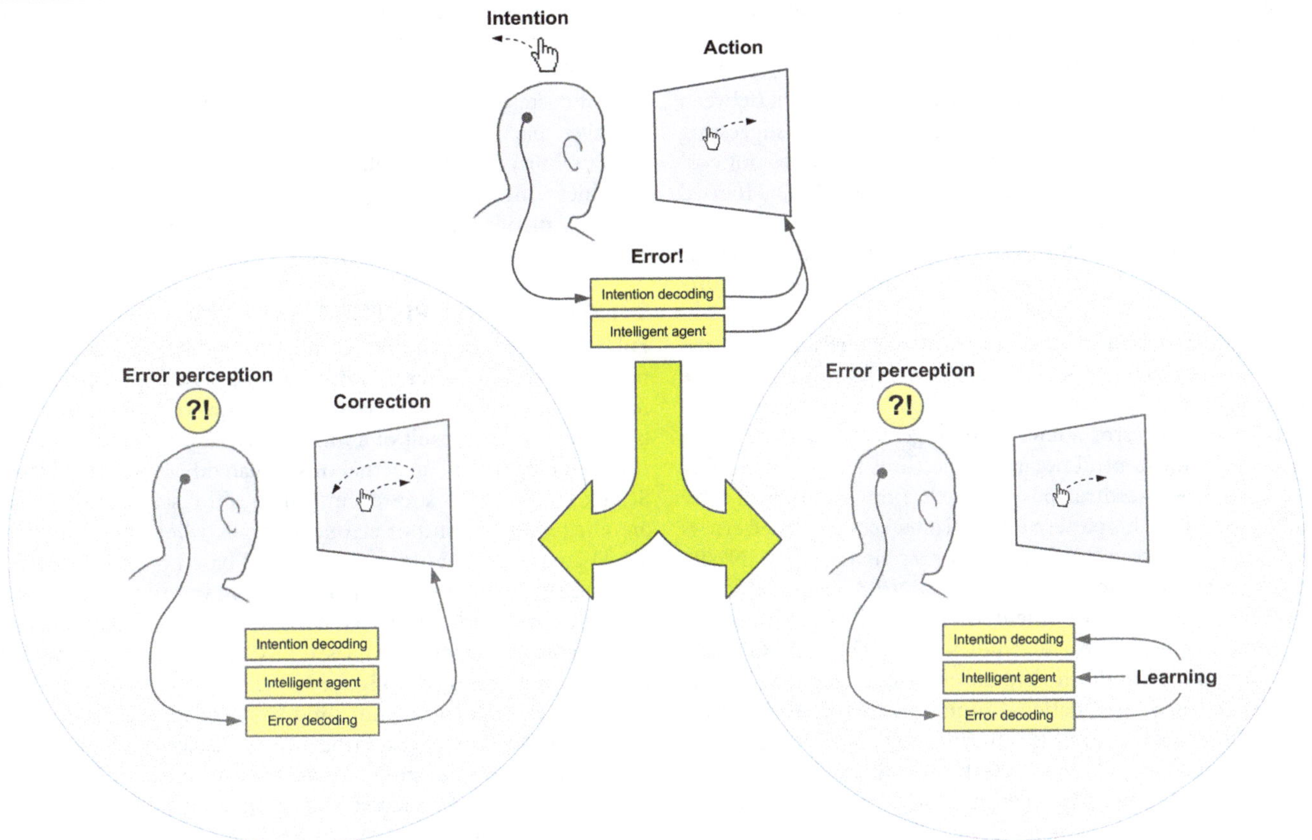

FIGURE 1 | Exploitation of error-related potentials to improve BMI performance. Left: Single trial detection of these potentials, indicating erroneous actions, is used to trigger a corrective action, e.g., preventing execution of the last BMI command. **Right:** ErrPs are used to update the BMI classifier or the device controller by means of reinforcement learning.

(2012), and Ullsperger et al. (2014). Here we focus on signals that have been mostly exploited for brain-machine interfacing and primarily discuss electroencephalographic signals found using non-invasive recording techniques (section 3). We go on to present different strategies that can be applied to increase the robustness of the BMI system by incorporating single-trial ErrP recognition in both able-bodied subjects and users with motor disabilities (sections 4 and 5). We also present recent efforts to integrate these signals into real-world applications (section 6). Finally, we review the techniques used for decoding these potentials (section 7) and discuss current challenges in the study and exploitation of these signals (section 8).

2. ERROR-RELATED BRAIN ACTIVITY

Early reports of error-related brain activity date back to the early 1990's (Falkenstein et al., 1991; Gehring et al., 1993). These studies showed a characteristic EEG event-related potential (ERP) elicited after subjects committed errors in a speed response choice task. This pattern is characterized by a negative potential deflection, termed the *error-related negativity* (ERN), appearing over fronto-central scalp areas at about 50–100 ms after a subject's erroneous response (Falkenstein et al., 2000). This negative component is followed by a centro-parietal positive deflection (Pe). Modulations of this latter component have been linked to the subject's awareness of the error. Interestingly, correlations have been found between the ERNs and behavioral adjustments following these errors, e.g., post-error response slowing (Debener et al., 2005; Frank et al., 2005; Themanson et al., 2012); supporting the idea that the signal indeed reflects an action monitoring process (Holroyd and Coles, 2002). This is further corroborated by the fact that the ERN amplitude seems to be modulated by the importance of errors in the given task (Frank et al., 2005; Taylor et al., 2007), as well as the subjective awareness of the error (Falkenstein et al., 2000; Wessel, 2012; Navarro-Cebrian et al., 2013). Regardless of such functional modulations, these signals are also influenced by individual differences and certain pathological conditions (Olvet and Hajcak, 2008). Importantly, however, these signals have been shown to be quite reliable over time (Olvet and Hajcak, 2009) and across different tasks (Riesel et al., 2013).

A similar medial-frontal EEG pattern has been reported to appear after presentation of "feedback," i.e., the delayed result of a choice or action. This *feedback-related negativity* (FRN), appearing between 200 and 300 ms after feedback onset, is modulated by choices leading to losing situations in strategic gambling tasks (Cohen et al., 2007), as well as subject-specific sensitivity to reinforcement signals (Frank et al., 2005). Interestingly, similar signals are also elicited in the absence of motor response or while observing errors committed by a different person or agent (van Schie et al., 2004; Yeung et al., 2005; Zander et al., 2008; Chavarriaga and Millán, 2010; Zander and Jatzev, 2012). Mounting evidence provides further support of the link between these signals and reward or utility prediction errors, suggesting that ErrPs are generated when the actual outcome does not correspond to the expected one (Holroyd and Coles, 2002; Holroyd et al., 2003; Nieuwenhuis et al., 2004; Yeung et al., 2005). Such information can be used for learning by adjusting the behavior to minimize errors, as proposed by the reinforcement learning theory (Sutton and Barto, 1998).

It is worth to notice that, although these signals are typically referred to as "negativities," the EEG correlates of performance monitoring comprise a uniform sequence of ERP components irrespective of the error source (Ullsperger et al., 2014). These include the fronto-central negative deflections related above, followed by a fronto-central positive deflection and then a later parietal positivity. This pattern is found after self-generated errors (i.e., the ERN/Pe complex), stimulus presentation (i.e., N2/P3 complex), and feedback errors (i.e., FRN/P3 complex). It is not entirely clear to what extent these signals share common underlying processes. Several studies using fMRI, EEG-based source localization, and intra-cranial recordings suggest that the fronto-central ERP modulations commonly involve the medial-frontal cortex, specifically the anterior cingulate cortex (ACC) (Ullsperger and von Cramon, 2001; Brázdil et al., 2002; van Veen and Carter, 2002; Herrmann et al., 2004; Taylor et al., 2007).

Lastly, ErrPs seen as distinct patterns in the temporal domain of electrophysiological signals are not an exhaustive description of the observable EEG phenomena. Accumulating invasive and non-invasive studies are also demonstrating frequency modulations, specifically with erroneous responses eliciting an increase of theta activity followed by a decrease of beta rhythm amplitude (Trujillo and Allen, 2007; Cohen et al., 2008; Koelewijn et al., 2008; Cavanagh et al., 2009, 2012). Moreover, connectivity studies reveal patterns of cross-regional synchronizations, pointing to influences from ACC to prefrontal areas (Cavanagh et al., 2009).

As already mentioned, several studies have reported an evoked response to errors in the user intention decoding when using BMI systems (c.f., **Figure 2**). This response exhibits the same pattern of modulations as described above. The difference waveform (error minus correct) over fronto-central areas is characterized by an initial positive peak at about 200 ms after feedback presentation, followed by a larger negative deflection at about 250 ms and a third larger positive peak at about 320 ms. Furthermore, estimation of the intracranial activity using sLoreta (Pascual-Marqui, 2002) indicated that the signals elicited during brain-machine interaction were generated in the ACC, consistent with other error-related EEG correlates (Ferrez and Millán, 2008a; Lopez-Larraz et al., 2010; Iturrate et al., 2013a). Notably, the term *error-related potential* (ErrP), has since become quite widespread within the BMI community, covering electrophysiological responses elicited in a number of paradigms. Resolving its relationship to ERP components, and their functional modulations, typically identified in basic cognitive neurosciences is beyond the scope of this BMI-focused review (although we refer to one relevant confound below). It can be considered as a useful umbrella term for application-driven research, albeit to a certain extent at the cost of correspondence with fundamental investigations. This is, however, partly justified by different research settings: closed-loop usability and practicalities of single-trial decoding are rarely the chief concern of basic neuroscience, while the latter's typical abstract, distilled experimental paradigms are not employed by engineering-oriented researchers.

3. ERROR-RELATED POTENTIALS FOR BMI

Following the basic neurophysiological findings described in the preceding section, several studies aimed at assessing whether similar signals were also to be found when the errors were produced by a machine as a result of a misclassification of the user's intention while operating an actual or simulated BMI. In a first report Schalk et al. (2000) showed in four healthy subjects that ErrPs are elicited at the end of erroneous trials when they controlled a 1-D cursor using a non-invasive BMI based on modulation of mu and beta EEG rhythms. This approach was further developed by Ferrez and Millán (2008a) in a study on five subjects using a 2-class motor-imagery (MI) based BMI controlling a cursor moving in discrete steps (c.f., **Figure 3A**). They showed that the ERPs elicited after each command could be decoded as corresponding to the error or correct condition with an accuracy of about 80%. Simultaneously, other studies tested the feasibility of decoding the error-related activity elicited after manual responses (Blankertz et al., 2003; Parra et al., 2003).

Further studies demonstrated other encouraging features of ErrPs for their use in BMI applications. Firstly, as with the ERN, they have been shown to be quite stable over time. ErrP classifiers maintained the same performance when tested several months after their calibration (Ferrez and Millán, 2008a; Chavarriaga and Millán, 2010). Furthermore, these signals seem to be mainly related to a general error-monitoring process, instead of specificities of the particular task that was performed. Iturrate et al. (2014) compared ErrPs elicited in three tasks in which subjects ($N = 6$) monitored the operation of devices of different degree of complexity: a 1-D cursor movement (**Figure 3A**), and a simulated (**Figure 3B**) and real robots (**Figure 3C**) moving in a 2-D space. Their results show that ErrPs across these tasks significantly differ in the latency of the peak modulations, but not in amplitude or overall waveform, thus suggesting the possibility of identifying task-independent markers of erroneous brain-machine interaction. Along the same lines, similar waveforms have been reported in tasks using different feedback modalities (Lehne et al., 2009; Perrin et al., 2010; López-Larraz et al., 2011; Chavarriaga et al., 2012).

An account of ErrP usage in BMI applications must indicate several specific confounds these signals may be susceptible to. Since –due to the nature of BMI– such applications often involve moving stimuli, there is the possibility that observed signals may be contaminated with electrooculographic (EOG) artifacts due to eye movements. This can bias the decoding particularly in application designs where direction of feedback movement is related to correctness of action. To counter this confound, researchers – especially in in proof-of-concept studies– may take care to ensure

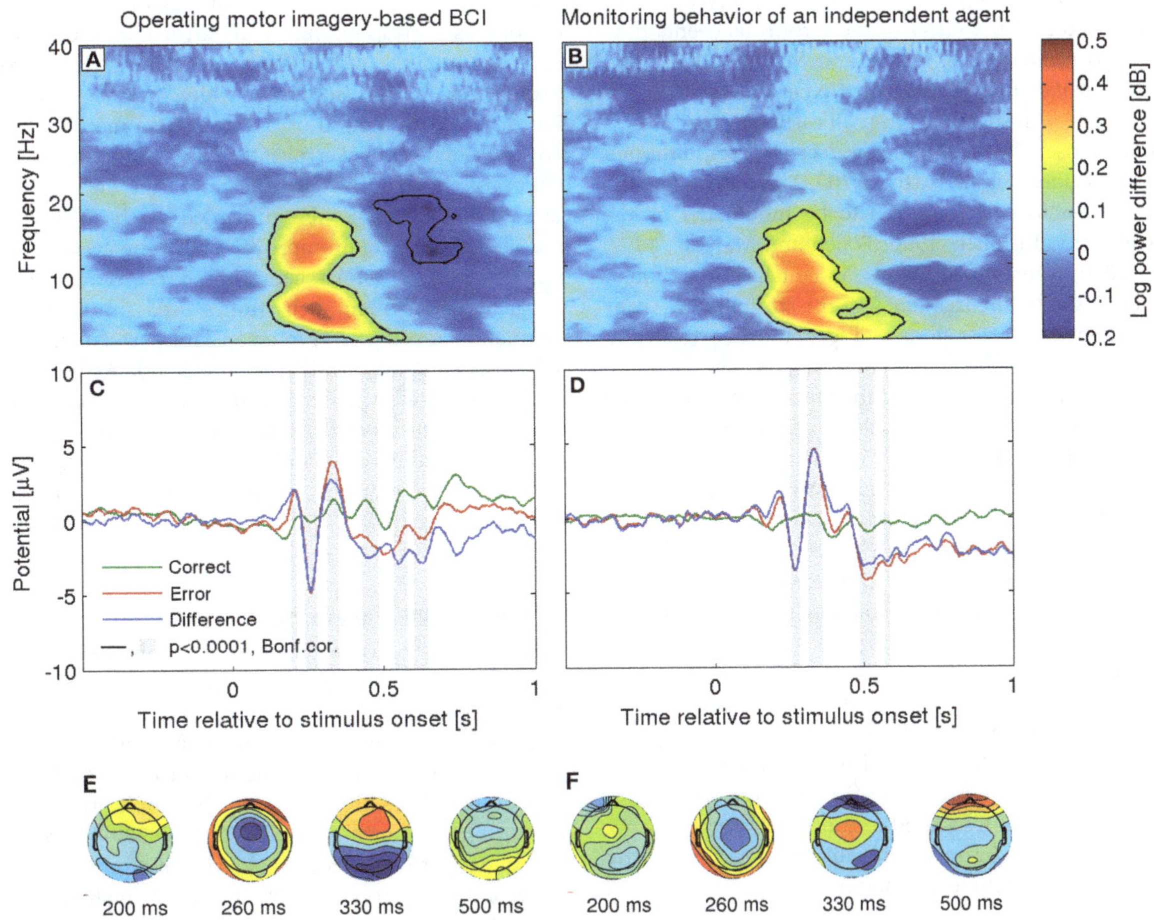

FIGURE 2 | Error-related potentials in a 2-class task used in BMI. Left column, Interaction ErrP. The cursor movement is controlled by a MI-based BMI (Ferrez and Millán, 2008a). Right column, Monitoring ErrP: The cursor moves automatically and the user is asked to evaluate whether it moves toward the target location (Chavarriaga and Millán, 2010). **(A,B)** Event-related spectral perturbation. **(C,D)** Grand-average ERP at electrode FCz for correct, error and difference (error minus correct) conditions. $t = 0$ corresponds to the stimulus presentation onset (i.e., cursor movement). **(E,F)** Topographical representation of the group average difference ERP for both the interaction ($N = 4$) and monitoring paradigms ($N = 6$). Activity is color coded from blue to red corresponding to the range [−5 5] uV.

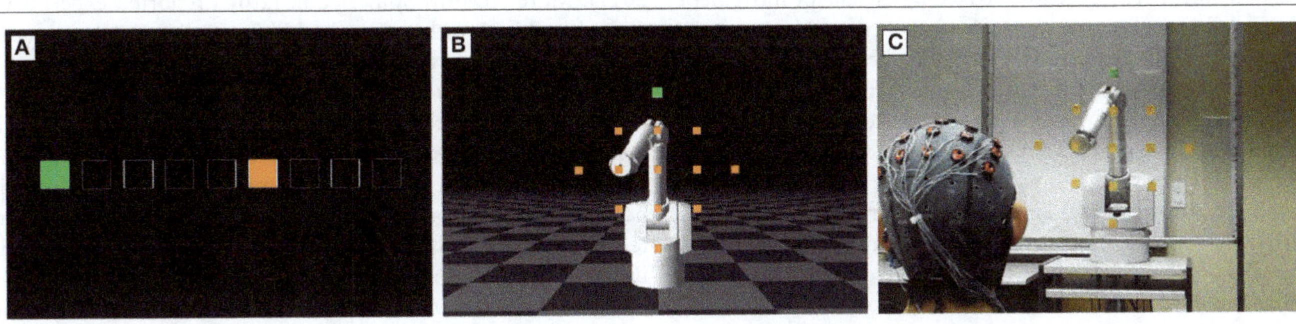

FIGURE 3 | Several experimental protocols used to study ErrPs during brain-machine interaction. (A) 1-D cursor control (Ferrez and Millán, 2008a; Chavarriaga and Millán, 2010; Tsoneva et al., 2010; Goel et al., 2011; Zhang et al., 2012; Iturrate et al., 2013a, 2014). The cursor (orange square) moves in discrete steps toward a target location (green square). **(B,C)** 2-D control of a simulated and real robotic arm (Omedes et al., 2013; Iturrate et al., 2014).

that the location or movement of target stimuli are balanced. Fortunately, it has consistently been found that ocular artifacts have little influence on the signals used for the decoding (Ferrez and Millán, 2008a; Chavarriaga and Millán, 2010; Iturrate et al., 2010; Artusi et al., 2011; Spüler et al., 2012): Nevertheless EOG artifacts remain an ever-present concern in EEG studies using moving stimuli and their potential impact should be systematically assessed.

A different possible confound is that the observed potentials are more related to the rarity of the erroneous events than their valence. To evaluate this, Ferrez and Millán (2008a) and Chavarriaga and Millán (2010) performed experiments with error rates of 50% and 40%, respectively. In both cases they report similar ErrPs than those obtained with lower error rates, although with lower amplitudes. Similarly, the N200/P300, as well as the FRN signals have also been reported to be modulated by the target/error likelihood (Polich, 1990; Polich and Margala, 1997; Jessup et al., 2010; Hauser et al., 2014). In conclusion, although ErrPs are modulated by the frequency of the stimulus they cannot be explained by this factor alone and seem more correlated to their meaning.

Another factor that can modulate the amplitude of the ErrP concerns the attention level of the subject and her/his engagement in the task (Hajcak et al., 2005). Subjects tend to have smaller ErrP amplitude when simply monitoring the device than when they are controlling it, c.f. **Figures 2C,D** (Ferrez and Millán, 2008a; Chavarriaga and Millán, 2010). This factor may influence the performance and, as with other BMI approaches, calls for efficient calibration methods, which could be used before online operation.

Overall, initial ErrP studies supported the idea that it was possible to identify erroneous responses–either manual or decoded through a BMI–and use them to correct these errors to improve the overall performance (c.f., **Figure 1** Left). They were based on offline analysis and did not assess the effect of these approaches during online operation, but fostered continued efforts to reliably decode such error-related brain activity and to integrate it in the framework of human–machine interaction.

4. ERROR-RELATED POTENTIALS AS A CORRECTIVE SIGNAL

4.1. ERROR CORRECTION IN MOTOR-RELATED BMI

Subsequent attempts at integration of ErrP-based correction into online BMI setups yielded generally positive results. Extending their previous protocol, Ferrez and Millán (2008b) used a two-class MI-based BMI to control one-dimensional step-wise movements of a cursor. The potential evoked by the cursor movement was decoded to indicate an erroneous or correct movement. In the former case, the cursor was returned to the previous position. Simultaneous real-time decoding of both ErrPs and MI-related activity in two subjects resulted in a three-fold increase in the information transfer rate. They report 80% accuracy in the ErrP recognition, which lead to a reduction of the MI decoding error from about 30% to less than 9%. Kreilinger et al. (2009) also reported performance improvement in a similar experimental protocol involving 13 healthy subjects. MI classification accuracy increased from about 70 to 80% using the online ErrP-based correction.

Other studies have provided further support to the feasibility of using such hybrid approaches, combining the use of one BMI signal to decode the action commands and the ErrP decoding to correct erroneous actions. For instance, Artusi et al. (2011) using offline analysis showed improvement in the decoding of movement-related potentials (i.e., preparatory EEG activity before actual movement performance) by introducing ErrP classification. In their approach, the outcome of the movement decoder was shown to the user and if the elicited EEG response was decoded as corresponding to the error condition, the trial was discarded and the task had to be repeated. Their experiment, involving six healthy subjects, yielded an average ErrP recognition of 80%. Simulation of this corrective mechanism showed a reduction of the global error rate in discriminating between imagination of slow and fast arm flexions from 26% to 14%. In this case, 20% of the trials were discarded based on the ErrP decoding. They estimated an improvement in the average information transfer rate of 76%. Altogether these results are indeed encouraging; however, often such studies used simulated initial BMI commands in order to keep a constant performance; e.g., Ferrez and Millán (2008a); Millán et al. (2009); Artusi et al. (2011). The purpose of such manipulation is to decouple the estimation of the benefits of ErrP-based detection from within-session variations of the command decoder. In consequence, further online tests are required to fully assess the actual performance of motor-related BMIs combined with ErrP-triggered corrective actions.

4.2. ERROR CORRECTION IN P300-BASED BMI

ErrP-based correction mechanisms have also been applied widely to P300-based spellers (Dal Seno et al., 2010; Takahashi et al., 2010; Combaz et al., 2012; Spüler et al., 2012; Schmidt et al., 2012). These systems exploit an event-related potential elicited by a rare, relevant stimulus: the so-called P300 ERP component (Farwell and Donchin, 1988). In this application, the interface can cancel a character selected with the P300-based speller upon subsequent ErrP detection or, alternatively, correct it by choosing the second most probable character according to the P300 decoding. Although, an early study showed little or no improvement by ErrP-based online correction for two subjects using a pseudo-random matrix speller (Dal Seno et al., 2010), later works showed advantage of integrating the ErrP detection into the BMI. Schmidt et al. (2012) reported an average increase of 40% in the writing speed of twelve healthy subjects using a speller interface designed to reduce the performance sensitivity to gaze shifts (Treder et al., 2011). More recently, Spüler et al. (2012) reported experiments with six subjects with motor disabilities (5 diagnosed with amyotrophic lateral sclerosis, ALS, and one with Duchenne muscular dystrophy) in which a performance increase was observed (0.37 bits per trial). For comparison, an age-matched group of eight able-bodied subjects showed an increase of 0.73 bits per trial, while a group of nine younger subjects had an increase of 0.44 bits per trial. Notably, patients with ALS exhibited similar ErrP patterns to those of healthy subjects, further supporting the potential use of error processing signals in such BMI applications, primarily meant for users with severe disabilities. Both studies found an inverse correlation between the performance improvement and the accuracy of the P300 decoder. However, conversely, a different study involving 16 healthy subjects reported larger improvement for users with higher spelling accuracy (Perrin et al., 2012). In this study, such subjects also showed a slightly higher specificity in the decoding of the ErrP signal. A potential issue to be taken into account in this approach is that both P300 and ErrPs are modulated by attentional processes (Yeung et al., 2005; Kleih et al., 2010). Therefore, factors that affect the level of engagement or motivation of the user (e.g., a BMI low accuracy, high mental workload) may be reflected in the elicited ERPs and, depending on the sensitivity of the decoder to these variations, be detrimental to the overall performance after integration of the ErrP-based correction in both able-bodied and users with disabilities.

4.3. CORRECTION OF MANUAL RESPONSES

Besides using ErrPs to correct commands generated by BMI systems, these signals can also be used in HCI applications requiring manual responses from the user. The first attempts to decode the ERN/Pe components date back to the early 2000s. Blankertz et al. (2003) reported decoding of error-related signals in eight able-bodied subjects using a modified d-2 attention task (Bates and Lemay, 2004). Then, Parra et al. (2003) analyzed ErrPs in a forced choice visual discrimination task, i.e., the Eriksen Flankers task. They reported single-trial classification accuracy of 91% averaged over seven healthy subjects. Furthermore, online correction of the manual responses using the decoded error-related EEG correlates reduced the discrimination error rate in 5 of the subjects (average error reduction was $21.4 \pm 21.7\%$). While in the above study users responded by pressing a key, Ventouras et al. (2011) also tested the decoding of the ERN/Pe in the Eriksen task using a joystick as input device. Their experiment included 16 healthy subjects, and classification performance was assessed using the leave-one-out procedure. They reported sensitivity and specificity values over 87.5%.

These signals have also been tested as a means to correct errors in typewriting tasks. Wang et al. (2011) decoded ErrPs elicited during a hear-and-type task where nine subjects had to type numbers dictated by a computer. They reported sensitivity and specificity values of 68.72 and 51.68% for classifiers trained and tested on the same subject. The performance for cross-subjects classifiers was 68.72 and 49.45%, respectively. A limitation of this study, and a potential reason for the low decoding performance, is the small number of keystroke errors made by the subjects, ranging from 0.42 to 3.58%. As discussed below, this limits the possibility of building proper models of the signals corresponding to errors.

Another interesting study evaluated both feedback and self-generated errors in a task involving visuo-tactile stimuli (Lehne et al., 2009). Eleven participants took part in the study where an array of vibrotactile stimulators provided information about a tactile cursor that should be directed toward a target location on the torso. Visual stimulus presented an intended direction of movement and upon its appearance, the user pressed a button to confirm or reject the proposed movement direction. Given the task difficulty, users made erroneous responses in 27.8% of the trials on average. Furthermore, in other trials machine errors were also introduced (i.e., the machine misinterpreted the button responses). Classification of both types of errors yielded accuracies of about 70%, with higher detection rates for the correct than the error trials (i.e., about 70 and 50%, respectively).

Overall, these works show the feasibility of decoding error-related information after user overt responses. In general the classification performance was higher for the correct condition, in particular when the complexity of the task increases.

5. ERROR-DRIVEN LEARNING

The studies presented above used ErrP detection to immediately correct erroneous decisions made by the BMI. An alternative use of these signals is error-driven learning. This approach, illustrated in **Figure 1** Right, has been applied to endow BMI systems with adaptive capabilities in two different manners. One possibility is to update the BMI classifier (Blumberg et al., 2007; Llera et al., 2011, 2012; Roset et al., 2013). For instance, Llera et al. (2011) used the decoding of error-related MEG activity to identify misclassification in a two-class covert visual attention paradigm ($N = 8$). The lateralization of alpha-band power in posterior channels was classified using logistic regression to infer which direction (i.e., left or right) the subject was covertly attending to. ErrP decoding was used to identify misclassifications and provide new labels for the incoming data in a semi-supervised manner. The labeled sample was then used to update the classifier parameters. Offline analysis showed that this approach can significantly increase the performance of the BMI classifier. Importantly, given that this is a binary task the intended target class can be easily inferred for the misclassified samples allowing the use of supervised learning techniques for the classifier adaptation. A similar strategy was adopted by Artusi et al. (2011) in the task described in section 4.1, i.e., decoding of imagery of fast vs slow movements. In their case, those trials that were considered as correct after ErrP classification were incorporated into a learning set that was used to perform online retraining of the MI classifier.

However, as long as the ErrP decoding is considered to be in essence binary, the overall performance will be substantially affected by the false positive rate (i.e., correct BMI actions misclassified as errors). A way to palliate this effect is to use methods relying on probabilistic error signals. In that way the reliability of the ErrP decoder (estimated from the training set) can be taken into account. Bayesian filtering or Expectation-Maximization have been put forward as possible approaches (Perrin et al., 2010; Artusi et al., 2011; Llera et al., 2012). A similar method was also proposed in a hybrid system for human-computer interaction where an acceleration-based gesture recognition system was updated using the decoding of the ErrP signal (Chavarriaga et al., 2010). However, as per our knowledge they have only been tested in offline experiments.

Besides adapting the BMI classifier, ErrPs can be used to improve the behavior of a semi-autonomous system. This approach is anchored in the concept of shared control, where intelligent devices can take care of low-level decisions while the user only provides high-level commands –using a BMI or another input modality– (Perrin et al., 2010). In this case, the user monitors the performance of the intelligent device and whenever an ErrP is detected, suggesting the action was perceived as erroneous, it is used to adapt the device controller to reduce the likelihood of committing the same error later on (Chavarriaga and Millán, 2010). In terms of the reinforcement learning algorithm, the detection of an ErrP corresponding to the error condition will be translated onto a negative reward value, effectively punishing the performed action when updating the control policy. This approach was first tested in a 1-D control task with six healthy subjects (c.f. **Figure 3A**). The offline analysis showed that it was possible for the device to learn optimal control policies even though the accuracy of the ErrP decoder was not perfect. An online evaluation of this approach on two subjects monitoring a simulated robot was demonstrated by Iturrate et al. (2010). In this work the subject had to choose the intended target location of the robot and then monitor its movements. The decoded ErrPs were used in a reinforcement learning paradigm to update the robot control policy. They reported that the learned policy converged toward the optimal one–i.e., taking the robot to the user's intended location–in 92% and 75% of the cases for each subject, respectively. Recent integration with shared control techniques suggests that further improvements in performance can be achieved (Iturrate et al., 2013b). In this case 4 subjects monitored a moving cursor in a 2D reaching task, and the ErrPs were used to select one control policy from a pre-defined repertoire; i.e., selecting the most suitable policy to reach the inferred target location.

6. ERROR-RELATED POTENTIALS IN REALISTIC APPLICATIONS

As summarized in section 2, a wealth of neuroscience literature has reported error-related neural correlates. These studies are typically performed in well-controlled laboratory conditions using abstract tasks and stimuli. This allows characterization of such correlates in recording conditions that yield higher signal-to-noise ratio and avoid confounds that may appear when allowing more behavioral freedom to the subject(user), or relaxing constraints of the operational setting.

Notably, several studies presented in previous sections corroborated the existence of similar correlates during complex scenarios or realistic interaction with complex devices. Wang et al. (2011) evaluated ErrPs when users performed a typewriting task, while Spüler et al. (2012); Schmidt et al. (2012) and others have tested these potentials while subjects use a P300-based speller. Moreover, it has been possible to observe and decode error-related potentials while people monitor the performance of a robotic arm (Kreilinger et al., 2012; Iturrate et al., 2014) or a mobile robot (Perrin et al., 2010; Chavarriaga et al., 2012), both using simulated and real platforms. Similar correlates were also found during simulated driving of an intelligent car (Zhang et al., 2013). Another study, assessing potential BMI applications to cope with the situational disability experienced by astronauts, reported similar ErrP waveforms and decoding performance under different gravity conditions in parabolic flights (Millán et al., 2009).

These studies suggest that these ErrPs can also be decoded in more complex tasks and scenarios. Nevertheless, it has to be noticed that the decoding performance is typically lower than in simpler, well-controlled experimental paradigms. The performance differences can be due to the decreased signal to noise ratio of the recorded signals, as well as the increased workload placed on the user in the complex tasks. As shown below, some works have attempted to identify and exploit common patterns between simple and complex tasks as a procedure to improve the training of the ErrP decoder in more challenging conditions (Kim and Kirchner, 2013; Iturrate et al., 2014).

7. CLASSIFICATION OF ERROR-RELATED POTENTIALS

A key factor for exploiting ErrPs to improve BMI performance is the ability to decode this signal in a single-trial. As it is the case for all BMI systems, they rely on the real-time processing of the neural signals and the use of machine learning techniques to relate the current activity pattern to a corresponding class (i.e., error or correct condition). This process involves the extraction of suitable features and the training of a classifier based on available labeled samples. Below we discuss the most common methods applied for decoding the error correlates. However, a comprehensive review of the machine learning methods applied in BMI is out of the scope of this paper. Interested readers can refer, among others, to introductory papers by Bashashati et al. (2007); Lotte et al. (2007) and Blankertz et al. (2011).

Studies presented in the previous sections show that it is possible to decode the ErrPs. Noticeably, they have often reported higher classification accuracy for correct trials than errors. This may be partly due to the protocols used to train the classifier. These typically involve a low error-rate (e.g., 20%) thus yielding a larger number of examples for the correct class. The use of an imbalanced number of samples per class may result in asymmetric costs for misclassification of each class and leads to classifiers that are biased toward one of the classes. Moreover, it is difficult to properly estimate the classifier parameters if only a limited number of examples is available.

Regarding the processing and classification techniques used to decode the ErrPs it can be observed that a vast majority of the reported studies are based on temporal features (i.e., waveform shape) computed from a few pre-selected electrodes in the fronto-central areas (e.g., FCz, Cz). Typically, EEG signals were low-pass filtered below 10 or 20 Hz and time-samples from a pre-defined window (usually between 200 and 600 ms) were used for classification (Blankertz et al., 2003; Ferrez and Millán, 2008a; Kreilinger et al., 2009; Chavarriaga and Millán, 2010; Dal Seno et al., 2010; Takahashi et al., 2010; Artusi et al., 2011; Spüler et al., 2012). In some cases, authors used automatic selection mechanisms over larger feature spaces, quantifying discriminant power of features with some metric, e.g., t-statistic, Fisher score or r^2 (Dal Seno et al., 2010; Goel et al., 2011; Iturrate et al., 2013a). These studies reported similar features than those manually selected but aimed at better capturing subject-dependent variations in the elicited signals. Alternative approaches to compute features have recently been proposed including the usage of spatiotemporal filters (Perrin et al., 2012; Rousseau et al., 2012; Iturrate et al., 2013a, 2014), as well as singular value decomposition (Hamner et al., 2011; Phlypo et al., 2011).

A few studies have tested the feasibility of exploiting features computed in the frequency domain (Bollon et al., 2009; Omedes et al., 2013) with generally encouraging results. Interestingly, Omedes et al. (2013) tested the use of theta power as a feature for classification in the three experiments shown in **Figure 3**. They evaluated which type of features generalize better across tasks by measuring the classifier performance in a different task than the one it was trained for. Offline tests of data from six subjects showed smaller performance degradation across tasks for classifiers using frequency features compared to those using temporal features. A separate study showed that ErrP variation across these tasks is mainly due to latency (Iturrate et al., 2014). This suggests that frequency-based features may be less sensitive to temporal jitter across individual ErrP trials.

Goel et al. (2011) tested the use of features computed on the intracranial EEG sources, which have been estimated using inverse solution methods. The hypothesis being that projection into the source space can act as a spatial filtering technique that increases the signal-to-noise ratio of neurophysiologically relevant discriminant features. Offline analysis in the monitoring protocol depicted in **Figure 3A**, showed improved performance– in terms of area under the curve, AUC (Fawcett, 2006)–with respect to previously reported results using surface EEG classifiers in the six subjects analyzed. Further online experiments confirmed the validity of using these features for classification although its potential advantages over standard methods is yet to be fully validated (Goel, 2013).

Taking into consideration the cross-regional interactions reported in neurophysiological studies (c.f., section 2), Zhang et al. (2012) evaluated the use of single-trial estimation of connectivity patterns for ErrP classification. They computed directional interaction across channels using a modified directed transfer function (DTF) method in different frequency bands (Kamiński and Blinowska, 1991). Offline analysis of data on 16 subjects using the same monitoring protocol as above, showed discriminant fronto-central interactions in the theta rhythm that yielded single-trial decoding above chance level. Furthermore, the combined use of connectivity and time-based features gave significantly better performance than temporal features alone, suggesting that the two feature sets convey complementary information.

The most common classification techniques used for the decoding include linear discriminant analysis (LDA) or its variations such as Fisher LDA or regularized LDA (Blankertz et al., 2003; Parra et al., 2003; Lehne et al., 2009; Ventouras et al., 2011; Iturrate et al., 2014), as well as Gaussian classifiers (Ferrez and Millán, 2008a; Kreilinger et al., 2009; Chavarriaga and Millán, 2010; Perrin et al., 2012) and support-vector machines (SVM) (Artusi et al., 2011; Ventouras et al., 2011; Wang et al., 2011; Spüler et al., 2012). In their study, Spüler et al. (2012) performed an offline comparison of LDA, step-wise LDA, and SVMs with linear and radial basis function (RBF) kernels. For this analysis they used previously recorded data of six patients with ALS. Using 10-fold cross-validation test they selected the RBF-kernel SVM as the best suitable for their application (P300-speller). Unfortunately, they did not report what specific criteria were used for this selection nor the performance of each method. Similarly, Ventouras et al. (2011) compared the performance of SVM and K-NN classifiers on the decoding of ErrPs elicited after manual responses. Their analysis using different feature selection mechanisms and leave-one-out cross-validation showed no significant differences between the two methods. Wang et al. (2011) also compared classifier performance when decoding those signals. Interestingly, they found little performance differences between the sensitivity obtained with LDA and SVM classifiers when training and testing on the same subject's data. In contrast, when the test was performed on a subject that was not part of the training set, the LDA yielded higher sensitivity. However, their results were close to chance level and may not be significant given that only a small number of trials were available for the error class.

A direct comparison of the performance obtained in these studies cannot be interpreted as a fair assessment of the advantages of a given decoding method. That is due to the differences in the pre-processing methods applied, the features selected for classification, and the reported performance metrics. Nevertheless, they often reported classification accuracies between 70 and 80%. As a tentative synthesis, one is under the impression that various classification methods reported in literature seem to obtain comparable results. Taking into account that most of these studies involve a rather small number of subjects, it is very likely that any performance differences are largely influenced by inter-subject variability.

In addition, efforts have been undertaken to design methods for fast training of the ErrP decoder. Some recent approaches rely on semi-supervised or unsupervised learning (Grizou et al., 2014; Zeyl and Chau, 2014). Another applied technique is the use of available data from other subjects to boost learning of a subject-dependent classifier (Iturrate et al., 2011; Putze et al., 2013). Alternatively, ErrPs have been shown to have common characteristics across tasks. In consequence, several methods have been proposed for online adaptation of classifiers trained in a previous protocol to the characteristics of the potentials elicited in the new task (Iturrate et al., 2013a; Kim and Kirchner, 2013; Iturrate et al., 2014). In this case, provided that an ErrP decoder has already been trained in a given task, the calibration time for a new task can be considerably reduced. Finally, as mentioned above, frequency features seemed less sensitive to task-dependent latency jitters in the neural response and were thus proposed as a potential means to implement task-independent classifiers (Omedes et al., 2013). These techniques have shown encouraging results, but have yet to be thoroughly tested to confirm their real advantages.

Lastly, besides direct single-trial classification problems, the ErrP detection process should take into account how this information will be later on utilized for interaction. In particular, there may be application-dependent requirements in terms of sensitivity and specificity that need to be considered when choosing the classification technique and parameters (Parra et al., 2003; Seno et al., 2010; Spüler et al., 2012).

8. DISCUSSION

The works reviewed in this paper strongly support the feasibility of decoding error-related potentials and using the information they carry to improve the performance of BMI and HCI systems. There are, however, several challenges that need to be overcome until efficient and fully working applications can be implemented in the real world.

First of all, there is a clear need for further evaluation of the online exploitation of ErrPs. Although there is an increasing amount of studies showing online decoding of error-related signals, in particular for P300 applications, they typically rely on a small number of subjects. These studies have already highlighted how individual differences may affect the overall performance of the error-correction mechanism (Perrin et al., 2012; Schmidt et al., 2012; Spüler et al., 2012). Therefore caution should be taken in the design of such studies. In particular, this includes the number of subjects involved in the study, the control conditions against which the performance will be evaluated, as well as the effects of subject learning and fatigue when testing over several sessions.

Further studies are also needed to evaluate the detection of these potentials in people with severe disabilities, which is the principal target user group of BMI today (one of the main potential applications of BMIs is the restoration or substitution of motor and communication capabilities). Spüler et al. (2012) reported encouraging results, showing that reliable ErrPs are elicited in patients with ALS and their decoding can improve performance of a P300-speller. Nonetheless, there is clearly a need for more studies characterizing these signals in different populations. Some studies have already pointed out age-related changes in the ERN (Davies et al., 2004; Wiersema et al., 2007), but it is yet to be assessed how these changes affect the discriminability between error and correct trials. Similarly, longitudinal studies may be necessary to identify how ErrPs change in the case of degenerative diseases. In addition, several works have pointed out that feedback modalities other than visual may be suitable for users in the locked-in state as they do not rely on volitional gaze control (Schreuder et al., 2010; Treder et al., 2011; Kaufmann et al., 2013). Preliminary evidence suggests that ErrPs can be elicited and, to some extent, decoded after tactile stimulation (Lehne et al., 2009; Chavarriaga et al., 2012) in healthy users. This possibility remains to be further tested, in particular in users with disabilities.

Another issue of interest concerns the evaluation of the performance of hybrid BMI systems exploiting ErrP-decoding. Typically, authors have reported changes using diverse metrics including accuracy, information transfer rate (Wolpaw et al., 2000), efficiency (Quitadamo et al., 2012) or utility value (Seno et al., 2010). This denotes a lack of a formal framework for performance assessment –a problem common to the overall BMI field– and prevents the comparison of results across different studies (Thomas et al., 2013; Thompson et al., 2014). It is advisable that future works provide a comprehensive evaluation of performance reporting different metrics to enable such comparisons. Moreover, performance can be affected by protocol-specific parameters. For instance, in the case of ErrP-based correction, each command correction will have a cost (e.g., time required to undo the last action), and the overall benefit of the correction mechanism will depend on both: this cost and the specificity of the ErrP decoder (Parra et al., 2003).

This is intrinsically linked to the sensitivity and specificity of the decoding performance. The impact of the falsely decoded trials will be highly dependent on the application and the actions taken upon error detection. A clear difference is observed between the corrective and learning use of the ErrPs. In the first case, ErrP classification errors are explicitly perceived by the user. This can be counterproductive if the false detections appear to impair proper use of the interface (e.g., by rejecting or changing correct commands), even if improved performance is achieved in the long-term. As an example, Perrin et al. (2012) reported that some users, despite having good ErrP decoding performance, still preferred the implementation of the P300 speller without the correction, since they perceived no benefit with respect to use of the P300 alone.

In contrast, the learning approach where the classifier or the device controller is updated according to the outcome of the ErrP decoding may mask these false detections. Moreover, it has been shown that reinforcement learning algorithms can converge toward optimal policies even in the case of noisy estimation of the reward signals, provided that the estimation performance is above chance level (Sutton and Barto, 1998). One can expect, thus, that the use of ErrPs for learning has lower requirements in terms of the minimal acceptable performance than immediate command correction. This holds, of course, provided that the initial performance of the control interface is already acceptable for the user. Future work assessing these requirements from a human factors perspective is certainly needed for effectively designing interaction systems that exploit these error-related signals.

Following basic studies on the ERN and FRN, BMI efforts of decoding error-related signals have so far mostly focused on the time-locked response generated by a discrete feedback stimulus. In consequence, exploitation of the ErrPs has been largely restricted to discrete tasks such as the P300-based speller or stepwise movements (c.f. section 3). Besides limiting the range of applications and their naturalness, this approach also limits the throughput of the system since after each command a time interval of several hundred milliseconds is required for evaluating the presence of an ErrP. Consequently, further research is required toward decoding in more continuous setups.

Although not an easy task, several lines of progress seem to be open. One alternative is to increase the pace at which the stimuli are presented. Typically, experiments exploiting ErrPs have an inter-stimulus interval of 2 s or more. In contrast, experiments using rapid serial visual presentation (RSVP) have shown single-trial decoding of EEG correlates of visual recognition with stimulus presentation rates higher than 4 Hz (Gerson et al., 2006). It still to be tested whether ErrPs can be detected in such fast-paced feedback presentations.

Another approach is combining usage of continuous feedback with additional discrete sensory events, used to time-lock ErrPs (Kreilinger et al., 2011, 2012). The first study used a game application where the decoding of MI-related patterns controlled lane changes in a continuously moving animated car. It provided feedback for correct or wrong changes in the form of multiple predictable collisions with point tokens (positioned on the correct lane) or barriers (on the wrong lane). The second work applied an interesting approach to the BMI-control of a robot arm, combining the performance of a continuous mental task with discrete feedback to elicit ErrPs. Subjects had to perform MI during a given period, then the robot arm moved and after that users should assess whether the robot's movement lasted the same amount of time as the MI task. Visual cues provided information of the robot movement duration. Offline analysis showed ErrP decoding above random level; however the performance in both studies was lower than those reported in purely discrete paradigms.

Besides the previous approaches employing, in essence, some strategy of circumvention of the continuous feedback problem, one can also try to directly tackle the possibility of decoding error-related signals in a purely asynchronous (non-time locked) manner. An example of such attempt with invasive electrocorticographic recordings (ECoG), benefiting from better signal-to-noise ratio than scalp EEG, demonstrated that error events can potentially be detected with good accuracy during a continuous task, given a temporal tolerance of several hundred milliseconds (Milekovic et al., 2013). For EEG, a potential avenue to explore is the use of the spectral content instead of temporal features. As shown in **Figure 2** the event-related ErrPs are characterized by positive theta modulations. Interestingly, it has been shown that erroneous manual responses elicit increases in both phase- and non-phase-locked theta activity (Trujillo and Allen, 2007). Moreover, the power increase in non-phase locked activity was higher than for the phase-locked activity. Noticeably, ErrP-decoding performance based on theta-power features was shown to be less sensitive to task changes (Omedes et al., 2013). As already mentioned the main ErrP changes across these tasks can be explained by latency shifts (Iturrate et al., 2014). Thus supporting the notion that oscillatory activity can allow asynchronous detection of erroneous events in continuous tasks.

To summarize, different studies have repeatedly demonstrated the feasibility of decoding error-related EEG signals on a single-trial basis. This has been achieved both when the errors are committed by the user, as well as when the errors are introduced by the interfacing device, in particular a BMI. The decoding accuracy of these signals is typically about 80%. This performance levels have been shown to usually be sufficient to improve the information transfer rate in different applications including motor-imagery based BMIs, P300 spelling and manual labeling of visual stimuli (c.f. section 4). Moreover, ErrPs can successfully be used as a learning signal to improve BMI decoders or the controller of an external device (c.f., section 5). All these results support the potential of error-related correlates to provide naturally elicited information about the user cognitive state that can be used to adjust the machine's behavior.

Despite these successful studies, several aspects remain to be further explored, as detailed above. These include improvement in decoding of these signals in more complex applications, as well as their further characterization in subjects with disabilities. More importantly, large scale evaluations involving end-users have to be performed from a user-centered perspective to identify performance requirements and design criteria that allow for optimal exploitation of these correlates in practical applications.

FUNDING

This work has been supported by the Swiss-funded SNSF NCCR Robotics. This paper only reflects the authors' view and funding agencies are not liable for any use that may be made of the information contained herein.

ACKNOWLEDGMENT

We thank H. Zhang, I. Iturrate, J. DiGiovanna, S. Rousseau, and J. Sanchez for useful discussions on this topic.

REFERENCES

Artusi, X., Niazi, I. K., Lucas, M.-F., and Farina, D. (2011). Performance of a simulated adaptive BCI based on experimental classification of movement-related and error potentials. *Emerg. Select. Topics Circ. Syst. IEEE J.* 1, 480–488. doi: 10.1109/JETCAS.2011.2177920

Bashashati, A., Fatourechi, M., Ward, R. K., and Birch, G. E. (2007). A survey of signal processing algorithms in brain-computer interfaces based on electrical brain signals. *J. Neural. Eng.* 4, R32–R57. doi: 10.1088/1741-2560/4/2/R03

Bates, M. E., and Lemay, E. P. (2004). The d2 test of attention: construct validity and extensions in scoring techniques. *J. Int. Neuropsychol. Soc.* 10, 392–400. doi: 10.1017/S135561770410307X

Blankertz, B., Dornhege, G., Schäfer, C., Krepki, R., Kohlmorgen, J., Müller, K., et al. (2003). Boosting bit rates and error detection for the classification of fast-paced motor commands based on single-trial EEG analysis. *IEEE Trans. Neural Sys. Rehab. Eng.* 11, 127–131. doi: 10.1109/TNSRE.2003.814456

Blankertz, B., Lemm, S., Treder, M., Haufe, S., and Müller, K. R. (2011). Single-trial analysis and classification of ERP components - a tutorial. *Neuroimage* 56, 814–825. doi: 10.1016/j.neuroimage.2010.06.048

Blumberg, J., Rickert, J., Waldert, S., Schulze-Bonhage, A., Aertsen, A., and Mehring, C. (2007). "Adaptive classification for brain computer interfaces," in *Engineering in Medicine and Biology Society, 2007. EMBS 2007. 29th Annual International Conference of the IEEE* (Lyon), 2536–2539. doi: 10.1109/IEMBS.2007.4352845

Bollon, J.-M., Chavarriaga, R., Millán, J. d. R., and Bessière, P. (2009). "EEG error-related potentials detection with a Bayesian filter," in *Proceedings of the 4th International IEEE/EMBS Conference on Neural Engineering NER '09* (Antalya), 702–705. doi: 10.1109/NER.2009.5109393

Brázdil, M., Roman, R., Falkenstein, M., Daniel, P., Jurák, P., and Rektor, I. (2002). Error processing–evidence from intracerebral ERP recordings. *Exp. Brain Res.* 146, 460–466. doi: 10.1007/s00221-002-1201-y

Cavanagh, J. F., Cohen, M. X., and Allen, J. J. B. (2009). Prelude to and resolution of an error: EEG phase synchrony reveals cognitive control dynamics during action monitoring. *J. Neurosci.* 29, 98–105. doi: 10.1523/JNEUROSCI.4137-08.2009

Cavanagh, J. F., Zambrano-Vazquez, L., and Allen, J. J. B. (2012). Theta lingua franca: a common mid-frontal substrate for action monitoring processes. *Psychophysiology* 49, 220–238. doi: 10.1111/j.1469-8986.2011.01293.x

Chavarriaga, R., Biasiucci, A., Förster, K., Roggen, D., Tröster, G., and Millán, J. d. R. (2010). "Adaptation of hybrid human-computer interaction systems using EEG error-related potentials," in *32nd Annual International Conference of the IEEE Engineering in Medicine and Biology Society (EMBC'10)* (Buenos Aires).

Chavarriaga, R., and Millán, J. d. R. (2010). Learning from EEG error-related potentials in noninvasive brain-computer interfaces. *IEEE Trans. Neural. Syst. Rehabil. Eng.* 18, 381–388. doi: 10.1109/TNSRE.2010.2053387

Chavarriaga, R., Perrin, X., Siegwart, R., and Millán, J. d. R. (2012). "Anticipation- and error-related EEG signals during realistic human-machine interaction: a study on visual and tactile feedback," in *34th International Conference of the IEEE Engineering in Medicine and Biology Society (EMBC'12)* (San Diego, CA). doi: 10.1109/EMBC.2012.6347537

Cohen, M. X., Elger, C. E., and Ranganath, C. (2007). Reward expectation modulates feedback-related negativity and EEG spectra. *Neuroimage* 35, 968–978. doi: 10.1016/j.neuroimage.2006.11.056

Cohen, M. X., Ridderinkhof, K. R., Haupt, S., Elger, C. E., and Fell, J. (2008). Medial frontal cortex and response conflict: evidence from human intracranial EEG and medial frontal cortex lesion. *Brain Res* 1238, 127–142. doi: 10.1016/j.brainres.2008.07.114

Combaz, A., Chumerin, N., Manyakov, N., Robben, A., Suykens, J., and Hulle, M. V. (2012). Towards the detection of error-related potentials and its integration in the context of a P300 speller brain-computer interface. *Neurocomputing* 80, 73–82. doi: 10.1016/j.neucom.2011.09.013

Dal Seno, B., Matteucci, M., and Mainardi, L. (2010). Online detection of P300 and error potentials in a BCI speller. *Comput. Intell. Neurosci.* 2010:307254. doi: 10.1155/2010/307254

Davies, P. L., Segalowitz, S. J., and Gavin, W. J. (2004). Development of error-monitoring event-related potentials in adolescents. *Ann. N.Y. Acad. Sci.* 1021, 324–328. doi: 10.1196/annals.1308.039

Debener, S., Ullsperger, M., Siegel, M., Fiehler, K., von Cramon, D. Y., and Engel, A. K. (2005). Trial-by-trial coupling of concurrent electroencephalogram and functional magnetic resonance imaging identifies the dynamics of performance monitoring. *J. Neurosci.* 25, 11730–11737. doi: 10.1523/JNEUROSCI.3286-05.2005

Falkenstein, M., Hohnsbein, J., Hoormann, J., and Blanke, L. (1991). Effects of crossmodal divided attention on late ERP components: II. Error processing in choice reaction tasks. *Electroencephalogr. Clin. Neurophysiol.* 78, 447–455. doi: 10.1016/0013-4694(91)90062-9

Falkenstein, M., Hoormann, J., Christ, S., and Hohnsbein, J. (2000). ERP components on reaction errors and their functional significance: A tutorial. *Biol. Psychol.* 51, 87–107. doi: 10.1016/S0301-0511(99)00031-9

Farwell, L. A., and Donchin, E. (1988). Talking off the top of your head: toward a mental prosthesis utilizing event-related brain potentials. *Electroencephalogr. Clin. Neurophysiol.* 70, 510–523. doi: 10.1016/0013-4694(88)90149-6

Fawcett, T. (2006). An introduction to ROC analysis. *Pattern Recogn. Lett.* 27, 861–874. doi: 10.1016/j.patrec.2005.10.010

Ferrez, P. W., and Millán, J. D. R. (2008a). Error-related EEG potentials generated during simulated brain-computer interaction. *IEEE Trans. Biomed. Eng.* 55, 923–929. doi: 10.1109/TBME.2007.908083

Ferrez, P. W., and Millán, J. d. R. (2008b). "Simultaneous real-time detection of motor imagery and error-related potentials for improved BCI accuracy," in *Proceedings of the 4th Intl. Brain-Computer Interface Workshop and Training Course* (Graz).

Frank, M. J., Woroch, B. S., and Curran, T. (2005). Error-related negativity predicts reinforcement learning and conflict biases. *Neuron* 47, 495–501. doi: 10.1016/j.neuron.2005.06.020

Gehring, W. J., Goss, B., Coles, M. G. H., Meyer, D. E., and Donchin, E. A. (1993). Neural system for error-detection and compensation. *Psychol. Sci.* 4, 385–390. doi: 10.1111/j.1467-9280.1993.tb00586.x

Gerson, A., Parra, L., and Sajda, P. (2006). Cortically-coupled computer vision for rapid image search. *IEEE Trans. Neural. Syst. Rehabil. Eng.* 14, 174–179. doi: 10.1109/TNSRE.2006.875550

Goel, M. K. (2013). *Inverse Solutions for Brain Computer Interface.* Ph.D thesis, Ecole Polytechnique Fédérale de Lausanne EPFL, Lausanne.

Goel, M. K., Chavarriaga, R., and Millán, J. d. R. (2011). "Cortical current density vs. surface EEG for event-related potential-based Brain-Computer interface," in *5th International IEEE EMBS Conference on Neural Engineering* (Cancún). doi: 10.1109/NER.2011.5910578

Grizou, J., Iturrate, I., Montesano, L., Oudeyer, P.-Y., and Lopes, M. (2014). "Calibration-free BCI based control," in *AAAI Conference on Artificial Intelligence* (Québec).

Hajcak, G., Moser, J. S., Yeung, N., and Simons, R. F. (2005). On the ERN and the significance of errors. *Psychophysiology* 42, 151–160. doi: 10.1111/j.1469-8986.2005.00270.x

Hamner, B., Chavarriaga, R., and Millán, J. d. R. (2011). "Learning dictionaries of spatial and temporal EEG primitives for brain-computer interfaces," in *Workshop on Structured Sparsity: Learning and Inference, ICML 2011* (Bellevue, WA).

Hauser, T. U., Iannaccone, R., Stämpfli, P., Drechsler, R., Brandeis, D., Walitza, S., et al. (2014). The feedback-related negativity (FRN) revisited: new insights into the localization, meaning and network organization. *Neuroimage* 84, 159–168. doi: 10.1016/j.neuroimage.2013.08.028

Herrmann, M. J., Römmler, J., Ehlis, A.-C., Heidrich, A., and Fallgatter, A. J. (2004). Source localization (LORETA) of the error-related-negativity (ERN/Ne) and positivity (Pe). *Brain Res. Cogn. Brain Res.* 20, 294–299. doi: 10.1016/j.cogbrainres.2004.02.013

Hoffmann, S., and Falkenstein, M. (2012). Predictive information processing in the brain: errors and response monitoring. *Int. J. Psychophysiol.* 83, 208–212. doi: 10.1016/j.ijpsycho.2011.11.015

Holroyd, C. B., and Coles, M. G. H. (2002). The neural basis of human error processing: reinforcement learning, dopamine, and the error-related negativity. *Psychol. Rev.* 109, 679–709. doi: 10.1037/0033-295X.109.4.679

Holroyd, C. B., Nieuwenhuis, S., Yeung, N., and Cohen, J. D. (2003). Errors in reward prediction are reflected in the event-related brain potential. *Neuroreport* 14, 2481–2484. doi: 10.1097/00001756-200312190-00037

Iturrate, I., Chavarriaga, R., Montesano, L., Minguez, J., and Millán, J. d. R. (2014). Latency correction of error potentials between different experiments reduces calibration time for single-trial classification. *J. Neural. Eng.* 11:036005. doi: 10.1088/1741-2560/11/3/036005

Iturrate, I., Montesano, L., Chavarriaga, R., Millán, J. d. R., and Minguez, J. (2011). "Minimizing calibration time of single-trial recognition of error potentials in brain-computer interfaces," in *Engineering in Medicine and Biology Conference (EMBC 2011)* (Boston, MA). doi: 10.1109/IEMBS.2011.6091572

Iturrate, I., Montesano, L., and Minguez, J. (2010). "Robot reinforcement learning using EEG-based reward signals," in *IEEE International Conference on Robotics and Automation (ICRA)*, (Alaska).

Iturrate, I., Montesano, L., and Minguez, J. (2013a). Task-dependent signal variations in EEG error-related potentials for brain-computer interfaces. *J. Neural. Eng.* 10:026024. doi: 10.1088/1741-2560/10/2/026024

Iturrate, I., Omedes, J., and Montesano, L. (2013b). "Shared control of a robot using EEG-based feedback signals," in *Proceedings of the 2nd Workshop on Machine Learning for Interactive Systems: Bridging the Gap Between Perception, Action and Communication*, MLIS '13 (New York, NY: ACM), 45–50.

Jessup, R. K., Busemeyer, J. R., and Brown, J. W. (2010). Error effects in anterior cingulate cortex reverse when error likelihood is high. *J. Neurosci.* 30, 67–3472. doi: 10.1523/JNEUROSCI.4130-09.2010

Kamiński, M. J., and Blinowska, K. J. (1991). A new method of the description of the information flow in the brain structures. *Biol. Cybern.* 65, 3–210. doi: 10.1007/BF00198091

Kaufmann, T., Holz, E. M., and Kübler, A. (2013). Comparison of tactile, auditory and visual modality for brain-computer interface use: a case study with a patient in the locked-in state. *Front. Neurosci.* 7:129. doi: 10.3389/fnins.2013.00129

Kim, S. K., and Kirchner, E. A. (2013). "Classifier transferability in the detection of error related potentials from observation to interaction," in *Systems, Man, and Cybernetics (SMC), 2013 IEEE International Conference on* (Manchester), 3360–3365. doi: 10.1109/SMC.2013.573

Kleih, S. C., Nijboer, F., Halder, S., and Kübler, A. (2010). Motivation modulates the P300 amplitude during brain-computer interface use. *Clin. Neurophysiol.* 121, 1023–1031. doi: 10.1016/j.clinph.2010.01.034

Koelewijn, T., van Schie, H. T., Bekkering, H., Oostenveld, R., and Jensen, O. (2008). Motor-cortical beta oscillations are modulated by correctness of observed action. *Neuroimage* 40, 767–775. doi: 10.1016/j.neuroimage.2007.12.018

Kreilinger, A., Neuper, C., and Müller-Putz, G. (2011). "Detection of error potentials during a car-game with combined continuous and discrete feedback," in *5th International BCI Conference 2011* (Graz).

Kreilinger, A., Neuper, C., and Müller-Putz, G. R. (2012). Error potential detection during continuous movement of an artificial arm controlled by brain-computer interface. *Med. Biol. Eng. Comput.* 50, 223–230. doi: 10.1007/s11517-011-0858-4

Kreilinger, A., Neuper, C., Pfurtscheller, G., and Müller-Putz, G. (2009). "Implementation of error detection into the Graz-brain-computer interface," in *Proceedings of AAATE09* (Florence).

Lehne, M., Ihme, K., Brouwer, A.-M., van Erp, J., and Zander, T. (2009). "Error-related EEG patterns during tactile human-machine interaction," in *Affective Computing and Intelligent Interaction and Workshops, 2009. ACII 2009. 3rd International Conference on* (Amsterdam), 1–9. doi: 10.1109/ACII.2009.5349480

Llera, A., Gómez, V., and Kappen, H. J. (2012). Adaptive classification on brain-computer interfaces using reinforcement signals. *Neural Comput.* 24, 2900–2923. doi: 10.1162/NECO_a_00348

Llera, A., van Gerven, M., Gómez, V., Jensen, O., and Kappen, H. (2011). On the use of interaction error potentials for adaptive brain computer interfaces. *Neural Netw.* 24, 1120–1127. doi: 10.1016/j.neunet.2011.05.006

López-Larraz, E., Creatura, M., Iturrate, I., Montesano, L., and Minguez, J. (2011). "EEG single-trial classification of visual, auditive and vibratory feedback potentials in brain-computer interfaces," in *Conference of the IEEE Engineering in Medicine and Biology Society* (Boston, MA), 4231–4234. doi: 10.1109/IEMBS.2011.6091050

Lopez-Larraz, E., Iturrate, I., Montesano, L., and Minguez, J. (2010). "Real-time recognition of feedback error-related potentials during a time-estimation task," in *32nd Annual International Conference of the IEEE Engineering in Medicine and Biology Society (EMBC'10).*

Lotte, F., Congedo, M., Lécuyer, A., Lamarche, F., and Arnaldi, B. (2007). A review of classification algorithms for EEG-based brain-computer interfaces. *J. Neural. Eng.* 4, R1–R13. doi: 10.1088/1741-2560/4/2/R01

Milekovic, T., Ball, T., Schulze-Bonhage, A., Aertsen, A., and Mehring, C. (2013). Detection of error related neuronal responses recorded by electrocorticography in humans during continuous movements. *PLoS ONE* 8:e55235. doi: 10.1371/journal.pone.0055235

Millán, J. d. R., Ferrez, P., and Seidl, T. (2009). Validation of brain-machine interfaces during parabolic flight. *Int. Rev. Neurobiol.* 86, 189–197. doi: 10.1016/S0074-7742(09)86014-5

Navarro-Cebrian, A., Knight, R. T., and Kayser, A. S. (2013). Error-monitoring and post-error compensations: dissociation between perceptual failures and motor errors with and without awareness. *J. Neurosci.* 33, 12375–12383. doi: 10.1523/JNEUROSCI.0447-13.2013

Nieuwenhuis, S., Yeung, N., Holroyd, C. B., Schurger, A., and Cohen, J. D. (2004). Sensitivity of electrophysiological activity from medial frontal cortex to utilitarian and performance feedback. *Cereb. Cortex* 14, 741–747. doi: 10.1093/cercor/bhh034

Olvet, D. M., and Hajcak, G. (2008). The error-related negativity (ERN) and psychopathology: toward an endophenotype. *Clin. Psychol. Rev.* 28, 1343–1354. doi: 10.1016/j.cpr.2008.07.003

Olvet, D. M., and Hajcak, G. (2009). Reliability of error-related brain activity. *Brain Res.* 1284, 89–99. doi: 10.1016/j.brainres.2009.05.079

Omedes, J., Iturrate, I., Montesano, L., and Minguez, J. (2013). Using frequency-domain features for the generalization of EEG error-related potentials among different tasks. *Conf. Proc. IEEE Eng. Med. Biol. Soc.* 2013, 5263–5266.

Parra, L. C., Spence, C. D., Gerson, A. D., and Sajda, P. (2003). Response error correction—A demonstration of improved human-machine performance using real-time EEG monitoring. *IEEE Trans. Neural. Syst. Rehabil. Eng.* 11, 173–177. doi: 10.1109/TNSRE.2003.814446

Pascual-Marqui, R. D. (2002). Standardized low-resolution brain electromagnetic tomography (sLORETA): technical details. *Methods Find. Exp. Clin. Pharmacol.* 24(Suppl. D), 5–12.

Perrin, M., Maby, E., Daligault, S., Bertrand, O., and Mattout, J. (2012). Objective and subjective evaluation of online error correction during P300-based spelling. *Adv. Hum. Comp. Inter.* 2012:578295.

Perrin, X., Chavarriaga, R., Colas, F., Siegwart, R., and Millán, J. d. R. (2010). Brain-coupled interaction for semi-autonomous navigation of an assistive robot. *Robot. Autonom. Syst.* 58, 1246–1255. doi: 10.1016/j.robot.2010.05.010

Pfurtscheller, G., Allison, B., Bauernfeind, G., Brunner, C., Solis Escalante, T., Scherer, R., et al. (2010). The hybrid BCI. *Front. Neurosci.* 4:42. doi: 10.3389/fnpro.2010.00003

Phlypo, R., Jrad, N., Rousseau, S., and Congedo, M. (2011). A non-orthogonal SVD-based decomposition for phase invariant error-related potential estimation. *Conf. Proc. IEEE Eng. Med. Biol. Soc.* 2011, 6963–6966.

Polich, J. (1990). Probability and inter-stimulus interval effects on the p300 from auditory stimuli. *Int. J. Psychophysiol.* 10, 163–170. doi: 10.1016/0167-8760(90)90030-H

Polich, J., and Margala, C. (1997). P300 and probability: comparison of oddball and single-stimulus paradigms. *Int. J. Psychophysiol.* 25, 169–176. doi: 10.1016/S0167-8760(96)00742-8

Putze, F., Heger, D., and Schultz, T. (2013). "Reliable subject-adapted recognition of EEG error potentials using limited calibration dataset," in *Neural Engineering (NER), 2013 6th International IEEE/EMBS Conference on*, 419–422. doi: 10.1109/NER.2013.6695961

Quitadamo, L. R., Abbafati, M., Cardarilli, G. C., Mattia, D., Cincotti, F., Babiloni, F., et al. (2012). Evaluation of the performances of different P300 based brain-computer interfaces by means of the efficiency metric. *J. Neurosci. Methods* 203, 361–368. doi: 10.1016/j.jneumeth.2011.10.010

Rabbitt, P. M. A. (1966). Errors and error correction in choice reaction tasks. *J. Exp. Psychol. Gen.* 71, 264–272. doi: 10.1037/h0022853

Riesel, A., Weinberg, A., Endrass, T., Meyer, A., and Hajcak, G. (2013). The ERN is the ERN is the ERN? convergent validity of error-related brain activity across different tasks. *Biol. Psychol.* 93, 377–385. doi: 10.1016/j.biopsycho.2013.04.007

Roset, S., Gonzalez, H., and Sanchez, J. (2013). "Development of an EEG based reinforcement learning brain-computer interface system for rehabilitation," in *Conference of the IEEE Engineering in Medicine and Biology Society* (Osaka), 1563–1566. doi: 10.1109/EMBC.2013.6609812

Rousseau, S., Jutten, C., and Congedo, M. (2012). "Designing spatial filters based on neuroscience theories to improve error-related potential classification," in *Machine Learning for Signal Processing (MLSP), 2012 IEEE International Workshop on* (Santander), 1–6.

Schalk, G., Wolpaw, J. R., McFarland, D. J., and Pfurtscheller, G. (2000). EEG-based communication: Presence of an error potential. *Clin. Neurophysiol.* 111, 2138–2144. doi: 10.1016/S1388-2457(00)00457-0

Schmidt, N. M., Blankertz, B., and Treder, M. S. (2012). Online detection of error-related potentials boosts the performance of mental typewriters. *BMC Neurosci.* 13:19. doi: 10.1186/1471-2202-13-19

Schreuder, M., Blankertz, B., and Tangermann, M. (2010). A new auditory multi-class brain-computer interface paradigm: spatial hearing as an informative cue. *PLoS ONE* 5:e9813. doi: 10.1371/journal.pone.0009813

Seno, B. D., Matteucci, M., and Mainardi, L. T. (2010). The utility metric: a novel method to assess the overall performance of discrete brain-computer interfaces. *IEEE Trans. Neural. Syst. Rehabil. Eng.* 18, 20–28. doi: 10.1109/TNSRE.2009.2032642

Spüler, M., Bensch, M., Kleih, S., Rosenstiel, W., Bogdan, M., and Kübler, A. (2012). Online use of error-related potentials in healthy users and people with severe motor impairment increases performance of a P300-BCI. *Clin. Neurophysiol.* 123, 1328–1337. doi: 10.1016/j.clinph.2011.11.082

Sutton, R., and Barto, A. G. (1998). *Reinforcement Learning - An Introduction.* Cambridge, MA:MIT Press.

Takahashi, H., Yoshikawa, T., and Furuhashi, T. (2010). "Reliability-based automatic repeat request with error potential-based error correction for improving P300 speller performance," in *Neural Information Processing. Models and Applications*, Vol. 6444 of *Lecture Notes in Computer Science*, eds K. Wong, B. Mendis, and A. Bouzerdoum (Springer Berlin / Heidelberg), 50–57.

Taylor, S. F., Stern, E. R., and Gehring, W. J. (2007). Neural systems for error monitoring: recent findings and theoretical perspectives. *Neuroscientist* 13, 160–172. doi: 10.1177/1073858406298184

Themanson, J. R., Rosen, P. J., Pontifex, M. B., Hillman, C. H., and McAuley, E. (2012). Alterations in error-related brain activity and post-error behavior over time. *Brain Cogn.* 80, 257–265. doi: 10.1016/j.bandc.2012.07.003

Thomas, E., Dyson, M., and Clerc, M. (2013). An analysis of performance evaluation for motor-imagery based BCI. *J. Neural Eng.* 10:031001. doi: 10.1088/1741-2560/10/3/031001

Thompson, D. E., Quitadamo, L. R., Mainardi, L., Laghari, K. U. R., Gao, S., Kindermans, P.-J., et al. (2014). Performance measurement for brain-computer or brain-machine interfaces: a tutorial. *J. Neural. Eng.* 11:035001. doi: 10.1088/1741-2560/11/3/035001

Treder, M. S., Schmidt, N. M., and Blankertz, B. (2011). Gaze-independent brain-computer interfaces based on covert attention and feature attention. *J. Neural. Eng.* 8:066003. doi: 10.1088/1741-2560/8/6/066003

Trujillo, L. T., and Allen, J. J. B. (2007). Theta EEG dynamics of the error-related negativity. *Clin. Neurophysiol.* 118, 645–668. doi: 10.1016/j.clinph.2006.11.009

Tsoneva, T., Bieger, J., and Garcia-Molina, G. (2010). Towards error-free interaction. *Conf. Proc. IEEE Eng. Med. Biol. Soc.* 2010, 5799–5802.

Ullsperger, M., Fischer, A. G., Nigbur, R., and Endrass, T. (2014). Neural mechanisms and temporal dynamics of performance monitoring. *Trends Cogn. Sci.* 18, 259–267. doi: 10.1016/j.tics.2014.02.009

Ullsperger, M., and von Cramon, D. Y. (2001). Subprocesses of performance monitoring: a dissociation of error processing and response competition revealed by event-related fMRI and ERPs. *Neuroimage* 14, 1387–1401. doi: 10.1006/nimg.2001.0935

van Schie, H. T., Mars, R. B., Coles, M. G. H., and Bekkering, H. (2004). Modulation of activity in medial frontal and motor cortices during error observation. *Nat. Neurosci.* 7, 549–554. doi: 10.1038/nn1239

van Veen, V., and Carter, C. S. (2002). The anterior cingulate as a conflict monitor: fMRI and ERP studies. *Physiol. Behav.* 77, 477–482. doi: 10.1016/S0031-9384(02)00930-7

Ventouras, E. M., Asvestas, P., Karanasiou, I., and Matsopoulos, G. K. (2011). Classification of error-related negativity (ERN) and positivity (Pe) potentials using kNN and support vector machines. *Comput. Biol. Med.* 41, 98–109. doi: 10.1016/j.compbiomed.2010.12.004

Wang, S., Lin, C.-J., Wu, C., and Chaovalitwongse, W. (2011). Early detection of numerical typing errors using data mining techniques. *Syst. Man . Cybern. A Syst. Hum. IEEE Trans.* 41, 1199–1212. doi: 10.1109/TSMCA.2011.2116006

Wessel, J. R. (2012). Error awareness and the error-related negativity: evaluating the first decade of evidence. *Front. Hum. Neurosci.* 6:88. doi: 10.3389/fnhum.2012.00088

Wiersema, J. R., van der Meere, J. J., and Roeyers, H. (2007). Developmental changes in error monitoring: an event-related potential study. *Neuropsychologia* 45, 1649–1657. doi: 10.1016/j.neuropsychologia.2007.01.004

Wolpaw, J. R., Birbaumer, N., Heetderks, W. J., McFarland, D. J., Peckham, P. H., Schalk, G., et al. (2000). Brain-computer interface technology: a review of the first international meeting. *IEEE Trans. Rehabi. Eng.* 8, 164–173. doi: 10.1109/TRE.2000.847807

Yeung, N., Holroyd, C. B., and Cohen, J. D. (2005). ERP correlates of feedback and reward processing in the presence and absence of response choice. *Cereb. Cortex* 15, 535–544. doi: 10.1093/cercor/bhh153

Zander, T. O., and Jatzev, S. (2012). Context-aware brain-computer interfaces: exploring the information space of user, technical system and environment. *J. Neural Eng.* 9:016003. doi: 10.1088/1741-2560/9/1/016003

Zander, T. O., and Kothe, C. (2011). Towards passive brain-computer interfaces: applying brain-computer interface technology to human-machine systems in general. *J. Neural Eng.* 8:025005. doi: 10.1088/1741-2560/8/2/025005

Zander, T. O., Kothe, C., Welke, S., and Roetting, M. (2008). "Enhancing human-machine systems with secondary input from passive brain-computer interfaces," in *Proceedings of the 4th International BCI Workshop and Training Course* (Graz), 144–149.

Zeyl, T. J., and Chau, T. (2014). A case study of linear classifiers adapted using imperfect labels derived from human event-related potentials. *Patt. Recogn. Lett.* 37, 54–62. doi: 10.1016/j.patrec.2013.05.020

Zhang, H., Chavarriaga, R., Gheorghe, L., and Millán, J. d. R. (2013). "Inferring driver's turning direction through detection of error related brain activity," in *Conference of the IEEE Engineering in Medicine and Biology Society* (Osaka), 2196–2199. doi: 10.1109/EMBC.2013.6609971

Zhang, H., Chavarriaga, R., Goel, M. K., Gheorghe, L., and Millán, J. d. R. (2012). "Improved recognition of error related potentials through the use of brain connectivity features," in *34th International Conference of the IEEE Engineering in Medicine and Biology Society (EMBC'12)* (San Diego, CA). doi: 10.1109/EMBC.2012.6347541

4

Classifying visuomotor workload in a driving simulator using subject specific spatial brain patterns

Chris Dijksterhuis[1]*, Dick de Waard[1], Karel A. Brookhuis[1,2], Ben L. J. M. Mulder[1] and Ritske de Jong[1]

[1] Department of Psychology, University of Groningen, Groningen, Netherlands
[2] Department of Infrastructure Systems and Services, Delft University of Technology, Delft, Netherlands

***Correspondence:**
Chris Dijksterhuis, Department of Psychology, University of Groningen, Grote Kruisstraat 2/1, 9712 TS Groningen, Netherlands
e-mail: c.dijksterhuis@rug.nl*

A passive Brain Computer Interface (BCI) is a system that responds to the spontaneously produced brain activity of its user and could be used to develop interactive task support. A human-machine system that could benefit from brain-based task support is the driver-car interaction system. To investigate the feasibility of such a system to detect changes in visuomotor workload, 34 drivers were exposed to several levels of driving demand in a driving simulator. Driving demand was manipulated by varying driving speed and by asking the drivers to comply to individually set lane keeping performance targets. Differences in the individual driver's workload levels were classified by applying the Common Spatial Pattern (CSP) and Fisher's linear discriminant analysis to frequency filtered electroencephalogram (EEG) data during an off line classification study. Several frequency ranges, EEG cap configurations, and condition pairs were explored. It was found that classifications were most accurate when based on high frequencies, larger electrode sets, and the frontal electrodes. Depending on these factors, classification accuracies across participants reached about 95% on average. The association between high accuracies and high frequencies suggests that part of the underlying information did not originate directly from neuronal activity. Nonetheless, average classification accuracies up to 75–80% were obtained from the lower EEG ranges that are likely to reflect neuronal activity. For a system designer, this implies that a passive BCI system may use several frequency ranges for workload classifications.

Keywords: passive brain computer interface, common spatial pattern, driving simulator, workload classification, adaptive automation, lateral control

INTRODUCTION

In contrast to an active Brain-Computer Interface (BCI) which allows users to engage in volitional thought control of a device, several BCI researchers have proposed to advance human-computer interaction by triggering machine actions based on inferences of the user's current mental state, known as passive BCI (Kohlmorgen et al., 2007; Cutrell and Tan, 2008; Zander et al., 2010; Zander and Kothe, 2011). For example, Kohlmorgen et al. (2007) showed that it is possible to classify mental workload elicited by a secondary task mimicking cognitive processes in a real driving environment. Moreover, these classifications were then used to switch on and off a tertiary task that mimicked an interaction with the vehicle's electrical devices that in turn improved performance on the secondary task.

In the human factors and ergonomics literature, which traditionally focuses on overall system performance and safety critical tasks, the potentially detrimental effects of both mental underload and overload have been a major research topic for decades. Mental workload can be defined as a "reaction to demand" and "the proportion of capacity that is allocated for task performance" (de Waard, 1996). Mental underload and overload both represent compromised functional states during which a breakdown of primary task performance is more likely (e.g., Hockey, 1997, 2003; see also Brookhuis and de Waard, 2010). Preventing these hazardous functional states by maintaining mental workload or task demand within an acceptable range in real-time has been the central goal of adaptive automation since the seventies (Chu and Rouse, 1979; Hancock and Chignell, 1988; Rouse, 1988; Parasuraman et al., 1992; Kaber and Prinzel, 2006).

A large part of adaptive automation literature is devoted to determining the right moment of providing or withdrawing task support, and several types of triggers may be available to optimize performance of a human-machine system (e.g., critical events and human task performance; see Parasuraman et al., 1992). Therefore, the question arises as to what physiological measures could offer in terms of improving the overall system's performance. The most important argument for the inclusion of physiological measures in a control loop is their potential for detecting user states that would otherwise remain hidden. Human beings may exhaust themselves to protect primary task performance in demanding situations. While performance protection is important for dealing with short bursts of task demand, when exposed to longer periods of high workload, it may have affective costs such as increases in anxiety, but also compensatory performance costs, such as neglecting secondary tasks (Hockey, 1997, 2003). Since straining effort expenditure has a neurophysiological base, the ability to reliably classify workload using physiological measures could be used to offload a person, before performance effects become apparent.

Traditional research approaches might not be well suited for uncovering the underlying neurophysiological mechanisms that could be used in a support system. As pointed out by Fairclough (2009), the fundamental problem of using physiological measures is the complex relationship between user states, such as mental overload, and their associated physiological variables. Specifically, four physiology-to-state mappings can be distinguished (Cacioppo et al., 2000). In the most straightforward case, there is a unique *one-to-one* mapping between a physiological variable and the psychological construct. Such a unique, one-to-one mapping would be ideal for an interactive system. However, a one-to-one mapping that holds true in both the laboratory and the field has to date not yet been found. A *many-to-one* mapping is more complicated as several signals are needed to infer a mental state. For example, heart rate, heart rate variability and blood pressure have been combined to infer mental workload (e.g., Mulder et al., 2009). In a *one-to-many* mapping, one physiological signal responds to a range of user states. For instance, systolic blood pressure information was found to be sensitive to excitement, frustration, and stress (Cacioppo and Gardner, 1999). Lastly, the most common finding is a *many-to-many* mapping where many signals are in fact sensitive to many mental states. Ultimately, in an implicit human-machine control loop, a one-to-one or a many-to-one relation is required. As briefly mentioned, another factor complicating the relationship between physiological measures and user state is lack of generalizability outside the laboratory setting where a mapping was found. Simply put, a relation between a physiological measure and a user state found in the laboratory may not hold true in a real world setting where environmental conditions are less controlled.

Furthermore, due to large individual differences in physiological responsiveness, traditional statistical tests might not be suitable to uncover relationships that are valuable for implicit machine control. Even in a repeated measures analysis of variance, where the variations due to individual differences are partly taken out of the error term, the directions of effects within the individuals need some consistency across individuals to reach statistical significance. While significant effects on a group level are interesting from a fundamental point of view, individual patterns are more relevant, when physiology is applied in human-machine systems. In this respect, the feature extraction and classification algorithms used by BCI researchers offer a promising way of dealing with these limitations.

As shown by Kohlmorgen et al. (2007), driver support may be linked to electroencephalogram (EEG) signals. Given the fact that the driving task is increasingly demanding, due to increased complexity of the road network, increased traffic intensity, and the availability of potentially distracting in-vehicle information systems, such as phones, (e.g., Carsten and Brookhuis, 2005), accurate assessment of user state while driving might be used to benefit driving performance. From driving behavior literature, it is clear that besides mental workload, other, related psychological constructs might be investigated for use in a support system. At this point there is no consensus about the exact psychological processes underlying driving behavior. Depending on the theoretical framework, the level of (subjective) risk, workload, or a general feeling of comfort is either maintained or avoided (e.g., risk homeostasis theory, the zero-risk theory, risk allostasis theory, safety margin model (Näätänen and Summala, 1976; Wilde, 1982; Fuller, 2005; Summala, 2005; see also: Lewis-Evans et al., 2011). To make it even more complex, drivers alter the level of workload in practice through behavioral adaptations. For example, in demanding situations with high information density (e.g., complex variable message signs), narrow lanes or a winding road, a driver may reduce speed, which will reduce the reaction time requirements, and thereby avoids high workload levels (Hockey, 2003; Lewis-Evans and Charlton, 2006).

Ultimately, we would like to provide a proof of concept for a passive brain-car interface that changes driving speed in response to visuomotor workload, thereby keeping workload levels within an acceptable range, similar to a human driver. However, in preparation for this, we have first investigated the feasibility of using EEG signals to classify between levels of lane keeping demand in a driving simulator. For this, we applied subject-specific Common Spatial Patterns (CSPs; e.g., Blankertz et al., 2008). The main advantage of using the CSP technique is that it maximizes the difference between two conditions by creating linear combinations of all included electrodes; spatial filters used to produce CSP components. In this way, some electrodes contribute more to the filtered signal(s) than others. These CSP components are determined per participant and therefore, individual differences are accounted for. The most discriminative components are then used to distinguish conditions.

Lane keeping demand was manipulated by changing driving speed, mimicking drivers' natural behavior. Driving speed was set relative to the participants' comfortable speed, since the effort that is required to keep the car safely on the road may vary between drivers for absolute driving speeds. A relative high driving speed is hypothesized to result in a relative high visuomotor workload. In addition, since the Standard Deviation of the car's Lateral Position (SDLP) reflects workload (e.g., Dijksterhuis et al., 2011), an individually set target SDLP was presented to the participants on the virtual windshield, urging drivers to show less swerving behavior in the driving lane. A relative low target SDLP is hypothesized to result in a relative high workload level.

MATERIALS AND METHODS

PARTICIPANTS

A total of 17 males and 17 females were recruited through social media and poster announcements throughout the University of Groningen and were paid 20 Euros for participation. A large part of the participants were either Dutch or German students at this university. Ages ranged from 21 to 34 years ($M = 24.0$; $SD = 3.0$) and the participants had held their driver's license for 3 to 15 years ($M = 5.3$; $SD = 2.8$). Self-reported total mileage ranged from 3000 to 350,000 km ($M = 53,000$; $SD = 76,000$), while the reported average annual mileage over the past 3 years ranged from 1000 to 50,000 km ($M = 9000$; $SD = 11,000$). None of the participants reported on using prescribed drugs that might affect driving behavior. The Ethical Committee of the Psychology

Department of the University of Groningen has approved the study.

SIMULATOR AND DRIVING ENVIRONMENT

The study was conducted using a fixed-base vehicle mock up with functional steering wheel, indicators, and pedals. The simulator runs on ST Software©which is capable of simulating fully interactive traffic. The three computers dedicated to the simulator compute the road environment and traffic which are displayed on three 32-inch plasma screens and provide a total view of the driving environment of 210°. In addition, three rear-view mirrors are projected on the screens. A detailed description of the driving simulator used can be found in Van Winsum and Van Wolffelaar (1993).

For the experiment a two-lane road (each 2.75 m wide) was prepared, without intersections and winding through rural scenery. The road consisted mainly of easy curves (about 80%) with a constant radius of 380 m and ranging in length from 120 to 800 m. The road surface was marked on the edges by a continuous line (0.20 m wide) and in the center by a discontinuous (dashed) line (0.15 m wide). Outside the edges a soft shoulder was present and there were no objects in the direct vicinity of the road. In the driving direction of the participants, no traffic was present. However, oncoming traffic, travelling between 76 and 84 km/h, was generated with a random interval gap between 1 and 2 s, resulting in 40 passing private vehicles per minute on average. The speed of the participant's vehicle was controlled by the simulator for all rides during the experimental session, except for the initial ride during which the participants drove the simulator car (width: 1.60 m) in automatic gear mode.

DESIGN AND PROCEDURE

Upon arrival at the experimental site of the University of Groningen, a participant was informed in general terms with respect to the experimental design, was requested to sign an informed consent form, and asked to fill in a short questionnaire mainly related to their driving experience. Hereafter, the participant was given some time (ca. 7 min) to practice driving in the simulator, before the sensors were attached. Next, a three minute baseline recording was made while the participant sat in the simulator car chair and an aquatic movie played on the center screen of the simulator.

After this baseline recording the participant completed 16 short rides. After each ride, the participant was requested to park the vehicle on the side of the road and to provide an answer to two brief questions (on subjective mental effort and estimated driving speed). During the initial ride (140 s) the participant exerted both longitudinal and lateral control over the vehicle and was asked to find and drive at a speed that felt most natural and comfortable in this situation while the speedometer was turned off to prevent rule-based speed setting. The speedometer remained turned off for the entire experiment. The mean speed and standard deviation of the vehicle's lateral position (SDLP) on the road during the last 110 s of the initial ride represented the participant's personal, comfortable driving style. These parameters were saved and used to set driving speed and target SDLP during the 15 remaining rides.

During these 15 rides (130 s each), speed was set relative to the participant's comfortable speed (either −40, −20, 0, +20, or +40 km/h). In addition, while speed was set at the comfortable driving speed, the participant was requested to keep SDLP at either 0, −0.05, or −0.10 m relative to the initial SDLP, which represent a normal, hard, or very hard task. For the other driving speeds, the target SDLP was determined as follows. From a pilot study ($n = 9$), using a similar roadway environment, it was found that SDLP naturally increases as a function of speed. To compensate for this effect and thereby creating five roughly comparable steering challenges across speeds, another 0.03 m per speed level was either added to or subtracted from the target SDLP. For example, when driving 40 km/h slower than the comfortable speed while the target SDLP condition was set at "very hard," the numerical target SDLP was set $0.10 + 2 \times 0.03 = 0.16$ m lower than the comfortable SDLP as established during the initial ride. Current values of SDLP were derived from a 15 s moving window which was updated every second and these were projected onto the bottom of the windshield of the simulator while driving, adjacent to the target SDLP. In this way a driver could monitor real SDLP and compare it to the target. Accounting for the time window and for the time the simulator needed to get to the required speed, only the last 110 s of each ride was used in subsequent analyses. To be clear, the data used for this analysis were the raw, not averaged, vehicle parameters. In total, the experimental manipulations resulted in a within-subject design consisting of two repeated measures factors with several levels: speed (5) and target SDLP (3). The participants were exposed to these driving conditions according to a randomized schedule.

After finishing the last ride, the baseline measurement was repeated once more before all physiological sensors were removed. Finally, the participants were debriefed and were paid upon leaving.

DEALING WITH COLLISIONS

Occasionally, the participants were challenged to the point that a collision with oncoming traffic could not be avoided. In total, six participants were involved in 10 collisions which is 1.8% of all experimental rides. Eight of these collisions occurred in a +40 km/h speed condition. When a collision occurred, that particular ride was repeated. Data acquired during the crash rides were not used for further analyses.

DATA ACQUISITION

Vehicle parameters

Driving speed and lateral position (LP) were sampled at 10 Hz. LP is defined as the difference in meters between the center of the participant's car and the middle of the (right hand) driving lane. Positive LP values correspond to deviations toward the right hand shoulder and negative values correspond to deviations toward the left hand shoulder. The sampled LP values were processed while driving and used to calculate mean LP and SDLP for each of the 16 rides. In addition, LP values were used to feed current values of SDLP back to the participant which were calculated by using moving, overlapping time windows (see Design and Procedure for more details), representing an indication of the participants lane keeping performance.

Subjective ratings

After each ride, a rating on the one-dimensional Rating Scale Mental Effort (RSME) was requested (Zijlstra, 1993). The RSME ranges from 0 to 150 and several effort indications are visible alongside the scale which may guide the participant in marking the scale. Indications start with "absolutely no effort" (RSME score of 2) and end with "extreme effort" (RSME score of 112). The participants, who did not receive speed information from the speedometer, were also asked to write down an estimate of the driving speed they just experienced.

Physiological measures

Physiological signals were sampled at 250 Hz. Firstly, the electrocardiogram (ECG) was registered using three Ag-AgCl electrodes, which were placed on the sternum (the ground electrode) and on the right and left side between the lower ribs. However, given the emphasis on brain activity in this paper, the ECG results are not reported here. Secondly, the electro-oculogram (EOG) was measured by Ag-AgCL electrodes attached next to the lateral canthus of each eye and above and below either the right or left eye. The EEG was measured using an electro-cap with 64 tin electrodes (at the following sites: FP1, FP2, Afz, F7, F5, Fz, F4, F8, T7, C5, C3, Cz, C4, T8, P7, P3, Pz, P4, P8, O1, and O2.) The amplifer was a REFA 8–72 (Twente Medical Systems International, Enschede, The Netherlands). Portilab 2 software was used to record all physiological signals. The ground electrode used for the ECG recording also served as the participant's ground for the EEG recording. EEG and EOG signals were amplified with a 1 s time constant (0.016 Hz high-pass). All EEG channels were referenced against the average activity of all channels during the registrations. In addition, a reference electrode was attached to each mastoid. Impedances were kept below 10 kΩ for all electrodes.

EEG DATA PROCESSING

Starting from the raw EEG signals, the sampled EEG and EOG data were first high-pass filtered (cutoff = 0.3 Hz, at 12 dB/Oct Butterworth filter) before the EEG data segments of the 15 experimental conditions (110 s each) were corrected for eye movements and blinks, using Brain Vision Analyzer (Gratton et al., 1983). The corrected data segments were then exported into binary files. No data epochs were removed before further processing.

The exported data files were processed using MATLAB R2010a (The MathWorks, Inc., USA, www.mathworks.com). After importing two data sets (two rides or conditions) of a particular participant, the EEG was band-passed filtered in the frequency domain (FFT filter) of interest, using an edge frequency of 1 Hz below and above the lower and upper frequency band limit respectively. The imported data (110 s for each condition) were then segmented into one second epochs and baselined relative to each mean activity. The first and last 10% of the epochs were omitted, leaving the 88 middle, non-overlapping, epochs per condition in the cross-validation design. This entailed a repeated (50 times) random portioning of two data classes (a condition pair) into a set of 66 training epochs (75%) and a set of 22 test epochs for each data class. The training sets were used to train the participant-specific classifier that was subsequently used to classify the testing epochs of each data class. This iteration process was carried out for each included participant, frequency band, EEG cap configuration, and data pair. The accuracies reported in the result section reflect the average accuracies across all 50 iterations and all included participants.

To improve discriminatory power of the data classifier, the contrast between two data classes was optimized by using the CSP technique. This technique determines CSP filters in such a way that they maximize the variances of spatially filtered signals for one training set while minimizing them for the other (Blankertz et al., 2008). A CSP filter is a coefficient vector by which the original channels can be transformed. This results in a new spatially filtered channel (a CSP component) which is a linear combination of all original channels, and the total number of filters and therefore, the number components, is equal to the number of original channels. The matrix of CSP filters is determined by solving a generalized eigen-value problem. The filter corresponding to the largest eigen-value yields a high variance signal in one condition, while producing a low variance signal in the other; and vice versa for the filters corresponding to the smallest eigen-value. The CSP filters are therefore ranked according to these eigen-values and the first and last filters in this sorted W matrix are usually used for further classification. To be more specific, in the current study, the two, four, or six filters (always an equal number from each side of the sorted W matrix) that resulted in the largest difference in variance between two training sets was used. Next, the total variance per training epoch and per CSP component was calculated and their logarithms were taken before entered into Fisher's linear discriminant analysis. This analysis again transforms the data by determining the linear weights of the discriminant function that combines data points of the two training sets in such a way that maximizes the distance between them. Finally, the CSP filters and classifier weights were used to classify the remaining testing epochs of the two conditions.

A wide range of EEG frequency bands were explored to investigate where useful discriminatory information might be present. Four frequency search strategies were deployed. The first frequency search strategy was characterized by both an increasing high pass cut-off point (increasing 1 Hz for each iteration) and an increasing frequency bandwidth (1.5 times the low frequency band limit). At the first iteration, frequencies between 3 and 4.5 Hz were passed. At the last iteration, frequencies between 72 and 108 Hz were passed. The second strategy entailed exploring all frequencies between 3 and 70 Hz using a fixed bandwidth of 1 Hz. For the third strategy, bandwidth was set to 4 Hz and iterations ran from 4 to 72 Hz. Lastly, data was filtered in broad bands to classify between conditions; 8–30, 32–54, 56–78, and 80–102 Hz.

In addition, several EEG cap configurations were explored. To start with, all 21 EEG channels were included. To explore whether classification accuracy may differ between scalp regions, several subsets were defined and tested. Firstly, a peripheral set was defined, consisting of 14 electrodes, (FP1, FP2, Afz, F7, F5, F4, F8, T7, C5, T8, P7, P8, O1, and O2). Secondly, a frontal set consisting of 7 electrodes (FP1, FP2, F7, F5, Fz, F4, and F8), which are associated with executive functions that are important in driving. Thirdly, a posterior set consisting of 7 electrodes (P7, P5, Pz,

P4, P8, O1, and O2), containing electrodes associated to visuomotor processing. Lastly, the electrode set identified by Prinzel III et al. (2001) (P3, Pz, P4, Cz), which has often been used in adaptive automation research to get the "engagement index" [defined as the ratio; beta/(alpha + theta)].

Lastly, five condition pairs were selected from a total of 105 possible combinations (15!/2!(15–2)!). An experimental condition can be defined in terms of its driving speed level and target SDLP difficulty level. To improve comparability one factor was kept constant for each condition pair. In this way, four speed differences for the normal target level were classified: −40 vs. +40 km/h, −20 vs. +20 km/h, −20 vs. 0 km/h, and 0 vs. +20 km/h. The normal target level was chosen since this target resembles the individuals' natural driving behavior. Focusing on classifying between speed differences in this way was done because of the envisioned application. A brain-based adaptive cruise control would change speeds and therefore, the effect of speed interventions has to be assessed. In addition, as it turned out, the very hard target conditions required more subjective effort compared to the normal target level, and therefore, these two conditions were compared in the 0 km/h relative speed condition.

Due to data anomalies such as missing channels, eight participants were excluded from the offline classification phase of this study. Despite a smaller participant pool, the number of condition pair comparisons is very large: 161 frequency bands × 5 condition pairs × 5 EEG cap configurations × 26 participants × 3 numbers of components = 313,950. Given these large numbers, only a selection of aggregated classification accuracy values can be reported (**Figures 2, 3**) next to examples of scalp topographies of CSP components (see **Figure 4** for an impression) reflecting how the information sources project to the scalp (retrieved from the inverse of W; see Blankertz et al., 2008).

RESULTS

VEHICLE PARAMETERS AND SUBJECTIVE RATINGS

Subjective ratings and vehicle parameters are shown in **Figure 1** and their test outcomes are listed in **Table 1**. To begin with, the participants' preferred speed during the initial ride ranged between 62 and 120 km/h, averaging at 90 km/h (see the black dot in **Figure 1A**). This is slightly faster than estimated for this ride ($M = 74$ km/h; **Figure 1B**). This pattern of underestimating driving speed is present for all speed levels (Pearson's product moment correlation =0.99 over all conditions).

The dimensions of the vehicle and driving lane allowed for 0.58 m of swerving margin on both sides of the vehicle. As can be seen in **Figure 1C**, the participants stayed well within their driving lane on average and positioned the vehicle slightly toward the right hand shoulder (0.07 m on average). As can be read in **Table 1**, there was a significant effect of speed on LP. The participants' mean position on the road curves toward the right-hand shoulder, both when driving slower and faster than the preferred speed (polynomial contrasts showed a quadratic trend; [$F_{(1,\ 33)} = 15.35$, $p < 0.001$, $\eta_p^2 = 0.317$]. Next, as speed increased, so did the participants' mean SDLP (see **Figure 1D**), representing swerving behavior, from 0.18 m during the slowest speed to 0.30 m during the fastest speed. This is mainly a linear increase [$F_{(1,\ 33)} = 182.81$, $p < 0.001$, $\eta_p^2 = 0.847$], although SDLP increases slightly more rapidly toward the higher speeds [quadratic trend; $F_{(1,33)} = 24.33$, $p < 0.001$, $\eta_p^2 = 0.424$]. Note that the factor; target SDLP, indicating the difficulty of keeping current SDLP values under the target SDLP while driving, had no effect on the actual SDLP.

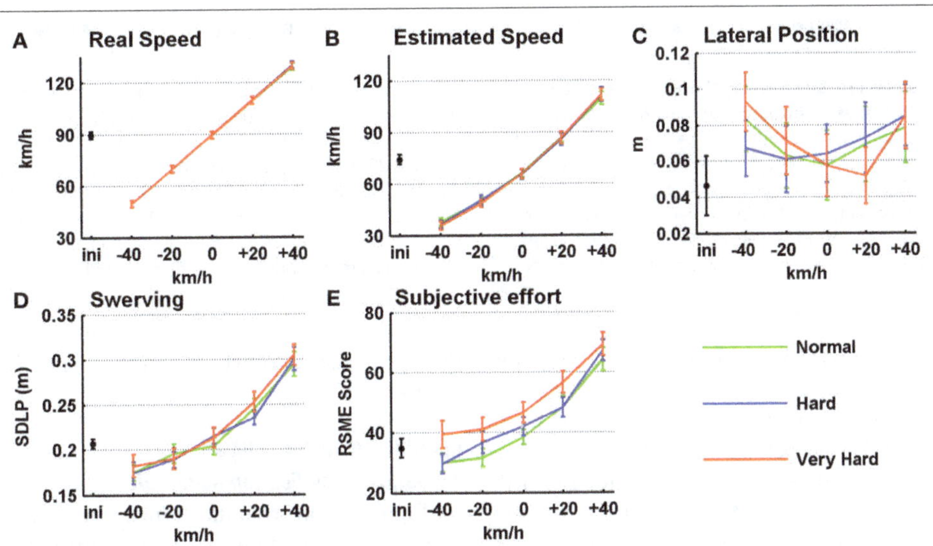

FIGURE 1 | Vehicle parameters and subjective ratings as a function of set driving speed condition. (A) Real driving speed. **(B)** Estimated driving speed. **(C)** Lateral Position (LP). **(D)** Standard Deviation of the Lateral Position (SDLP). **(E)** Rating Scale Mental Effort (RSME). On the x-axes, values for the initial ride (black dots) are shown in addition to five driving speeds that were set, relative to the individual's preferred driving speed established during the initial ride. Error bars represent the standard error. LP values represent the middle of the car (car width = 1.60 m) in relation to the middle of the right (driving) lane (width = 2.75 m). Normal, hard, and very hard indicate the difficulty of keeping current SDLP values under the target SDLP: see section Design and Procedure for details. Positive LP values indicate a position to the right hand of the lane mid. Maximum score for mental effort is 150. $n = 34$.

Table 1 | Multivariate test results for vehicle parameters and subjective effort ratings (Figure 1).

	Vehicle parameters and subjective ratings								
Effect	**LP**			**SDLP**			**RSME score**		
	$F_{(df1,df2)}$	p	η_p^2	$F_{(df1,df2)}$	p	η_p^2	$F_{(df1,df2)}$	p	η_p^2
Speed (S)	**4.46 (4,30)**	**0.006**	**0.373**	**45.40 (4,30)**	**<0.001**	**0.858**	**21.10 (4,30)**	**<0.001**	**0.748**
Target (T)	0.26 (2,32)	0.974	0.002	1.32 (2,32)	0.283	0.076	**08.49 (2,32)**	**0.001**	**0.347**
S ×T	0.77 (8,26)	0.633	0.191	1.22 (8,26)	0.324	0.274	1.25 (8,26)	0.309	0.278

LP, Lateral Position; SDLP, Standard Deviation Lateral Position; RSME, Rating Scale Mental Effort. Significant effects (p < 0.05) are shown in bold. Speed effect relates to speed condition, Target to SDLP target.

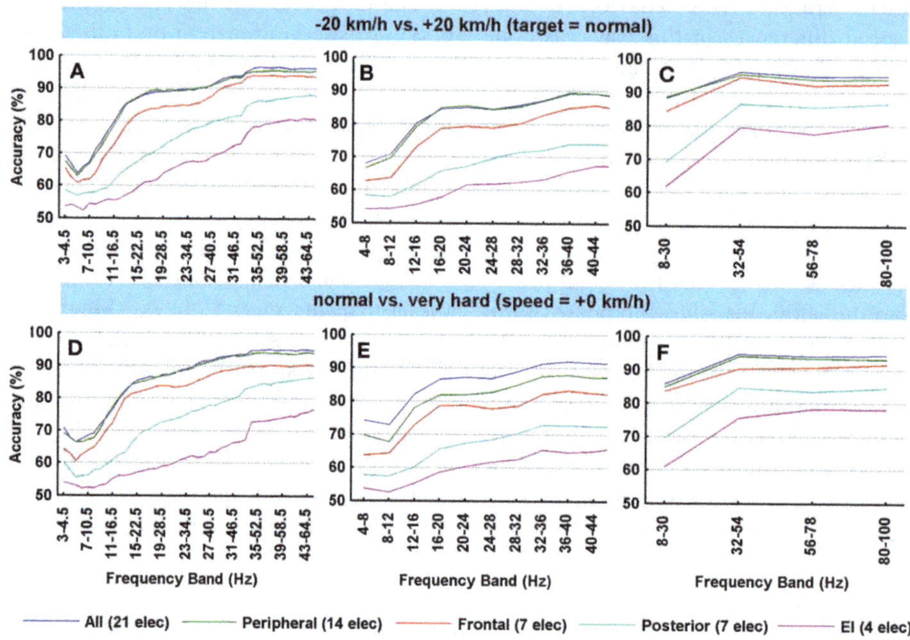

FIGURE 2 | Average classification accuracies of the Fisher's linear discriminant analyses after spatial filtering for several condition pairs. (A–F) The accuracy values represent the average subject-specific classification accuracy over all participants that resulted from the cross-validation scheme. Classifications were based on applying the two most contrasting CSP components to the EEG channels. $N = 26$. For each row of subfigures, a different EEG cap configuration was used. For the left column **(A,D)**, the frequency bandwidth is 1.5 times the start frequency (step size 1 Hz), starting at 3–4.5 Hz and ending at 43–64.5 Hz. For the middle column **(B,E)**, 4 Hz bands were used and a stepsize of 4. For the right column **(C,F)**, a broad band frequency search (22 Hz) was deployed. All electrodes: FP1, FP2, Afz, F7, F5, Fz, F4, F8, T7, C5, C3, Cz, C4, T8, P7, P3, Pz, P4, P8, O1, O2. Peripheral set: FP1, FP2, Afz, F7, F5, F4, F8, T7, C5, T8, P7, P8, O1, O2. Frontal set: FP1, FP2, F7, F5, Fz, F4, F8. Posterior set: P7, P5, Pz, P4, P8, O1, O2. Engagement index (EI) set: P3, Pz, P4, Cz.

In addition, interactions between speed and target SDLP are not present in the data.

Figure 1E shows that the mental effort ratings increased from between "a little effort" and "some effort" (a mean RSME score of 33) for the slowest speeds to between "rather much effort" and "considerable effort" (a mean RSME score of 34) for the fastest speeds [linear trend; $F_{(1,\,33)} = 88.48$, $p < 0.001$, $\eta_p^2 = 0.728$]. Also, similar to SDLP, this increase is stronger toward the faster speeds [quadratic trend; $F_{(1,\,33)} = 86.04$, $p < 0.001$, $\eta_p^2 = 0.327$]. In addition, even though target SDLP did not have an effect on vehicle parameters, there was a main effect on mental effort ratings. Bonferroni corrected pairwise comparisons revealed that the "very hard" level was perceived as more difficult than the other two, while "normal" and "hard" did not show a difference.

CLASSIFICATION RESULTS

Averages classification accuracies

In **Figure 2**, the classification accuracies for several condition pairs are shown. **Figure 2** (and **Figure 3**) only shows the average classification accuracies for two data pairs (−20 km/h vs. +20 km/h and normal performance target vs. very hard performance target). Although more extreme driving speed conditions could have been shown (e.g., 40 vs. +40 km/h), we feel that more similar speed conditions better reflect real driving circumstances and are therefore more relevant. Also, accuracy levels

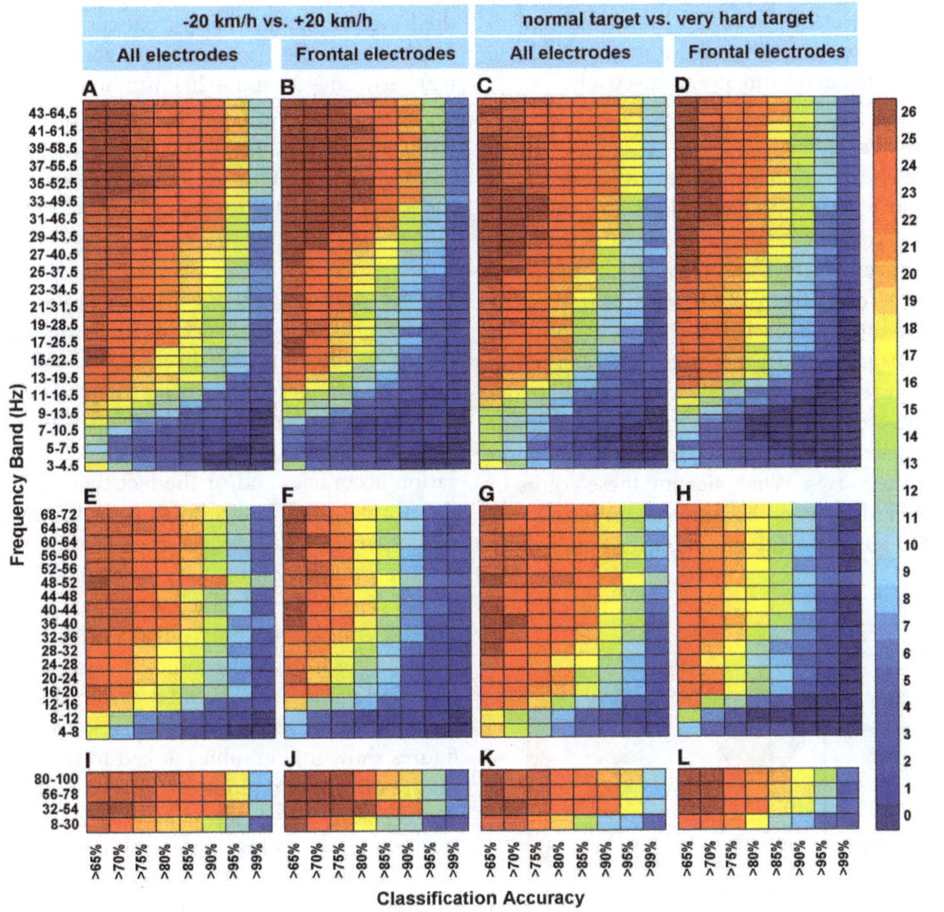

FIGURE 3 | The cumulative frequencies of classification accuracies. **(A–L)** Colors represent the number of participants for whom a particular accuracy was found or better (max = 26 participants) in the accuracy category displayed on the x-axes. Subfigure columns are arranged by EEG cap configuration (all electrodes or the frontal set) and by classified condition pair. All electrodes: FP1, FP2, Afz, F7, F5, Fz, F4, F8, T7, C5, C3, Cz, C4, T8, P7, P3, Pz, P4, P8, O1, and O2. Frontal electrodes: FP1, FP2, F7, F5, Fz, F4, and F8. "−20 km/h vs. +20 km/h" indicate set driving speeds relative to the participants' preferred speed as determined during the initial ride (at normal target level). "Normal target vs. hard target" indicate performance target difficulty (at relative speed = 0 km/h). For each row of subfigures, a different frequency search strategy was used. **(A–D)** For the top row of subfigures, the frequency bandwidth is 1.5 times the begin frequency (step size 1 Hz), starting at 3–4.5 Hz and ending at 44–66 Hz. **(E–H)** For the middle row of subfigures, 4 Hz bands were used and a step size of 4. **(I–L)** For the bottom row, a broad band frequency (22 Hz) search was deployed.

across condition pairs tended to be similar, and therefore the number of shown condition pairs was limited.

The graphs in **Figure 2** reveal several general trends. Firstly, accuracy tends to increase as frequency increases. This can be seen across electrode sets and condition pairs with accuracies reaching levels of 95% on average over all participants when a relative high number of electrodes is included (21 and 14). This increase is most pronounced in the frequencies from 5 to 20 Hz, after which it continues to rise more gradually indicating a ceiling effect (see for example **Figure 2A**). This ceiling is about 5–10% lower for the middle column of subplots in **Figure 2** (displaying the 4 Hz search strategy). Secondly, a broader frequency band tends to yield higher accuracies, which is most apparent when comparing the middle column (**Figures 2B,E**; 4 Hz frequency bands) to the right column (**Figures 2C, 3F**; 22 Hz frequency bands). For example, when including all electrodes, the 4 Hz frequency bands in the 8–32 Hz range in **Figure 2B** range produced about 15% less accuracy when compared to the first broad band (8–30 Hz) in **Figure 2C**. Thirdly, there are distinct differences in accuracies as a result of using different channel sets. For example, the larger electrode sets (21 and 14 electrodes) yielded very comparable high accuracies, while the smallest (4 electrodes) consistently resulted in lower classification accuracies (about 15–25% less, depending on frequency band). Such differences can be understood in part from the fact that more channels provide a richer, higher-dimension database for the CSP technique to extract useful discriminatory power. Note however, that the seven frontal electrodes outperformed the seven posterior electrodes by about 5–15%, again depending on frequency band. The shape of the frontal curve in all subfigures (the red lines) reflect the upper two curves (all electrodes and 14 peripheral electrodes), while the posterior curves resemble the bottom EI curves. Finally, when focusing on the somewhat lower EEG frequency of **Figures 2A,D** ranges (e.g., 10–21 Hz), which are more likely to reflect neuronal activity, the mean accuracy in that range over both subfigures is 80% for the larger two electrode sets. The frontal set led to a classification of 76% on average, while the posterior and the engagement index set resulted in 62 and 55% respectively.

Cumulative classification accuracies

In **Figure 3**, cumulative classification accuracies are shown for a selection of classification results. This figure indicates the consistency of classification accuracies across all 26 included participants. For instance, **Figure 3A** shows that in the high frequency range (e.g., 43–64.5 Hz), test data from 10 participants were accurately classified 99% of the time or better. **Figure 4** confirms that higher frequencies usually yield better accuracies as the top frequencies in all subfigures display more red/yellow than the bottom frequencies. The green/yellow colors indicate that about half to two third of the participants were above the classification threshold indicated on the x-axes. When viewing these colors in **Figure 3** through the eyelashes, it can be seen that, especially for the larger electrode set (**Figures 3A,E,I** and **3C,G,K**), data from a substantial number of participants still yielded 85% + accuracy in the lower (alpha and beta) frequency ranges (e.g., 10–20/30 Hz). For instance, the classifier could accurately classify (85% or better) between −20 and +20 km/h in the 16–20 Hz frequency range for 16 out of 26 participants (**Figure 3G**). For the smaller, frontal electrode set (**Figures 3B,F,J** and **3D,H,L**) the number of participants yielding highly accurate classifications is somewhat less in the lower frequency range; as indicated by the larger presence of blue colors.

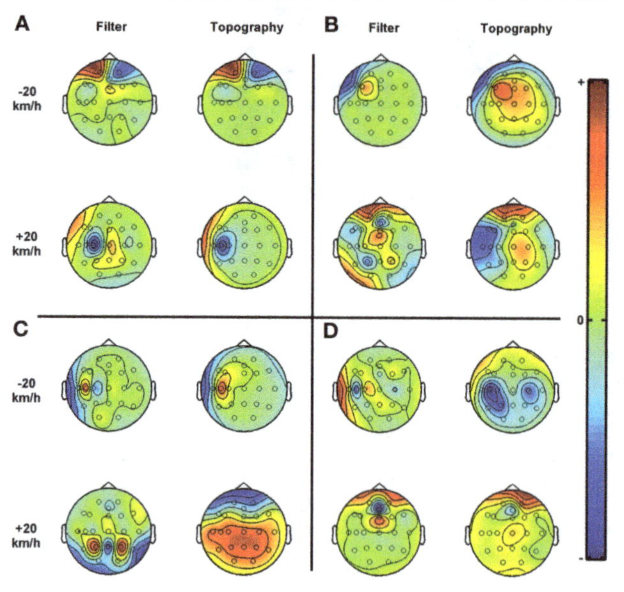

FIGURE 4 | Examples of CSP analyses. (A–D) The scalp topography of the components illustrate how the physiological sources project to the scalp. The components are determined such that projected signals are optimally discriminative. The filters and topographies correspond to the first and last vector of the sorted W matrix and its inverse respectively (see section Design and Procedure for more details). Absolute coloring is arbitrary, however, dense red or blue areas show where the greatest differences in the projected signals' amplitudes were found, between the −20 km/h and the +20 km/h set driving speed (at normal target level). These driving speeds were set relative to the participants' preferred speed as determined during the initial ride. Included electrodes: FP1, FP2, Afz, F7, F5, Fz, F4, F8, T7, C5, C3, Cz, C4, T8, P7, P3, Pz, P4, P8, O1, and O2. **(A)** Subject = 13, frequency band = 72–108 Hz, classification accuracy = 100%. **(B)** Subject = 27, frequency band = 8–12 Hz, classification accuracy = 98%. **(C)** Subject = 21, frequency band = 24–28 Hz, classification accuracy = 82%. **(D)** Subject = 25, frequency band = 8–30 Hz, classification accuracy = 74%. Please note that in the CSP literature, a scalp topography of a component is usually referred to as a spatial pattern.

Example common spatial pattern analysis

Figure 4 displays several CSP filter-topography pairs which are meant to illustrate the diversity of CSP scalp topographies. A common topography across participants, reflecting how the neurological sources project to the scalp, was not identified. However, we selected these topographies based on their resulting classification accuracies and/or the fact that the frequencies are within the normal EEG range. To start with, **Figure 4A** shows that for participant 13, the perfect classification accuracy in the broad 72–108 frequency range originates mainly from the frontal electrodes (Fp1 and Fp2) which were highly specific for the -20 km/h driving condition, and from C5 which was highly specific for the +20 km/h driving condition. This is illustrative for the general finding that the frontal electrodes were often the main contributors to very high classification accuracies. The other subfigures show topographies linked to frequencies below 30 Hz. In **Figure 4B**, topographies are shown that resulted in an unusually accurate classification for this relative low frequency band (98% in the 8–12 Hz, alpha, frequency band). In this case, the topographies are more distributed over the scalp, although the left temporal and frontal regions were important physiological sources for discriminating between the two data classes. The scalp topography for the +20 km/h condition in **Figure 4C** shows a central-parietal distribution, illustrating that the EI electrodes: P3, Pz, and P5 contributed to the 82% classification accuracy in the high beta range of participant 21. The −20 km/h topography suggests that C5 was by far the most distinctive electrode when maximizing the variance of the projected signals in this data class while minimizing it for the other. Finally, **Figure 4D** shows the CSP resulting in 74% classification accuracy for subject 25 in the broad 8–30 (alpha plus beta) Hz frequency band. These topographies suggest that discriminative power was distributed over the posterior electrodes in the −20 km/h condition and more evenly distributed over the scalp in the +20 km/h condition.

DISCUSSION

The aim of the study was to investigate the feasibility of using EEG for monitoring the level of visuomotor workload in a driving environment, which can potentially be used by an user adaptive driver support system. To manipulate workload, we exposed drivers to five levels of driving speed that were set relative to their preferred driving speed. In addition, since increasing steering effort normally decreases swerving behavior within the driving lane given a particular speed, participants were presented with three explicit swerving performance targets represented as the standard deviation of the lateral position of the car with respect to the driving lane. To distinguish between workload levels, subject-specific CSP and linear discriminant analysis based classification models were used.

To begin with, subjective mental effort data show that driving at a higher speed is indeed experienced as requiring more effort. Furthermore, estimated driving speed was slightly lower than the real driving speed. Previous research has shown that driving speed in a simulator, when driving on straight roads or easy curves, tends to be higher than it would be on real roads (e.g., Bella, 2008). This effect could be caused by a difference in speed perception between the real world and (fixed-base) driving simulators due to the absence of several speed cues, such as car movements and stereoscopic depth perception. During the current study these factors may also have contributed to misjudging driving speed, especially since the speedometer was hidden from view at all times. The standard deviation of the lateral position (SDLP), indicating lane keeping performance, increased as function of speed, which is normal (e.g., Peng et al., 2013). However, the performance target (target SDLP) did not have an effect on vehicle parameters, suggesting that this manipulation failed since a decrease of SDLP was expected if participants were exposed to more difficult target SDLPs. However, participants did rate the "very hard" target SDLP condition as the most difficult, perhaps demonstrating that participants were trying hard but could not manage. Also, EEG data from the very hard SDLP condition could be accurately discriminated from data acquired during the normal SDLP condition which is another indication that participants did not simply ignore the instructions. Since other task manipulations aimed at increasing steering difficulty, such as decreasing lane width, have proven to affect SDLP (e.g., Dijksterhuis et al., 2011), the absence of an effect on SDLP may be explained by this particular manipulation. In contrast to the automatic nature of the steering task during normal driving participants had to actively engage themselves in transferring numerical information about their lane keeping behavior, as presented on their windshield, to steering wheel movements.

EEG activities during the experimental conditions were classified, yielding several interesting results. Firstly, applying CSP to a variety of frequencies and frequency band widths revealed that, overall, broader bands and higher frequencies result in higher classification accuracies. This could be taken to suggest that neuronal gamma synchronization correlated with the task manipulations in which case these results are in line with other research suggesting that activity in the gamma frequencies reflects sensory-motor coordination (Schoffelen et al., 2005; see also Fries et al., 2007). However, this conclusion should be drawn with caution since muscle activity as represented in the EMG has power in the same frequencies, which is picked up by EEG electrodes as well (Whitham et al., 2007; Muthukumaraswamy and Singh, 2013). This view of muscular activities contributing to high classification accuracies in the gamma band is confirmed by graphs showing the projections of the CSP components. **Figure 4A** demonstrates just one case where the perfect classification for high frequencies can mostly be traced to the EEG electrodes close to the eyes. However, a relative high contribution of the peripheral electrodes for extremely high classification accuracies is an emerging pattern. Moreover, when performing a semi-real task, such as driving in a simulator, EMG activity can be expected to be more dominantly present compared to more controlled laboratory tasks, making classifications based on neuronal gamma activities less likely.

High accuracies were also found for a substantial number of participants in the lower frequency ranges, as shown in **Figures 2** and **3**, and these are unlikely to be confounded by EMG activity. As shown by Whitham et al. (2007), who recorded EEG during paralysis by neuromuscular blockade, EMG activity is largely absent from frequencies below 20 Hz. Therefore, we suggest that classifications in the lower frequency ranges were likely determined by underlying neuronal activity.

CSP component topographies showed no readily discernible degree of consistency across participants, as illustrated in **Figure 4**. This indicates that the effects of changes in psychological construct such as mental workload on electrical activities on the scalp is very subject dependent, which confirms that individually tuned classification approaches are required for accurate classifications. In case of high frequencies this implies that the, perhaps subconsciously produced muscular activities, show large inter-individual variations. In case of the lower frequencies, it is likely that also on a neurological level, there are large variations. Finding consistent topographies would have been promising for future applications. For example, it could lead to a theory-driven pre-selection of scalp locations, thereby excluding possible irrelevant information from the classification model. Yet, it may be expected to find a large inter-individual variability when classifying rather abstract mental states compared to, for example, classifying the difference between left and right hand motor imagery for which the neuroanatomical base is much clearer.

A limitation of the current study is that the experimental conditions (rides) could not be randomized within each participant. e.g., changing speed conditions every couple of seconds would have resulted in a highly unnatural driving experience. The drawback of the used approach is that there was an average of about 15 min between one condition and the other within each condition pair that was used for the classifications. Since neighboring epochs can be similar to each other, a difference in time may have led to an inflation of the classification accuracies. For future research, it is advised to repeat conditions within subjects to assess the potential effects of time dependencies. For example, by training the classifier on one condition pair and validating it on the other, identical condition pair. While it is important to realize that time dependencies cannot be ruled out, it should also be noted that it probably did not affect other effects, such as the accuracy difference between the parietal and frontal electrode set or the difference between low and high EEG frequencies.

Overall, these findings imply that the subject-specific CSP approach provides very good discriminatory power between visuomotor workload conditions over a large range of frequency bands. With respect to the high (gamma) frequency ranges it is important to realize that major contributions from muscular activities cannot be ruled out. Moreover, this will probably be true for most passive BCI applications as real life tasks, such as driving a car, usually require a lot of motor activity. A workload classification strategy based on EMG activity would therefore be worthwhile investigating in future research, which requires a relative low number of electrodes. However, high classification accuracies were also found for the lower EEG frequencies, implying a large contribution of neurological activities. These high accuracies are promising for future applications, however, several issues need to be addressed before a system is working from the user's point of view. Some of these issues will be further discussed below.

Even if classification accuracies of up to 80% may be considered quite high for 1-s epochs, it raises the issue of applicability; especially when performing a safety-critical task, this seems insufficient. However, depending on the temporal responsiveness requirements of an application, these accuracy levels might suffice. For example, using longer data epochs can be expected to result in more accurate classifications, since more information is available to the classifier (e.g., Brouwer et al., 2012). Although not further reported in the result section, increasing the epoch length from 1 to 2 s was found to increase accuracies with about 3% for the lower frequency ranges. Another option would be to combine several successive small data epochs. As an illustration, assuming that successive classifications are independent and applying a simple binomial chance distribution, then combining five successive epochs, each having a 80% chance of accurately being classified, would lead to a 94% accuracy when using a majority vote (i.e., three or more epochs are classified correctly). This would decrease the negative effects of small periods of noisy data which may be expected in real life tasks and which should improve a system's behavior from the users point of view.

Another important issue that needs to be solved before reliable applications can be build are the so-called non-stationarities in EEG signals, which refer to shifts in EEG signals between the initial calibration session during which a model is trained and online application. Non-stationarities negatively impact the transfer of classification accuracies between calibration and application of a model (e.g., Shenoy et al., 2006). One solution to this issue could be to update the classification model from time to time by adding additional calibration periods when the task at hand allows for it. Another solution are adaptive classifiers, which use data that are acquired while the user is interacting with the system in real-time (Shenoy et al., 2006). The drawback of using an adaptive classifier is that it requires immediate labeling of new, incoming data while the user is engaged in task performance. In some active BCI systems, for example, when controlling a game, it is plausible that the required information is available. In case of a passive BCI system however, this is most likely not the case. Again, using longer periods of time may offer a solution to this problem. For example, assuming that mental workload does not vary every second, all EEG data measured over a somewhat longer period reflect one particular level of workload. If the classifier therefore classifies most epochs as data class A, then all epochs in that period could be labeled as such and subsequently used to update the classification model. Finding acceptable and robust methods of updating the classification model is likely to be a necessary development before (passive) BCI systems can be applied to task situations.

For the viability of future applications it is also important that the binary approach of discriminating between two data classes is expanded to the multiclass situation. For instance, workload levels during task performance may be either too high, too low or within an acceptable range. In an adaptive system, where support may be changed, activated, or deactivated based on workload classifications it is therefore of equal importance that the conditions for no change are defined. Thus, in terms a passive BCI application, a homeostatic system aimed at keeping workload at or around optimal levels, must also "know" when not to initiate changes. One way to accomplish multi-class analyses is to combine several pairwise classifications through voting procedures (Friedman, 1996; see also Dornhege et al., 2004; Grosse-Wentrup and Buss, 2008).

In conclusion, depending on temporal responsiveness requirements, a system's designer may have the option to either focus on high EEG frequencies and accept that muscular activities likely contribute to classification accuracies, or to focus on lower EEG frequencies that mainly reflect neurological activities but accept slightly lower accuracies. Although it is clear that the very high classification accuracies found in this offline study by themselves do not guarantee a well-functioning online system, it is a promising start in realizing a CSP based passive BCI system that can reliably be used to monitor visuomotor load in real-time.

ACKNOWLEDGMENTS

Firstly, the authors would like to thank graduate students Lucas van Assen and Camilla de Jong for their contributions in recruiting participants, carrying out the experiment, and data processing. Secondly, the technical support given by Mark Span is greatly appreciated. Thirdly, the reviewers are thanked for their helpful suggestions during the publication process. Finally, this research was supported by the European Commission Project No. 215893 REFLECT, Responsive Flexible Collaborating Ambient, within the 7th framework programme. The REFLECT project investigated ways of realizing pervasive-adaptive environments.

REFERENCES

Bella, F. (2008). Driving simu-lator for speed research on two-lane rural roads. *Accid. Anal. Prev.* 40, 1078–1087. doi: 10.1016/j.aap.2007.10.015

Blankertz, B., Tomioka, R., Lemm, S., Kawanabe, M., and Muller, K. R. (2008). Optimizing spatial filters for robust EEG single-trial analysis. *IEEE Signal Process. Mag.* 25, 41–56. doi: 10.1109/MSP.2008.4408441

Brookhuis, K. A., and de Waard, D. (2010). Monitoring drivers' mental workload in driving simulators using physiological measures. *Accid. Anal. Prev.* 42, 898–903. doi: 10.1016/j.aap.2009. 06.001

Brouwer, A. M., Hogervorst, M. A., Van Erp, J. B., Heffelaar, T., Zimmerman, P. H., and Oostenveld, R. (2012). Estimating work- load using EEG spectral power and ERPs in the n-back task.

Kohlmorgen, J., Dornhege, G., Braun, M., Blankertz, B., Müller, K.-R., Curio, G., et al. (2007). "Improving human performance in a real operating environment through real-time mental workload detec- tion," in *Toward Brain–Computer Interfacing*, eds G. Dornhege, J.

D. R. Millán, T. Hinterberger, D. McFarland, and K.-R. Müller (Cambridge, MA: MIT press), 409–422.

Lewis-Evans, B., and Charlton, S. G. (2006). Explicit and implicit processes in behavioural adap- tation to road width. *Accid. Anal. Prev.* 38, 610–614. doi: 10.1016/j.aap.2005.12.005

Lewis-Evans, B., de Waard, D., and Brookhuis, K. A. (2011). Speed maintenance under cognitive load - implications for theo- ries of driver behavior. *Accid. Anal. Prev.* 43, 1497–1507. doi: 10.1016/j.aap.2011.02.030

J. Neural Eng. 9, 045008. doi: 10.1088/1741-2560/9/4/045008 Cacioppo, J. T., and Gardner, W.

L. (1999). Emotion. *Annu. Rev. Psychol.* 50, 191–214. doi: 10.1146/annurev.psych.50.1.191

Cacioppo, J. T., Tassinary, L. G., and Berntson, G. G. (2000). "Psychophysiological science," in *Handbook of Psychophysiology*, eds T. Cacioppo, L. G. Tassinary, and G. G. Berntson (Cambridge: Cambridge University Press), 3–26.

Carsten, O. M. J., and Brookhuis, (2005). Issues arising from the HASTE experiments. *Trans. Res. Part F Traffic Psychol. Behav.* 8, 191–196. doi: 10.1016/j.trf.2005.04.004

Chu, Y., and Rouse, W. B. (1979). Adaptive allocation of decision making responsibility between human and computer in multitask situations. *IEEE Trans. Syst. Man Cybern.* 9, 769–778. doi: 10.1109/TSMC.1979.4310128

Cutrell, E., and Tan, D. (2008). "BCI for passive input in HCI," in *Proceedings of CHI*, Vol. 8. (New York, NY: ACM Press).

de Waard, D. (1996). *The Measurement of Drivers' Mental Workload*. Doctoral dissertation, University of Groningen, Haren.

Dijksterhuis, C., Brookhuis, K. A., and de Waard, D. (2011). Effects of steering demand on lane keeping behaviour, self-reports, and phys- iology. a simulator study. *Accid. Anal. Prev.* 43, 1074–1081. doi: 10.1016/j.aap.2010.12.014

Dornhege, G., Blankertz, B., Curio, G., and Muller, K. R. (2004). Boosting bit rates in noninvasive EEG single-trial classifications by feature combination and mul- ticlass paradigms. *IEEE Trans. Biomed. Eng.* 51, 993–1002. doi: 10.1109/TBME.2004.827088

Gratton, G., Coles, M. G., and Donchin, E. (1983). A new method for off-line removal of ocular artifact. *Electroencephalogr. Clin. Neurophysiol.* 55, 468–484. doi: 10.1016/0013-4694(83)90135-9

Grosse-Wentrup, M., and Buss, M. (2008). Multiclass common spa- tial patterns and information theo- retic feature extraction. *IEEE Trans. Biomed. Eng.* 55, 1991–2000. doi: 10.1109/TBME.2008.921154

Fairclough, S. H. (2009). Fundamentals of physiological computing. *Interact. Comput.* 21, 133–145. doi: 10.1016/j.intcom.2008.10.011

Friedman, J. (1996). *Another Approach to Polychotomous Classication*. Technical report, Department of Statistics, Stanford University.

Fries, P., Nikolic, D., and Singer, W. (2007). The gamma cycle. *Trends Neurosci.* 30, 309–316. doi: 10.1016/j.tins.2007.05.005

Fuller, R. (2005). Towards a gen- eral theory of driver behaviour. *Accid. Anal. Prev.* 37, 461–472. doi: 10.1016/j.aap.2004.11.003

Hancock, P. A., and Chignell, M. H. (1988). Mental workload dynam- ics in adaptive interface design. *IEEE Trans. Syst. Man Cybern.* 18, 647–658. doi: 10.1109/21.17382

Hockey, G. R. J. (1997). Compensatory control in the regulation of human performance under stress and high workload: a cognitive-energetical framework. *Biol. Psychol.* 45, 73–93. doi: 10.1016/S0301-0511(96) 05223-4

Hockey, G. R. J. (2003). "Operator functional state as a framework for the assessment of perfor-(Amsterdam: IOS Press), 8–23.

Kaber, D. B., and Prinzel, L. J. III. (2006). *Adaptive and Adaptable Automation Design: A Critical Review of the Literature and Recommendations for Future Research*. Report No. NASA/TM- 2006-214504. Available online at: http://ntrs.nasa.gov/search.jsp? R=20060053373

Mulder, L. J. M., Dijksterhuis, C., Stuiver, A., and de Waard, D. (2009). Cardiovascular state changes during performance of a simulated ambulance dispatchers' task: potential use for adaptive support. *Appl. Ergon.* 40, 965–977. doi: 10.1016/j.apergo.2009.01.009

Muthukumaraswamy, S. D., and Singh, K. D. (2013). Visual gamma oscillations: the effects of stimulus type, visual field coverage and stimulus motion on MEG and EEG record- ings. *Neuroimage* 69, 223–230. doi: 10.1016/j.neuroimage.2012.12.038

Näätänen, R., and Summala, H. (1976). *Road-User Behavior and Traffic Accidents*. Amsterdam: North-Holland.

Parasuraman, R., Bahri, R., Deaton, T., Morrison, J., and Barnes, M. (1992). *Theory and Design of Adaptive Automation in Aviation Systems* (Progress Report No. NAWCADWAR-92033- 60). Warminster, PA: Naval Air Warfare Center, Aircraft Division.

Peng, Y., Boyle, L. N., and Hallmark, S. L. (2013). Driver's lane keep- ing ability with eyes off road: insights from a naturalistic

Prinzel III, L. J., Pope, A. T., Freeman, F. G., Scerbo, M. W., and Mikulka, P. J. (2001). *Empirical Analysis of EEG and ERPs for Psychophysiological Adaptive Task Allocation*. Report No. NASA/TM- 2001-211016. Hampton, VA: NASA.

Available online at: http://nix.nasa. gov/search.jsp?R=20010060403

Rouse, W. B. (1988). Adaptive aiding for human/computer control. *Hum. Factors* 30, 431–443.

Schoffelen, J. M., Oostenveld, R., and Fries, P. (2005). Neuronal coherence as a mechanism of effective corticospinal interac- tion. *Science* 308, 111–113. doi: 10.1126/science.1107027

Shenoy, P., Krauledat, M., Blankertz, B., Rao, R. P., and Müller, K. R. (2006). Towards adaptive classifica- tion for BCI. *J. Neural Eng.* 3, R13. doi: 10.1088/1741-2560/3/1/R02

Summala, H. (2005). "Traffic psychology theories: towards understanding driving behaviour and safety efforts," in *Traffic and Transport Psychology, 1st Edn.*, ed G. Underwood (Amsterdam: Elsevier), 383–394.

Van Winsum, W., and Van Wolffelaar, P. C. (1993). "GIDS small world simulation," in *Generic Intelligent Driver Support*, ed J. A. Michon, (London: Taylor and Francis), 175–191.

Whitham, E. M., Pope, K. J., Fitzgibbon, S. P., Lewis, T., Clark, C. R., Loveless, S., et al. (2007). Scalp electrical recording during paralysis: quantitative evidence that EEG frequencies above 20Hz are contaminated by EMG. *Clin. Neurophysiol.* 118, 1877–1888. doi: 10.1016/j.clinph.2007.04.027

Wilde, G. J. S. (1982). The the-ory of RHT: implications for safety and health. *Risk Anal.* 2, 209–226. doi: 10.1111/j.1539-6924.1982.tb01384.x

Zander, T. O., and Kothe, C. (2011). Towards passive brain–computer interfaces: applying brain- computer interface technology to human–machine systems in general. *J. Neural Eng.* 8:025005. doi: 10.1088/1741-2560/8/2/025005

Zander, T. O., Kothe, C., Jatzev, S., and Gaertner, M. (2010). "Enhancing human–computer interaction with input from active and passive brain–computer interfaces," in *The Human in Brain–Computer Interfaces and the Brain in Human– Computer Interaction*, eds D. S. Tan and A. Nijholt (Berlin: Springer), 181–199.

Zijlstra, F. R. H. (1993). *Efficiency in Work Behavior. A Design Approach for Modern Tools*. Doctoral disserta- tion, Delft University of Technology, Delft: Delft University Press.

5

Developing an EEG-based on-line closed-loop lapse detection and mitigation system

Yu-Te Wang[1,2], Kuan-Chih Huang[3], Chun-Shu Wei[2,4], Teng-Yi Huang[3], Li-Wei Ko[5], Chin-Teng Lin[3], Chung-Kuan Cheng[1,6] and Tzyy-Ping Jung[2,4,6]*

[1] Department of Computer Science and Engineering, Jacobs School of Engineering, University of California San Diego, La Jolla, CA, USA
[2] Swartz Center for Computational Neuroscience, Institute for Neural Computation, University of California San Diego, La Jolla, CA, USA
[3] Department of Electrical Engineering, National Chiao-Tung University, Hsinchu, Taiwan
[4] Department of Bioengineering, Jacobs School of Engineering, University of California San Diego, La Jolla, CA, USA
[5] Department of Biological Science and Technology, National Chiao-Tung University, Hsinchu, Taiwan
[6] Center for Advanced Neurological Engineering, Institute of Engineering in Medicine, University of California San Diego, La Jolla, CA, USA

***Correspondence:**
Tzyy-Ping Jung, Swartz Center for Computational Neuroscience, Institute for Neural Computation, University of California San Diego, La Jolla, CA 92092, USA
e-mail: jung@sccn.ucsd.edu

In America, 60% of adults reported that they have driven a motor vehicle while feeling drowsy, and at least 15–20% of fatal car accidents are fatigue-related. This study translates previous laboratory-oriented neurophysiological research to design, develop, and test an On-line Closed-loop Lapse Detection and Mitigation (OCLDM) System featuring a mobile wireless dry-sensor EEG headgear and a cell-phone based real-time EEG processing platform. Eleven subjects participated in an event-related lane-keeping task, in which they were instructed to manipulate a randomly deviated, fixed-speed cruising car on a 4-lane highway. This was simulated in a 1st person view with an 8-screen and 8-projector immersive virtual-reality environment. When the subjects experienced lapses or failed to respond to events during the experiment, auditory warning was delivered to rectify the performance decrements. However, the arousing auditory signals were not always effective. The EEG spectra exhibited statistically significant differences between effective and ineffective arousing signals, suggesting that EEG spectra could be used as a countermeasure of the efficacy of arousing signals. In this on-line pilot study, the proposed OCLDM System was able to continuously detect EEG signatures of fatigue, deliver arousing warning to subjects suffering momentary cognitive lapses, and assess the efficacy of the warning in near real-time to rectify cognitive lapses. The on-line testing results of the OCLDM System validated the efficacy of the arousing signals in improving subjects' response times to the subsequent lane-departure events. This study may lead to a practical on-line lapse detection and mitigation system in real-world environments.

Keywords: electroencephalogram (EEG), drowsiness, fatigue, driving, smartphone, cell-phone, brain computer interface (BCI)

INTRODUCTION

Fatigue-related performance decrements such as lapses in attention and slowed reaction time could lead to catastrophic incidents in occupations ranging from ship navigators to airplane pilots, railroad engineers, truck and auto drivers, and nuclear plant monitors. Fatigue (or drowsiness) "concerns the inability or disinclination to continue an activity, generally because the activity has been going on for too long," defined by European Transport Safety Council (Croo et al., 2001). Sixty percent of American adults reported that they have been driving a motor vehicle when feeling drowsy (National Sleep Foundation, 2005). Furthermore, studies have concluded that at least 15–20% of fatal car accidents are fatigue-related (The Royal Society for the Prevention of Accidents, 2001; Connor et al., 2002; National Highway Traffic Safety Administration, 2003). Therefore, an earlier detection of driving fatigue is a crucial issue for preventing catastrophic incidents.

In order to detect the driving fatigue, several approaches have been proposed in scientific literature. (1) Computer vision-based systems (Bergasa et al., 2006; D'Orazio et al., 2007; Golz et al., 2010). Bergasa et al. (2006) used a real-time image-acquisition system to monitor drivers' visual behaviors that revealed a drivers' alertness level. Six parameters: percentage of eye closure, eye closure duration, blink frequency, nodding frequency, face position, and fixed gaze were included in a fuzzy classifier for identifying a driver's vigilance level. D'Orazio et al. (2007) proposed a neural classifier to recognize the eye activities from images without being constrained to head rotation or partially occluded eyes. (2) Driving behavior counter-measurements (Lin et al., 2009, 2010a, 2013). Lin et al. (2009) performed an event-related, lane-keeping driving task in an immersive virtual-reality environment. Subjects were asked to steer the stimulated car back to the middle of the cruising lane once they perceived the randomized lane-departure events. The results showed that the reaction time (RT), defined as the time interval between the onset of the simulated car deviation and the user response, could be improved by providing arousing auditory warning to the subjects combating with fatigue.

A Brain Computer Interface (BCI) translates neural activities into control signals to provide a direct communication pathway between the human brain and an external device (Wolpaw et al., 2002). Broadly speaking, BCIs can be grouped into three categories: active, passive and reactive BCIs (Zander and Kothe, 2011). Electroencephalogram (EEG)-based passive BCIs measure brain electrical activities from the scalp and enrich a human–machine interaction with implicit information on the actual user state without conscious effort from the user (Lehne et al., 2009; Zander et al., 2009, 2010; Zander and Jatzev, 2012). Given appropriate signal-processing algorithms in the passive BCIs, meaningful information can be directly extracted from the EEGs. For instance, time-domain analysis such as averaging across different channels, moving average with a specific window length, standard deviation, linear correlation and so on are useful approaches to extract information from EEGs (Dong et al., 2011). In a frequency-domain analysis, the short-time Fourier transform (STFT) is often applied to the EEG data to estimate the power spectral density in distinct frequency bands, including delta (1–3 Hz), theta (4–7 Hz), alpha (8–13 Hz), beta (14–30 Hz), and gamma (31–50 Hz). Many studies have shown that the brain dynamics linked to fatigue and behavioral lapses can be assessed by EEG power spectra (Kecklund and Akerstedt, 1993; Makeig and Inlow, 1993; Jung and Makeig, 1995; Makeig and Jung, 1996; Jung et al., 1997; Lal and Craig, 2002; Campagne et al., 2004; Horne and Baulk, 2004; Debener et al., 2005; Peiris et al., 2006; Davidson et al., 2007; Eichele et al., 2010, 2008; Golz et al., 2010; Lin et al., 2010a), combinations of EEG band power (Jap et al., 2011), alpha spindle parameters (Simon et al., 2011) and autoregressive features (Rosipal et al., 2007). These studies provided solid evidence for the neurophysiological correlates of fatigue and behavioral lapses. In short, while the physical- and behavioral symptom-based methods indirectly measure drivers' cognitive states, the neurophysiology-based methods offer a more direct path to assess the brain dynamic linked to fatigue and behavioral lapses with a high temporal resolution.

Efforts have also been made to assist individuals in combating fatigue and/or preventing lapses in concentration. For instance, Dingus et al. (1997) and Spence and Driver (1998) proposed using warning signals to maintain drivers' attention. The types of warning signals could be auditory (Spence and Driver, 1998; Lin et al., 2009), visual (Liu, 2001), tactile (Ho et al., 2005) or mixed (Liu, 2001). Empirical results showed that auditory warning could reduce the number of lapses in sustained-attention tasks (Spence and Driver, 1998), and could help subjects to maintain driving performance (Lin et al., 2009). More recent studies demonstrated that arousing auditory signals presented to individuals experiencing momentarily behavioral lapses could not only agitate their behavioral responses but also change their EEG theta and alpha power in a sustained-attention driving task (Jung et al., 2010; Lin et al., 2010a, 2013). However, the studies also showed that sometimes subjects did not respond to the arousing signals, and more importantly the EEG activity of these non-responsive episodes showed little or no changes following the ineffective warning (Jung et al., 2010; Lin et al., 2010a, 2013). Lin et al. (2013) later demonstrated the feasibility of using the post-warning EEG power spectra to predict the (in)efficacy of the arousing warning. A caveat of their studies was that the arousing warning was delivered to subjects after they behaviorally failed to respond to lane-departure events. In reality, the delivery of arousing warning could have been too late because the behavioral lapse might have led to catastrophic consequences. A truly EEG-based lapse monitoring system needs to continuously and non-invasively observe EEG dynamics to predict fatigue-related lapses, deliver arousing signal to arouse the user, and assess the efficacy of the arousing signal to trigger a repeated or secondary warning signal if necessary. Furthermore, all of the aforementioned studies were conducted with traditional bulky and tethered EEG systems and were performed in well-controlled laboratories. However, it is argued that there might be fundamentally dynamic differences between laboratory-based and naturalistic human behavior in the brain (McDowell et al., 2013). It thus remains unclear how well the current laboratory-oriented knowledge of EEG correlates of cognitive-state changes can be translated into the highly dynamic real world.

This study aims to extend previous studies to design, develop and test a truly On-line Closed-loop Lapse Detection and Mitigation (OCLDM) System that can continuously monitor EEG dynamics, predict fatigue-related lapses based on EEG signals, arouse the fatigued users by delivering arousing signals, and assess the efficacy of the arousing signal based on EEG spectra. This study hypothesized that (1) EEG spectral values would differ under different arousal states; (2) it is feasible to predict lapses based on the spectral changes in the spontaneous EEG; (3) arousing warning delivered to cognitively challenged subjects would mitigate cognitive lapse, and (4) the rectified performance would be accompanied by the changes in EEG power spectra. This study conducted an off-line experiment to explore the neurophysiological correlates of lapses, which tested the above-mentioned hypotheses and guided the development of a truly OCLDM system. The system was then validated by an on-line driving experiment. Furthermore, to be practical for routine use in a car or workplace by freely moving individuals, the EEG-based lapse monitoring system must be non-invasive, non-intrusive, lightweight, battery-powered, and easily to put on and take off (Lin et al., 2008a,b). This study thus also investigates the feasibility of using a practical, low-density, lightweight dry EEG headgear and a smartphone-based EEG-processing platform (Wang et al., 2012) to build a truly mobile and wireless OCLDM System for real-life applications.

MATERIALS AND METHODS

SUBJECTS

Eleven healthy and naive subjects (10 males and one female) with normal hearing and aged 20–28 years old participated in this study. All of them were free of neurological and psychological disorders. They were introduced how to manipulate the car and practiced ~10 min to get acquainted before the experiment started. None of them worked night shifts or traveled across multiple time zones in the previous 2 months. All participants were asked to read and sign the informed consent form before participating in the studies. After the experiments, subjects were asked to complete the questionnaire for assessing their cognitive states during the experiments.

EXPERIMENTAL EQUIPMENT

Experiments of this study were conducted in an 8-screen and 8-projector immersive virtual-reality (VR) environment that simulates the 1st person view scene of highway driving. This study adapted an event-related lane-departure driving paradigm originally proposed by Huang et al. (2006, 2007a,b, 2009) that allowed objective and quantitative measures of momentary event-related brain dynamics following lane-departure events and driving-performance fluctuations over longer periods. The VR scenes simulated driving at a constant speed (at ~100 km/h) on a highway with the simulated car randomly drifting away from the center of the cruising lane to simulate driving on non-ideal road surfaces or with poor alignment (Huang et al., 2007a,b, 2009; Lin et al., 2008b, 2009). The scene was updated according to the land-departure events and the subject's manipulation. The vehicle trajectory, user's input, and lane-departure events could be accurately logged and time-synchronized to the EEG recordings (Huang et al., 2007a,b, 2009; Lin et al., 2008b). There were no traffic or distractive objects other than 4-lane roads and dark sky appeared in the VR while the simulated car was cruising on the highway.

Thirty-two channel EEG data were collected from participants by the NuAmp system (32-channels Quick-Cap, Compumedics Ltd., VIC, Australia). The electrodes were placed according to a modified international 10–20 system with a unipolar reference at the right earlobe. The EEG activities were recorded with 500 Hz sampling rate and 16-bit quantization level.

EXPERIMENTAL PARADIGM

Figure 1A shows the experimental paradigm of this study. The simulated car starts cruising at a fixed speed (~100 km/h) on the 3rd lane and drifting to either right or left with equal probability within 8–10 s. Subjects were instructed to steer the simulated car back to the 3rd lane as soon as they noticed the lane drift. The simulated car keeps cruising on the right (or left) most lane if the subjects failed to respond to lane drift. The baseline period of each lane-departure epoch is defined as the 3 s before the onset of a lane-drifting event. The empty circle in **Figure 1A** represents the unexpected lane-departure events marked as the "deviation

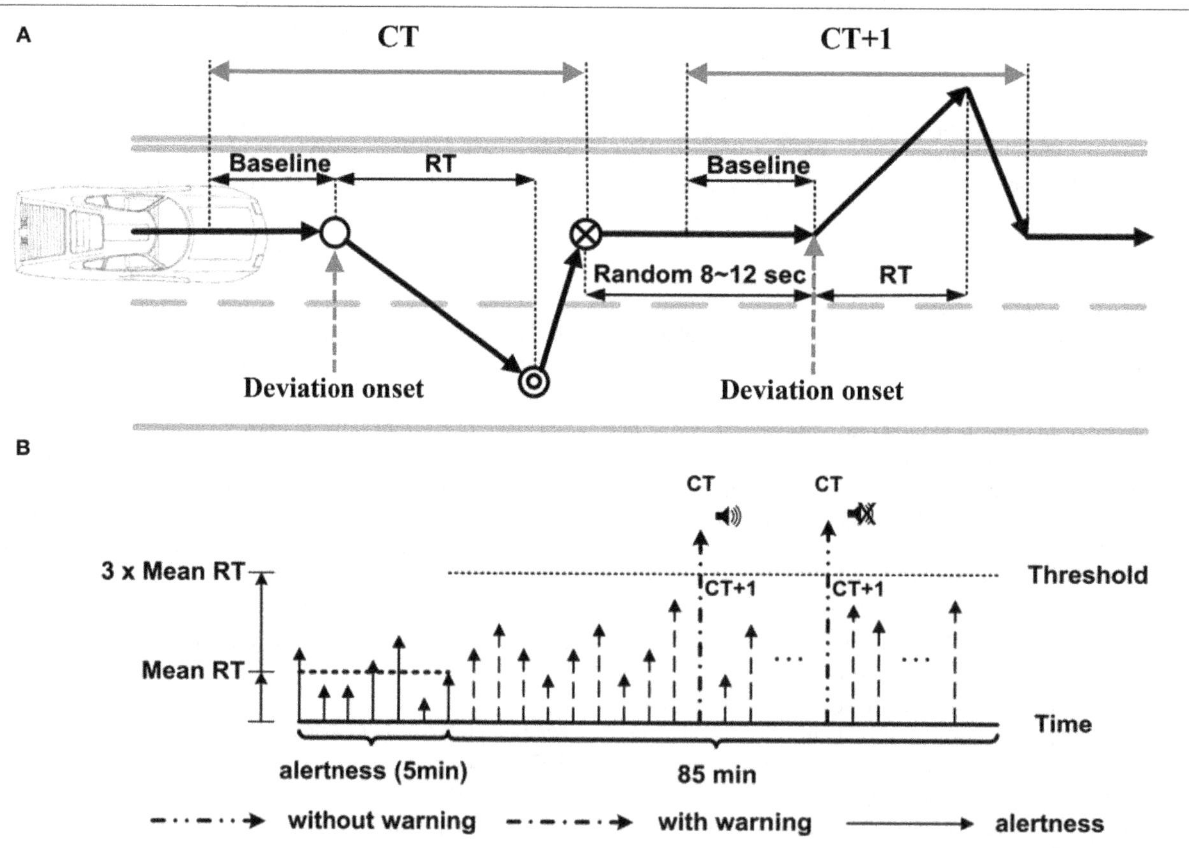

FIGURE 1 | Experiment paradigm. (A) Event-related lane-departure driving tasks. The solid arrows represent the driving trajectory. The empty circle represents the deviation onset. The double circle represents the response onset. The circle with the cross represents the response offset. The baseline is defined as the 3 s period prior to deviation onset. The response time (RT) of a driver is the interval from the deviation (empty circle) to the response onset (the double circle). A trial starts at deviation onset and ends at response offset (circle with a cross). The next deviation begins 8–12 s after response offset. **(B)** Criterion for delivering auditory warning during driving tasks. The height of an arrow represents the response time in a single trial. The warning was delivered to the subject when the RT in the trial exceeded three times the mean RT of trials in the first 5 min of the task, when the subject was presumably alert and fully attended to lane-departure events. In this figure is adapted with permission from Figure 1 of Lin et al. (2010a).

onset." After the deviation onset, subjects were instructed to steer the simulated car back to the center of the cruising lane immediately (double circle), and the time when the subjects started steering was marked as the "response onset." The moment that the simulated car reached the center of the cruising lane (circle with cross) was marked as the "response offset." A subject's response time (RT) was defined as the time between the deviation onset and the response onset. At the first 5 min of the experiment, subjects were asked to be fully alert, verified by the vehicle trajectory and the video from a surveillance camera, to obtain an averaged alert RT (aRT) for each subject (1.51~2.54 s), which is a threshold for the entire experiment. The entire experiment consisted of 5 min training and 85 min driving periods.

Figure 1B shows the criterion of delivering auditory warnings in the experiment. When a subject failed to respond within three times the aRT, the system treated the trials as a behavioral lapse and triggered a 1750 Hz tone-burst to arouse the subject from fatigue-related lapse in half (50%) of these drowsy trials (marked as the "current trial (CT)" in **Figure 1A**). The very next trial is defined as CT + 1, and so on. The lapse trials that were randomly selected to receive arousing warning were referred to as CT with warning, whereas the remaining half of trials that did not receive auditory warning were referred to as CT without warning. Note that our previous studies showed that in some trials subjects remained non-responsive following the arousing warning, which was analogous to sleeping through an alarm clock (Jung et al., 2010; Lin et al., 2013). If the RT of the following trial (CT + 1) was shorter than the double of the averaged aRT, the warning signal delivered in the CT trial was defined as an "effective warning." On the other hand, if the RT of the CT + 1 trial was longer than triple of the averaged aRT, the warning was defined as an "ineffective warning." This study did not include the trials with RTs between 2 and 3 aRT to define the alert vs. fatigue spectral thresholds because the cognitive states of the subjects during those trials were unclear. Note that, subjects didn't know about the warning before the experiments.

DATA ANALYSIS

The 32-channel EEG data were first down-sampled to 250 Hz, and a low-pass filter of 50 Hz and a high-pass filter of 0.5 Hz were applied. Channels or trials with severe artifacts (such as body movements or muscle activities) were manually removed (less than three channels and 20% trials per subject in general). The remaining EEG data were segmented into several 115 s trials, each of them consisting of 15 s before and 100 s after the lane-deviation onsets. Independent Component Analysis (ICA, Bell and Sejnowski, 1995; Makeig et al., 1997) implemented in EEGLAB (Delorme and Makeig, 2004) was then applied to decompose the ~32-channel EEG into ~32 independent components (ICs), based on the assumption that the collected EEG data from the scalp were a weighted linear mixture of electrical potentials projected instantaneously from temporally ICs accounting for distinct brain sources. The comparable ICs across subjects were grouped into component clusters based on their scalp maps, equivalent dipole locations and baseline power spectra of component activations (Jung et al., 2001; Delorme and Makeig, 2004). Across 11 subjects, there were 155 trials with warning (30 trials were ineffective and 125 trials were effective) and 192 trials without warning.

Since the RT and EEG power were not normally distributed, non-parametric statistic tests were performed for the data analysis (Delorme and Makeig, 2004). The Wilcoxon rank-sum test (Matlab statistical toolbox, Mathworks) was used to assess the effects of warning on RTs. Bootstrapping (EEGLAB toolbox, University of California, San Diego) was used to test the statistical significance of EEG power changes at specific frequency bins from 2 to 30 Hz with a 0.25 Hz resolution. To test group statistics, the intrinsic inter-subject RT differences were reduced by dividing RTs by the mean RT. The EEG spectra were normalized by dividing the spectral power by the standard deviation of the spectral distribution.

RESULTS: NEUROPHYSIOLOGICAL CORRELATES OF BEHAVIORAL LAPSES

EFFICACY OF AROUSING AUDITORY SIGNALS FOR RECTIFYING LAPSES

This study first explored the efficacy of the delivery of arousing auditory signals by measuring the change in subjects' reaction time. **Figure 2A** shows the boxplots of RTs of three trial groups:

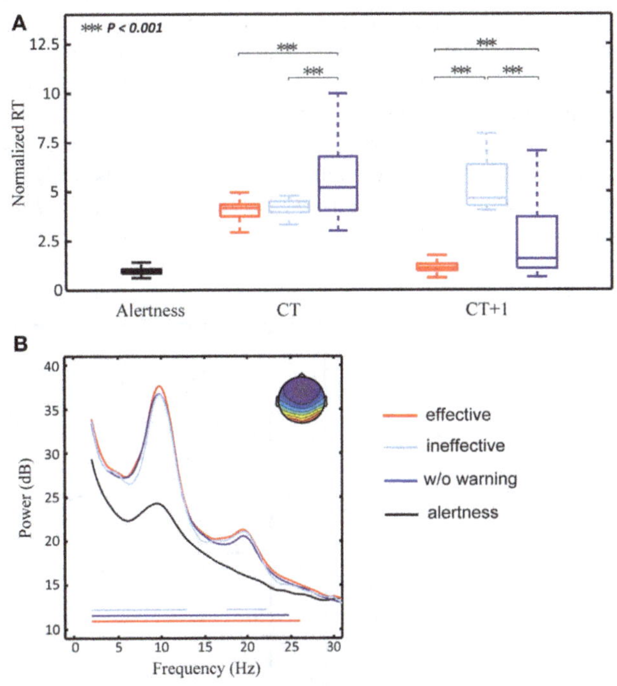

FIGURE 2 | Experiment results. (A) The boxplot for the RT distribution of trials with effective warning, ineffective warning, and without warning among CTs and CTs + 1. Note that middle horizontal line is the median of the distribution, and the top and bottom of the rectangle are the third and first quartile, and the dash line ends are the maximum and minimum after outlier removal. **(B)** The component spectra of the alert CTs (black curve), with an effective warning (red curve), with an ineffective warning (light blue curve) and without warning (dark blue curve). The red, light blue and blue horizontal lines mark the spectral differences between the alert trials and trials with an effective warning, with an ineffective warning, and without warning, respectively. All the spectral plots were calculated from the activity of the bilateral occipital components separated by ICA.

Alertness, CT, and CT + 1 (left to right). The averaged aRT of trials within the Alertness group across 11 subjects was ~676 ms. The RTs of the CT group with arousing warning (red and light blue) were statistically significantly shorter than those of trials without receiving arousing warning (dark blue). The RTs of the CT + 1 group with effective vs. ineffective warning differed while the RTs of the preceding group (CT) were comparable. Even though the subjects responded to the arousing warning by immediately steering the simulated car back to the cruising position, they could well be totally non-responsive to the very next lane-departure event (~10 s later). In other words, the arousing signals reliably rectified human behavioral lapses, but did not guarantee that subjects were fully awake, alert, or attentive. This suggests an analogous regime of snooze after an alarm is turned off.

EEG DYNAMICS PRECEDING BEHAVIORAL LAPSES

Figure 2B shows the mean scalp map of the bilateral occipital cluster (upper-right corner) and its component baseline power of drowsy trials without auditory warning (dark blue), with either effective (red) or ineffective warning (light blue). First, among the resultant ICA clusters, bilateral occipital components exhibited statistically significant spectral differences between trials with and without auditory warning. Second, the component power spectra exhibited tonic increases in theta (4–7 Hz), alpha (8–12 Hz), and beta (13–30 Hz) bands in drowsy trials (red, dark blue, and light blue), compared to the alert trials (black). Horizontal lines mark the frequency bins under which the spectral differences between alert trials and drowsy trials with either (in)effective warning, or without warning were statistically significant (alpha = 0.05, Bonferroni adjusted *p*-value of 0.05/(112 frequency bins) = 0.0004 for multiple comparisons). Note that the spectra shown here were calculated from the component activities prior to the lane-deviation onset. The nearly identical pre-lapse spectra of these three groups of non-responsive trials demonstrate the robustness of the broadband spectral augmentation preceding the behavioral lapses, suggesting the feasibility of using theta and alpha power from the lateral occipital areas to predict behavioral lapses in this sustained-attention driving task.

EFFECTS OF AROUSING AUDITORY SIGNALS ON THE EEG

Next, this study explored temporal spectral dynamics preceding, during and following fatigue-related behavioral lapses and following arousing warning. **Figure 3** shows time courses of spectral changes in the bilateral occipital area following ineffective warning (light blue trace), effective warning (red trace), and without warning (dark blue trace), compared to those of the alert trials (black trace). **Figure 3** shows that both theta- an alpha-band power steadily increased prior to the lane-departure onset (at time 0 s). Again, the trends of steady increasing theta- and alpha-band power leading to behavioral lapses in the three groups of drowsy trials were nearly identical, indicating the robustness of the theta and alpha augmentation preceding the behavioral lapses.

Figure 3 also shows that after the lane-departure onset (at time 0 s), the alpha (top panel), and theta (bottom panel) power abruptly decreased by over 10 and 5 dB to nearly the alert (black trace) baseline, respectively. More importantly, following the subjects' responses, the spectra of trials with ineffective warning (light blue trace) and without warning (dark blue trace) rapidly rose from the alert baseline to the drowsy level in 5–15 s. The theta and alpha power of trials with effective warning, however, remained low for ~40 s. The green horizontal lines mark the time points when the difference between the spectra of trials with

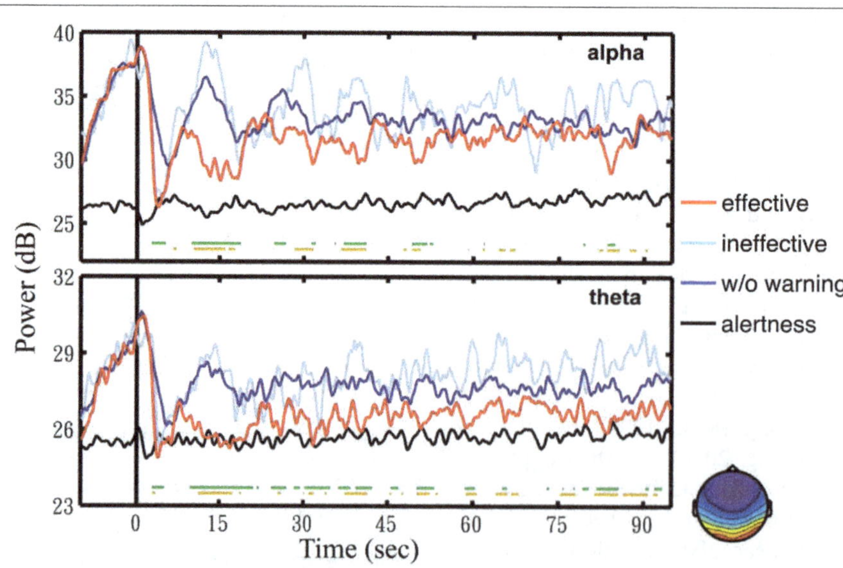

FIGURE 3 | Average component EEG power changes in alpha (top panel) and theta (bottom panel) bands from the bilateral occipital components (lower right corner). All the trials are aligned to the lane-deviation onsets at time 0 s (vertical solid black line). The red, light blue, dark blue, and black traces are the averaged spectra of trials with effective feedback, with ineffective feedback, without feedback, and in alertness, respectively. The green horizontal line indicates the statistically significant differences ($p < 0.01$) between trials with effective feedback and without feedback. The brown indicates the statistically significant differences ($p < 0.01$) between trials with effective feedback and ineffective feedback.

effective warning and without warning were statistically significant ($p < 0.01$). The spectral difference between the trials with effective warning and without warning was significant from 7 to 18 s in alpha band and from 7 to 21 s in the theta band ($p < 0.01$). Furthermore, the spectral difference between the trials with effective and ineffective warning was significant from 7 to 16 s in both alpha and theta bands (brown horizontal lines).

In sum, these results provided invaluable insights into the optimal electrode locations (lateral occipital region) and EEG features (theta- and alpha-band power) for a practical OCLDM system detailed below. The EEG and behavioral data collected from this experiment were used to assess the EEG correlates of fatigue-related lapses and build a lapse prediction model for the second experiment.

DEVELOPING A OCLDM SYSTEM

Our previous study (Wang et al., 2012) proposed a cellphone based drowsiness monitoring and management system to continuously and wirelessly monitor brain dynamics using a lightweight, portable, and low-density EEG acquisition headgear. The system was designed to assess brain activities over the forehead, detect drowsiness, and deliver arousing warning to users experiencing momentary cognitive lapses, and assess the efficacy of the warning in near real-time. However, the system was not fully implemented nor experimentally validated in humans. Furthermore, according to the neurophysiological results in section Results: Neurophysiological Correlates of Behavioral Lapses, EEG signals collected over the lateral occipital regions were more informative for lapse detection. This study extends the previous work to design, develop, and test an OCLDM System.

SYSTEM ARCHITECTURE

Figure 4A shows the system diagram of the proposed OCLDM System. The system consists of two major components: (1) a mobile platform featuring the OCLDM algorithm, and (2) a mobile and wireless 4-channel headgear measuring EEG signals over the hair-bearing occipital regions with dry EEG sensors (Liao et al., 2011). The OCLDM System was implemented as an App on an Android-based platform (e.g., Samsung Galaxy S3). The smartphone has a Bluetooth module, 16 GB RAM, an ARM Cortex-A9 processor, Android (Ice Cream Sandwich) OS, and other components. When the App is launched, it can automatically search and connect to a nearby EEG headgear to receive data from the EEG acquisition headgear. In the mean time, the App opened an USB port to receive the events from a four-lane highway scene to synchronize the EEG data and scene events. The build-in speaker (or plug-in a ear set) of the smartphone delivers auditory warning signal once the OCLDM System detects that the subject is experiencing a cognitive lapse. Both the EEG data and scene-generated events could be logged onto either smartphone's build-in memory or an external microSD card for further analysis.

The mobile and wireless EEG acquisition headgear features a 4-channel lightweight portable bio-signal acquisition device powered by a 3.7 v Li-ion battery (Lin et al., 2010b). It consists of a TI MSP430 microprocessor, a pre-amplifier, a battery-charging circuit, a 24 bit ADC, a Bluetooth module, and dry spring-loaded EEG sensors (Liao et al., 2011). The spring-loaded probes of the sensor can penetrate the hair to provide good electrical conductivity with the scalp. The microprocessor controls all the components including the amplifiers, digitizers, and transmits the digitalized EEG data to the Bluetooth module. The 4-channel EEG data are then transmitted to the authorized receiver of the OCLDM System. Depending on the applications, the system's sampling rate can be programmed at 128, 256, or 512 Hz. An experienced subject can easily put on this EEG acquisition device within 1–3 min without any help from a technician. **Figure 4B** shows a photo of a subject wearing a 4-channel EEG headgear and performing the simulated driving experiment.

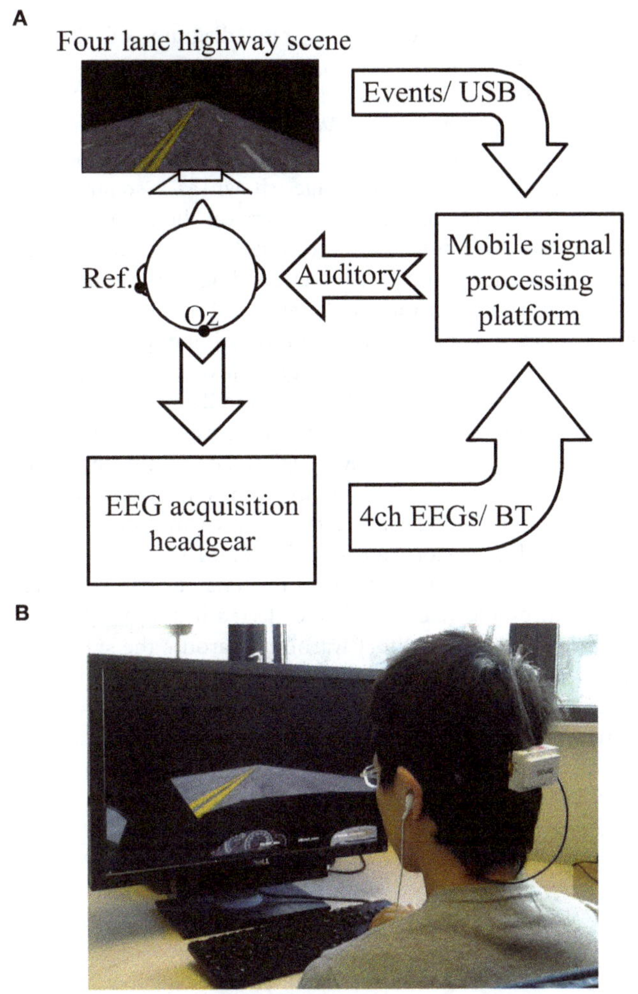

FIGURE 4 | The system diagram of the proposed OCLDM System. (A) The EEG headgear collected 4-channel brain activities from the lateral occipital area while a subject was performing the lane-drifting experiment. The mobile signal-processing platform received the acquired EEG raw data through Bluetooth, and the event markers generated from the lane-departure scene through an USB interface. Finally, the auditory feedback was delivered to the subject when the averaged EEG power across four channels was 3 dB over the alert baseline. **(B)** A photo of a subject performing the on-line driving experiment while wearing a 4-channel EEG headgear (the white small box attached on a flexible band) over the lateral occipital area.

SYSTEM SOFTWARE DESIGN

Figure 5 shows the program's state diagram of the proposed OCLDM System. Three major states, including Baseline Collecting (BC), Driving Performance Monitoring (DPM), and Warning Efficacy Assessment (WEA), were implemented in the program. When the program is launched, one can modify the parameters in the SETTING page, shown as a square box in the figure. For instance, the parameters can be the duration of baseline data collection, or the threshold of auditory warning delivering for the other two states. Depending on the applications, the lapse threshold in the DPM state can be calculated accordingly. For example, one can use a combination of power of alpha, beta, theta, and delta bands to detect cognitive lapse. The program then enters the next (DPM) state after the Baseline (calibration) data collection has completed. The DPM module continuously monitors the driver's neurophysiological data. The program stays in the DPM state until the lapse threshold is met, which depends on the neurophysiological results as shown in section Results: Neurophysiological Correlates of Behavioral Lapses. For instance, when the subject's power spectrum in alpha band is 3 dB higher than the threshold (alert baseline collected in the BC state), the program delivers an auditory warning to arouse the subject and enters the FEA state. The current value is stored as the lapse reference in the FEA module. The system repeatedly delivers auditory warning until the EEG power decreases to another threshold.

ON-LINE EXPERIMENTAL PARADIGM

Three new male subjects (who did not participated in the first experiment) with normal hearing and aged 25–30 years old participated in the on-line closed-loop lane-departure driving experiments to evaluate the OCLDM System in a more naturalistic setting (in a regular office without any electromagnetic shielding). All of them were asked to read and sign the informed consent form before participating in the studies.

The entire experiment consisted of a 1 min training and a ~60 min driving periods. During the training session, subjects were asked to stay fully alert. The averaged alpha power collected in the BC session was used as an alert baseline to determine whether a subject is experiencing cognitive lapses in the driving task. The subject performed the lane-departure driving experiments following the protocol below:

(1) Subjects seated in an armchair and the driving scene was displayed on a 27″ monitor, placed at ~60 cm in front of the subject.
(2) Subjects used a keyboard to control a vehicle cruising on a high way, i.e., a left key turns the simulated car to the left while a right key turns to the right.
(3) Four electrodes were placed over the lateral occipital area to collect EEG data non-invasively. The data were transmitted to a smartphone for processing via Bluetooth.
(4) When the averaged power spectra in alpha band met a certain criterion, arousing auditory warning (~65 dB 1750 Hz tone-burst) would be delivered in half of these lapse episodes through an ear set to the subjects. Note that, the subjects didn't know the warning before the experiments.
(5) The arousing tone-burst would be continuously delivered to the subjects until the averaged power spectra in the alpha band has dropped 3 dB from the lapse power.

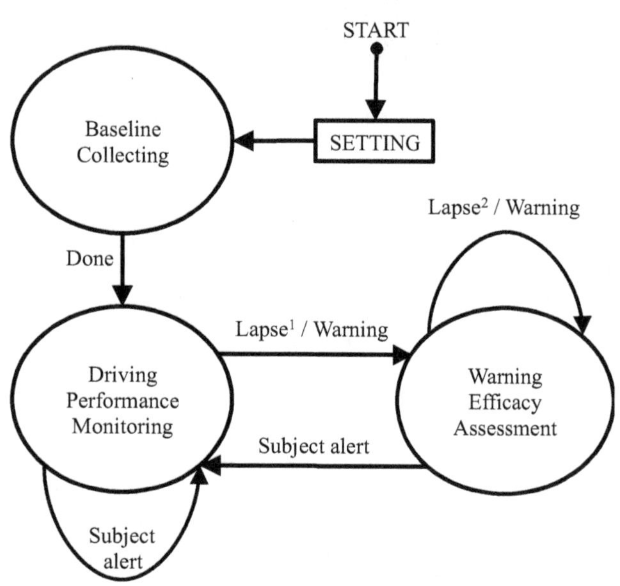

FIGURE 5 | The software state diagram of the OCLDM System. The program first goes through SETTING and Baseline collecting state. Then, the system continuously detects and monitors subjects' driving performance until the EEG spectra indicate cognitive lapse. Note that, Lapse^1 represents the averaged EEG power across four channels is 3 dB over the alert baseline. Lapse^2 represents that the averaged EEG power across four channels has not yet dropped 3 dB from the lapse power.

The cognitive lapses were detected when the subject's alpha-band power (Jung et al., 2010; Lin et al., 2010a, 2013), calculated by a moving-averaged STFT with a 256-point sliding window advanced at 1 s step running on the smartphone, was 3 dB over the alert baseline power (Lin et al., 2010a, 2013 and Results in section Results: Neurophysiological Correlates of Behavioral Lapses). This study used the alpha power fluctuations to monitor cognitive lapses because (1) a recent study showed that the alpha augmentation was sensitive to the transition from full alertness to mediate drowsiness, while the theta augmentation was more sensitive to the transition from mediate to deep drowsiness (Chuang et al., 2012); (2) the empirical results of this study showed that the augmentation of alpha-band power changes was greater than that of the theta-band power (**Figure 2**). The system would repeatedly deliver auditory warning until the alpha-band power amplitude has dropped to 3 dB below the power level when the cognitive lapse was identified.

RESULTS FROM THE OCLDM SYSTEM

The numbers of detected cognitive lapses varied across subjects. **Table 1** lists the numbers of trials with effective, ineffective warning and without warning, respectively. Here, the way we defined the effective trials was based on the RT in response to the lane-departure event immediately following the arousing signal (CT + 1 whose RT was shorter than two times aRT); while the ineffective trials had RT longer than three times aRT.

Table 1 | Number of trials collected from the on-line experiment.

	With auditory warning		Without auditory warning
	Effective	Ineffective	
Subject 1	20	2	21
Subject 2	17	1	24
Subject 3	23	0	27

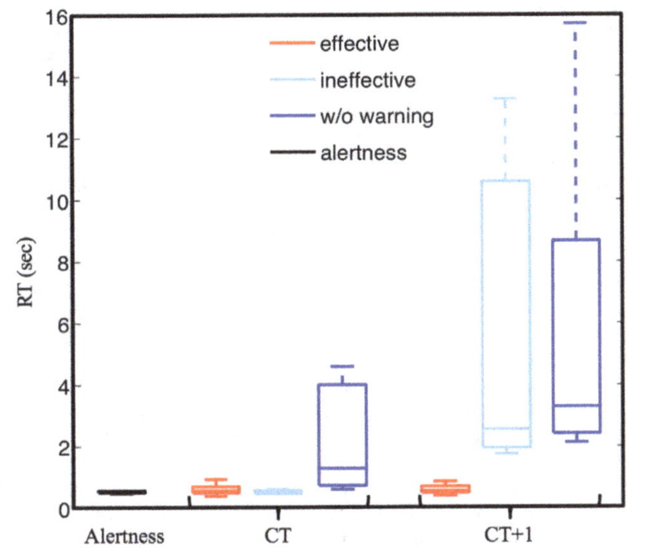

FIGURE 6 | The behavioral performance comparison for the trials of with effective feedback (red), with ineffective feedback (light blue), and without feedback (blue), compared to alert trials (black) after removing the outliers.

Figure 6 shows the boxplot of behavioral performance (RTs) of trials with effective trials (red), ineffective trials (light blue), and without warning (dark blue), compared to the averaged aRT (black) during the on-line experiments. The effective trials had RTs comparable to the averaged aRT (less than 1 s) in both CT and CT + 1. Note that the RTs of CT + 1 with effective vs. ineffective warning differed largely because that was how the effective and ineffective trials were defined. However, the RTs of CT trials (red and light blue) of these two groups of trials were very comparable. That is, even though the subjects responded to the arousing warning by steering the simulated car immediately back to the cruising position, they could well be totally non-responsive to the very next lane-departure event. This finding is consistent to our off-line study reported in section Results: Neurophysiological Correlates of Behavioral Lapses in which the arousing warning was delivered to the subjects who just had a behavioral lapse.

Figure 7 showed the averaged alpha-band spectral time courses across subjects and trials with effective warning (red trace), with ineffective warning (light blue trace), and without warning (dark blue trace), compared to averaged aRT (black trace). All spectral time courses were aligned to the user response onset (thick vertical black line at time 0 s), and the auditory warning for effective- and ineffective-trials were delivered ~5 s before

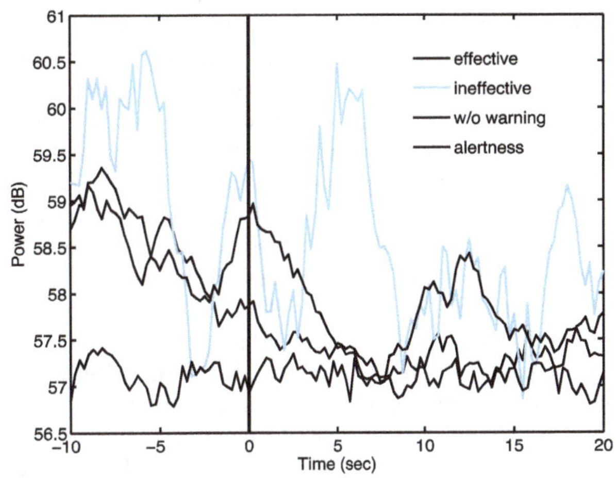

FIGURE 7 | The averaged alpha power time course plotting time-locked to subject response onset (vertical solid line at time 0 s). Averaged alpha power of trials with effective feedback (red trace), with ineffective feedback (light blue), and without feedback (blue trace), compared to trial with aRT (black). The time course of power was estimated by short time Fourier transform with 256 points of time window and 224 points overlapping.

the user response. In the trials following effective auditory warning, the alpha power decreased steadily and reached the averaged aRT in ~7 s. The power spectra remained as low as that of the alert baseline from 7 to 20 s after response onset. In the trials with ineffective auditory warning, the spectral time series fluctuated fierously due to the small number of trials. In the trials without warning, the alpha power fluctuated before response onset and steadily dereased until ~7 s. Thereafter, the alpha power increased again from ~7 to 13 s, suggesting the subjects might be partially arouse by the lane-departure event and their own bebavioral reposense temportally but returned to the fatigue state rapidly thereafter.

DISCUSSIONS

Many studies have shown that the brain dynamics correlated with behavioral lapses can be assessed from EEG data. Recent studies have also shown auditory signals can arouse drowsy subjects and affect EEG activities (Lin et al., 2010a, 2013). However, in these studies, the arousing warning was delivered to subjects after they displayed behavioral lapses, which in reality may be too late because the behavioral lapse might have already had catastrophic consequences. Therefore, a system that features real-time lapse detection and delivers warnings to the drowsy subjects is desirable in preventing catastrophic incidents while driving.

The first experiment of this study showed that EEG power changes in either alpha or theta band can be used as an indicator for assessing the subjects' fatigue (cf. **Figure 3**), and auditory warning temporarily reduces the alpha and theta band power and mitigates the behavioral lapses (cf. **Figure 2A**). In addition, EEG changes after delivery of auditory warning are a good indicator of the efficacy of arousing warning. More importantly and interestingly, empirical results of the first study showed that arousing auditory signals could always reliably mitigate human behavioral lapses, but these immediate behavioral responses could not guarantee the subjects were fully awake, alert, or attentive, similar to snooze after an alarm is turned off. This finding may open a new research direction of how to accurately confirm a subject's cognitive level for some sustained-attention tasks, such as an aircraft navigator or a long-haul truck driver. In other words, further studies to explore the brain changes in this sleep inertia period may provide valuable insights of brain dynamics during a transitional state of lowered arousal occurring immediately after awakening from sleep. Based on previous studies (Lin et al., 2010a, 2013) and the results of the first experiment, this study further developed a truly OCLDM system to detect/predict cognitive lapse based on the EEG spectra, deliver arousing warning on the occurrence of cognitive lapse, and assess the efficacy of the arousing warning, again, based on the EEG spectra. Most importantly, the EEG spectra changes within ~10 s after delivering arousing warning were closely monitored, such that any false-awake situations could be decreased. This study then documented the design, development, and on-line evaluation of the proposed OCLDM System that featured a lightweight wireless EEG acquisition headgear and a smartphone-based signal-processing platform. Experimental results showed that subjects' EEG power could almost remain at the alert state without bouncing back to the drowsy level (cf. **Figure 7**). These results suggest that the proposed system could prevent potential behavioral lapses based solely on the EEG signals, and this demonstration could lead to a real-life application of the dry and wireless EEG technology and smartphone-based signal-processing platform. An interesting question is if the neural correlates of fatigue could be generalized across different sustained-attention tasks and different recording conditions. In the past few years, we have conducted several sustained-attention tasks, including auditory target detection tasks (Makeig and Jung, 1995, 1996; Jung et al., 1997), visual compensatory tracking tasks (Huang et al., 2008), and simulated driving tasks (Lin et al., 2005, 2006, 2008b) and found that performance-related EEG dynamics were comparable across tasks (Huang et al., 2007b). Results of these studies also showed the fatigue-related brain dynamics were quite consistent across different recording environments (within a well-controlled EEG laboratory vs. a 6-degree-of-freedom motion platform) and responding methods (using a button press or a steering wheel). Therefore, it is reasonable to believe the methods developed under this study could be translated from laboratory settings to real-world environments.

In sum, this study demonstrated the feasibility of translating a laboratory-based passive BCI system to a neuroergonomic device that is capable of continuously monitoring and mitigating operator neurocognitive fatigue using a pervasive smartphone in real-world environments. The passive BCI technologies might also be applicable to other real-world cognitive-state monitoring, such as attention, distraction, comprehension, confusion, and emotion. We thus believe more real-world passive BCI implementations will emerge in the foreseeable future.

ACKNOWLEDGMENT

This work was supported in part by US Office of Naval Research, Army Research Office (W911NF-09-1-0510), Army Research Laboratory (W911NF-10-2-0022), and DARPA (DARPA/USDI D11PC20183). This work was also supported in part by the UST-UCSD International Center of Excellence in Advanced Bioengineering sponsored by the Taiwan National Science Council I-RiCE Program under Grant Number: NSC-102-2911-I-009-101, and the Aiming for the Top University Plan of National Chiao Tung University sponsored by the Ministry of Education of Taiwan, under Grant Number 103W963. The authors also appreciate Melody Jung's editorial assistance.

REFERENCES

Bell, A. J., and Sejnowski, T. J. (1995). An information-maximization approach to blind separation and blind deconvolution. *Neural Comput.* 7, 1129–1159. doi: 10.1162/neco.1995.7.6.1129

Bergasa, L. M., Nuevo, J., Sotelo, M. A., Barea, R., and Lopez, M. E. (2006). Real-time system for monitoring driver vigilance. *IEEE Trans. Intell. Transport. Syst.* 7, 63–67. doi: 10.1109/TITS.2006.869598

Campagne, A., Pebayle, T., and Muzet, A. (2004). Correlation between driving errors and vigilance level: influence of the driver's age. *Physiol. Behav.* 80, 515–524. doi: 10.1016/j.physbeh.2003.10.004

Chuang, C.-H., Huang, C.-S., Lin, C.-T., Ko, L.-W., Chang, J.-Y., and Yang, J.-M. (2012). "Mapping information flow of independent source to predict conscious level: a granger causality based brain-computer interface," in *International Symposium on Computer, Consumer and Control (IS3C)* (Taichung: IEEE), 813–816. doi: 10.1109/IS3C.2012.209

Connor, J., Norton, R., Ameratunga, S., Robinson, E., Civil, I., and Dunn, R. (2002). Driver sleepiness and risk of serious injury to car occupants: population based case control study. *BMJ* 324:1125. doi: 10.1136/bmj.324.7346.1125

Croo, H. D., Bandmann, M., Mackay, G. M., Rumar, K., and Vollenhoven, P. V. (2001). *The Role of Driver Fatigue in Commercial Road Transport Crashes.* Etterbeek: European Transport Safety Council.

Davidson, P. R., Jones, R. D., Peiris, M., and Davidson, T. R. (2007). EEG-based lapse detection with high temporal resolution. *IEEE Trans. Biomed. Eng.* 54, 832–839. doi: 10.1109/TBME.2007.893452

Debener, S., Ullsperger, M., Siegel, M., Fiehler, K., Von Cramon, D. Y., and Engel, A. K. (2005). Trial-by-trial coupling of concurrent EEG and fMRI identifies the dynamics of performance monitoring. *J. Neurosci.* 25, 11730–11737. doi: 10.1523/JNEUROSCI.3286-05.2005

Delorme, A., and Makeig, S. (2004). EEGLAB: an open source toolbox for analysis of single-trial EEG dynamics including independent component analysis. *J. Neurosci. Methods* 134, 9–21. doi: 10.1016/j.jneumeth.2003.10.009

Dingus, T. A., McGehee, D. V., Manakkal, N., Jahns, S. K., Carney, C., and Hankey, J. M. (1997). Human factors field evaluation of automotive headway maintenance/collision warning devices. *Hum. Factors* 39, 216–229. doi: 10.1518/001872097778543930

Dong, Y., Hu, Z., Uchimura, K., and Murayama, N. (2011). "Driver inattention monitoring system for intelligent vehicles: a review," in *2009 IEEE Intelligent Vehicles Symposium* (Xi'an), 875–880.

D'Orazio, T., Leo, M., Guaragnella, C., and Distante, A. (2007). A visual approach for driver inattention detection. *J. Pattern Recogn.* 40, 2341–2355. doi: 10.1016/j.patcog.2007.01.018

Eichele, H., Juvodden, H. T., Ullsperger, M., and Eichele, T. (2010). Mal-adaptation of event-related EEG responses preceding performance errors. *Front. Hum. Neurosci.* 4:65. doi: 10.3389/fnhum.2010.00065

Eichele, T., Debener, S., Calhoun, V. D., Specht, K., Engel, A. K., Hugdahl, K., et al. (2008). Prediction of human errors by maladaptive changes in event-related brain networks. *Proc. Natl. Acad. Sci. U.S.A.* 105, 6173–6178. doi: 10.1073/pnas.0708965105

Golz, M., Sommer, D., Trutschel, U., Sirois, B., and Edwards, D. (2010). Evaluation of fatigue monitoring technologies. *Somnologie Schlafforschung und Schlafmedizin* 14, 187–199. doi: 10.1007/s11818-010-0482-9

Ho, C., Tang, H. Z., and Spence, C. (2005). Using spatial vibrotactile cues to direct visual attention in driving scenes. *Transp. Res. F Traffic Psychol. Behav.* 8, 397–412. doi: 10.1016/j.trf.2005.05.002

Horne, J. A., and Baulk, S. D. (2004). Awareness of sleepiness when driving. *Psychophysiology* 41, 161–165. doi: 10.1046/j.1469-8986.2003.00130.x

Huang, R.-S., Jung, T.-P., Delorme, A., and Makeig, S. (2008). Tonic and phasic electroencephalographic dynamics during continuous compensatory tracking. *Neuroimage* 39, 1896–1909. doi: 10.1016/j.neuroimage.2007.10.036

Huang, R.-S., Jung, T.-P., Delorme, A., and Makeig, S. (2009). "Tonic and phasic brain dynamics during responses to simulated driving challenges," in *15th Annual Meeting, Organization of Human Brain Mapping, NeuroImage 47, Supplement 1, S103* (San Francisco, CA).

Huang, R.-S., Jung, T.-P., Duann, J.-R., and Makeig, S. (2006). *Imaging Brain Dynamics during Continuous Driving using Independent Component Analysis, in Human Brain Mapping.* Florence: Wiley Periodicals Inc.

Huang, R.-S., Jung, T.-P., and Makeig, S. (2007a). "Multi-scale EEG brain dynamics during sustained attention tasks," in *Acoustics, Speech and Signal Processing, 2007, ICASSP 2007, IEEE International Conference* (Honolulu, HI), 1173–1176.

Huang, R.-S., Jung, T.-P., and Makeig, S. (2007b). "Event-related brain dynamics in continuous sustained-attention tasks," in *Foundations of Augmented Cognition*, eds D. Schmorrow and L. Reeves (Berlin; Heidelberg: Springer), 65–74.

Jap, B. T., Lal, S., and Fischer, P. (2011). Comparing combinations of EEG activity in train drivers during monotonous driving. *Expert Syst. Appl.* 38, 996–1003. doi: 10.1016/j.eswa.2010.07.109

Jung, T.-P., Huang, K.-C., Chuang, C.-H., Chen, J.-A., Ko, L.-W., Chiu, T.-W., et al. (2010). "Arousing feedback rectifies lapse in performance and corresponding EEG power spectrum," in *Engineering in Medicine and Biology Society (EMBC), 2010 Annual International Conference, IEEE)* (Buenos Aires), 1792–1795.

Jung, T.-P., and Makeig, S. (1995). "Prediction failures in auditory detection from changes in the EEG spectrum," in *Proceeding of the 17th Annual International Conference of the IEEE Engineering in Medicine and Biology Society* (Montreal, QC), 927–928.

Jung, T.-P., Makeig, S., Stensmo, M., and Sejnowski, T. J. (1997). Estimating alertness from the EEG power spectrum. *IEEE Trans. Biomed. Eng.* 44, 60–69. doi: 10.1109/10.553713

Jung, T.-P., Makeig, S., Westerfield, M., Townsend, J., Courchesne, E., and Sejnowski, T. J. (2001). Analysis and visualization of single-trial event-related potentials. *Hum. Brain Mapp.* 14, 166–185. doi: 10.1002/hbm.1050

Kecklund, G., and Akerstedt, T. (1993). Sleepiness in long-distance truck driving: an ambulatory EEG study of night driving. *Ergonomics* 36, 1007–1017. doi: 10.1080/00140139308967973

Lal, S. K., and Craig, A. (2002). Driver fatigue: electroencephalography and psychological assessment. *Psychophysiology* 39, 313–321. doi: 10.1017/S0048577201393095

Lehne, M., Ihme, K., Brouwer, A. M., van Erp, J., and Zander, T. O. (2009). "Error-related EEG patterns during tactile human-machine interaction," in *Affective Computing and Intelligent Interaction and Workshops, 2009. ACII2009. 3rd International Conference* (Los Alamitos, CA), 1–9.

Liao, L.-D., Wang, I.-J., Chen, S.-F., Chang, J.-Y., and Lin, C.-T. (2011). Design, fabrication and experimental validation of a novel dry-contact sensor for measuring electroencephalography signals without skin preparation. *Sensors* 11, 5819–5834. doi: 10.3390/s110605819

Lin, C.-T., Chen, Y.-C., Huang, T.-Y., Chiu, T.-T., Ko, L.-W., Liang, S.-F., et al. (2008a). Development of wireless brain computer interface with embedded multitask scheduling and its application on real-time driver's drowsiness detection and warning. *IEEE Trans. Biomed. Eng.* 55, 1582–1591. doi: 10.1109/TBME.2008.918566

Lin, C.-T., Huang, K.-C., Chao, C.-F., Chen, J.-A., Chiu, T.-W., Ko, L.-W., et al. (2010a). Tonic and phasic EEG and behavioral changes induced by arousing feedback. *Neuroimage* 52, 633–642. doi: 10.1016/j.neuroimage.2010.04.250

Lin, C.-T., Huang, K.-C., Chao, C.-F., Chuang, C.-H., Ko, L.-W., and Jung, T.-P. (2013). Can Arousing feedback rectify lapses in driving? Prediction from EEG power spectra. *J. Neural Eng.* 10:056024. doi: 10.1088/1741-2560/10/5/056024

Lin, C.-T., Huang, T.-Y., Liang, W.-C., Chiu, T.-T., Chao, C.-P., Hsu, S.-H., et al. (2009). Assessing effectiveness of various auditory warning signals in maintaining drivers' attention in virtual reality-based driving environments. *Percept. Mot. Skills* 108, 825–835. doi: 10.2466/pms.108.3.825-835

Lin, C.-T., Ko, L.-W., Chang, M.-H., Duann, J.-R., Chen, J.-Y., Su, T.-P., et al. (2010b). Review of wireless and wearable electroencephalogram systems and brain–computer interfaces—a mini-review. *Gerontology* 56, 112–119. doi: 10.1159/000230807

Lin, C.-T., Ko, L.-W., Chiou, J.-C., Duann, J.-R., Chiu, T.-W., Huang, R.-S., et al. (2008b). Noninvasive neural prosthesis using mobile and wireless EEG. *Proc. IEEE* 96, 1167–1183. doi: 10.1109/JPROC.2008.922561

Lin, C.-T., Ko, L.-W., Chung, I.-F., Huang, T.-Y., Chen, Y.-C., Jung, T.-P., et al. (2006). Adaptive EEG-based alertness estimation system by Using ICA-based fuzzy neural networks. *IEEE Trans. Circuits Syst. I* 53, 2469–2476. doi: 10.1109/TCSI.2006.884408

Lin, C.-T., Wu, R.-C., Liang, S.-F., Huang, T.-Y., Chao, W.-H., Chen, Y.-J., et al. (2005). EEG-based drowsiness estimation for safety driving using independent component analysis. *IEEE Trans. Circuits Syst.* 52, 2726–2738. doi: 10.1109/TCSI.2005.857555

Liu, Y.-C. (2001). Comparative study of the effects of auditory, visual and multimodality displays on drivers' performance in advanced traveller information systems. *Ergonomics* 44, 425–442. doi: 10.1080/00140130010011369

Makeig, S., and Inlow, M. (1993). Lapses in alertness: coherence of fluctuations in performance and EEG spectrum. *Electroencephalogr. Clin. Neurophysiol.* 86, 23–35. doi: 10.1016/0013-4694(93)90064-3

Makeig, S., and Jung, T.-P. (1995). Changes in alertness is principal component of variance in the EEG spectrum. *Neuroreport* 7, 213–216, doi: 10.1097/00001756-199512000-00051

Makeig, S., and Jung, T.-P. (1996). Tonic, phasic, and transient EEG correlates of auditory awareness in drowsiness. *Brain Res. Cogn. Brain Res.* 4, 15–25. doi: 10.1016/0926-6410(95)00042-9

Makeig, S., Jung, T.-P., Bell, A. J., Ghahremani, D., and Sejnowski, T. J. (1997). Blind separation ofauditory event-related brain responses into independent components. *Proc. Natl. Acad. Sci. U.S.A.* 94, 10979–10984.

McDowell, K., Lin, C.-T., Oie, K. S., Jung, T.-P., Gordon, S., Whitaker, K. W., et al. (2013). Real-world neuroimaging technologies. *IEEE Access* 1, 131–149. doi: 10.1109/ACCESS.2013.2260791

National Highway Traffic Safety Administration. (2003). *Drowsy Driving and Automobile Crashes.* New Jersey, NJ: N.H.T.S. Administration.

National Sleep Foundation. (2005). *Summary Findings of the 2005 Sleep in America Poll.* Arlington, VA. Available online at: http://sleepfoundation.org/sites/default/files/2005_summary_of_findings.pdf

Peiris, M. T. R., Jones, R. D., Davidson, P. R., Carroll, G. J., and Bones, P. J. (2006). Frequent lapses of responsiveness during an extended visuomotor tracking task in non-sleep-deprived subjects. *J. Sleep Res.* 15, 291–300. doi: 10.1111/j.1365-2869.2006.00545.x

Rosipal, R., Peters, B., Kecklund, G., Akerstedt, T., Gruber, G., Woertz, M., et al. (2007). "EEG-based drivers'drowsiness monitoring using a hierarchical Gaussian mixture model," in *Foundations of Augmented Cognition*, eds D. Schmorrow and L. Reeves (Berlin; Heidelberg: Springer), 294–303.

Simon, M., Schmidt, E. A., Kincses, W. E., Fritzsche, M., Bruns, A., Aufmuth, C., et al. (2011). EEG alpha spindle measures as indicators of driver fatigue under real traffic conditions. *Clin. Neurophysiol.* 122, 1168–1178. doi: 10.1016/j.clinph.2010.10.044

Spence, C., and Driver, J. (1998). Inhibition of return following an auditory cue. The role of central reorienting events. *Exp. Brain Res.* 118, 352–360. doi: 10.1007/s002210050289

The Royal Society for the Prevention of Accidents. (2001). *Driver Fatigue and Road Accidents. A Literature Review and Position Paper.* Birmingham. Available online at: http://www.rospa.com/roadsafety/info/fatigue.pdf

Wang, Y.-T., Cheng, C.-K., Huang, K.-C., Lin, C.-T., Wang, Y., and Jung, T.-P. (2012). "Cell-phone based drowsiness monitoring and management system," in *2012 IEEE on Biomedical Circuits and Systems Conference (BioCAS)* (Hsinchu), 200–203.

Wolpaw, J. R., Birbaumer, N., McFarland, D. J., Pfutscheller, G., and Vaughan, T. M. (2002). Brain-computer interfaces for communication and control. *Clin. Neurophysiol.* 113, 767–791. doi: 10.1016/S1388-2457(02)00057-3

Zander, T. O., and Jatzev, S. (2012). Context-aware brain–computer interfaces: exploring the information space of user, technical system and environment. *J. Neural Eng.* 9:016003. doi: 10.1088/1741-2560/9/1/016003

Zander, T. O., and Kothe, C. (2011). Towards passive brain–computer interfaces: applying brain–computer interface technology to human–machine systems in general. *J. Neural Eng.* 8:025005. doi: 10.1088/1741-2560/8/2/025005

Zander, T. O., Kothe, C., Jatzev, S., and Gaertner, M. (2010). "Enhancing human-computer interaction with input from active and passive brain-computer interfaces," in *Brain-Computer Interfaces*, eds D. S. Tan and A. Nijholt (London: Springer), 181–199.

Zander, T. O., Kothe, C., Welke, S., and Roetting, M. (2009). "Utilizing secondary input from passive brain-computer interfaces for enhancing human-machine interaction," in *Foundations of Augmented Cognition. Neuroergonomics and Operational Neuroscience*, eds D. Schomorrow, I. Estabrooke, and M. Grootjen (Berlin; Heidelberg: Springer), 759–771.

6

Knowledge-based identification of sleep stages based on two forehead electroencephalogram channels

Chih-Sheng Huang[1,2], Chun-Ling Lin[1,3], Li-Wei Ko[1,4,5]*, Shen-Yi Liu[1,6], Tung-Ping Su[1,6] and Chin-Teng Lin[1,2]*

[1] *Brain Research Center, National Chiao-Tung University, Hsinchu, Taiwan*
[2] *Institute of Electrical Control Engineering, National Chiao-Tung University, Hsinchu, Taiwan*
[3] *Department of Electrical Engineering, Ming Chi University of Technology, New Taipei City, Taiwan*
[4] *Institute of Bioinformatics and Systems Biology, National Chiao-Tung University, Hsinchu, Taiwan*
[5] *Department of Biological Science and Technology, National Chiao-Tung University, Hsinchu, Taiwan*
[6] *Department of Psychiatry, Taipei Veterans General Hospital, Taipei, Taiwan*

***Correspondence:**
Li-Wei Ko, Brain Research Center, Institute of Bioinformatics and Systems Biology, and Department of Biological Science and Technology, National Chiao-Tung University, 416 MIRC., 1001 University Rd., Hsinchu 300, Taiwan
e-mail: lwko@mail.nctu.edu.tw;
Chin-Teng Lin, Brain Research Center and Institute of Electrical Control Engineering, National Chiao-Tung University, 416 MIRC., 1001 University Rd., Hsinchu 300, Taiwan
e-mail: ctlin@mail.nctu.edu.tw

Sleep quality is important, especially given the considerable number of sleep-related pathologies. The distribution of sleep stages is a highly effective and objective way of quantifying sleep quality. As a standard multi-channel recording used in the study of sleep, polysomnography (PSG) is a widely used diagnostic scheme in sleep medicine. However, the standard process of sleep clinical test, including PSG recording and manual scoring, is complex, uncomfortable, and time-consuming. This process is difficult to implement when taking the whole PSG measurements at home for general healthcare purposes. This work presents a novel sleep stage classification system, based on features from the two forehead EEG channels FP1 and FP2. By recording EEG from forehead, where there is no hair, the proposed system can monitor physiological changes during sleep in a more practical way than previous systems. Through a headband or self-adhesive technology, the necessary sensors can be applied easily by users at home. Analysis results demonstrate that classification performance of the proposed system overcomes the individual differences between different participants in terms of automatically classifying sleep stages. Additionally, the proposed sleep stage classification system can identify kernel sleep features extracted from forehead EEG, which are closely related with sleep clinician's expert knowledge. Moreover, forehead EEG features are classified into five sleep stages by using the relevance vector machine. In a leave-one-subject-out cross validation analysis, we found our system to correctly classify five sleep stages at an average accuracy of 76.7 ± 4.0 (*SD*) % [average kappa 0.68 ± 0.06 (*SD*)]. Importantly, the proposed sleep stage classification system using forehead EEG features is a viable alternative for measuring EEG signals at home easily and conveniently to evaluate sleep quality reliably, ultimately improving public healthcare.

Keywords: sleep quality, sleep stages, polysomnography (PSG), electroencephalogram (EEG), sleep stage classification system

INTRODUCTION

Monitoring human physiology during sleep is essential for individual health. Sleep is increasingly viewed as playing an important role in restitution (Akerstedt et al., 2007). As an important aspect of well-being, sleep quality is closely related to overall quality of life, life satisfaction, secretion of the stress hormone, cortisol, and inadequate immunity (Gallagher et al., 2010). Evaluating of sleep quality is especially relevant, owing to a considerable number of pathologies linked to the sleep. Sleep stages are also recorded for clinical diagnosis and the treatment of sleep disorders. Sleep quality is most closely related to the distribution of depth of sleep; indeed, sufficient sleep quality must reach adequate deep sleep. The depth of sleep is characterized by different cortical electrical activities. Several sleep stages can be defined by variations of cortical electrical activities and other physiological signals, i.e., muscle activity and eye movement. According to Rechtschaffen and Kales rules (R&K rules), sleep stage can be segmented into wakefulness, movement time (MT), REM and sleep stages S1, S2, S3, and S4 based on features of EEG, EOG, and EMG (Kales and Rechtschaffen, 1968). In addition to modifying the standard guidelines for sleep classification by R&K, the American Academy of Sleep Medicine (AASM) developed guidelines for terminology, recording method, and scoring rules for sleep-related phenomena (Iber et al., 2007). In the AASM guidelines, sleep stages S1 to S4 are referred to as NREM stage 1 (N1), NREM stage2 (N2), and NREM stage3 (N3). N3 reflects slow wave sleep (SWS, R&K stages S3 + S4).

As the reference standard clinical multi-parametric system, polysomnography (PSG) (Holland et al., 1974) is used in sleep studies to define the different physiological sleep stages and diagnose many sleep disorders, including narcolepsy, restless legs syndrome, rapid eye movement (REM) behavior disorder, parasomnias, and sleep apnea. The PSG system requires a minimum of 11 channels, including electroencephalogram (EEG), electromyogram (EMG), electrooculogram (EOG), oxygen saturation (SpO2), and electrocardiogram (ECG). However, assessing a complete PSG has several limitations. First, PSG is not a portable device and typically placed in a sleep center, which is unfamiliar environment for patients. Second, PSG requires many physiological electrodes and wires placed on the scalp and body, possibly affecting their sleep further. Third, a standard sleep diagnosis in clinical practice is time-consuming and expensive (Zoubek et al., 2007). These processes are monotonous, and time consuming and unproductive. A simpler EEG acquisition and analysis system must be operable by patients for home use, as well as solve current PSG problems.

Recent studies have adopted bioelectrical signals (i.e., EEG, ECG, EMG, and EOG signals), which allow subjects to operate at home in order to develop sleep stage scoring methods, while attempting to obtain results similar to those of experts involved in visual scoring (Park et al., 2000; Anderer et al., 2005; Tian and Liu, 2005; Berthomier et al., 2007; Doroshenkov et al., 2007; Virkkala et al., 2007; Wang et al., 2009; Güneş et al., 2010; Jo et al., 2010; Yılmaz et al., 2010; Eiseman et al., 2011). The classification structure of most of sleep stage classifications consists of feature extraction and classification schemes. The references differ from each other not only in the presented feature extractions and the corresponding classification schemes, but also in different bioelectrical signals used, such as EEG, EOG, or ECG. Feature extraction is a highly efficient means of achieving a satisfactory classification performance in order to develop a sleep stage classification approach. Certainly, if extracted features can achieve a high separability in distinguishing between different classes, classifiers can perform satisfactorily. In recent studies (Berthomier et al., 2007; Doroshenkov et al., 2007; Güneş et al., 2010; Jo et al., 2010), the signal process procedure regards an entire 30-s epoch as a processing unit to extract spectral and temporal information directly. The specific characteristics of sleep stages are smoothened easily within an entire 30-s signal process. For instance, the k-complex and sleep spindle only appear suddenly in a short period with 0.5–1.5 s in a 30-s epoch. Therefore, a short-term signals process should be incorporated when a developing feature extraction approach. Compared with EEG measurement, despite overcoming the hair problem, EOG and ECG still have certain limitations. For instance, EOG and ECG requires adhesive electrode pads, and the locations of EOG (or ECG) and corresponding amplifier are divergent from each other. A subject's sleep position may interfere with the wire, thereby degrading the EOG and ECG signal quality. Despite the persistent hair and conductive gel problems associated with EEG measurement, recent developments to resolve these problems include a headband and portable EEG recording device, as well as a dry polymer foam electrode for long-term EEG measurement (Lin et al., 2008, 2011). Additionally, physiological characteristics during sleep are more easily identified by EEG than by EOG and ECG, explaining why the former is preferred when classifying sleep stages.

Berthomier et al. (2007) assessed an automatic sleep scoring software (ASSEEGA). The system adopts a 3-step procedure for automatic sleep scoring, based on a single EEG channel. In classifying five sleep stages, the agreements between ASSEEGA and two expert manual scorings are 76.0% (kappa = 0.67) and 78.2% (kappa = 0.69). Although highly promising for diagnostic and automatic ambulant scoring. This system still requires 2 bipolar channels (Cz-Pz, international 10–20 standard system), which are located at the back of the skull and hair site, conductive gel, and a laboratory EEG recording device to achieve a high resolution. The connection between hair and conductive gel, and subject's sleep position may also worsen the EEG quality, further lowering the estimation accuracy of the sleep stage.

This work develops a sleep stage classification system via two forehead EEGs, i.e., FP1 and FP2. FP1 and FP2 EEG measurements have the following advantages: non-hairy site EEG recording is performed; the two signals also contain eye movement information; and the system is easily self-adhesive and self-applicable for homecare users and long-term monitoring. The proposed classification system incorporates a novel feature extraction approach, capable of extracting spectral information while considering manual scoring rules. The proposed system further incorporates the relevance vector machine (RVM) as the basic classifier. Importantly, the proposed system provides preliminary results for diagnostic assistance and automatic ambulant scoring to determine whether a patient requires detailed testing with the PSG system in a sleep laboratory. Furthermore, the headband and portable EEG device as well as dry EEG electrodes (Lin et al., 2008, 2011) greatly facilitate the implementation of the proposed system in homecare setting for long-term monitoring of sleep quality, as well as for large-scale population studies.

MATERIALS AND METHODS

SUBJECTS AND DATA ACQUISITION

Ten right-handed adults participated in our study (ten males; mean age 24 ± 6 years). None of the participants reported having a history of psychological disorders. Following a detailed explanation of the experimental procedure, all participants completed a consent form before the experiment. To avoid influences from other external factors, all subjects were instructed not to consume alcoholic or caffeinated drinks or sleeping pills beforehand. The experiments were performed at night (10:00 p.m.–08:00 a.m.). All experimental procedures received approval from the local ethics committee (Institutional Review Board of Taipei Veterans General Hospital, Taiwan).

The sleep PSG signals were recorded with a sampling rate of 128 Hz using Sandman Elite (Sandman Elite, Nellcor Puritan Bennett [Melville] Ltd., Kanata, Ontario, Canada) (**Figure 1D**). All subjects were required to sleep for a single night in the sleep laboratory of National Chiao-Tung University (**Figure 1A**) and wore all PSG electrodes during sleep. The complete PSG recording contains six channels EEG (F3, F4, C3, C4, O1, O2), two channels EOG, chin EMG, leg EMG, airflow signals, lead-II ECG, oximetry, nasal pressure, snoring sounding, and body position (**Figure 1B**). Forehead EEG signals from FP1 and FP2 were also recorded by the same PSG system simultaneously (**Figure 1C**). All of the EEG signals were re-referenced to the opposite lateral mastoids (A1

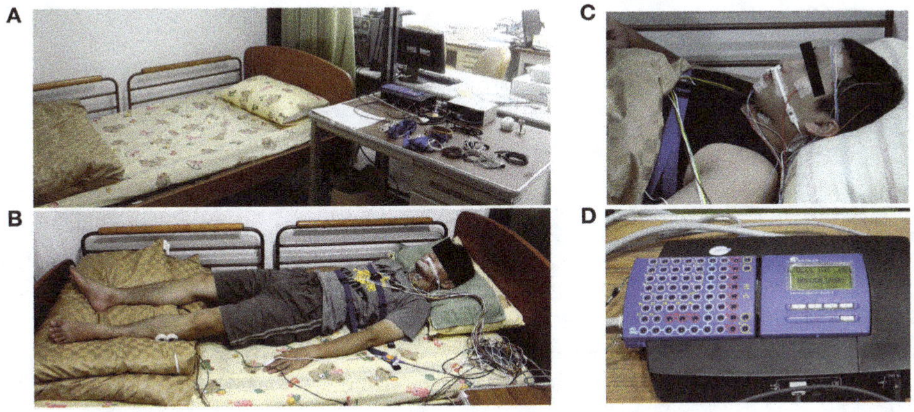

FIGURE 1 | Experiment environment and the polysomnography recording device (Holland et al., 1974). (A) The experiment environment in the sleep laboratory of National Chiao-Tung University. **(B)** The real situation with complete PSG recording. **(C)** The FP1 and FP2 EEG channels are also recorded by the same PSG system simultaneously. **(D)** The PSG amplifier (Sandman Elite, Nellcor Puritan Bennett [Melville] Ltd., Kanata, Ontario, Canada).

Table 1 | Distribution of sleep stages for each subject.

SC	W	N1	N2	N3	REM
S01	286	132	263	117	92
S02	138	46	356	69	81
S03	214	85	182	111	14
S04	88	120	356	156	154
S05	98	124	265	99	87
S06	102	122	267	145	99
S07	301	94	239	148	100
S08	117	105	364	136	189
S09	71	135	336	170	275
S10	103	121	491	132	156
Ratio	18.4%	13.1%	37.8%	15.6%	15.1%

The number in each lattice represents the number of corresponding sleep stages. SC refers to the subject code.

and A2). The contact impedance between all of the electrodes and scalp was controlled to be lower than 5 kΩ. No adjustment or artificial removal techniques were applied to the data. Each data set contained 5–8 h of forehead EEG signals and complete PSG signals.

SLEEP STAGE MANUAL SCORING

Sleep data for each subject were scored visually based on the manual scoring rules of AASM to five sleep stages by an experienced sleep expert. The five sleep stages are W, N1, N2, N3, and REM, and each 30 s sequential epochs was assigned to a sleep stage. **Table 1** summarizes the distribution of sleep stage belonging to subjects.

PROPOSED AUTOMATIC SLEEP STAGES CLASSIFICATION SYSTEM

Visual manual scoring often identifies the different sleep stages based on EEG activities. While attempting to incorporate the advantages of EEG activities of manual scoring rule, this work presents a novel sleep stage classification system embedded with a feature extraction approach, which is inspired by the sleep clinician's expert knowledge in translating two forehead EEG signals to the relevant features, and relevance vector machine (RVM) in order to classify the sleep stages automatically. **Figure 2** displays the flowchart of the proposed sleep stage classification system. As per AASM recommendations, a 30-s sequential EEG recording should function as a unit to assign a sleep stage. In the preprocessing step, all of the 30-s EEG signals are filtered by a band pass filter within 0.5–50 Hz. The following sections described the proposed feature extraction, normalization, and RVM procedures in detail. After RVM, the input 30-s EEG recording assigns a sleep stage. When the recording procedure stops, the final sleep stage results for the whole recording can be estimated.

Feature extraction

Previous studies extracted frequency-domain features by fast Fourier transform (FFT) within the entire30-s signals. However, the previous studies regarded the entire 30-s signals as a processing unit to directly extract frequency-domain features by FFT. Under this circumstance, the specific characteristics of power spectrum density of 30 s signals are easily smoothened, and the corresponding sleep spectral activities are lost, when the characteristics of sleep appear only at a short period in the time signals. The entire 30 s signals contain a significant amount of information, and the spectral information obtained from FFT directly cannot accurately reflect the advantages of the manual scoring rules. To resolve this problem, this work presents a novel feature extraction approach to extract spectral features by short-time Fourier transform and manual scoring knowledge, which retain the properties of temporal manual scoring rules and represent the spectral response in power spectral density. According to the manual scoring rules of AASM (Iber et al., 2007), the EEG activities include alpha rhythm, theta rhythm, K complex, sleep spindle and slow waves. For instance, the epoch is scored the wakefulness when more than 50% of the epoch has alpha (8–12 Hz) rhythm. The epoch is scored as the N1 when alpha rhythm is attenuated and replaced by low amplitude, predominantly theta (5–7 Hz) rhythm for more than 50% of the epoch. The epoch is scored as N2 when the K complex or sleep spindle (12–14 Hz) occurs

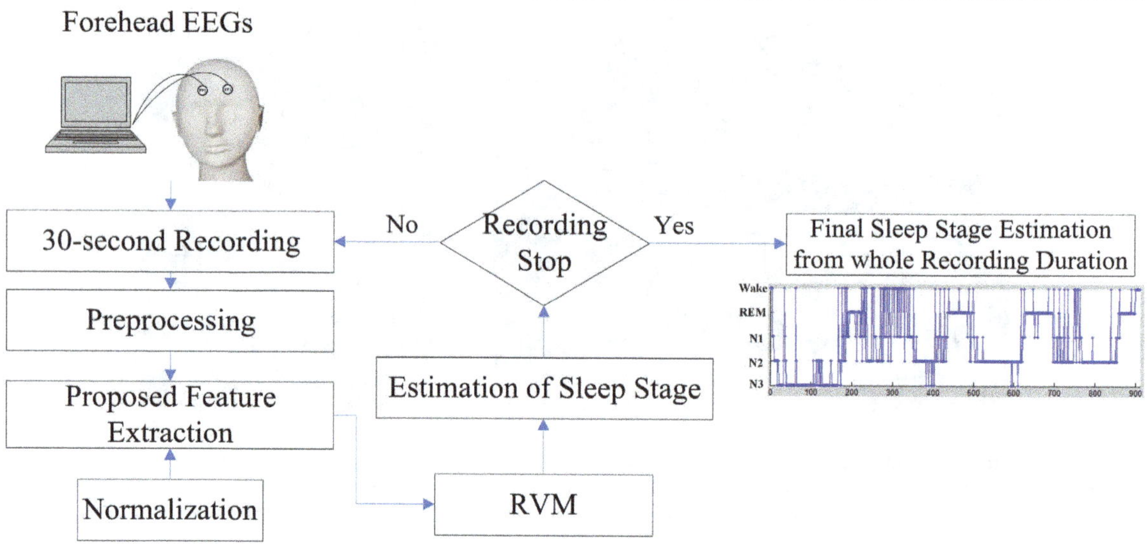

FIGURE 2 | Flowchart of the proposed sleep stage classification system based on the forehead EEG channels (FP1 and FP2).

with the theta background rhythm. The epoch is scored as N3 when more than 20% of the epoch has high amplitude slow wave activity. If a single epoch contains 2 or more stages, the stage that contains the greatest portion of the epoch is assigned.

Figure 3 describes the proposed feature extraction for each 30-s EEG signal. Following the expert knowledge of manual scoring rules, the short-time Fourier transform (STFT) with a 1 s Hamming window overlapped with a 0.5 s window is used rather than using FFT within the entire 30-s signals (**Figure 3A**). Power spectrum densities (PSD) of fifty-nine segments are calculated after using STFT in entire 30-s EEG signals. Following STFT, the PSD of each segment is normalized to avoid individual differences. PSD of each frequency bin of each segment is divided by the total PSD of each segment (**Figure 3B**). Proposed features are identified in the following definition.

The slow wave activity (0.5–2 Hz and amplitude of greater than 75 microvolt) refers to an important index to score N3, and the ratio of slow wave activity has to be greater than 20% visually. Therefore, PSD in lower delta (0.5–2 Hz, denoted as ↓Delta, **Figure 3C**) is chosen to represent the feature of the slow wave activity. Moreover, the average PSDs of the lower delta of upper and lower 80% of 59 segments are viewed as the features of slow wave activity.

As the most important characteristics in visually identifying N2, and K complex and sleep spindle occur spontaneously and roughly every two epochs. K complex is a well-delineated negative sharp wave in EEG immediately followed by a positive component with total duration at least 0.5 s; in addition, sleep spindles are oscillations of sigma (12–14 Hz) with duration of 0.5–1.5 s. Hence, the maximum PSD of sigma band among 59 segments and the average PSD of sigma band of the remaining 58 segments is represented as features of sleep spindle. Moreover, the maximum PSD of delta band (1–4 Hz) among 59 segments and the average PSD of delta band of the remaining 58 segments are represented as features of K complex (**Figure 3C**).

While tending to appear during drowsy, meditative, and sleep onset, theta rhythm scores the epoch as N1, N2, and REM. The average PSDs of theta of upper and lower 50% of 59 segments represent the features of light sleep (N1+N2) (**Figure 3C**).

Movement time, normal resting waking consciousness and wakeful relaxation with eyes closed are accompanied by gamma rhythm (30–50 Hz), beta rhythm (15–30 Hz) and alpha rhythm, respectively. Experts score the epoch as stage wakefulness, when beta and alpha rhythm appear more than 50% of epoch. Thus, the average PSDs of beta and alpha band of upper and lower 50% of 59 segments are represented as the features of stage wakefulness. Movement time stage is mainly accompanied by muscle artifacts obscuring the EEG for more half an epoch. Hence, the average PSD of gamma of 59 segments is represented as the feature of movement time stage (**Figure 3C**).

As mentioned earlier, for FP1 and FP2 EEG channels, sixteen features are extracted, respectively. Two features are extracted as ↓delta activity; two features are extracted as delta activity; two features are extracted as theta activity; two features are extracted as alpha activity; two features are extracted as sigma activity; two features are extracted as beta activity; and one feature is extracted as gamma activity.

For investigating the influence of the proposed feature extraction approach, the conventional PSD feature extraction approach is compared with the proposed one. The conventional PSD feature extraction approach is calculated by the fast Fourier transformation directly for each entire 30-s EEG signal. Notably, this work does not further consider the feasibility of integrating the frequency bins to the specific frequency bands such as delta and theta. The PSD activity ranging from 1 to 50 Hz is used here as input features. Also, for FP1 and FP2 EEG channel, fifty features are extracted, respectively.

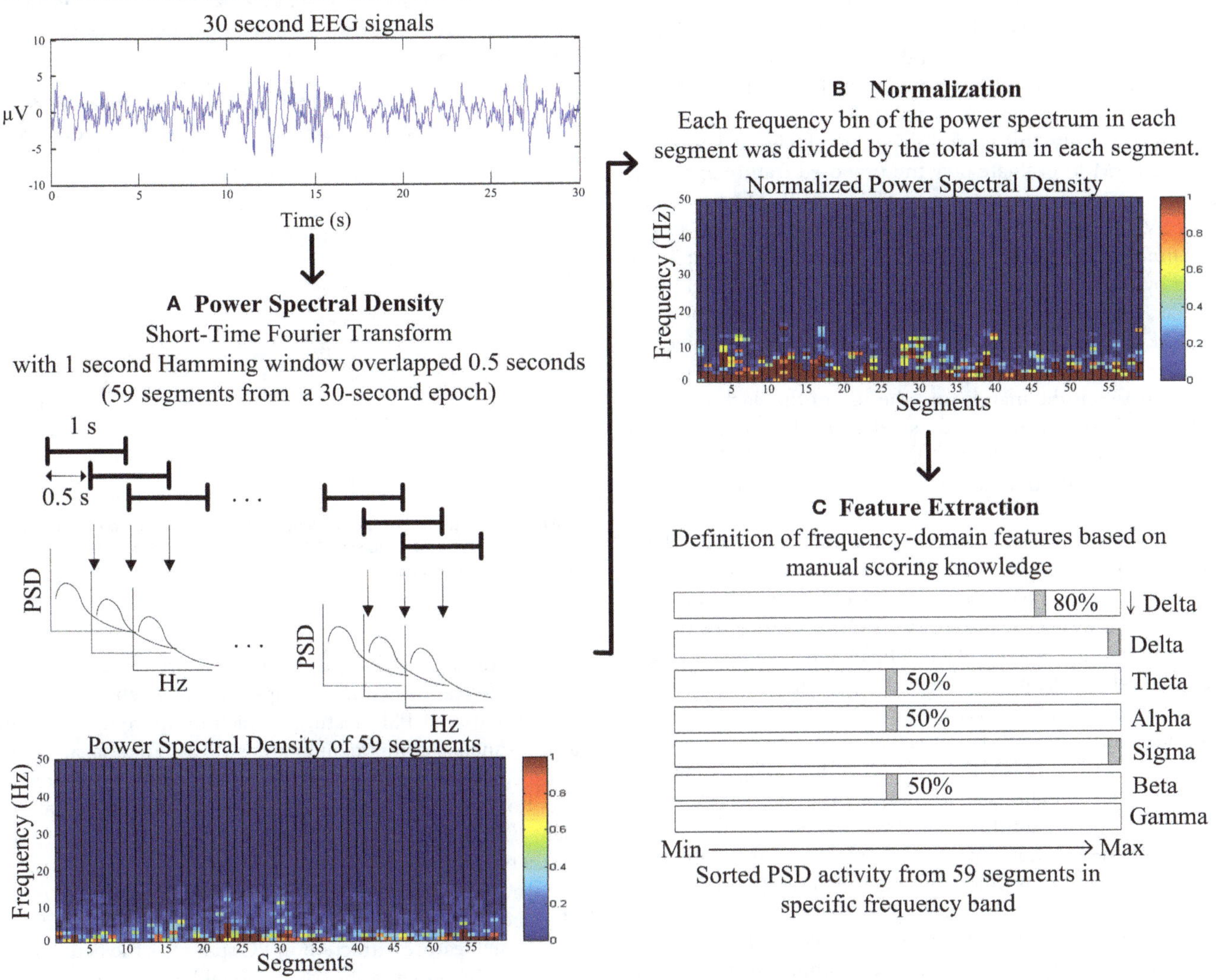

FIGURE 3 | Flowchart of the proposed feature extraction. (A) The power spectral density (PSD) by the short-time Fourier transform (STFT) with a 1 s Hamming window overlapped with a 0.5 s window. **(B)** The normalization for PSD of each frequency bin of each segment is divided by the total PSD of each segment. **(C)** The frequency-domain feature extraction based on the manual scoring knowledge.

Relevance vector machine

Relevance vector machine (RVM) is a learning algorithm based on Bayesian framework and support vector machine (SVM) (Tipping, 2001). RVM has a form similar to that of SVM; they differ in the measurement between binary classes. SVM learns the maximal distance of margins between binary classes, while RVM learns the maximal probability of margins between binary classes. In contrast with RVM, SVM has the following disadvantages: the number of support vectors (SVs) grows with an increasing number of training patterns; the overfitting problem may occur if SVM selects too many SVs; the decision value is derived from the hyperplane function of SVM in the feature space, making its formation as the probability degree impossible; and the penalty parameter of SVM must be set; this penalty parameter significantly influences the classification results. This parameter is generally determined by the cross-validation approach. Further details of RVM and SVM can be found in Tipping (2001).

SYSTEM PERFORMANCE VALIDATION

To illustrate the efficiency of the proposed feature extraction approach, this work evaluates the separability of different feature extraction approaches by using the Fisher criteria (Fukunaga, 1990). Two Fisher criteria are expressed as follow:

$$J_1 = \frac{tr(S_b)}{tr(S_w)}$$

$$J_2 = tr(S_w^{-1} S_b)$$

where S_b and S_w denote the between-class and within-class scatter matrix, and $tr\ (A)$ refers to the trace of square matrix A. A larger J_1 and J_2 imply a larger separability of the presented features in feature space.

Under the extracted feature approaches, this work compares the classification performances of linear discriminate analysis

(LDA) (Fukunaga, 1990), k-nearest neighbor classifier (k-NN) (Fukunaga, 1990), SVM (Chang and Lin, 2011; Li et al., 2012), and RVM (Tipping, 2001). Several trials are performed for k-NN, in which the value of k is varied from 1 to 20, to determine the value that maximizes the accuracy. The selected k in k-NN is 13. For simplicity, this work only adopts the linear kernel for SVM and RVM to evaluate how the proposed feature approach influences. From the perspective of SVM and RVM, the advantage of SVM and RVM is the extension of feature space by the kernel function. The feature space of SVM and RVM is implicitly defined by the kernel function. Hence, two popular kernel functions, i.e., linear and radial basis function (RBF) kernel of SVM and RVM, are more closely examined. As for the SVM, a penalty parameter (also called slack variable) C of SVM, in which the trade-off between the margin and the size of the slack variables in this experiment is controlled, is determined by a grid search within given set {0.1, 0.5, 1, 10, 50, 100, 500, 1000, 1500}. Here, the C selected from the grid search is 50. A grid search is also performed to derive the proper parameter of RBF kernel within a set {0.1, 0.25, 0.5, 0.75, 1, 2, 5, 10, 50, 100, 1000}. Here, the selected parameter of RBF for both SVM and RVM is 0.5.The multiclass strategy in SVM and RVM adopted in this work is a one-against-all strategy (Bottou et al., 1994; Li et al., 2012).

In this work, the sleep PSG data of ten subjects are collected. To evaluate the performance of the proposed classification system, the classification performance is evaluated using leave-one-subject-out cross validation (LOSO). Implementing LOSO involves taking the data from one subject as the testing set and the data from other remaining subjects as the training set; the same procedure is repeated until all subjects are including in the testing set. As is well known, the training data and the testing data should be independent of each other. Restated, the testing information should not be used in the training step. The k-fold cross validation approach is the conventional means of evaluating the classification performance. However, this approach cannot ensure that the training data and testing data are independent. Because the training data and testing data are from different subjects, the training data and the testing data in LOSO are independent. Hence, LOSO is less subjective than the normally adopted k-fold cross validation within the single subject.

This system performance is evaluated using three valid indices, i.e., overall accuracy, sensitivity, and Cohen's kappa coefficient. Overall accuracy refers to proximity of measurement results to the actual value and precision to the repeatability or reproducibility of the measurement. Sensitivity is performed to reflect the ability to identify positive results for each class. Cohen's kappa is a statistical measure of inter-rater agreement or inter-annotator agreement for qualitative (categorical) items (Cohen, 1960). As is generally assumed this measurement is more robust than simple percent agreement calculation since kappa takes into account the agreement occurring coincidentally.

EXPERIMENTAL RESULTS

Performance of the proposed feature extraction approach is evaluated by using Fisher criteria, i.e., J_1 and J_2, to demonstrate the separability. **Table 2** lists the values of J_1 and J_2. Both of J_1 and J_2 in the proposed feature extraction approach are larger than

Table 2 | Separability measurements by using Fisher criterion for the conventional PSD feature extraction and the proposed feature extraction approach.

	Conventional PSD feature extraction	Proposed feature extraction
J_1	0.69	0.74
J_2	1.82	4.57

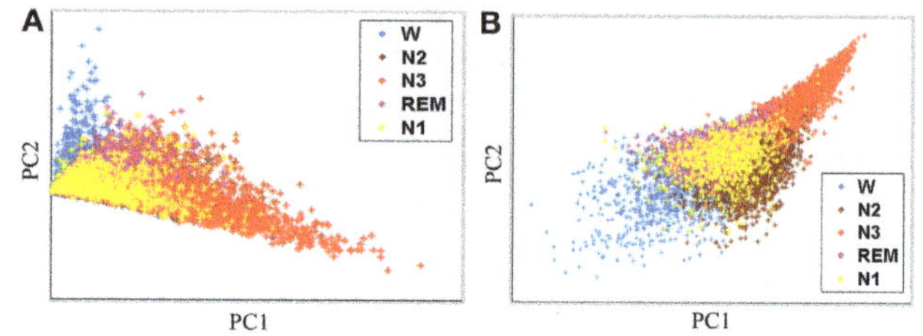

FIGURE 4 | Feature scatter plots with first two principal components (PCs) by (A) the conventional PSD feature extraction, and (B) the proposed feature extraction.

the conventional PSD feature extraction approach, implying that the proposed feature extraction approach has a better separability than conventional PSD feature extraction approach. For illustration, principal component analysis (PCA, Fukunaga, 1990) is performed to decompose the proposed extracted features and conventional frequency PSD features to first two principal components (PCs), respectively. **Figures 4A,B** show the scatter plot of the first two PCs from the conventional PSD feature extraction approach and the proposed feature extraction approach, respectively. These figures clearly reveal that the spatial distribution of the proposed feature extraction in PC space has the better scatter distribution than that of the conventional PSD feature extraction one. The scatter plot of the proposed feature extraction approach presents the scatter points from different groups, i.e., wakefulness, N2, N3, and REM, which are leading ones in their own industries. However, the conventional PSD feature extraction approach can not verify this observation. Most data points from the conventional PSD feature extraction approach are mixing in PC space. Additionally, regardless of in which feature extraction approaches, most of the data points of N1overlap with N2, and REM, because the EEG characteristics of N1 in manual scoring rules closely resemble that of N2, REM.

Figure 5 and **Table 3** display the average classification performances from two feature extraction approaches and four classifiers. The performances, both in terms of overall accuracy and kappa coefficient, of the proposed feature extraction more significantly improves ($p < 0.05$, paired t-test) than the conventional frequency PSD features. The proposed feature extraction approach has an approximately 20% greater increase in overall accuracy and kappa coefficient than the conventional frequency PSD extraction approach. The overall accuracy and kappa coefficient can reach as high as 76.7 and 68.2% by RVM, respectively.

Figure 4 shows scatter plots of the sleep pattern, while **Table 2** lists the separability values of Fisher criteria, which compare the

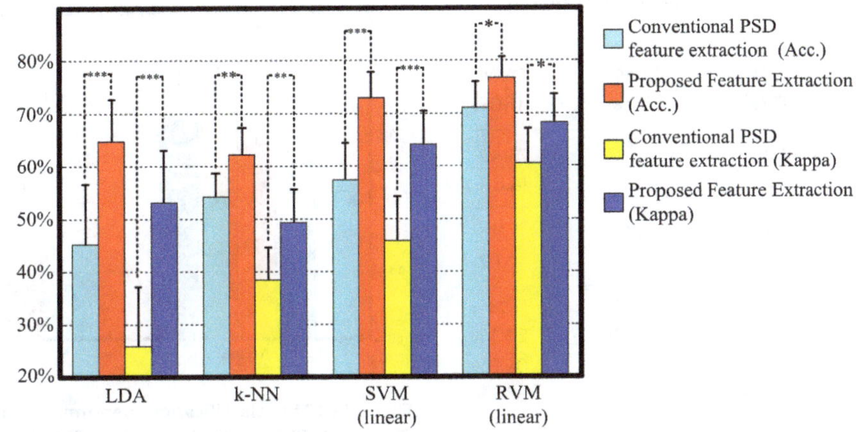

FIGURE 5 | The classification performance comparison between conventional frequency PSD feature extraction and the proposed feature extraction with LDA, k-NN, SVM, and RVM. Acc. and kappa represents overall accuracy and Cohen's kappa coefficient, respectively. Error bars indicate standard deviations. For better visualization, the kappa values have been scaled with the factor 100. $^{*}p < 0.05$, $^{**}p < 0.01$, $^{***}p < 0.001$.

Table 3 | Comparison of feature extraction approaches in terms of classification performance.

		Conventional PSD feature extraction				Proposed feature extraction			
		LDA	k-NN	SVM (linear)	RVM (Linear)	LDA	k-NN	SVM (linear)	RVM (Linear)
Acc.		45.2% (11.4%)	54.2% (4.4%)	57.4% (7.0%)	71.1% (4.8%)	64.7% (7.9%)	62.3% (4.9%)	73.0% (4.9%)	76.7% (4.0%)
Kappa		0.26 (0.11)	0.39 (0.06)	0.46 (0.08)	0.60 (0.07)	0.53 (0.10)	0.49 (0.06)	0.64 (0.06)	0.68 (0.06)
Sensitivity	W	95.7%	61.4%	62.6%	72.7%	58.9%	58.4%	77.2%	79.1%
	N1	8.0%	20.9%	49.3%	14.8%	56.2%	21.4%	41.1%	23.2%
	N2	59.9%	60.5%	47.5%	82.2%	78.2%	70.6%	73.4%	85.6%
	N3	7.1%	56.3%	83.0%	77.7%	83.7%	78.1%	91.3%	87.9%
	REM	10.4%	50.3%	47.2%	80.7%	14.5%	57.6%	63.8%	77.6%

Each lattice represents the mean value of the validation index from ten subjects, and the corresponding bracket is the standard deviation. Acc. and kappa represents overall accuracy and Cohen's kappa coefficient, respectively. Highlighted parts display the optimum performance of all comparison results.

features of the conventional extracted PSD with those of the proposed approach. According to the above results and Fisher criteria, the proposed feature extraction approach has a better separability than the conventional PSD feature extraction approach, as also verified by the classification performance in **Table 3**. The rise in classification performance depends on the proposed feature extraction approach while considering the manual scoring criteria. In particular, the kappa coefficient in the proposed feature extraction approach is increasing significant implying that the proposed method improves both the overall performance of classification and its accuracy for each class with a balance trade-off. For instance, the sensitivity for wakefulness in LDA (conventional PSD feature extraction approach) is 95.7%, i.e., the highest sensitivity of a single class; however, the sensitivity of the other classes is extremely low.

Table 4 and **Figure 6** summarize the results of SVM and RVM with RBF kernel and liner kernel. The optimum result is RVM with linear kernel, in which the accuracy and kappa can reach 76.7% and 0.68, respectively. Next, RVM and SVM are compared, revealing a significant increase in both linear kernel function (over accuracy, $p = 0.012$, paired t-test; kappa coefficient, $p = 0.024$, paired t-test) and RBF kernel function (over accuracy, $p = 0.033$, paired t-test; kappa coefficient, $p = 0.069$, paired t-test). Two kernel functions in SVM and RVM are also compared. Applying the RBF kernel in SVM has a ~1.5% improvement in overall accuracy and kappa coefficient. However, it does not reach a statistically significant level (over accuracy, $p = 0.071$, paired t-test; kappa coefficient, $p = 0.089$, paired t-test). In terms of RVM, applying the RBF kernel in RVM also does not reach a statistically significant level (over accuracy, $p = 0.582$, paired t-test; kappa coefficient, $p = 0.658$, paired t-test).

In terms of SVM, although the number of SVs is normally less than the training patterns, the number of SVs grows larger with an increasing number of training patterns. However, the overfitting problem occasionally occurs in SVM with a large number of SVs. The number of SVs of SVM is generally larger than that of RVs

Table 4 | Performance comparison of different kernel functions in SVM and RVM.

		SVM (Linear)	SVM (RBF)	RVM (Linear)	RVM (RBF)
Acc.		73.0% (4.9%)	74.4% (4.9%)	76.7% (4.0%)	76.4% (4.8%)
Kappa		0.64 (0.06)	0.66 (0.06)	0.68 (0.06)	0.68 (0.07)
Sensitivity	W	77.2%	71.3%	79.1%	79.3%
	N1	41.1%	37.9%	23.2%	24.1%
	N2	73.4%	76.3%	85.6%	84.9%
	N3	91.3%	89.8%	87.9%	86.7%
	REM	63.8%	76.0%	77.6%	77.6%

Each lattice represents the mean value of the validation index from ten subjects, and the corresponding bracket is the standard deviation. Acc. and kappa represents the overall accuracy and Cohen's kappa coefficient, respectively.

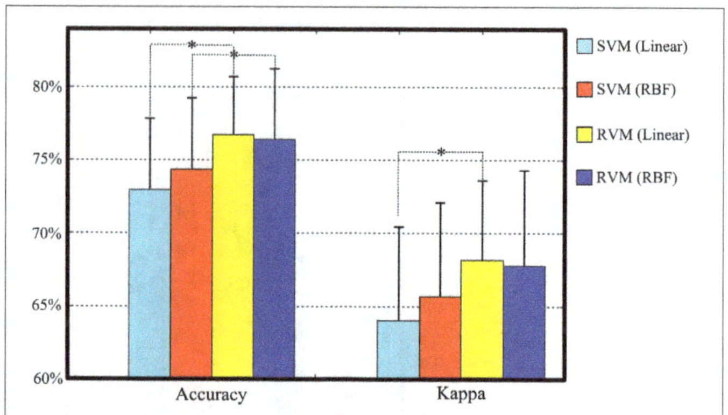

FIGURE 6 | The classification performance comparison between SVM and RVM with linear and RBF kernel functions. Acc. and kappa represents overall accuracy and Cohen's kappa coefficient, respectively. Error bars indicate standard deviations. For better visualization, the kappa values have been scaled with the factor 100. $*p < 0.05$.

in RVM. The number of support vectors (SVs) is also compared with that of relevance vectors (RVs). RVM is characterized by the fewer number of RVs than that of SVs in SVM.

Fewer RVs can avert the overfitting problem. For each subject, the training patterns come from the remained nine subjects, explaining the variation in the number of training patterns. This work adopts the one-against-all multiclass strategy, which is a "one class vs. all others" method, for SVM and RVM. Therefore, the train population is considered from all classes. In the one-against-all multiclass strategy, SVM and RVM train individual decision hyperplane (formula of SVs or RVs and corresponding coefficients) for each class. From ten subjects, the mean of number of train pattern is 7425.9, and standard deviation is 131.4. **Table 5** shows the mean of number of SVs and RVs from linear kernel and RBF kernel. Regardless of whether linear kernel or RBF kernel is adopted, the number of RVs is significantly less than the number of SVs (all p-values are less than 0.0001 with Student's t-test). Although the number of trained SVs is in the thousands, the number of trained RVs only ranges less than several hundred, thus representing a significant difference between RVs and SVs.

To investigating how class imbalance prior influences the classification performance, this work describes the confusion matrix between the proposed sleep classification approach, in which RVM is used with linear kernel function and expert manual scoring (**Table 6**). The overall accuracy and kappa coefficient, as computed from this confusion matrix, are 76.7% and 0.69, respectively. **Table 6** and the performance in **Table 4** demonstrate that the reported validation indices are not biased.

Figure 7 shows the estimation results, based on the proposed classification approach and the manual scoring results for one subject (S07). The top plot is the distribution of the estimated sleep stages from proposed classification, and the below plot is the distribution of the sleep stages from the sleep expert. For this subject, the accuracy between the proposed classification approach and the sleep expert's scoring is 82.5% (kappa = 0.77). The proposed classification approach with only forehead EEG can reach a quite similar performance with the sleep expert.

Table 5 | Number of support vectors in SVM and number of relevance vectors in RVM.

	W vs. others	N1 vs. others	N2 vs. others	N3 vs. others	REM vs. others
SVM (Linear)	1503.0 (105.5)	5276.9 (150.9)	3096.8 (86.8)	921.9 (46.9)	1988.4 (46.3)
RVM (Linear)	18.7 (1.1)	15.9 (1.3)	20 (1)	16.5 (2.1)	22.4 (1.5)
SVM (RBF)	7425.9 (131.4)	7425.9 (131.4)	7425.9 (131.4)	7425.9 (131.4)	7425.9 (131.4)
RVM (RBF)	19.7 (1.4)	22.9 (6.5)	37.1 (2.7)	11.3 (2.0)	41.5 (1.4)

Each block is the mean from all ten subjects, and the corresponding bracket is the standard deviation.

Table 6 | Confusion matrix: proposed sleep classification approach vs. expert manual scoring.

		Proposed Classification					
		W	**N1**	**N2**	**N3**	**REM**	**Sensitivity (%)**
Expert manual scoring	W	1276	103	83	6	50	84.1
	N1	187	243	392	6	256	22.4
	N2	49	117	2652	196	105	85.0
	N3	4	0	154	1117	8	87.1
	REM	28	100	77	4	1038	83.2

DISCUSSION

Based on the scatter plot and Fisher criteria, this work demonstrates that the proposed feature extraction approach can achieve a better separability than the conventional PSD feature extraction approach. The classification performance also demonstrates that the proposed feature extraction approach is more effective

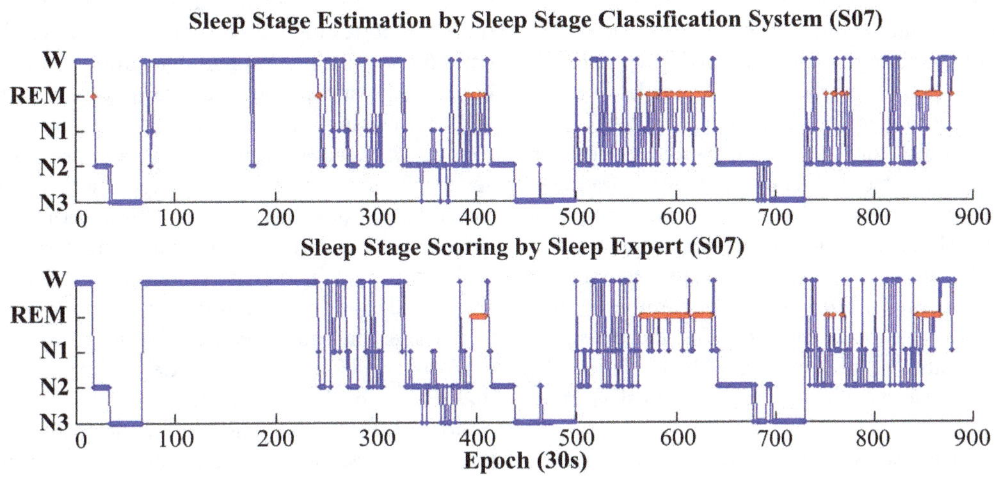

FIGURE 7 | Hypnograms obtained from the proposed sleep stage classification system (top plot) and the sleep expert with manual scoring rules (bottom plot). For this subject (S07), the overall accuracy is 82.5% (kappa 0.77).

than the conventional PSD feature extraction approach in distinguishing between different sleep stages. The proposed feature extraction approach is considered with the sleep stage manual scoring knowledge. Additionally, time-frequency analysis is performed to extract the spectral activities in a short segment window signal not whole 30-s signals. The proposed feature extraction approach characterizes not only by its temporal information of manual scoring, but also by its spectral response. Sleep experts distinguish between the different sleep stages by counting the rhythm and the amplitude of EEG visually by per-second EEG signals from whole 30-s signals. The proposed feature extraction approach applies the short-time Fourier transform with a one second window and overlap 0.5 s. Also, the PSD activity is transferred from STFT to several specific frequency bands, e.g., low delta (1–2 Hz), delta (1–4 Hz), theta (5–7 Hz), alpha (8–12 Hz), sigma (12–14 Hz), beta (15–30 Hz), and gamma (30–50 Hz). With the entire 30-s data, 59 segments are extracted. To overcome the individual differences, the PSD of each segment is divided by the total sum of the PSD of each segment. Hence, the PSD activity in the proposed feature extraction approach is the proportion response of PSD. Based on the expert's manual scoring knowledge, several features are extracted from these specific frequency bands of 59 segments. STFT can achieve the spectral activity of specific frequency response which may be more or less resonant in the spectral space. For instance, the sleep spindle is a sigma rhythm lasting from 0.5 to 1 s, and occurring suddenly. If the fast Fourier transfer is applied to a N2 epoch with one spindle of whole 30-s EEG signals, the specific sigma frequency response cannot be identified clearly. The principal spectral response might be a background spectral response, i.e., theta spectral response, and the amplitude of PSD within the sigma band might be extremely low. However, STFT can separate the signals into several segments in order to calculate the PSD individually. If the spindle occurs, STFT can enhance the corresponding spectral activity more than that of FFT with whole signals. Moreover, in addition, to using STFT to transfer the signals to PSD, this work also proposes sorted power activities to extract the manual rules' properties for the specific frequency spectral activity as the sleep features. The corresponding specific frequency spectral activities are extracted by following the manual scoring rules. For instance, the maximum power of sorted sigma power activities can represent the feature of the sleep spindle. If the current epoch is N2, the value of the maximum power of sorted sigma power activities is higher than that of the maximum power of sorted sigma power activities from the other sleep stages.

The value extracted by average PSDs of alpha and beta of upper 50% of 59 segments from wake stage is higher than that of sleep. The value extracted by the average PSDs of the slow wave of upper 80% of 59 segments from N3 stage is higher than that of other stages. Similarly, the other features from different frequency bands can represent the other sleep stages. Berthomier et al. (2007) characterized several contrast functions, which are feature extraction approaches, as defined by the EEG power activity calculating from whole epoch directly. Although Berthomier et al. (2007) considered the baseline resting EEG frequency of each individual to adjust the spectral criteria, the extracted features were still calculated from the whole 30-s EEG signals. The specific frequency activity still diminishes, when the frequency activity is calculated within the whole 30-s signals. Hence, the proposed feature extraction approach is a more effective means of extracting the sleep characteristics.

SVM has recently achieved higher empirical accuracy and better generalization capabilities than other standard supervised classifiers (Fatma Guler and Ubeyli, 2007; Lotte et al., 2007; Xu et al., 2009; Li et al., 2012). However, as mentioned earlier, SVM is limited in the number of SVs and the selection of penalty parameter. The penalty parameter in SVM is adjusts the generalization capability. RVM is an extension algorithm that eliminates the disadvantages of SVM. SVM learns the maximal distance of margins between binary classes while, in contrast, RVM learns the maximal probability of margins by exploiting a probabilistic Bayesian learning framework between binary classes. The penalty parameter in SVM is usually determined by the cross-validation approach. The chosen penalty parameter depends on the setting candidate set. Too much training time is expended when selecting the penalty parameter in SVM, if the setting candidate set has a wide range. The chosen penalty parameter is a local optimum parameter, depending on the setting candidate set, not the global optimum parameter. The chosen penalty parameter, which affects the number of SVs, incurs the overfitting problem in training phase. RVM can estimate penalty parameters automatically. Additionally, RVM can improve the problem in the number of SVs. Accounting to our results, the number of SVs can significantly decrease in the number of RVs; the classification performance can also be improved by RVM. Hence, the RVM is applied as the basic classifier in the proposed sleep stage classification system.

The detection of N1 is always the most problematic aspect of the sleep stages (Virkkala et al., 2007). Identifying a significant feature in EEG that could separate N1 from wakefulness, N2, and REM, is rather difficult because N1 is a transition phase in the changes of wakefulness and other sleep stages (Virkkala et al., 2007). The sleep EEG characteristics of N1 closely resemble those of N2, REM, and resting wakefulness. Our results demonstrate that the extracted features from PSDs in N1 resemble to N2, REM and resting wakefulness (**Figure 4**). Moreover, many epochs of N1 are misclassified to Wake, N2, and REM (**Table 6**), explaining the difficulty in automatically identifying N1 by a computer. Efforts are underway in our laboratory to address this problem.

Recent efforts have attempted to develop a more reliable sleep system with few bioelectrical channels, i.e., one EEG, one ECG, or two EOGs, in order to simplify the complex PSG inspection (Berthomier et al., 2007; Virkkala et al., 2007; Yılmaz et al., 2010). Virkkala et al. (2007) devised an automatic sleep stage classification via two EOGs. The performances (Virkkala et al., 2007) with 5 sleep stages are 72.5% epoch-to-epoch agreement and 0.63 Cohen's kappa, and the sensitivity of Wake, REM, N1, N2, and SWS are 74.10, 72.7, 39.2, 79.1, and 73%, respectively. Although this work applies two channel signals, the FP1 and FP2 EEGs, which can reflect the eye movement, have more information in classifying sleep stages. Hence, both the characteristics of sleep EEG and eye movement are captured. Additionally, the proposed classification system accurately estimates sleep stages. Yılmaz et al. (2010) presented a sleep stage and obstructive apneic epoch classification via single-lead ECG. The performances (Yılmaz et al., 2010) with 6 sleep stages are 73.1% epoch-to-epoch agreement, and the sensitivities of Wake, REM, NREM1, NREM 2,NREM 3, and NREM 4 are 95.6, 84.9, 98.5, 61.8, 94.3, and 87.4%, respectively.

Performance of the classification (Yılmaz et al., 2010) is satisfactory, even the sensitivity of NREM 1 (98.5%), which is the most difficult sleep stage to be identified automatically (Berthomier et al., 2007; Virkkala et al., 2007). Yılmaz et al. (2010) applied the 10-fold cross validation within a single subject data, which totally separates a subject's self-data as the training data and also as the testing data. For instance, for a subject with total 800 epochs, partitioning produces 10 subsets with 80 epochs each. Therefore, the training set (720 epochs) and testing set (80 epochs) include totally separate sets of data. The training set and testing set originate from a specific subject. Moreover, the properties of training and testing data resemble each other, the corresponding with the over-fitting problem in training phase. Notably, attempting to use a subject-dependence model by a specific subject in order to classify another independent dataset may cause worst results. LOSO cross-validation is a more objective evaluation approach for machine learning experiment involving human subjects to allow for subject-to-subject variation. The testing data are subject-independent to the training data. Hence, the performance evaluation by LOSO is more effective and reliable than k-fold cross validation in developing a general model involving human subjects. As mentioned earlier, the right and left EOG signals are recorded by placing two electrodes at the nasal and temporal canthal regions of the eye, in which one electrode is attached to the middle of the forehead as ground electrode while another electrode is placed on the left mastoid M1 as reference electrode. ECG signals are acquired by two electrodes in a modified leads II configuration (Malmivuo and Plonsey, 1995). The positive and negative leads are placed on the fourth inter costal space and the left of the sternum. Also, both of the EOGs and ECG still require adhesive electrode pads, and the locations of EOGs (or ECG) and corresponding amplifier diverge from each other. The sleep position may affect the recording quality of physiological signals. Berthomier et al. (2007) presented an ASSEEGA based on an EEG channel. In terms of performance, the proposed sleep stage classification system is nearly equivalent to the ASSEEGA. However, ASSEEGA still requires 2 bipolar channels (Cz-Pz, international 10–20 standard system), making it infeasible for homecare applications. First, the position of electrodes is not easily identified, self-adhesive, and self-applicable for a self-operating user. Second, the conductive gel and a laboratory EEG recording device are still required in the recording signals. Although several portable EEG devices (e.g., Mindo-4S (Mindo, Hsinchu, Taiwan), MindWave Mobile (NeuroSky, CA, USA), and Emotiv epoc headset (Emotiv, Eveleigh NSW, Australia), as well as dry sensors) can overcome this problem, the comfort of dry electrodes of Cz and Pz is still a major challenge during sleep.

Anderer et al. (2005) recently developed and optimized an automatic classification system based on a central EEG channel, two EOG channels and a chin EMG channel; in addition, the final validation of overall epoch-by-epoch agreement is 80% (Cohen's kappa is 0.72) between the proposed automatic classification system and human expert scoring. Obviously, the data-rich recordings have more information, e.g., sleep brain electrical activity from EEG, muscle activity from EMG, and eye movement from EOGs. Such information-rich physiological data provide more important indices to classify the difference between REM and light sleep, i.e., the rapid eye movement and the lowest mandible muscle activity. Hence, the data-rich recording can achieve an excellent performance. Although the performance in this work is not equivalent to that of the classification system (Anderer et al., 2005), the proposed system attempts to reduce the number of full PSG signals to fewer physiological channels, as well as further classify the sleep stages effectively. Therefore, the proposed system uses forehead EEGs, i.e., FP1 and FP2. FP1 and FP2 have the following advantages: the physiological data include information from sleep brain electrical activity and eye movement; and adopting the forehead EEGs makes it feasible for self-application for a self-operating user. With the portable EEG device (Lin et al., 2008) and dry sensors (Lin et al., 2011), home-based users can easily to wear the EEG headband to record the sleep forehead EEG signals by self-applicable. Furthermore, we can further analyze with the collected data can be analyzed further, even leading to the development of on-line sleep stage classification software.

Despite its contributions, this work has certain limitations. The collected data are limited to young and healthy study participants. The sleep stages in normal person are expected to diverge from the norm and to be more heterogeneous than those of older or younger, healthy individuals or patients. The sleep stage manual scoring rules are based on counting the rhythm of different frequency activities. The proposed system attempts to comply with this criterion in order to extract the sleep features. The system also uses STFT as temporal and visual rules, i.e., processing the signal within one-second window, and further extracts features by PSDs representing different rhythms of different frequency activities. This system is created by the healthy subjects, and does not have obvious evidence to verify that the proposed sleep stage classification is reliable in older individuals or patients. Therefore, efforts are underway in our laboratory to study the relation between patients and the proposed sleep stage classification system.

CONCLUSION

This work presents a novel sleep stage classification system, consisting of a novel feature extraction method and RVM classifier, based on only two forehead EEG channels. Also, the classification performance is consistent with the sleep clinician's expert knowledge. Experimental results demonstrate the feasibility of using the proposed system as the preliminary screening results for a preclinical diagnosis to assist clinicians in making a diagnosis (rather having a depth testing with PSG system in a sleep laboratory) to reduce time for the procedure. Moreover, the proposed system only uses two forehead EEG signals, allowing us to apply the wearable and wireless EEG recording device (Lin et al., 2008; Liao et al., 2012) [e.g., Mindo-4S (Mindo, Hsinchu, Taiwan) and MindWave Mobile (NeuroSky, CA, USA)] in order to record the patient's EEG signals at home. Importantly, the proposed system provides an easier way for large population studies, long-term sleep monitoring, and home-based daily care. Efforts are underway in our laboratory to integrate the wearable and wireless EEG recording device and the proposed sleep stage classification system. As an important aspect of performance, the automatic artifact detection might be a possible way to improve the efficacy of the proposed system. Hence, the efficacy of the automatic artifact detection should be considered in the proposed system in the future work.

ACKNOWLEDGMENTS

This work was supported in part by the Aiming for the Top University Plan of National Chiao Tung University, the Ministry of Education, Taiwan, under Contract 102W9633, and in part by UST-UCSD International Center of Excellence in Advanced Bioengineering sponsored by the Ministry of Science and Technology I-RiCE Program under Grant Number: NSC-102-2911-I-009-101. Research was sponsored by the Army Research Laboratory and was accomplished under Cooperative Agreement Number W911NF-10-2-0022. The views and the conclusions contained in this document are those of the authors and should not be interpreted as representing the official policies, either expressed or implied, of the Army Research Laboratory or the U.S Government. The U.S Government is authorized to reproduce and distribute reprints for Government purposes notwithstanding any copyright notation herein.

REFERENCES

Akerstedt, T., Kecklund, G., and Gillberg, M. (2007). Sleep and sleepiness in relation to stress and displaced work hours. *Physiol. Behav.* 92, 250–255. doi: 10.1016/j.physbeh.2007.05.044

Anderer, P., Gruber, G., Parapatics, S., Woertz, M., Miazhynskaia, T., Klösch, G., et al. (2005). An E-health solution for automatic sleep classification according to Rechtschaffen and Kales: validation study of the Somnolyzer 24× 7 utilizing the Siesta database. *Neuropsychobiology* 51, 115–133. doi: 10.1159/000085205

Berthomier, C., Drouot, X., Herman-Stoica, M., Berthomier, P., Prado, J., Bokar-Thire, D., et al. (2007). Automatic analysis of single-channel sleep EEG: validation in healthy individuals. *Sleep* 30, 1587–1595. Available online at: http://www.journalsleep.org/ViewAbstract.aspx?pid=26998

Bottou, L., Cortes, C., Denker, J. S., Drucker, H., Guyon, I., Jackel, L. D., et al. (1994). "Comparison of classifier methods: a case study in handwritten digit recognition," in *Proceedings of the 12th IAPR International. Conference on Pattern Recognition - Conference B: Computer Vision & Image Processing*, (Jerusalem), 77–82.

Chang, C.-C., and Lin, C.-J. (2011). LIBSVM: a library for support vector machines. *ACM Trans. Intell. Syst. Technol.* 2, 1–27. doi: 10.1145/1961189.1961199

Cohen, J. (1960). A coefficient of agreement for nominal scales. *Educ. Psychol. Meas.* 20, 37–46. doi: 10.1177/001316446002000104

Doroshenkov, L., Konyshev, V., and Selishchev, S. (2007). Classification of human sleep stages based on EEG processing using hidden Markov models. *Biomed. Eng.* 41, 25–28. doi: 10.1007/s10527-007-0006-5

Eiseman, N. A., Westover, M. B., Mietus, J. E., Thomas, R. J., and Bianchi, M. T. (2011). Classification algorithms for predicting sleepiness and sleep apnea severity. *J. Sleep Res.* 21, 101–112. doi: 10.1111/j.1365-2869.2011.00935.x

Fatma Guler, N., and Ubeyli, E. D. (2007). Multiclass support vector machines for EEG-signals classification. *IEEE Trans. Inf. Technol. Biomed.* 11, 117–126. doi: 10.1109/TITB.2006.879600

Fukunaga, K. (1990). *Introduction to Statistical Pattern Recognition, 2nd Edn.* San Diego, CA: Academic Press Professional, Inc.

Gallagher, S., Phillips, A. C., and Carroll, D. (2010). Parental stress is associated with poor sleep quality in parents caring for children with developmental disabilities. *J. Pediatr. Psychol.* 35, 728–737. doi: 10.1093/jpepsy/jsp093

Güneş, S., Polat, K., and Yosunkaya, Ş. (2010). Efficient sleep stage recognition system based on EEG signal using k-means clustering based feature weighting. *Expert Syst. Appl.* 37, 7922–7928. doi: 10.1016/j.eswa.2010.04.043

Holland, J. V., Dement, W. C., and Raynal, D. M. (1974). "Polysomnography: a response to a need for improved communication," in *14th Annual Meeting of the Association for the Psychophysiological Study of Sleep* (Jackson Hole, WY), 121–122.

Iber, C., Ancoli-Israel, S., Chesson, A., and Quan, S. (2007). *The AASM Manual for the Scoring of and Associated Events: Rules, Terminology and Technical Specifications.* Westchester, IL: American Academy of Sleep Medicine.

Jo, H. G., Park, J. Y., Lee, C. K., An, S. K., and Yoo, S. K. (2010). Genetic fuzzy classifier for sleep stage identification. *Comput. Biol. Med.* 40, 629–634. doi: 10.1016/j.compbiomed.2010.04.007

Kales, A., and Rechtschaffen, A. (1968). *A Manual of Standardized Terminology, Techniques, and Scoring System for Sleep Stages of Human Subjects.* Los Angeles, CA: Brain Information Service. Brain Research Institute, University of California.

Li, C.-H., Kuo, B.-C., Lin, C.-T., and Huang, C.-S. (2012). A spatial-contextual support vector machine for remotely sensed image classification. *IEEE Trans. Geosci. Remote Sens.* 50, 784–799. doi: 10.1109/TGRS.2011.2162246

Liao, L.-D., Chen, C.-Y., Wang, I.-J., Chen, S.-F., Li, S.-Y., Chen, B.-W., et al. (2012). Gaming control using a wearable and wireless EEG-based brain-computer interface device with novel dry foam-based sensors. *J. Neuroeng. Rehabil.* 9:5. doi: 10.1186/1743-0003-9-5

Lin, C.-T., Ko, L.-W., Chiou, J.-C., Duann, J.-R., Huang, R.-S., Liang, S.-F., et al. (2008). Noninvasive neural prostheses using mobile and wireless EEG. *Proc. IEEE* 96, 1167–1183. doi: 10.1109/JPROC.2008.922561

Lin, C. T., Liao, L. D., Liu, Y. H., Wang, I. J., Lin, B. S., and Chang, J. Y. (2011). Novel dry polymer foam electrodes for long-term EEG measurement. *IEEE Trans. Biomed. Eng.* 58, 1200–1207. doi: 10.1109/TBME.2010.2102353

Lotte, F., Congedo, M., Lécuyer, A., Lamarche, F., and Arnaldi, B. (2007). TOPICAL REVIEW: a review of classification algorithms for EEG-based brain computer interfaces. *J. Neural Eng.* 4, R1–R13. doi: 10.1088/1741-2560/4/2/R01

Malmivuo, J., and Plonsey, R. (1995). *Bioelectromagnetism: Principles and Applications of Bioelectric and Biomagnetic Fields.* New York, NY: Oxford University Press.

Park, H. J., Oh, J. S., Jeong, D. U., and Park, K. S. (2000). Automated sleep stage scoring using hybrid rule-and case-based reasoning. *Comput. Biomed. Res.* 33, 330–349. doi: 10.1006/cbmr.2000.1549

Tian, J. Y., and Liu, J. Q. (2005). "Automated sleep staging by a hybrid system comprising neural network and fuzzy rule-based reasoning," in *Engineering in Medicine and Biology Society. IEEE-EMBS* 2005. *27th Annual International Conference* (Shanghai), 4115–4118.

Tipping, M. E. (2001). Sparse bayesian learning and the relevance vector machine. *J. Mach. Learn. Res.* 1, 211–244. doi: 10.1162/15324430152748236

Virkkala, J., Hasan, J., Värri, A., Himanen, S. L., and Müller, K. (2007). Automatic sleep stage classification using two-channel electro-oculography. *J. Neurosci. Methods* 166, 109–115. doi: 10.1016/j.jneumeth.2007.06.016

Wang, B., Sugi, T., Kawana, F., Wang, X., and Nakamura, M. (2009). Expert knowledge-based automatic sleep stage determination by multi-valued decision making method. *IEEJ Trans. Electron. Inf. Syst.* 129, 614–619. doi: 10.1541/ieejeiss.129.614

Xu, Q., Zhou, H., Wang, Y., and Huang, J. (2009). Fuzzy support vector machine for classification of EEG signals using wavelet-based features. *Med. Eng. Phys.* 31, 858–865. doi: 10.1016/j.medengphy.2009.04.005

Yılmaz, B., Asyalı, M. H., Arıkan, E., Yetkin, S., and zgen, F. (2010). Sleep stage and obstructive apneaic epoch classification using single-lead ECG. *Biomed. Eng. Online* 9:39. doi:10.1186/1475-925X-9-39

Zoubek, L., Charbonnier, S., Lesecq, S., Buguet, A., and Chapotot, F. (2007). Feature selection for sleep/wake stages classification using data driven methods. *Biomed. Signal Process. Control* 2, 171–179. doi: 10.1016/j.bspc.2007.05.005

7

Brain fingerprinting classification concealed information test detects US Navy military medical information with P300

Lawrence A. Farwell[1]*, Drew C. Richardson[2], Graham M. Richardson[3] and John J. Furedy[4]

[1] *Brain Fingerprinting Laboratories, Inc./Brain Fingerprinting, LLC, Seattle, WA, USA*
[2] *Federal Bureau of Investigation, FBI Laboratory, Quantico, VA, USA (at the time of the research)*
[3] *Department of Cell and Developmental Biology, Vanderbilt University, Nashville, TN, USA*
[4] *Department of Psychology, University of Toronto, Toronto, ON, Canada*

Correspondence:
Lawrence A. Farwell, Brain Fingerprinting Laboratories, Inc., 14220 37th Ave. NE, Seattle, WA 98125, USA
e-mail: brainwave@larryfarwell.com

A classification concealed information test (CIT) used the "brain fingerprinting" method of applying P300 event-related potential (ERP) in detecting information that is (1) acquired in real life and (2) unique to US Navy experts in military medicine. Military medicine experts and non-experts were asked to push buttons in response to three types of text stimuli. Targets contain known information relevant to military medicine, are identified to subjects as relevant, and require pushing one button. Subjects are told to push another button to all other stimuli. Probes contain concealed information relevant to military medicine, and are not identified to subjects. Irrelevants contain equally plausible, but incorrect/irrelevant information. Error rate was 0%. Median and mean statistical confidences for individual determinations were 99.9% with no indeterminates (results lacking sufficiently high statistical confidence to be classified). We compared error rate and statistical confidence for determinations of both information present and information absent produced by classification CIT (Is a probe ERP more similar to a target or to an irrelevant ERP?) vs. comparison CIT (Does a probe produce a larger ERP than an irrelevant?) using P300 plus the late negative component (LNP; together, P300-MERMER). Comparison CIT produced a significantly higher error rate (20%) and lower statistical confidences: mean 67%; information-absent mean was 28.9%, less than chance (50%). We compared analysis using P300 alone with the P300 + LNP. P300 alone produced the same 0% error rate but significantly lower statistical confidences. These findings add to the evidence that the brain fingerprinting methods as described here provide sufficient conditions to produce less than 1% error rate and greater than 95% median statistical confidence in a CIT on information obtained in the course of real life that is characteristic of individuals with specific training, expertise, or organizational affiliation.

Keywords: P300, concealed information test, brain fingerprinting, P300-MERMER, ERP, LNP, event-related potential, detection of concealed information

INTRODUCTION

THE CLASSIFICATION CIT

The concealed information test (CIT) or guilty knowledge test (GKT) has been used to detect concealed information since Lykken (1959). Until the 1980s, the dependent measures were autonomic nervous system (ANS) responses. The ANS-based CIT is a *comparison* CIT (Lykken, 1959). The comparison CIT compares the responses to crime- or situation-relevant and irrelevant items. If the responses to the relevant items are larger, then the determination is made that the subject knows the relevant information. ("Larger" is variously defined.) Otherwise, the determination is made that the subject does not know the information.

Farwell and Donchin (1991) introduced three innovations in the CIT (Farwell, 2013). They (1) applied a classification CIT, rather than the conventional comparison CIT; (2) used event-related brain potentials (ERPs) as the dependent measure; and (3) computed a statistical confidence for each individual determination using the technique of bootstrapping. (Farwell and Donchin, 1991 was preceded by abstracts on the same studies, Farwell and Donchin, 1986, 1988a). Several researchers subsequently applied ERPs and bootstrapping in a comparison CIT (e.g., Johnson and Rosenfeld, 1992; Rosenfeld et al., 2004, 2008; Meixner and Rosenfeld, 2014). This is a fundamentally different paradigm (see Discussion and Appendix 2).

In the classification CIT, three types of stimuli are presented. (1) "Probes" are relevant to the investigated situation. Probes contain information that the subject has no way of knowing other than participation in the investigated situation (and, in field cases, that the subject denies knowing or recognizing as being crime-relevant). (2) "Targets" also may be relevant to the investigated situation. (In all our recent applications including the study reported here, they are.) Experimental protocols ensure that the subject knows the targets, for reasons other than participation in the investigated situation. The response to targets provides a template for the subject's response to known, situation-relevant information. (3) "Irrelevants" contain irrelevant information. The response to irrelevants provides a template for the subject's response to irrelevant information. If the ERP response to the probes is mathematically classified as being more similar to the ERP response to the known, relevant target information than to the irrelevants, the subject is determined to be "information present" with respect to the information contained in the probes. If the ERP response to the probes is more similar to the ERP response to the irrelevant information than to the targets, the subject is determined to be "information absent." If the probe ERP response cannot be classified with a high statistical confidence as being more similar to either the target or the irrelevant response, no determination is made; the outcome is "indeterminate."

The classification CIT with ERPs can be applied in two different types of tests. Specific issue tests detect knowledge of a specific event such as a crime. Specific screening or focused screening tests detect knowledge relevant to specific training or expertise, or inside knowledge of a particular organization or group. This study is a specific screening test conducted in collaboration with the US Central Intelligence Agency (CIA) and the US Navy. The information detected is military medical knowledge in US Navy military medical experts.

We compared the classification CIT with the comparison CIT by analyzing our data with both methods. Farwell and Donchin (1991) used the classification CIT with the P300, an electrically positive event-related potential (ERP) maximal at the parietal midline area of the head that is elicited when a subject recognizes and takes note of a stimulus that is significant in the current context. In this research we compared the results of using the P300 alone vs. the P300 plus the late negative component (LNP; together, P300-MERMER, memory and encoding related multifaceted electroencephalographic response)[1] . We compared error rate and statistical confidences produced by the classification CIT with the results of analysis applying the comparison CIT on the same data. We investigated whether the classification CIT provides significantly lower error rate and higher statistical confidences than the comparison CIT.

PREVIOUS RESEARCH ON SUFFICIENT AND NECESSARY CONDITIONS FOR A VIABLE CIT FOR REAL-WORLD FIELD USE

In our view, in order to be considered reliable, an ERP-based CIT must reliably produce less than 1% error rate and median statistical confidences of greater than 95% for individual determinations, including median statistical confidences greater than 90% for both information-present and information-absent determinations, across different field and laboratory conditions. These same criteria, in our view, are the minimum criteria required to effectively and ethically apply a technique in criminal investigations or any application with non-trivial consequences.

Farwell and Donchin's (1991) method provided the sufficient conditions to meet these requirements. They only established sufficient conditions, and did not investigate which conditions were necessary. Since then, research has progressed substantially in two parallel, largely non-overlapping series of studies. One series of studies has investigated the sufficient conditions to meet these criteria under varying field and laboratory conditions. Another series of studies has investigated the necessary conditions.

Eight previous peer-reviewed studies conducted by six researchers in four laboratories have applied a specific set of methods in the ERP-based CIT [Farwell and Donchin, 1991 (two studies); Allen and Iacono, 1997; Farwell and Smith, 2001; Farwell et al., 2013 (four studies); see also Iacono, 2008]. These specific methods are the only methods that have reliably produced less than 1% error rate and median 95% statistical confidences for individual determinations, including over 90% for both information-present and information-absent determinations, in the laboratory and the field. These same error rates and statistical confidences have been achieved with countermeasures, without countermeasures, and in field conditions where it is unknown whether countermeasures are being used or not (Farwell et al., 2013). (Countermeasures are physical or mental procedures that a subject may practice in an attempt to influence the outcome of a test. They were not studied in this research).

The methods applied in these studies are the same as in the original Farwell and Donchin studies, with several improvements based on the more demanding requirements of field applications, as described below. Farwell (2012) documented these methods (or rules or recommendations) as 20 brain fingerprinting scientific standards (Appendix 1). Farwell (1994, 2012) defined "brain fingerprinting" as the classification-CIT technique incorporating the 20 standards. These methods are applied here[2]. We have focused our previous research primarily on establishing the sufficient conditions because this provides a technique we can use, and have successfully used, in the field. Previous studies by others investigated the necessary conditions to obtain low error rates and high statistical confidences (Farwell, 2012, 2014; Appendix 2).

P300 AND LNP

Farwell and Donchin (1991) used the classification CIT with the P300. In this research we compared the results of using the P300 alone vs. the P300 plus the LNP. Our rationale for this is as follows.

Early P300 research (e.g., Sutton et al., 1965) used very simple stimuli, such as auditory clicks and tones. As the sophistication of experimental designs progressed, more complex stimuli were used, including simple words and phrases presented visually. The latency of P300 was found to increase with stimulus complexity

[1]To obtain statistical confidences for each individual determination, Farwell, Donchin, Wasserman, and Bockenholt collaborated to introduce the statistical technique of bootstrapping in the field of psychophysiology. This first was published in conference abstracts by Farwell and Donchin (1986, 1988a), and full papers by Wasserman and Bockenholt (1989) and Farwell and Donchin (1991), which reported the same studies as the abstracts. Wasserman and Bockenholt used Farwell and Donchin's application of bootstrapping in the classification CIT as an example of the correct use of the technique.

[2]The study reported here appeared first as a conference abstract, Farwell and Richardson (2006).

and the concomitant stimulus evaluation time (Magliero et al., 1984). With simple words and phrases, an inter-stimulus interval (ISI) of 1000–1500 ms or less was adequate for the subject to process the stimuli and to capture the entire ERP response (Farwell and Donchin, 1988b). Farwell and Donchin (1991), for example, used phrases consisting of two, one-syllable words, and an ISI of 1500 ms.

In conducting research at the FBI in 1993, however, Farwell et al. (2013; Farwell, 1994, 1995a,b) had the task of developing text stimuli that accurately represented knowledge unique to FBI agents. This required some stimuli to be several long words. To give subjects time to fully process the stimuli, we extended the ISI to 3000 ms. Under these conditions, we found that the positive P300 peak was followed by a negative peak with a peak latency of up to 1200 ms, which we termed the late negative potential (LNP).

The stimuli we used in this study and in previous research (Farwell and Smith, 2001; Farwell et al., 2013) were more personally significant than the stimuli presented in most previous P300 research. LNP may be driven at least in part by this personal significance. Compared to many previous P300 studies, our stimuli may also be more salient, be more related to previous memories, require more complex processing, and involve a task more important to the subject. They are also presented with a longer ISI than that applied in most previous P300 studies. Further research is necessary to identify the antecedent conditions and delineate the functional significance of the LNP.

We called the overall pattern of the P300 followed by the LNP in the time domain, along with concomitant changes in the frequency domain and other putative changes measurable by other mathematical methods, a P300-MERMER. Although the P300-MERMER—and for that matter, the P300—may be comprised of additional features that are not visible in the time domain (Farwell, 2012; Farwell et al., 2013), the time-domain pattern is sufficient to define and to detect the response. This pattern consists of a positive peak followed by a negative peak (or a negative-positive-negative pattern if the N200, a well-known negative component that generally precedes the P300, is included).

We compared results obtained using the P300 alone with results obtained by including the P300 plus the LNP. Our computations consider only the conventional, time-domain characteristics of the signals. The difference between our two epoch-related analyses is the length of the epoch analyzed, and therefore the inclusion or exclusion of the LNP and its amplitude, morphology, and latency.

In the early 1990s, when Farwell et al. (2013) first encountered the LNP that follows the P300, we initially hypothesized that LNP was an artifact, perhaps generated by the analog filters and the return of the P300 to baseline. The data contradicted this hypothesis, however. If the LNP were an artifact produced by the filter's effect on the P300, then similar P300s with identical filters would produce similar LNPs. We found that the latency, amplitude, and morphology of the LNP varied independently of the P300. Also, the scalp distribution of the LNP was more frontal than that of the P300. Moreover, the negative peak persisted when we varied our filter settings (Farwell, 1994, 2012). Even recording without analog filters did not eliminate the LNP, or substantially change its characteristics. This definitively disproved the filter-generated-artifact hypothesis (Farwell et al., 2013).

The data we recorded with filters also contradict the hypothesis that the LNP is an artifact. We used the same recording equipment for all subjects and all scalp sites. If the LNP were an artifact produced by the equipment, the same equipment would produce identical effects in different scalp sites and different subjects. The features of the LNP would be a function of the features of the P300. This was not observed. For different scalp sites in one subject, and for different subjects, the relative amplitude, latency, and morphology of the LNP and the P300 were very different. Sometimes there was a difference of hundreds of milliseconds in the latency, and amplitude differences of a factor of two or more, in LNPs that followed virtually identical P300s recorded from different subjects (Farwell et al., 2013). In some cases the LNP was considerably larger than the P300 at one scalp site (Fz) and considerably smaller than the P300 at another (Pz) for the same subject. In short, the data contradict the hypothesis that the LNP (or the latter part of the P300-MERMER) is an artifact produced by some combination of the P300, the return to baseline after the P300, and the filters and other equipment.

In the current paradigm, a negative peak (the N200) precedes the P300 positive peak, and another negative peak (the LNP) follows the P300. Our first observation of this tri-phasic negative-positive-negative morphology in the ERP response was in the early 1990s (Farwell, 1994, 2012; Farwell and Smith, 2001; Farwell et al., 2013). Others applying intracranial recordings have observed this same negative-positive-negative pattern in a number of brain structures (Halgren et al., 1998; Linden, 2005). These include dorsolateral and orbital frontal cortices, anterior cingulate (Baudena et al., 1995), amygdala and hippocampus (Halgren et al., 1986; Stapleton and Halgren, 1987), superior temporal sulcus (Halgren et al., 1995), and inferior parietal lobe/supramarginal gyrus (Smith et al., 1990).

Others investigating the ERP-based CIT, including Meijer et al. (2007), have also reported the LNP. Brouwer et al. (2010) observed the LNP and investigated its utility in brain-computer interfaces. Several other studies (Matsuda et al., 2009; Gamer and Berti, 2010, 2012) reported a difference in the N200 in responses to relevant stimuli in ERP-based CITs. Virtually all researchers conducting research on ERP-based CITs now include in their data-analysis algorithms both the P300 and the LNP (for reviews, see Farwell, 2012, 2014), although some refer to the entire response including both positive and negative peaks as "P300" (e.g., Rosenfeld et al., 2008) and some refer to the positive peak as "P300" and the entire response as "P300-MERMER" or "P300 + LNP" (e.g., Sutton et al., 1965; Farwell, 2012, 2014; Farwell et al., 2013).

Changes in the frequency domain and other changes in the dimensionality and other characteristics of the signal may be included in the term "P300-MERMER." The positive and negative time-domain changes constituting the P300 and the LNP are sufficient to detect and characterize the response, and are all that are measured in this research, although they undoubtedly do not constitute a complete and comprehensive description of all the patterns of electrophysiological activity that manifest the underlying information-processing brain activity (Farwell, 1994, 2012; Farwell and Smith, 2001).

We compared the error rate and statistical confidences produced by data analysis including the P300 plus the LNP with the results of analysis using the P300 alone. We investigated whether the classification-CIT analysis with the P300 plus the LNP provides significantly lower error rate and/or higher statistical confidences than the analysis with the P300 alone.

SUMMARY OF RESEARCH QUESTIONS

Our primary research questions are as follows:

(1) Does the classification CIT provide significantly (a) lower error rate and/or (b) higher statistical confidences than the comparison CIT.
(2) Does the classification-CIT analysis with the P300 + LNP provide significantly (a) lower error rate and/or (b) higher statistical confidences than the analysis with the P300 alone.

MATERIALS AND METHODS

SUBJECTS

We tested 16 experts (information present) and 14 non-experts (information absent) in military medicine. Experts were students and faculty at Uniformed Services University of the Health Sciences (USUHS) possessing professional knowledge of military medicine. Non-experts lacked this specific expertise and training. Mean age of 30 subjects was 26; standard deviation was 2.9. Mean ages of information-present and information-absent subjects were 27 and 25, respectively; standard deviations were 3.2 and 2.6, respectively. 15 subjects (8 information present) were female.

Experimental procedures were approved by the Brain Fingerprinting Laboratories, Inc., ethics committee and performed in accordance with the ethical standards of the 1964 Declaration of Helsinki, including written informed consent prior to participation.

STIMULI

Three types of stimuli consisting of words or phrases were presented on a computer screen: probes, targets, and irrelevants. Probes contain specific information relevant to the investigated situation. The test is designed to detect the subject's knowledge or lack of knowledge of the information contained in the probes as relevant in the context of the investigated situation.

In this specific screening study, the relevant information detected was known only to experts in military medicine. Information was obtained from interviews with USUHS military medical experts. Individuals interviewed were not tested. Probe stimuli contained the relevant information to be detected. We presented two additional types of stimuli. Responses to target stimuli provide a template for the subject's brain response to known information relevant to the investigated situation. Responses to irrelevant stimuli provide a template for the subject's brain response to irrelevant information. Target stimuli present information relevant to the investigated situation that is known to be known to the subject. There are significant, proven advantages to using targets that are relevant to the investigated situation rather than inherently irrelevant targets that are made relevant only by task instructions (Farwell, 2012; Farwell et al., 2013), although we and others have successfully used the latter (Farwell and Donchin, 1991). Target stimuli, unlike probes, were identified as such to the subject in experimental instructions. Subject instructions also conveyed the significance of each target in the context of the investigated situation, and required a different behavioral response to targets than to probes and irrelevants, as described in the next section.

For each probe (and each target) comparable irrelevants were structured that contained similar, plausible, but incorrect information about the investigated situation. For a subject lacking the relevant knowledge contained in the probes, the irrelevants and probes were equally plausible as correct, relevant details. Each probe and its comparable irrelevants were indistinguishable for a subject lacking the information that the test was structured to reveal. Each probe contained correct, relevant information fitting the description of that probe. The two irrelevants comparable to each probe contained incorrect information that would be plausible as fitting that same description for an individual lacking the information contained in the probes. For example, a probe stimulus could be the technical name of a military medical procedure in which experts are trained. Corresponding irrelevants could be technical terms that do not name any real procedure. For security reasons, the exact stimuli cannot be given. Subjects were provided with a description of each probe that specified the significance of the probe in the context of the investigated situation, but were not informed which was the correct, situation-relevant probe and which were the corresponding irrelevants.

Similarly, each target stimulus contained correct, situation-relevant information, and the two irrelevant stimuli comparable to each target contained comparable, incorrect but plausible information. Unlike probes, targets were identified as such in instructions to the subjects.

Stimuli were constructed in groups of six: one probe, one target, and four irrelevants. For each probe there were two comparable irrelevants. For each target there were two comparable irrelevants. We used a ratio of 1/6 targets, 1/6 probes, and 2/3 irrelevants so targets and probes were relatively rare, which is known to enhance P300 amplitude (Farwell and Donchin, 1991).

Our prediction was that targets would elicit a large P300 + LNP (or P300-MERMER) in all subjects, irrelevants would not elicit a large P300 + LNP, and probes would elicit a large P300 + LNP only in information-present subjects. Thus, for information-present subjects, ERP responses to probes would be similar to ERPs for targets. For information-absent subjects, ERP responses to probes would be similar to ERPs for irrelevants.

There were 32 unique probes, 32 unique targets, and 128 unique irrelevants, a total of 192 unique stimuli. These comprised 32 groups of stimuli, each consisting of one probe, one target, and four irrelevants. 20 probes were words or phrases embodying the relevant knowledge; 12 were acronyms. The same stimuli were presented to all subjects. Each unique stimulus was presented more than once, so the total number of stimulus presentations was greater than the total number of unique stimuli.

PROCEDURE

Before the test, we made certain that the subject understood the significance of the probes. We described the significance of each probe to the subject. We then showed the subject the probe and the corresponding irrelevants, in the context of the description of the significance of the probe, without revealing which was the probe. Thus, subjects were informed of the significance of each probe stimulus, but were not told which stimulus was the probe and which were corresponding irrelevants. For example, subjects were told, "One of these three items is the term for a medical technique applied to burn victims in battlefield situations" followed by a list of one probe and two irrelevants (in alphabetical order). Although the descriptions of the probes were made known to subjects, the probe stimuli themselves were never identified as probes.

Targets were explicitly identified to the subjects. Experimental instructions ensured that the subject knew the targets and their significance in the context of the investigated situation. We described the significance of each target to the subject. We showed the subject each target and the corresponding irrelevants, in the context of the description of the significance of the target. We also showed subjects a list of the targets, and noted that subjects would be required to recognize the targets during the test. We instructed subjects to press a button with one thumb in response to targets, and another button with the other thumb in response to "all other stimuli." The subject's task was to read and comprehend each stimulus, and then to indicate by a button press whether the stimulus was a target stimulus or not.

For a subject possessing the knowledge embodied in the probes, "all other stimuli" consisted of two types of stimuli: probes containing the known situation-relevant information, and irrelevant stimuli. For a subject lacking the tested knowledge, "all other stimuli" appeared equally irrelevant. Probes were indistinguishable from irrelevants. For "all other stimuli" (that is, everything except targets), the subject was instructed to push the opposite button from the one pushed in response to targets. This instruction applied whether the subject perceived these as a single category (all equally irrelevant, if the subject was information absent) or as two categories (irrelevant, and relevant to the concealed information being tested, if the subject was information present).

The differential button-press task in response to every stimulus presentation ensured that the subject was required to read and comprehend every stimulus, including the probe stimuli, and to prove behaviorally that he had done so on every trial. This allowed us to avoid depending on detecting brain responses to assigned tasks that the subject could covertly avoid doing, while performing the necessary overt responses (see Appendix 2).

Testing was divided into separate blocks. In each block the computer display presented 72 stimulus presentations or trials. In blocks 1–3, four stimulus groups were presented in each block, that is, in each block there were four unique probes, four unique targets, and 16 unique irrelevants. Each stimulus was presented three times in a block to make the total of 72 stimulus presentations per block. Stimuli were presented in random order. In blocks 4–7, five stimulus groups were presented in each block in random order until 72 trials had been presented. (Since the total of 72 trials is not divisible by 5, some randomly selected stimuli were presented 3 times and some 4.) In blocks 1–3, stimuli were acronyms. In blocks 4–7, stimuli were words and phrases.

Immediately before each block, we repeated the description of the significance of each of the probes and targets that were to appear in each block (but not the actual stimuli). For example, "In this test you will see the term for a medical technique applied to burn victims in battlefield situations, a medical instrument applied in field wound treatments, a type of injury sustained from exposure to chemical weapons, and the name of the individual who developed the preferred treatment for exposure to sarin gas."

Stimuli were presented for 300 ms at an ISI of 3000 ms. A fixation point ("X") was presented for 1000 ms prior to each stimulus. For each trial, the sequence was a fixation point for 1000 ms, the stimulus (target, probe, or irrelevant) for 300 ms, a blank screen for 1700 ms, and then the next fixation point.

Trials contaminated by artifacts generated by eye movements or muscle-generated noise were rejected on-line, and additional trials were presented until 72 artifact-free trials were obtained. Trials with a range of greater than 97.7 microvolts in the EOG channel were rejected. Data for "rejected" trials were collected and recorded, but rejected trials did not contribute to the count of trials presented, so each rejection resulted in an additional stimulus presentation. In 7 blocks, a total of 84 probe, 84 target, and 336 irrelevant artifact-free trials were collected, for a grand total of 504 trials. (Previous research, e.g., Fabiani et al., 1987 has shown that repeating the stimuli does not substantially affect the relevant brain response.)

Brain responses were recorded from the midline frontal, central, and parietal scalp locations (Fz, Cz, and Pz, International 10–20 system) referenced to linked mastoids, and from a location on the forehead to track eye movements. Med Associates silver-silver chloride disposable electrodes were held in place by a custom headband.

Data were digitized at 333 Hz, and resampled at 100 Hz off-line for analysis. Electroencephalograph (EEG) data were amplified at a gain of 50,000 using custom amplifiers. Electro-oculograph (EOG/eye movement) data were amplified at a gain of 10,000. Impedance did not exceed 10 kilohm. Analog filters passed signals between 0.1 and 30 Hz. Data were stored on disk for off-line analysis.

DATA ANALYSIS

We analyzed ERP data from the Pz scalp site. Data were digitally filtered using a 49-point, equal-ripple, zero-phase-shift, optimal, finite impulse response, low-pass filter with a passband cutoff frequency of 6 Hz and a stopband cutoff frequency of 8 Hz (Farwell et al., 1993). Trials with a range of greater than 97.7 microvolts in the EOG channel were excluded from analysis. We decided on this threshold based on our previous experience (Farwell and Donchin, 1991; Farwell et al., 2013). In exploratory data analysis, we have varied this threshold considerably, and the results are robust even if we change this parameter within quite a wide range.

For each subject's data we conducted two separate classification-CIT analyses applying bootstrapping as described below. One analysis used the positive P300 peak followed by the LNP, a later negative peak (together also known as the

P300-MERMER). A second analysis included only the positive P300. The P300 + LNP epoch was defined as 300–1800 ms after stimulus onset. The P300 epoch was 300–900 ms after stimulus onset. The two analyses were identical except for the epoch analyzed. A third analysis applied bootstrapping with the comparison CIT on the full P300 + LNP epoch, as in previous ERP studies with the comparison CIT.

The data analysis produced three sets of results for each subject: (1) a determination of information present or information absent along with a statistical confidence for the determination using the classification CIT and the full P300 + LNP epoch; (2) a comparable determination and statistical confidence using the P300 alone with the classification CIT; and (3) a comparable determination and statistical confidence using the comparison CIT on the full epoch. This allowed us to compare the error rate/accuracy and statistical confidence provided by (a) the P300 + LNP vs. the P300 alone in a classification CIT, and (b) the classification CIT vs. the comparison CIT.

BOOTSTRAPPING

Classification-CIT bootstrapping method

The primary data-analysis task was to determine whether the ERP responses to the probe stimuli contained a large P300 and LNP similar to that elicited by the targets, or whether the probe responses lacked a large P300 and LNP, like the irrelevants.

We used bootstrapping (Wasserman and Bockenholt, 1989; Farwell and Donchin, 1991; Farwell et al., 2013) to determine whether the probe responses were more similar to the target responses or to the irrelevant responses, and to compute a statistical confidence for this determination for each individual subject. The metric for similarity was double-centered correlation.

The bootstrapping procedure accomplished two goals: (1) to take into account the variability across single trials, while also maintaining the smooth and relatively noise-free shape provided by signal averaging; (2) to isolate the critical variable—knowledge of the information embodied in the probes—by classifying the responses to the probe stimuli as being either more similar to the target responses or to the irrelevant responses. We conducted two classification-CIT analyses, one using only the P300 and one using the P300 plus the LNP (together also known as the P300-MERMER).

Briefly, the bootstrapping procedure for the classification CIT is as follows. We repeat the following procedure 1000 times. Randomly sample P probes, T targets, and I irrelevants, with P, T, and I equal to the total number of probe, target, and irrelevant trials in the data set, respectively. In each iteration, compare the probe-target correlation with the probe-irrelevant correlation. Count the number of times that the probe-target correlation is greater than the probe-irrelevant correlation, and convert this to a percentage. This is the probability that the probe response is more similar to the target response than to the irrelevant response, or the probability that information present is the correct determination. 100% minus this is the probability that the probe response is more similar to the irrelevant response, or the probability that information absent is the correct determination.

We set an *a priori* bootstrapping probability criterion of 90% for an information-present determination and 70% (in the opposite direction) for an information-absent determination. If the probability was greater than 90% that the probe response was more similar to the target response than to the irrelevant response, we classified the subject as information present. The bootstrap probability is the statistical confidence for this determination.

The probability that information absent is the correct determination is 100% minus the probability that information present is the correct determination. For example, if there is a 90% probability that the probe response is more similar to the target than to the irrelevant response (information present is correct), then there is a 10% probability that the probe response is more similar to the irrelevant response (information absent is correct). If the probability was greater than 70% that the probe response was more similar to the irrelevant response than to the target response (equivalent to a 30% probability that the probe response was more similar to the target response), we classified the subject as information absent. The bootstrap probability is the statistical confidence for this determination.

If the results did not meet either criterion, we did not classify the subject in either category. The outcome would then be indeterminate (although there were no indeterminates).

For each subject, each data analysis method produced a determination and a statistical confidence, e.g., information present, 99.9% statistical confidence. The statistical confidence is the probability that the determination is correct, based on the within-subjects statistical computation taking into account the size of the effect and the variability in the data.

Figure 1 illustrates example stimuli, ERP responses, bootstrapping probabilities, and determinations for a hypothetical classification CIT to determine if an individual has information regarding US political history.

Error rate is the percentage of incorrect information-present (false positive) and information-absent (false negative) determinations. Accuracy is 100% minus the error rate. In reporting error rates and/or accuracy, indeterminates must be reported as such. In reporting "accuracy," some authors have confounded indeterminates with false positives and/or false negatives, reporting "accuracy" as the percentage of tests that result in a correct determination, and hiding the number of indeterminates. This irretrievably hides the true error rate if there are indeterminates, and makes it impossible to make a meaningful comparison with studies that report the true error rate. In any meaningful reporting, indeterminates if any must be identified as such, and not confounded with false positive or false negative errors. (Some legitimate techniques such as Bayesian analysis do not allow indeterminates, in which case this must also be reported).

We restricted our conclusions to a determination as to whether or not a subject knew the specific situation-relevant knowledge embodied in the probes at the time of the test. Our procedures recognize the fact that the ERP-based classification CIT detects only presence or absence of information—not guilt, innocence, honesty, lying, deception, or any past action or non-action.

Comparison-CIT bootstrapping method

The comparison CIT uses bootstrapping in an entirely different way. The comparison CIT ignores the target responses and applies

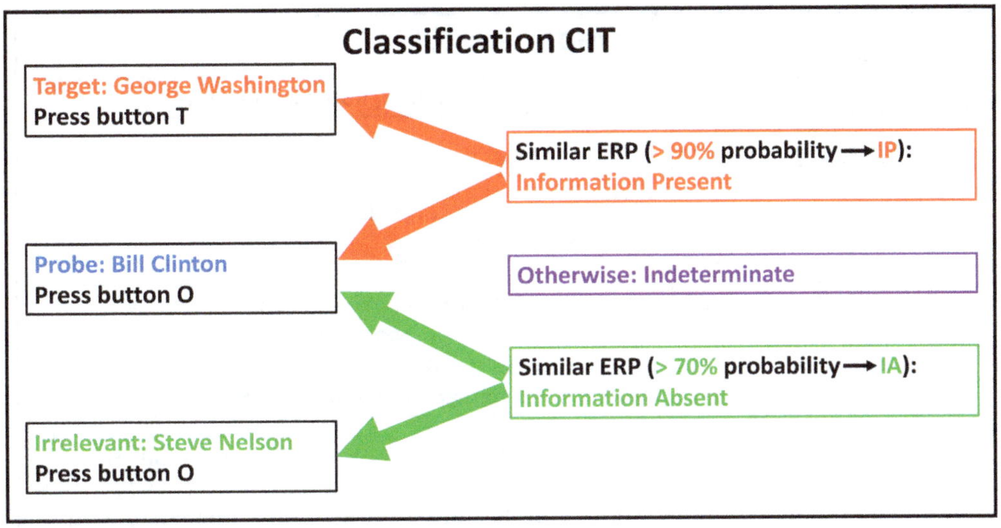

FIGURE 1 | Classification CIT: stimuli, responses, and determinations. Example of a classification CIT to determine whether an individual has information about US political history. Subject instructions: "You will view names of former US presidents. Some of these are on this list: George Washington, John Adams, Ronald Reagan. Press button T [target] for any name on this list. Otherwise press button O [other]. George Washington was a US president on the list, so then you should press T." Since Bill Clinton was not on the list and was not identified to the subject as a US president, the subject will press button O for Bill Clinton, whether he recognizes him as a US president (information present) or not (information absent). IP, Information Present; IA, Information Absent.

bootstrapping to compute the probability that the amplitude of the probe ERP is larger than the amplitude of the irrelevant ERP. The amplitude of the ERP response is defined as the difference between the highest voltage in the P300 window (300–900 ms) and the lowest voltage in the LNP window (900–1800 ms). (This is essentially the sum of the peak amplitudes of the P300 and the LNP.) This is in accord with the metric used in previous applications of the comparison CIT (e.g., Rosenfeld et al., 2008).

Trials are randomly sampled with replacement and averaged as described above for the classification CIT, except that only probe and irrelevant trials are sampled and averaged. In each of 1000 iterations, the amplitude of the ERP in the sampled probe average is compared with the amplitude of the ERP in the sampled irrelevant average. The percentage of times that the sampled probe ERP is larger than the sampled irrelevant ERP provides an estimate of the probability that the probe ERP is larger than the irrelevant ERP. If the probability that the probe ERP is larger than the irrelevant ERP is greater than 90%, then the subject is determined to be information present. If the probability that the probe ERP is larger than the irrelevant ERP is less than 90%, then the subject is determined to be information absent. (The comparison CIT does not have an indeterminate category.) A probability of 90% that information present is correct (that is, probe ERP is larger than irrelevant ERP) is equivalent to a probability of 10% (that is, 100%–90%) that information absent is correct. Therefore, any subject with a probability of over 10% that information absent is correct is determined to be information absent. This results in subjects being determined to be information *absent* when the computed bootstrap probability is as high as 89.9% that information *present* would be the correct determination, that is, as low as a 10.1% statistically computed probability that the selected information-absent determination is correct. Information-absent statistical confidences range from 10.1% to 99.9% and average 50% (chance) (see Appendix 2).

Correct information-absent determinations are of two types, valid and invalid. Valid determinations are those that have a greater than 50% (chance) statistical confidence, i.e., a greater than chance computed probability of being correct. An invalid determination is a (correct) determination where the statistical confidence is less than chance (50%); that is, the computed probability that the determination is correct is less than 50%. Such a result is invalid because clearly one cannot validly report that "Our statistical procedure determined that the individual is information absent; the statistics computed a probability of [15%] that the determination is correct." (This also applies to any other percentage lower than 50%.) Such a statement is not statistically meaningful or logically tenable. To be valid, the computed statistical confidence for a result must at least be better than chance (see **Figure 2** and Appendix 2). To be scientifically meaningful and practically useful, it must be considerably better than chance.

There are serious scientific, mathematical, logical, and statistical flaws with the ERP-based comparison-CIT data-analysis procedure, as described in Farwell (2012, 2014), Farwell et al. (2013), and Appendix 2. These flaws cannot be corrected by simply changing the criterion for information present/absent determinations. We have implemented this procedure, however, because this is the way that the bootstrapping statistical confidence has been computed in all or virtually all of the comparison-CIT studies that have previously applied bootstrapping (e.g., Rosenfeld et al., 2008).

Figure 2 illustrates example stimuli, ERP responses, bootstrapping probabilities, and determinations for a hypothetical comparison CIT to determine if an individual has information regarding US political history.

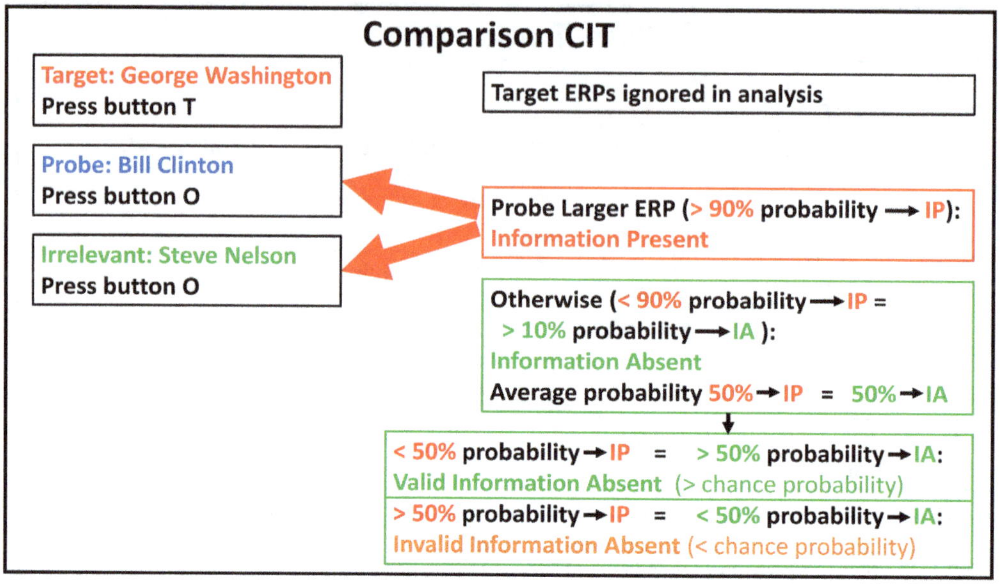

FIGURE 2 | Comparison CIT: stimuli, responses, and determinations. Example of a comparison CIT to determine whether an individual has information about US political history. Subject instructions and button presses are the same as in **Figure 1**. IP, Information Present; IA, Information Absent.

RESULTS

The results are delineated in **Tables 1–4** and illustrated in **Figures 3** and **4**. **Table 1** presents the error rate/accuracy of the results of the classification CIT, for both P300 + LNP and P300 analysis methods. Both P300 + LNP and P300 analysis methods produced 0% error rate, 100% accuracy. Both also produced no indeterminates.

Table 2 presents the error rate/accuracy of the comparison CIT. (Only correct determinations and errors are tabulated: the comparison CIT does not have an indeterminate category).

Table 3 presents the individual determinations and the statistical confidences for each subject whose true state was information present. It compares the results obtained with the classification CIT with P300 + LNP with the other two methods: classification CIT with P300 and comparison CIT.

Figure 3 presents the brain responses to probe, target, and irrelevant stimuli for each of the information-present subjects, averaged across all trials for each subject.

Table 4 presents the individual determinations and the statistical confidences for each subject whose true state was information absent. It compares the results obtained with the classification CIT with P300 + LNP with the other two methods: classification CIT with P300 and comparison CIT.

Figure 4 presents the brain responses to probe, target, and irrelevant stimuli for each of the information-absent subjects, averaged across all trials for each subject.

RESULTS OF THE CLASSIFICATION CIT WITH P300 + LNP ANALYSIS

All classification-CIT determinations with the P300 + LNP analysis were correct. Error rate was 0%: there were no false positives and no false negatives. Accuracy was 100%. Also, there were no indeterminates. Grier's A' (Grier, 1971) was 1.0.

Table 1 | Classification CIT error rate/accuracy of determinations with P300 + LNP and P300.

Classification CIT: error rate/accuracy with P300 + LNP and P300			
Information-present subjects	Tests	16	100%
	Correct positives	16	100%
	False negatives	0	0%
	Indeterminates	0	0%
Information-absent subjects	Tests	14	100%
	Correct negatives	14	100%
	False positives	0	0%
	Indeterminates	0	0%
All subjects	Tests	30	100%
	Correct determinations	30	100%
	Errors	0	0%
	Indeterminates	0	0%
	Accuracy	30/30	100%
	Error rate	0/30	0%

All information-present statistical confidences were above the *a priori* criterion of 90%. All information-absent determinations were above the *a priori* criterion of 70% (in the opposite direction). Median statistical confidence was 99.9% with the P300 + LNP. Mean statistical confidence was 95.1% with the P300 + LNP.

All of the information-present determinations were made with a statistical confidence of at least 99%, and all but one were made with a statistical confidence of 99.9%. Median statistical confidence for information-present determinations was 99.9%, and mean statistical confidence was also 99.9%.

All information-present determinations exceeded the *a priori* criterion of 90% statistical confidence by at least 9 percentage points in the bootstrap probability computation. No information-present determinations were close to an indeterminate outcome. All information-present determinations were extremely far from a false negative. The lowest information-present determination was separated by a buffer of 69 percentage points in the bootstrap probability computation from the criterion for a false negative. (Exceeding the 70% probability for an information-absent determination would result in a false negative. This is equivalent to 100 – 70% = 30% probability for an information-present determination. Lowest information-present probability obtained was 99.3%, and 99.3 – 30% = 69.3%).

All of the information-absent determinations also exceeded the corresponding *a priori* criterion of 70% statistical confidence for information-absent determinations. Median information-absent statistical confidence with the P300 + LNP was 91.8%. Mean information-absent statistical confidence with the P300 + LNP was 89.7%.

All information-absent determinations were far from a false positive. The least statistically confident information-absent determination was separated by a buffer of 64 percentage points in the bootstrap probability computation from the criterion for a false positive. (Exceeding the 90% probability for an information-present determination would result in a false positive. This is equivalent to 100 – 90% = 10% probability for an information-absent determination. Lowest information-absent probability obtained is 74.2%, and 74.2 – 10% = 64.2%).

Statistical confidences for information-absent determinations were lower than for information-present determinations, however, and some were close to an indeterminate outcome. 9 information-absent determinations had statistical confidences of less than 95%. 6 had statistical confidences of less than 90%. 2 statistical confidences were less than 75% and were within 5

Table 2 | Comparison CIT error rate/accuracy.

Comparison CIT: error rate/accuracy			
Information-present subjects	Tests	16	100%
	Correct positives	13	81%
	False negatives	3	19%
Information-absent subjects	Tests	14	100%
	Correct negatives	11	79%
	False positives	3	21%
All subjects	Tests	30	100%
	Correct determinations	24	80%
	Errors	6	20%
	Accuracy	24/30	80%
	Error rate	6/30	20%

Table 3 | Determinations and statistical confidences for information-present subjects.

Determinations and statistical confidences, information-present subjects								
	Classification CIT					Comparison CIT		
	P300 + LNP analysis		P300 analysis					
Subject #	Determination	Statistical confidence (%)	Determination	Statistical confidence (%)	P300 + LNP vs. P300 (%)	Determination	Statistical confidence (%)	Classification CIT vs. comparison CIT (%)
1	Info present	99.9	Info present	99.9	0.0	Info present	99.9	0.0
2	Info present	99.9	Info present	99.9	0.0	Info present	99.8	0.1
3	Info present	99.3	Info present	92.0	7.3	Info absent	17.3	n/a
4	Info present	99.9	Info present	99.5	0.4	Info absent	34.3	n/a
5	Info present	99.9	Info present	99.7	0.2	Info present	99.9	0.0
6	Info present	99.9	Info present	99.4	0.5	Info present	99.9	0.0
7	Info present	99.9	Info present	91.8	8.1	Info present	96.2	3.7
8	Info present	99.9	Info present	96.8	3.1	Info present	98.8	1.1
9	Info present	99.9	Info present	99.9	0.0	Info present	99.9	0.0
10	Info present	99.9	Info present	99.8	0.1	Info absent	28.0	n/a
11	Info present	99.9	Info present	96.6	3.3	Info present	99.9	0.0
12	Info present	99.9	Info present	99.9	0.0	Info present	99.9	0.0
13	Info present	99.9	Info present	99.9	0.0	Info present	91.4	8.5
14	Info present	99.9	Info present	99.9	0.0	Info present	99.9	0.0
15	Info present	99.9	Info present	95.5	4.4	Info present	99.9	0.0
16	Info present	99.9	Info present	99.1	0.8	Info present	99.9	0.0

Errors are underlined.

Table 4 | Determinations and statistical confidences for information-absent subjects.

Determinations and statistical confidences, information-absent subjects								
	Classification CIT					Comparison CIT		
	P300 + LNP analysis		P300 analysis					
Subject #	Determination	Statistical confidence (%)	Determination	Statistical confidence (%)	P300 + LNP vs. P300 (%)	Determination	Statistical confidence (%)	Classification CIT vs. comparison CIT (%)
17	Info absent	74.9	Info absent	74.9	0.0	Info present	92.4	n/a
18	Info absent	75.0	Info absent	72.3	2.7	*Info absent*	*22.5*	52.5
19	Info absent	90.5	Info absent	70.6	19.9	*Info absent*	*35.1*	55.4
20	Info absent	74.2	Info absent	74.2	0.0	Info absent	58.0	16.2
21	Info absent	87.0	Info absent	72.7	14.3	*Info absent*	*11.7*	75.3
22	Info absent	85.0	Info absent	72.8	12.2	*Info absent*	*37.7*	47.3
23	Info absent	96.9	Info absent	94.8	2.1	*Info absent*	*39.2*	57.7
24	Info absent	89.0	Info absent	71.7	17.3	*Info absent*	*18.9*	70.1
25	Info absent	93.0	Info absent	93.0	0.0	Info present	95.2	n/a
26	Info absent	97.6	Info absent	97.6	0.0	*Info absent*	*12.6*	85.0
27	Info absent	99.9	Info absent	99.9	0.0	Info present	93.3	n/a
28	Info absent	94.1	Info absent	94.1	0.0	*Info absent*	*28.9*	65.2
29	Info absent	99.9	Info absent	99.6	0.3	*Info absent*	*47.4*	52.5
30	Info absent	98.7	Info absent	98.7	0.0	*Info absent*	*11.6*	87.1

Errors are underlined; invalid determinations, i.e., correct determinations made with less than 50% (chance) statistical confidence, are in italics.

percentage points of an indeterminate outcome. Possible reasons for this are discussed below.

RESULTS OF THE CLASSIFICATION CIT WITH P300 ANALYSIS

As with the classification-CIT P300 + LNP-based analysis, all determinations with the classification-CIT P300-based analysis were correct. Error rate was 0%: there were no false positives and no false negatives. Accuracy was 100%. Also, there were no indeterminates. Grier's A' (Grier, 1971) was 1.0. All information-present statistical confidences were above the *a priori* criterion of 90%. All information-absent determinations were above the *a priori* criterion of 70% (in the opposite direction). Median statistical confidence was 97.2% with the P300 alone. Mean statistical confidence was 91.9% with the P300 alone. For information-present subjects, median statistical confidence was 99.6%, and mean statistical confidence was 98.1%. For information-absent subjects, median statistical confidence was 84.0%, and mean statistical confidence was 84.8%. With the P300 analysis, 12 subjects (2 information present and 10 information absent) had statistical confidences of less than 95%, and 7 (all information absent) had statistical confidences of less than 75% and were within 5 percentage points of an indeterminate outcome. All determinations were very far from a false negative or false positive error.

COMPARING CLASSIFICATION-CIT P300 + LNP ANALYSIS vs. P300 ANALYSIS

The classification-CIT P300 + LNP-based analysis produced significantly higher statistical confidences for individual determinations than the classification-CIT P300-based analysis ($p < 0.0001$, Wilcoxon matched-pairs signed rank test). The statistical confidence for the P300 + LNP-based analysis was an average of 3.2% higher than the statistical confidence for the P300-based analysis. In every case where there was a difference, the statistical confidence produced by the P300 + LNP was higher than that produced by the P300 alone. The P300 yielded a greater number of determinations with relatively low statistical confidence, close to an indeterminate outcome, than the P300 + LNP.

RESULTS OF THE COMPARISON CIT

Error rate with the comparison CIT was 20% overall, 19% false negatives for information-present subjects and 21% false positives for information-absent subjects. (The comparison CIT does not have an indeterminate category.) Mean statistical confidence for correct determinations was 67.0%. The lowest statistical confidence for a correct determination was 11.6%. Median statistical confidence for correct determinations was 93.8%. For information-present subjects, statistical confidences for correct determinations were all over 90%, as required by the criterion of 90% probability for information-present determinations; median was 99.9%; mean was 98.9%. As predicted by the statistical model, statistical confidences for correct information-absent determinations were on average not better than chance (50%). Median was 28.9%; mean was 29.4%. Most of the correct information-absent determinations were invalid, i.e., made with less than a 50% (chance) statistical confidence.

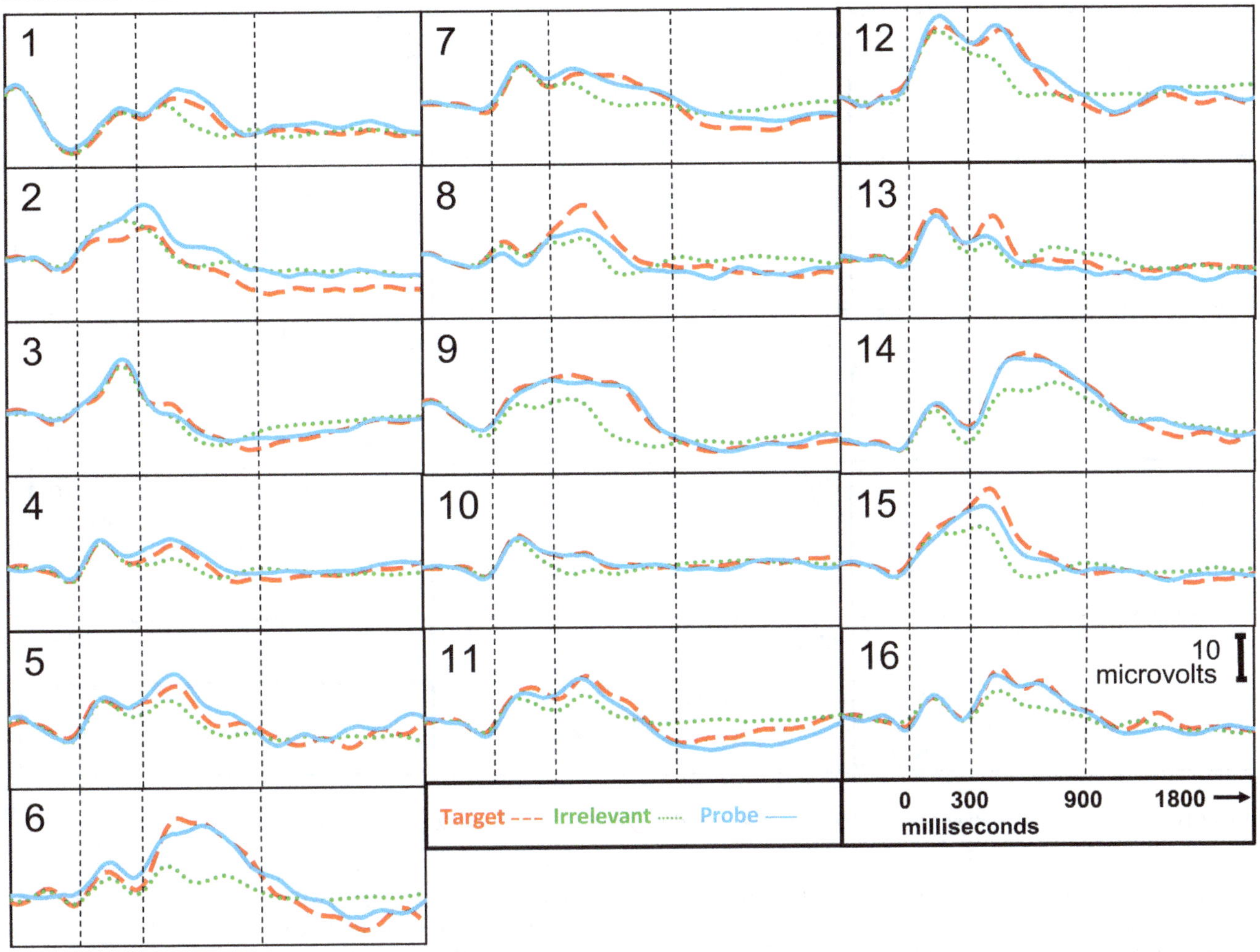

FIGURE 3 | ERP responses, information-present subjects. Stimulus onset is at 0 ms. P300 epoch is 300–900 ms. P300 + LNP epoch is 300–1800 ms.

CLASSIFICATION CIT (P300 + LNP ANALYSIS) vs. COMPARISON CIT

Even if we conservatively consider the 0% error rate of the classification CIT to be "less than 1%" for the sake of avoiding the anomalies of 0%, the comparison CIT produced more than an order of magnitude higher error rate than the classification CIT. This difference was significant ($p < 0.05$, sign test). Moreover, the comparison CIT produced significantly lower statistical confidences for correct determinations than the classification CIT ($p < 0.0007$, Wilcoxon matched-pairs signed rank test). On average, the comparison CIT produced statistical confidences 28.2 percentage points lower than those of the classification CIT in the bootstrap probability computation (for correct determinations). As predicted by the statistical model, this difference was particularly striking for information-absent subjects: comparison-CIT statistical confidences averaged 60.4 percentage points lower than classification-CIT statistical confidences for information-absent subjects. Correct statistical confidences for information-absent subjects with the comparison CIT averaged 29.4%, which is less than chance (50%).

DISCUSSION

CONCLUSIONS

Our results suggest the following:

(1) The classification CIT applying the brain fingerprinting methods and scientific standards described herein produces (a) significantly lower error rates (less than 1%; actually 0%) and (b) significantly higher statistical confidences than the comparison CIT.
(2) Classification-CIT data analysis with the P300 plus the LNP produces significantly higher statistical confidences than analysis with the P300 alone. Error rates were less than 1% (actually 0%) for both methods.

Our results suggest that the classification CIT, when practiced according the methods and standards described here, is a reliable and valid method for detecting concealed information obtained in the course of real life that is characteristic of individuals with

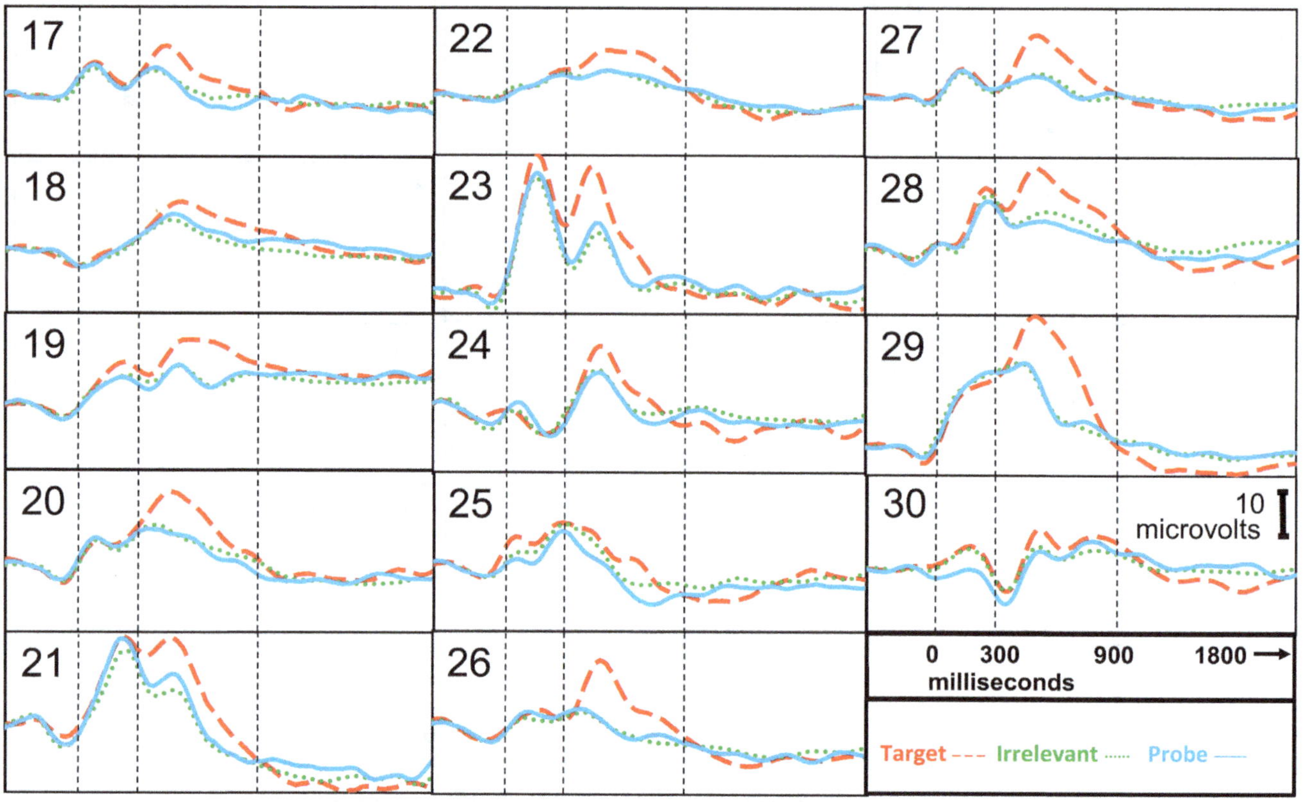

FIGURE 4 | ERP responses, information-absent subjects. Stimulus onset is at 0 ms. P300 epoch is 300–900 ms. P300 + LNP epoch is 300–1800 ms.

specific training, expertise, and/or affiliation with a particular agency or organization.

In our view, the minimum criteria for valid, reliable, and ethical field use for an ERP-based CIT are an error rate of less than 1% along with median statistical confidences of greater than 95%, including greater than 90% for both information-present and information-absent determinations. Our results, taken together with the results of our previous research and independent replications by others (see Farwell, 2012, 2014), suggest that the classification-CIT methods reported herein provide sufficient conditions to meet these criteria in the laboratory and the field. In our view, the methods applied in this research are sufficiently valid and reliable to be ethically applied in field use with substantial consequences to the outcome. These methods can be (and have been) reliably and effectively applied in field criminal cases.

Our results and those of all previous studies taken together (see Farwell, 2012, 2014) suggest that the comparison CIT with ERPs falls far short of these performance criteria for both error rate and statistical confidence. They also suggest that including the P300 + LNP in data analysis provides higher statistical confidences than P300 alone, but it is not a necessary condition for low error rate and high statistical confidences.

The most striking feature of the data reported to date, including the data of this study, is that there is a sharp bimodal distribution of error rates and statistical confidences, based on the following. One set of methods, as described here, applies the classification CIT and always has produced less than 1% error rate and greater than 95% median statistical confidences. Alternative methods, exemplified by Rosenfeld et al. (2008), Dietrich et al. (2014), and Meixner and Rosenfeld (2014), apply the comparison CIT and have produced an order of magnitude higher error rates, as well as statistical confidences averaging no better than 50% (chance) for information-absent determinations. Two reviews including all previous publications in English, Farwell (2012, 2014), documented that only the specific methods that substantially incorporate the 20 brain fingerprinting standards have so far reliably produced less than 1% error rate and greater than 95% median statistical confidences in the laboratory and the field. These are the methods applied in this research. The results of this research suggest that the differences in statistical methods between the classification CIT and the comparison CIT are responsible, at least in large measure, for the extremely large differences between the statistical confidences achieved empirically by the respective techniques.

Our experiment is a specific screening test where the information detected was relevant to expertise and experience in a particular field. Subjects obtained the tested information in the course of real life over a period of years, completely unconnected to any experimental procedures at the time the information was gained by the subjects. The results contribute to the accumulating evidence [e.g., the FBI and bomb-maker studies in Farwell et al. (2013)] that these methods provide a reliable and accurate technique for such applications.

In a few previous studies, real-life information has been detected for real-world crimes with life-changing consequences [the real crime study of Farwell et al. (2013)], and other real-life specific events [experiment 2 of Farwell and Donchin (1991), Farwell and Smith (2001), and people (Meijer et al., 2007)]. Almost all other ERP-based CIT studies have detected information obtained by the subjects in the course of a laboratory information-imparting procedure such as a mock crime (Farwell, 2012, 2014). Meixner and Rosenfeld (2014) conducted a comparison CIT in detecting information regarding unscripted activities that subjects had videotaped the previous day in conjunction with the experiment. Such activities are different from real-life activities; no one would commit an actual crime under such circumstances. Meixner and Rosenfeld failed to cite the previous peer-reviewed publications reporting field studies on real-world crimes and other real-life events, and falsely claimed to be the first study investigating information obtained in real life. Their results were similar to those of other comparison-CIT studies, including the results reported here (Appendix 2).

FIELD APPLICATIONS IN REAL-WORLD CRIMES

These results complement the results of previous studies (Farwell and Smith, 2001; Farwell et al., 2013) in which the classification CIT was applied to detect concealed information regarding specific events, including field applications involving real-world major crimes. Field applications with life-changing or life-threatening consequences to the outcome involve more demanding conditions, including high motivation and other emotional factors, complexities, logistical challenges, uncontrolled context, and other factors that are difficult to bring under experimental control. We have conducted classification-CIT tests in real-world situations in which all of these demanding conditions were present, for example, tests on both innocent and guilty individuals who were facing the death penalty for murder as well as individuals who had already been convicted of murder and were attempting to establish their innocence. In such situations, low error rate and high statistical confidence are obviously of paramount importance.

The low error rate produced by the classification-CIT methods applied was one of the key features considered when brain fingerprinting was ruled admissible in court in the Harrington murder case (Harrington v. State, 2001; Farwell and Makeig, 2005; Roberts, 2007) in which a falsely convicted man was ultimately exonerated and freed. Extremely low error rates and high statistical confidences were equally important for using the ERP-based classification CIT to bring perpetrators such as serial killer J. B. Grinder to justice (Farwell, 2012; Farwell et al., 2013).

WHAT ARE THE PRIMARY METHODS THAT MAY HAVE CONTRIBUTED TO THE LOW ERROR RATE AND HIGH STATISTICAL CONFIDENCES REPORTED HEREIN?

The following features of the methods practiced in this research may have contributed to the low error rate and high statistical confidences obtained here and in previous studies with these methods. The primary difference between this research and various studies that produced an order of magnitude higher error rates and average 50% (chance) statistical confidence for information-absent determinations is that we used the classification CIT, rather than the comparison CIT. The comparison CIT was used in virtually all of the studies that have reported high error rates and low statistical confidences (Farwell, 2012, 2014). We applied a classification statistical algorithm, rather than a comparison algorithm, in data analysis. We used each subject's response to situation-relevant target stimuli as a template for that subject's brain response to known, situation-relevant information. We used the subject's response to irrelevant stimuli as a template for that subject's brain response to unknown or irrelevant information. We then used bootstrapping to classify the subject's brain response to the probe stimuli as being more similar to his response to known information relevant to the investigated situation (targets) or to her response to unknown, irrelevant information (irrelevants). This allowed us to make both information-present and information-absent determinations with a high statistical confidence that the determination made is in fact correct in light of the effect size and variability in this subject's data, and that the opposite determination would be incorrect (see Appendix 2).

By contrast, the comparison CIT ignores the target responses and compares only the probe and irrelevant responses, resulting in lower accuracy and statistical confidences averaging 50% (chance) for information-absent determinations, as described in Appendix 2 and in Farwell (2012, 2014) and Farwell et al. (2013).

One previous error and resulting misrepresentation (we presume inadvertent) has caused considerable confusion in this regard (see Appendix 2). Rosenfeld et al. (2004) purported to be a replication of Farwell and Donchin (1991), but in fact did not use the two-tailed classification CIT of Farwell and Donchin, but rather a one-tailed method similar to the comparison CIT of Rosenfeld's other studies (see Appendix 2). The high error rates and low statistical confidences of Rosenfeld et al. (2004) have been mistakenly cited (Rosenfeld et al., 2008) as evidence that Farwell and Donchin's classification-CIT methods are inaccurate (and susceptible to countermeasures), whereas in fact those results only demonstrate that Rosenfeld et al.'s fundamentally different methods are inaccurate (and susceptible to countermeasures) (Farwell, 2011).

Our current results demonstrate once again that the comparison CIT produces higher error rates and lower statistical confidences than the classification CIT, even when the other brain fingerprinting scientific standards (Appendix 1) are substantially met.

WHAT METHODS ARE NECESSARY TO PRODUCE HIGH STATISTICAL CONFIDENCES WITH BOOTSTRAPPING?

To produce high statistical confidences with bootstrapping, first of all the methods applied must be effective in producing the predicted experimental effects in the brain responses. Given that, what else is necessary in the statistical methods?

The statistical model of the classification CIT predicts high statistical confidences for both information-present and information-absent determinations, and this is what has been consistently reported. The statistical model of the comparison CIT predicts average statistical confidences no better than chance (50%) for information-absent determinations, and this also is what has been reported in the studies to date (Farwell, 2012, 2014; Appendix 2).

The bootstrapping technique applied here, and in all studies implementing the 20 standards, uses a classification CIT. It computes the probability that the probe responses are more similar to the target responses than to the irrelevant responses. 100% minus this is the probability that the probe responses are more similar to the irrelevant responses. This allows for a result of a high statistical confidence for both information-present and information-absent determinations. The comparison CIT computes the probability that the probe responses are larger than the irrelevant responses. This probability is expected to be high for information-present subjects. For information-absent subjects, probe and irrelevant responses are expected to be identical, so the expected value of the probability that the probe response is larger is 50%. This is the expected bootstrap probability that information present is the correct determination, the expected information-present statistical confidence. This makes the expected information-absent probability or statistical confidence also 50% (i.e., 100-50% = 50%). Thus, the expected statistical confidence for an information-absent determination with the comparison CIT is 50% (chance), assuming that the methods and statistics work as predicted. This is described in detail in Appendix 2.

Statistical confidences for information-absent determinations reported for the comparison CIT to date have in every study averaged approximately 50% (or less). Approximately half of the information-absent statistical confidences reported have been invalid, that is, less than 50% (chance) (Farwell, 2012, 2014). In approximately half of the cases, authors reported less than a 50% probability that the chosen (information-absent/"innocent") determination was correct, according to the statistics used to arrive at the determination. For example, in Meixner et al. (2009, p. 215; Table 2; "innocent" subject 11) the subject was determined to be "innocent" (information absent) when the computed probability was 85% that "guilty" was the correct determination (i.e., that the probe P300 was larger than the irrelevant P300). Statistical confidence for this (correct) determination was 15%, far less than chance. 60% of subjects correctly determined to be "innocent" in this condition had statistical confidences of less than 50% (chance) that this determination was correct (i.e., had invalid results).

The comparison CIT in this research, as in previous comparison CIT studies (e.g., Rosenfeld et al., 2008; Dietrich et al., 2014; Meixner and Rosenfeld, 2014; see Appendix 2), produced markedly higher error rates and lower statistical confidences than those of the classification CIT. The results of this research, along with the results of all previous research (Farwell, 2012, 2014), suggest that applying the classification CIT rather than the comparison CIT is not only a sufficient condition, but is also a necessary condition for obtaining median 95% statistical confidences, and in particular for obtaining greater than 90% median statistical confidences for information-absent subjects—or even for obtaining greater than chance (50%) median statistical confidences for information-absent subjects (see Appendix 2).

WHAT ADDITIONAL METHODS MAY HAVE CONTRIBUTED TO THE LOW ERROR RATE AND HIGH STATISTICAL CONFIDENCES REPORTED?

We used double-centered correlation as a measure of the similarity of the probe response to the target or irrelevant response (see Appendix 2). This metric has the advantage of including the entire response, not just a single point (or average of a few points) such as the peak amplitude or the difference between the positive P300 peak and the negative LNP peak. It inherently takes into account not only the peak amplitude, but also the latency and morphology of the full ERP. With the correlation metric, latency differences between probe, target, and irrelevant responses, as well as individual differences in latency and morphology of the ERP, contribute to the characterization of the response and hence to the accuracy and statistical confidence of the result. The information contained in such differences is lost when the P300 is characterized by a single number such as peak amplitude, as applied in, for example, Rosenfeld et al. (2008) and Meixner and Rosenfeld (2014). Our more comprehensive characterization of the waveform may be one reason for the low error rate and high statistical confidence of this research and the previous studies that have used this method.

The term "brain fingerprinting" arises from an analogy to fingerprints that has several facets. Fingerprinting matches prints from the crime scene with prints on the fingers. DNA "fingerprinting" matches biological samples from the crime scene with biological samples from the suspect. "Brain fingerprinting" matches information from the crime scene with information stored in the brain of the subject. Moreover, fingerprints calculate a match based on multiple characteristics. In the autonomic skin conductance response (SCR) as well as in comparison-CIT P300 measurements, the response is generally defined in terms of a single parameter. With SCR this may be the maximum conductance increase that occurs following stimulus onset. With the P300 this is usually peak-to-post-(negative)-peak amplitude, defined as a single number. Brain fingerprinting, like fingerprinting, uses multiple facets of the response to compute a match between known patterns and the pattern tested, taking into account not only the peak amplitude but also the morphology and time course of both the positive and negative peaks in the response.

We used situation-relevant targets. Target stimuli, like probes, were relevant to the information detected. This makes the targets more similar to the probes for the subjects who possess the relevant information, and thus may increase accuracy and statistical confidence (Farwell et al., 2013). The difference between the targets and the probes was that the targets were identified to the subject in subject instructions and required a special button press, and probes were not identified in instructions and required the same button press as irrelevants.

WHAT ARE THE POSSIBLE SHORTCOMINGS OF THE CURRENT STUDY?

Despite the 0% error rate, the results of this research have certain shortcomings when considered in light of the rigorous requirements demanded by field applications with major consequences. Although all determinations were correct and very far from a false positive or false negative error, the statistical confidence of some determinations was low enough to be close to an indeterminate. This contrasts with previous studies (Farwell and Smith, 2001; Farwell et al., 2013), where all determinations were correct and also far from an indeterminate result.

One reason for this shortcoming may be the relatively low number of trials presented in this research, and consequently a lower signal-to-noise ratio. [This does not, however, explain why the FBI agent study (Farwell et al., 2013) produced higher statistical confidences than this research, without more trials. Further research may identify other differentiating factors]. This research used only 84 probe trials and 84 target trials in the averages. In previous studies where we have used at least 100 probe trials and an equal number of targets, statistical confidences have been considerably higher. Moreover, the results of these two studies demonstrate that while brain fingerprinting standard 13 (use at least 100 probe trials—see Appendix 1) has been shown to be useful for producing optimal results, it is not absolutely requisite for achieving high levels of accuracy or statistical confidence. In other words, standard 13 is part of the well-established set of sufficient conditions, but is not a necessary condition for low error rate and high statistical confidences.

SUMMARY

We used the classification CIT to detect information gained by subjects in the course of real life. They gained the tested information in real-life events over a period of years before, and completely unrelated to, the experimental procedures. This was a specific screening or focused screening test, rather than a specific issue test. That is, rather than detecting information obtained at a particular place and time (such as while committing a crime), we detected information known to people with specific training, expertise, and organizational affiliation, specifically knowledge of military medicine by US Navy military medical experts. Subjects obtained this knowledge through a variety of experiences at different times and places for different individuals.

In detecting this concealed information, the classification CIT with the P300 + LNP produced 0% error rate and median 99.9% statistical confidence for individual determinations, a significantly lower error rate and higher statistical confidences than those produced by the comparison CIT.

Although the classification-CIT methods using both the P300 and the P300 + LNP produced the same 0% error rate, the P300 + LNP produced significantly higher statistical confidences for individual determinations. In continued field use, with the concomitant demanding conditions, eventually errors (or at least indeterminates) may occur with these methods. If so, then the higher statistical confidences produced by the P300 + LNP (rather than the P300 alone) can be expected to result in lower error rates when the error rate is non-zero.

In our view, to reliably produce the predicted experimental effect and to be viable for field use, a technique must consistently produce less than 1% error rate, along with high statistical confidences for both information-present and information-absent determinations.

The results of this study, together with the results of similar studies such as the FBI agent study and the bomb-maker study of Farwell et al. (2013), suggest that the classification CIT methods specified here, when the full P300 + LNP epoch is employed in data analysis, can be used effectively in specific screening tests to detect knowledge characteristic of individuals with specific training, expertise, and/or affiliation with a particular agency or organization. In our current study, this was accomplished in a specific screening test under controlled conditions, with the limitations inherent thereto. Prior research has applied these same methods in field conditions in a specific issue test in investigating actual crimes, with the concomitant complications related to motivation, emotions, logistics, experimental control, and other uncontrollable factors. Taken together with previous successful field applications in real-world criminal investigations, our results suggest that these methods may have application in both national security and law enforcement, for instance in identifying trained terrorists, bomb makers, members of a terrorist cell, hostile intelligence agents, members of an organized crime organization, and others with specific knowledge, expertise, training, and/or affiliations of interest.

ACKNOWLEDGMENTS

Funding was provided by the US Central Intelligence Agency (CIA), Contract No. 92-F138600-000. We are grateful to the US Navy and USUHS for providing subjects and facilities. We are grateful to Dr. Christine Furedy (York University) for assistance in editing the manuscript. Study design; collection, analysis, and interpretation of data; and writing of this report were undertaken solely by the authors. The views expressed herein are solely the views of the authors.

REFERENCES

Allen, J., and Iacono, W. G. (1997). A comparison of methods for the analysis of event-related potentials in deception detection. *Psychophysiology* 34, 234–240. doi: 10.1111/j.1469-8986.1997.tb02137.x

Baudena, P., Halgren, E., Heit, G., and Clarke, J. M. (1995). Intracerebral potentials to rare target and distractor auditory and visual stimuli. III. Frontal cortex. *Electroencephalogr. Clin. Neurophysiol.* 94, 251–264. doi: 10.1016/0013-4694(95)98476-O

Brouwer, A. M., van Erp, J. B. B., Aloise, F., and Cincotti, F. (2010). Tactile, visual, and bimodal P300s: could bimodal P300s boost BCI performance? *SRX Neurosci.* 2010:967027. doi: 10.3814/2010/967027

Dietrich, A. B., Hu, X., and Rosenfeld, J. P. (2014). The effects of sweep numbers per average and protocol type on the accuracy of the P300-based concealed information test. *Appl. Psychophysiol. Biofeedback* 39, 67–73. doi: 10.1007/s10484-014-9244-y

Fabiani, M., Gratton, G., Karis, D., and Donchin, E. (1987). "Definition, identification, and reliability of measurement of the P300 component of the event-related brain potential," in *Advances in Psychophysiology*, Vol. 2, eds P. K. Ackles, J. R. Jennings, and M. G. H. Coles (Greenwich, CT: JAI Press, Inc.), 1–78.

Farwell, L. A. (1994). *Method and Apparatus for Multifaceted Electroencephalographic Response Analysis (MERA)*. US Patent #5,363,858. Washington, DC: United States Patent and Trademark Office.

Farwell, L. A. (1995a). *Method and Apparatus for Truth Detection*. US Patent #5,406,956. Washington, DC: United States Patent and Trademark Office.

Farwell, L. A. (1995b). *Method for Electroencephalographic Information Detection*. US Patent #5,467,777. Washington, DC: United States Patent and Trademark Office.

Farwell, L. A. (2011). Brain fingerprinting: corrections to Rosenfeld. *Sci. Rev. Mental Health Pract.* 8, 56–68.

Farwell, L. A. (2012). Brain fingerprinting: a comprehensive tutorial review of detection of concealed information with event-related brain potentials. *Cogn. Neurodyn.* 6, 115–154. doi: 10.1007/s11571-012-9192-2

Farwell, L. A. (2013). "Lie detection," in *Encyclopedia of Forensic Sciences, 2nd Edn.*, eds J. A. Siegel and P. J. Saukko (Waltham: Academic Press), 144–149. doi: 10.1016/B978-0-12-382165-2.00025-8

Farwell, L. A. (2014). "Brain fingerprinting: detection of concealed information," in *Wiley Encyclopedia of Forensic Science*, eds A. Jamieson and A. A. Moenssens (Chichester: John Wiley). doi: 10.1002/9780470061589.fsa1013

Farwell, L. A., and Donchin, E. (1986). The "brain detector": P300 in the detection of deception. *Psychophysiology* 23, 434.

Farwell, L. A., and Donchin, E. (1988a). Event-related brain potentials in interrogative polygraphy: analysis using bootstrapping. *Psychophysiology* 25, 445.

Farwell, L. A., and Donchin, E. (1988b). Talking off the top of your head: toward a mental prosthesis utilizing event-related brain potentials. *Electroencephalogr. Clin. Neurophysiol.* 70, 510–513. doi: 10.1016/0013-4694(88)90149-6

Farwell, L. A., and Donchin, E. (1991). The truth will out: interrogative polygraphy ("lie detection") with event-related brain potentials. *Psychophysiology* 28, 531–547. doi: 10.1111/j.1469-8986.1991.tb01990.x

Farwell, L. A., and Makeig, T. H. (2005). Farwell brain fingerprinting in the case of Harrington v. State. *Open Court* X[10]:(3), 7–10.

Farwell, L. A., Martinerie, J. M., Bashore, T. R., Rapp, P. E., and Goddard, P. H. (1993). Optimal digital filters for long-latency components of the event-related brain potential. *Psychophysiology* 30, 306–315. doi: 10.1111/j.1469-8986.1993.tb03357.x

Farwell, L. A., and Richardson, D. C. (2006). Brain fingerprinting in field conditions. *Psychophysiology* 43, S38.

Farwell, L. A., and Richardson, D. C. (2013). Brain fingerprinting: let's focus on the science—a reply to Meijer, Ben-Shakhar, Verschuere, and Donchin. *Cogn. Neurodyn.* 7, 159–166. doi: 10.1007/s11571-012-9238-5

Farwell, L. A., Richardson, D. C., and Richardson, G. M. (2013). Brain fingerprinting field studies comparing P300-MERMER and P300 brainwave responses in the detection of concealed information. *Cogn. Neurodyn.* 7, 263–299. doi: 10.1007/s11571-012-9230-0

Farwell, L. A., and Smith, S. S. (2001). Using brain MERMER testing to detect concealed knowledge despite efforts to conceal. *J. Foren. Sci.* 46, 135–143.

Gamer, M., and Berti, S. (2010). Task relevance and recognition of concealed information have different influences on electrodermal activity and event-related brain potentials. *Psychophysiology* 47, 355–364. doi: 10.1111/j.1469-8986.2009.00933.x

Gamer, M., and Berti, S. (2012). P300 amplitudes in the concealed information test are less affected by depth of processing than electrodermal responses. *Front. Hum. Neurosci.* 6:308. doi: 10.3389/fnhum.2012.00308

Grier, J. B. (1971). Non-parametric indexes for sensitivity and bias: computing formulas. *Psychol. Bull.* 75, 424–429. doi: 10.1037/h0031246

Halgren, E., Baudena, P., Clarke, J. M., Heit, G., Liegeois, C., Chauvel, P., et al. (1995). Intracerebral potentials to rare target and distractor auditory and visual stimuli. I. Superior temporal plane and parietal lobe. *Electroencephalogr. Clin. Neurophysiol.* 94, 191–220. doi: 10.1016/0013-4694(94)00259-N

Halgren, E., Marinkovic, K., and Chauvel, P. (1998). Generators of the late cognitive potentials in auditory and visual oddball tasks. *Electroencephalogr. Clin. Neurophysiol.* 106, 156–164. doi: 10.1016/S0013-4694(97)00119-3

Halgren, E., Stapleton, J. M., Smith, M. E., and Altafullah, I. (1986). "Generators of the human scalp P3(s)," in *Evoked Potentials, Frontiers of Clinical Neuroscience,* Vol. 3, eds R. Q. Cracco and I. Bodis-Wollner (New York, NY: Alan R. Liss), 269–286.

Harrington v. State. (2001). *Case No. PCCV 073247, Iowa District Court for Pottawattamie County.* Council Bluffs, IA.

Iacono, W. G. (2008). The forensic application of "brain fingerprinting": why scientists should encourage the use of P300 memory detection methods. *Am. J. Bioeth.* 8, 30–32. doi: 10.1080/15265160701828550

Johnson, M. M., and Rosenfeld, J. P. (1992). Oddball-evoked P300-based method of deception detection in the laboratory II: utilization of non-selective activation of relevant knowledge. *Int. J. Psychophysiol.* 12, 289–306. doi: 10.1016/0167-8760(92)90067-L

Linden, D. (2005). The P300, where in the brain is it produced and what does it tell us? *Neuroscientist* 11, 563–576. doi: 10.1177/1073858405280524

Lykken, D. T. (1959). The GSR in the detection of guilt. *J. Appl. Psychol.* 43, 385–388. doi: 10.1037/h0046060

Magliero, A., Bashore, T. R., Coles, M. G. H., and Donchin, E. (1984). On the dependence of P300 latency on stimulus evaluation processes. *Psychophysiology* 21, 171–186. doi: 10.1111/j.1469-8986.1984.tb00201.x

Matsuda, I., Nittono, H., Hirota, A., Ogawa, T., and Takasawa, N. (2009). Event-related brain potentials during the standard autonomic-based concealed information test. *Int. J. Psychophysiol.* 74, 58–68. doi: 10.1016/j.ijpsycho.2009.07.004

Meijer, E. H., Smulders, F. T. Y., Merckelbach, H. L. G. J., and Wolf, A. G. (2007). The P300 is sensitive to face recognition. *Int. J. Psychophysiol.* 66, 231–237. doi: 10.1016/j.ijpsycho.2007.08.001

Meixner, J. B., Haynes, A., Winograd, M. R., Brown, J., and Rosenfeld, P. J. (2009). Assigned versus random, countermeasure-like responses in the p300 based complex trial protocol for detection of deception: task demand effects. *Appl. Psychophysiol. Biofeedback* 34, 209–220. doi: 10.1007/s10484-009-9091-4

Meixner, J. B., and Rosenfeld, J. P. (2014). Detecting knowledge of incidentally acquired, real-world memories using a P300-based concealed-information test. *Psychol. Sci.* 25, 1994–2005. doi: 10.1177/0956797614547278

Roberts, A. J. (2007). Everything new is old again: brain fingerprinting and evidentiary analogy. *Yale J. Law Technol.* 9, 234–270.

Rosenfeld, J. P., Labkovsky, E., Lui, M. A., Winograd, M., Vandenboom, C., and Chedid, K. (2008). The complex trial protocol (CTP): a new, countermeasure-resistant, accurate P300-based method for detection of concealed information. *Psychophysiology* 45, 906–919. doi: 10.1111/j.1469-8986.2008.00708.x

Rosenfeld, J. P., Soskins, M., Bosh, G., and Ryan, A. (2004). Simple effective countermeasures to P300-based tests of detection of concealed information. *Psychophysiology* 41, 205–219. doi: 10.1111/j.1469-8986.2004.00158.x

Smith, M. E., Halgren, E., Sokolik, M., Baudena, P., Musolino, A., Liegeois-Chauvel, C., et al. (1990). The intracranial topography of the P3 event-related potential elicited during auditory oddball. *Electroencephalogr. Clin. Neurophysiol.* 235–248. doi: 10.1016/0013-4694(90)90018-F

Stapleton, J. M., and Halgren, E. (1987). Endogenous potentials evoked in simple cognitive tasks: depth components and task correlates. *Electroencephalogr. Clin. Neurophysiol.* 67, 44–52. doi: 10.1016/0013-4694(87)90162-3

Sutton, S., Braren, M., Zubin, J., and John, E. R. (1965). Evoked potential correlates of stimulus uncertainty. *Science* 150, 1187–1188. doi: 10.1126/science.150.3700.1187

Wasserman, S., and Bockenholt, U. (1989). Bootstrapping: applications to psychophysiology. *Psychophysiology* 27, 208–221. doi: 10.1111/j.1469-8986.1989.tb03159.x 76,

APPENDIX 1

BRAIN FINGERPRINTING SCIENTIFIC STANDARDS

1. Use equipment and methods for stimulus presentation, data acquisition, and data recording that are within the standards for the field of cognitive psychophysiology and event-related brain potential research. These standards are well documented elsewhere. For example, the standard procedures Farwell introduced as evidence in the Harrington case were accepted by the court, the scientific journals, and the other expert witnesses in the case (Harrington v. State, 2001; Farwell, 2012, 2014). Use a recording epoch other expert witnesses in the case. Use a recording epoch long enough to include the full P300 + LNP (i.e., P300-MERMER). For pictorial stimuli or realistic word stimuli, use at least a 1,800-millisecond recording epoch. (Shorter epochs may be appropriate for very simple stimuli).
2. Use correct electrode placement. The P300 and P300-MERMER are universally known to be maximal at the midline parietal scalp site, Pz in the standard International 10–20 system.
3. Apply brain fingerprinting tests only when there is sufficient information that is known only to the perpetrator and investigators. Use a minimum of six probes and six targets.
4. Use stimuli that isolate the critical variable: the subject's knowledge or lack of knowledge of the probe stimuli as significant in the context of the investigated situation. Obtain the relevant knowledge from the criminal investigator (or for laboratory studies from the knowledge-imparting procedure such as a mock crime and/or subject training session). Divide the relevant knowledge into probe stimuli and target stimuli. Probe stimuli constitute information that has not been revealed to the subject. Target stimuli contain information that has been revealed to the subject after the crime or investigated situation.
5. If initially there are fewer targets than probes, create more targets. Ideally, this is done by seeking additional known information from the criminal investigators. Note that targets may contain information that has been publicly disclosed. Alternatively, some potential probe stimuli can be used as targets by disclosing to the subject the specific items and their significance in the context of the investigated situation.
6. For each probe and each target, fabricate several stimuli of the same type that are unrelated to the investigated situation. These become the irrelevant stimuli. Use stimuli that isolate the critical variable. For irrelevant stimuli, select items that would be equally plausible for an information-absent subject. The stimulus ratio is approximately one-sixth probes, one-sixth targets, and two-thirds irrelevants.
7. Ascertain that the probes contain information that the subject has no known way of knowing, other than participation in the investigated situation. This information is provided by the criminal investigator for field studies, and results from proper information control in laboratory studies.
8. Make certain that the subject understands the significance of the probes, and ascertain that the probes constitute only information that the subject denies knowing, as follows. Describe the significance of each probe to the subject. Show him the probe and the corresponding irrelevants, without revealing which is the probe. Ask the subject if he knows (for any non-situation-related reason) which stimulus in each group is situation-relevant/crime-relevant. Describe the significance of the probes and targets that will appear in each test block immediately before the block.
9. If a subject has knowledge of any probes for a reason unrelated to the investigated situation, eliminate these from the stimulus set. This provides the subject with an opportunity to disclose any knowledge of the probes that he may have for any innocent reason previously unknown to the scientist. This will prevent any non-incriminating knowledge from being included in the test.
10. Ascertain that the subject knows the targets and their significance in the context of the investigated situation. Show him a list of the targets. Describe the significance of each target to the subject.
11. Require an overt behavioral task that requires the subject to recognize and process every stimulus, specifically including the probe stimuli, and to prove behaviorally that he has done so on every trial. Detect the resulting brain responses. Do not depend on detecting brain responses to assigned tasks that the subject can covertly avoid doing while performing the necessary overt responses.
12. Instruct the subjects to press one button in response to targets, and another button in response to all other stimuli. Do not instruct the subjects to "lie" or "tell the truth" in response to stimuli. Do not assign different behavioral responses or mental tasks for probe and irrelevant stimuli.
13. In order to obtain statistically robust results for each individual case, present a sufficient number of trials of each type to obtain adequate signal-to-noise enhancement through signal averaging. Use robust signal-processing and noise-reduction techniques, including appropriate digital filters and artifact-detection algorithms. The number of trials required will vary depending on the complexity of the stimuli, and is generally more for a field case. In their seminal study, Farwell and Donchin (1991) used 144 probe trials. In the Harrington field case, a murder case wherein brain fingerprinting and Farwell's testimony in it were admitted as scientific evidence, Farwell used 288 probe trials (Harrington v. State, 2001; Farwell et al., 2013). In any case, use at least 100 probe trials and an equal number of targets. Present three to six unique probes in each block.
14. Use appropriate mathematical and statistical procedures to analyze the data. Do not classify the responses according to subjective judgments. Use statistical procedures properly and reasonably. At a minimum, do not determine subjects to be in a category where the statistics applied show that the determination is more likely than not to be incorrect, i.e., statistical confidence is less than 50%.
15. (a) Use a mathematical classification algorithm, such as bootstrapping on correlations, that isolates the critical variable by classifying the responses to the probe stimuli as being either more similar to the target responses or to the irrelevant responses. (b) In a forensic setting, conduct two analyses: one using only the P300 (to be more certain of meeting the

standard of general acceptance in the scientific community), and one using the P300 + LNP (P300-MERMER) to provide the current state of the art.

16. Use a mathematical data-analysis algorithm that takes into account the variability across single trials, such as bootstrapping.
17. Set a specific, reasonable statistical criterion for an information-present determination and a separate, specific, reasonable statistical criterion for an information-absent determination. Classify results that do not meet either criterion as indeterminate. Recognize that an indeterminate outcome is not an error, neither a false positive nor a false negative. Error rate is the percentage of information-present or information-absent determinations that are false positives and false negatives respectively; accuracy is 100% minus the error rate.
18. Restrict scientific conclusions to a determination as to whether or not a subject has the specific situation-relevant knowledge embodied in the probes stored in his brain. Recognize that brain fingerprinting detects only presence or absence of information – not guilt, honesty, lying, deception, or any action or non-action. Do not offer scientific opinions on whether the subject is lying or whether he committed a crime or other act. Recognize that the question of guilt or innocence is a legal determination to be made by a judge and jury, not a scientific determination to be made by a scientist or a computer.
19. Evaluate error rate/accuracy based on actual ground truth. Ground truth is the true state of what a scientific test seeks to detect. Brain fingerprinting is a method to detect information stored in a subject's brain. Ground truth is whether the specific information tested is in fact stored in the subject's brain. Establish ground truth with certainty through post-test interviews in laboratory experiments and in field experiments wherein subjects are cooperative. Establish ground truth insofar as possible through secondary means in real-life forensic applications with uncooperative subjects. Recognize that ground truth is the true state of what the subject in fact knows, not what the experimenter thinks the subject should know, not what the subject has done or not done, and not whether the subject is guilty, or deceptive.
20. Make scientific determinations based on brain responses. Do not attempt to make scientific determinations based on overt behavior that can be manipulated, such as reaction time.

APPENDIX 2

PREVIOUS RESEARCH ON SUFFICIENT AND NECESSARY CONDITIONS FOR CRITERION LOW ERROR RATES AND HIGH STATISTICAL CONFIDENCES

Summary of previous results

The most striking feature of the data reported to date, including this research, is the sharp bimodal distribution of error rates and statistical confidences. So far, the only proposed explanation for this bimodal distribution is that a specific set of classification-CIT methods, as described here and in the 20 brain fingerprinting standards (Appendix 1), have consistently produced less than 1% error rate and greater than 95% median statistical confidences for individual determinations (Farwell, 2012, 2014; Farwell et al., 2013). Alternative methods, exemplified by Rosenfeld et al. (2004, 2008), Dietrich et al. (2014), and Meixner and Rosenfeld (2014), have produced an order of magnitude higher error rates, as well as statistical confidences averaging no better than chance (50%) for information-absent ("innocent"/"nonknowledgeable") determinations. By applying two different data-analysis methods to the same data, our research directly addresses a fundamental difference in methods: the classification CIT vs. comparison CIT. This fundamental difference in methods accounts for a major difference in the results reported by previous studies applying the respective methods.

Previous results can be summarized as follows. All data are consistent with the hypothesis that standards 1–20 (Appendix 1) provide sufficient conditions for an ERP-based CIT to obtain less than 1% error rate and greater than 95% median statistical confidence, including greater than 90% statistical confidence for both information-present and information-absent determinations. At least some of these standards constitute necessary conditions. Several previous studies (e.g., Johnson and Rosenfeld, 1992; Rosenfeld et al., 2008; Dietrich et al., 2014; Meixner and Rosenfeld, 2014) demonstrated that applying comparison-CIT methods that fail to meet Standards 3–6, 8–15, and 17–20 resulted in high error rates, low statistical confidences, and invalid results. For reviews of all relevant studies in English to date, including a detailed discussion of which of the 20 standards were found to be necessary conditions in which studies, see Farwell (2012, 2014). Among the necessary conditions are standards 14, 15a, and 17, which describe the classification CIT and distinguish it from the comparison CIT. Standard 11, which requires subjects to read and process each stimulus and prove with a differential button press that they have done so, is a necessary condition for tests on motivated subjects in field conditions with major consequences to the outcome, but not for tests with accommodating subjects in the absence of non-trivial consequences. Standard 13, which requires a minimum number of probe trials in the average, is not a necessary condition, but does contribute to higher statistical confidences and potentially to higher accuracy.

Why the classification CIT (standards 14, 15a, and 17) is a necessary condition for high statistical confidences

In the classification CIT, probes and targets are both relevant details about the investigated situation. For information-present subjects, both are expected to result in essentially the same ERP, containing a large P300 and LNP. For an information-absent subject, the irrelevants and (unrecognized) probes are indistinguishable and equally irrelevant, and are expected to elicit identical ERPs lacking a large P300 and LNP. Classification-CIT bootstrapping asks the statistical question, "What is the probability that the probes are more similar to the targets than to the irrelevants?" 100% minus this is the probability that the probes are more similar to the irrelevants. The expected value of this statistic is 100% in the information-present direction (probes resemble targets) for information-present subjects, and 100% in the information-absent direction (0% in the information-present direction; probes resemble irrelevants) for information-absent subjects (see **Figure 1**). Thus, if the data are as predicted, the classification CIT provides a high statistical confidence for both information-present and information-absent determinations.

The comparison CIT ignores targets and asks the statistical question, "What is the probability that the probe ERPs are larger than the irrelevant ERPs?" For an information-present subject, the expected value is 100%. If the ERPs are as predicted, this method can deliver a high statistical confidence for information present subjects. That is, it can provide a high probability that information present is the correct determination. If the bootstrap probability that information present is correct is over 90%, the subject is determined to be information present (see **Figure 2**). If the bootstrap probability that information present is correct is less than 90%—equivalent to a probability of greater than 10% (i.e., 100–90%) that information absent is correct—the subject is determined to be information absent. Subjects are determined to be information absent with as low as a 10.1% statistically computed probability that this determination is correct. For an information-absent subject, probe and irrelevant ERPs are expected to be identical, so the expected value of the probability that probes are larger is 50%. This is the expected information-present statistical confidence, which makes the expected information-absent statistical confidence also 50% (i.e., 100% − 50% = 50%). This means that if the ERPs are as predicted and the statistics work as designed, the average statistical confidence for information-absent determinations will be 50% (chance). In all comparison-CIT studies reported to date (Farwell, 2012, 2014), the average statistical confidence for information-absent subjects has been approximately 50% (or less), and subjects have been determined to be information absent with as low as 10.1% statistical confidence or computed probability that this determination is correct. In summary, the comparison CIT, in accord with the predictions of the statistical model, has in every study to date produced statistical confidences averaging no better than chance for information-absent determinations. Thus, applying the classification CIT rather than the comparison CIT is a necessary condition for obtaining high statistical confidences, or even better-than-chance statistical confidences for information-absent subjects[3].

Corrections regarding previous studies

Two major errors have led to considerable confusion and misinformation in the literature. Johnson and Rosenfeld (1992) cited Farwell and Donchin (1988a, 1991) and Wasserman and Bockenholt (1989) as the origin of the bootstrapping method, but they did not apply the classification-CIT method introduced by Farwell, Donchin, Wasserman, and Bokenholt. They applied a comparison CIT. Several other subsequent studies by the same group and others have cited Farwell and Donchin and Wasserman and Bockenholt as the source of their bootstrapping method, but have applied the comparison CIT instead. This has led to confusion and misinformation because the results of these two methods are substantially different. In particular, the high error rates and low statistical confidences characteristic of the comparison CIT have sometimes been falsely attributed to the classification CIT (e.g., Rosenfeld et al., 2004, 2008) or to all ERP-based CITs (see Farwell, 2012, 2014; Farwell and Richardson, 2013). Our data demonstrate that these two methods are substantially different not only in experimental design but also in results, for both error rate and statistical confidence.

Another error and consequent (good faith) misrepresentation has led to some apparently (but not actually) highly anomalous results in the literature. Rosenfeld et al. (2004) reported the high error rates and low statistical confidences that are typical of comparison-CIT studies that did not implement the 20 brain fingerprinting scientific standards, but mistakenly characterized their study as a replication of Farwell and Donchin (1991), the original classification-CIT study substantially implementing the standards. The error rate in the "FIT" condition, which was mistakenly described as a replication of Farwell and Donchin, was 46% in one group and 31% in another (without countermeasures), and even higher with countermeasures. Both of these are obviously higher than the less-than-1% error rate that has been achieved (both with and without countermeasures) in all instances in which the Farwell and Donchin methods were actually applied. The reason for this discrepancy is that, although Rosenfeld et al. characterized their methods as a replication of Farwell and Donchin, the actual methods they applied, as in that group's other studies, did not implement over half of the 20 brain fingerprinting standards, specifically standards 3–6, 8–10, 12–15, and 17–20 (Farwell, 2012, 2014; Farwell and Richardson, 2013). Among many other fundamental differences, they did not use the classification-CIT bootstrapping method of Farwell and Donchin and Wasserman and Bockenholt (1989). Thus, the high error rates Rosenfeld et al. reported are consistent with the high error rates of the other studies that did not implement many of the same standards. Rosenfeld et al. erroneously concluded that their results showed that the Farwell and Donchin method was inaccurate and susceptible to countermeasures (Rosenfeld et al., 2008), whereas in fact their results showed that their fundamentally different method is inaccurate and susceptible to countermeasures.

When the distinction between the classification CIT and the comparison CIT, and the other standards, are taken into account, the pattern of results in the literature is clear. Two different sets of methods produce two different sets of results. One set of methods, the classification CIT implementing the 20 standards, always has produced low error rates and high statistical confidences. Another, different set of methods implementing the comparison CIT has produced high error rates and low statistical confidences. In light of this distinction, the bimodal distribution of error

[3]We report the bootstrap probability that information present is correct for information-present determinations and the probability that information absent is correct for information-absent determinations. Some previous publications (e.g., Rosenfeld et al., 2004, 2008) report the probability that information present ("guilty") is correct for information-absent ("innocent") as well as information-present determinations. Such papers report bootstrap statistics ranging from 0.01% to 89.9% for information-absent determinations (i.e., the probabilities that information present is correct), with a lower bootstrap figure corresponding to a higher statistical confidence. In such terminology, a determination of "information absent (or innocent), bootstrap index 80%" actually means "information absent, bootstrap probability of being correct 20%." In such terminology, any bootstrap index for a correct information-absent determination that is higher than 50% is an invalid result (although Rosenfeld et al. and some other researchers do not clearly identify such results as invalid). In our terminology, any bootstrap index for a correct information-absent determination that is lower than 50% is an invalid result.

rates and statistical confidences is explicable and even predictable. When this fundamental distinction is ignored or blurred, the literature inexplicably appears to contain two strikingly different groups of results for implementations of one undifferentiated method. Our experiment and results contribute to the clarification of this distinction in methods and the concomitant difference in results.

Why a required button-press discrimination for all stimuli (standard 11) is a necessary condition

The comparison CIT has been implemented in two different experimental designs for stimulus presentation and subject responses. One is the same as the three-stimulus target-probe-irrelevant design applied in the classification CIT and in our comparison-CIT experiment. The difference between the classification and comparison CITs with this design is in the data analysis: *classifying* the probe ERPs as being more similar to the target ERPs or the irrelevant ERPs (or neither—indeterminate) vs. ignoring the targets and *comparing* the probe ERPs with the irrelevant ERPs to determine whether the probe ERPs are significantly larger. Another version of the comparison CIT uses a four-stimulus "complex trial protocol" design (Rosenfeld et al., 2008). Each trial presents two stimuli. The first is always either a target or a non-target. The second is always either a probe or an irrelevant. Targets and non-targets are a completely different type of stimuli from probes and irrelevants, e.g., meaningless numbers (target: "six," nontargets "one" through "five"). Thus, the targets do not provide a template for an information-present response, and without such a template the classification CIT cannot be used. The four-stimulus design must use the comparison-CIT data-analysis algorithm.

In the three-stimulus design, subjects are required to read and process every stimulus, decide if it is a target or not, and push the appropriate button. All subjects, regardless of motivation, are required to perform the same information-processing and button-press tasks. Subject strategies for responding to the four-stimulus complex trial protocol comparison-CIT design, by contrast, differ substantially depending on the motivation of the subject. Subjects are required to distinguish by a button press between targets and non-targets, so they must read and process them, regardless of motivation. After they have pushed the correct button in response to the target/nontarget, they know that no discrimination will be required in response to the next stimulus. They know for certain that either a probe or an irrelevant will appear, and they simply push the same button whatever appears. Accommodating laboratory subjects read and process the probe/irrelevant stimuli as instructed, push the button, and respond with different ERPs to probes and irrelevants, resulting in better-than-chance accuracy of the test (Meixner and Rosenfeld, 2014). Motivated subjects with life-changing consequences to the outcome recognize that they do not need to read and process the probe/irrelevant stimuli in order to push a button whenever something appears on the screen shortly after the target/nontarget discrimination and button press. Thus, motivated subjects do not read and process the probe/irrelevant stimuli. They simply press the single required probe/irrelevant button when something appears on the screen after the target/nontarget, without reading and processing that probe/irrelevant stimulus. Thus, for motivated subjects with life-changing consequences to the outcome, there is no processing of the information content of probes and irrelevants, there are no differences between probe and irrelevant ERPs, and accuracy rate is 0% for the four-stimulus complex trial protocol (Farwell et al., 2013). By contrast, the required button-press discrimination on every trial in the three-stimulus CIT ensures that the subjects read and process every stimulus, resulting in the predicted ERPs to targets, probes, and irrelevants and reliable results of the test. This behaviorally required button-press discrimination in response to every stimulus, including when a probe or irrelevant is presented, may not be necessary for tests with accommodating subjects and lacking any non-trivial consequences, as several studies (e.g., Rosenfeld et al., 2008; Dietrich et al., 2014; Meixner and Rosenfeld, 2014) have shown. It is, however, a necessary condition for reliable results in field use or any application when subjects are highly motivated not to reveal the concealed information, e.g., when they are facing major life-changing consequences to the outcome (Farwell et al., 2013).

Recent comparison-CIT publications provide additional evidence for necessary conditions

Several recent comparison-CIT studies have provided additional evidence for the necessary conditions for low error rates and high statistical confidences. Dietrich et al. (2014) conducted a four-stimulus comparison-CIT test and obtained results similar to those of other previous comparison-CIT studies, including ours. They varied the number of trials in the analysis, and concluded that "even procedures that utilize as few as 33 trials can reliably detect the presence of concealed information." This is in accord with our finding that standard 13 is not a necessary condition. The statement that the four-stimulus complex trial protocol method of Dietrich et al. can "reliably detect…" depends on one's definition of "reliably." Dietrich et al.'s results are indeed no less reliable than those of previous comparison-CIT studies. They are, however, much less reliable than the results obtained with the classification CIT in this research and all previous studies meeting the same standards. In separate experiments Dietrich et al. applied two different comparison CITs: the three-stimulus method and the four-stimulus method. Their subjects were accommodating college students who presumably read and processed the probe and irrelevant stimuli as instructed, despite the fact that the behavioral (button-press) demands of the task did not require them to do so in the four-stimulus method. Thus the probe and irrelevant waveforms were significantly different. They also found that subjects later recalled stimuli in both the three-stimulus and four-stimulus experiments. All of this is expected behavior and results for accommodating subjects when there are no non-trivial consequences to the outcome. Their study does not address the phenomenon described above that with the four-stimulus method, motivated subjects in situations with life-changing consequences to the outcome of the test do not read and process the probe and irrelevant stimuli because the button-press task does not require it in the four-stimulus method, and therefore the four-stimulus complex trial protocol has 100% error rate (0% accuracy) with highly motivated subjects and life-changing consequences to the outcome (Farwell et al., 2013).

Meixner and Rosenfeld (2014) conducted a comparison CIT. They published only bootstrap probabilities and failed to identify a specific criterion for distinguishing between information present ("knowledgeable") and information absent ("nonknowledgeable") subjects[4]. Applying the usual 90% criterion that was applied in all of their previous studies (and in virtually all others), Meixner and Rosenfeld's results are as follows. With one of their two analysis techniques, 25% of determinations for information-present subjects are false negatives, and only 33% of the information-absent determinations are valid, i.e., 67% are invalid, having a computed bootstrap probability of less than chance (50%) of being correct. Their other analysis technique correctly classifies only 33% of the information-present subjects, with 67% false negatives. (Any higher criterion would produce even more errors; any lower criterion would produce unacceptably low statistical confidences for both information-present and information-absent determinations). Their results contribute to establishing the necessary conditions for a viable ERP-based CIT. Their results are comparable to those of the other comparison-CIT studies published to date, including the research we report here. They provide additional data in support of the hypothesis that the application of the classification CIT, rather than the comparison CIT, is a necessary condition for obtaining low error rates, high statistical confidences, reliability, and validity.

[4]Note that Meixner and Rosenfeld (2014), unlike our reports, report only the probability that information present (or "knowledgeable") is correct (or the corresponding number of bootstrap iterations), for all subjects, even if the determination would be information absent (or "nonknowledgeable").

8

EEG sensorimotor correlates of translating sounds into actions

Jaime A. Pineda[1,2]*, Mark Grichanik[1], Vanessa Williams[1], Michelle Trieu[1], Hailey Chang[1] and Christian Keysers[3,4]

[1] *Department of Cognitive Science, University of California, San Diego, La Jolla, CA, USA*
[2] *Neurosciences Group, University of California, San Diego, La Jolla, CA, USA*
[3] *Netherlands Institute for Neuroscience, KNAW, Amsterdam, Netherlands*
[4] *Department of Neuroscience, University Medical Center Groningen, University of Groningen, Netherlands*

***Correspondence:**
Jaime A. Pineda, Department of Cognitive Science, University of California, 9500 Gilman Drive, San Diego, La Jolla, CA 92093-0515, USA
e-mail: pineda@cogsci.ucsd.edu

Understanding the actions of others is a necessary foundational cornerstone for effective and affective social interactions. Such understanding may result from a mapping of observed actions as well as heard sounds onto one's own motor representations of those events. To examine the electrophysiological basis of action-related sounds, EEG data were collected in two studies from adults who were exposed to auditory events in one of three categories: action (either hand- or mouth-based sounds), non-action (environmental sounds), and control sounds (scrambled versions of action sounds). In both studies, triplets of sounds of the same category were typically presented, although occasionally, to ensure an attentive state, trials containing a sound from a different category were presented within the triplet and participants were asked to respond to this oddball event either covertly in one study or overtly in another. Additionally, participants in both studies were asked to mimic hand- and mouth-based motor actions associated with the sounds (motor task). Action sounds elicited larger EEG mu rhythm (8–13 Hz) suppression, relative to control sounds, primarily over left hemisphere, while non-action sounds showed larger mu suppression primarily over right hemisphere. Furthermore, hand-based sounds elicited greater mu suppression over the hand area in sensorimotor cortex compared to mouth-based sounds. These patterns of mu suppression across cortical regions to different categories of sounds and to effector-specific sounds suggest differential engagement of a mirroring system in the human brain when processing sounds.

Keywords: auditory mirror neuron system, action comprehension, mu rhythm, sensorimotor cortex, mu suppression

INTRODUCTION

The discovery of motor neurons in the primate premotor cortex that also exhibit visual "mirroring" properties has spurred a significant amount of research into how we understand the actions of others both within and across species having similar biological effectors (di Pellegrino et al., 1992; Rizzolatti and Craighero, 2004; Iacoboni and Dapretto, 2006). Such visuomotor neurons fire both when a monkey performs a motor action and when it observes another conspecific or human agent perform a similar goal-directed action (Rizzolatti and Craighero, 2004; Iacoboni and Dapretto, 2006; Rizzolatti and Sinigaglia, 2010). Evidence for the existence of a human mirror neuron system (MNS) has been obtained through a variety of indirect population-level measures (Iacoboni et al., 1999; Fadiga et al., 2005) including transcranial magnetic stimulation (TMS) (Fadiga et al., 1999; Maeda et al., 2002), positron emission tomography (PET) (Parsons et al., 1995), functional magnetic resonance imaging (fMRI) (Grezes et al., 2003; Buccino et al., 2004; Iacoboni and Dapretto, 2006), and electroencephalography (EEG) (Cochin et al., 1998, 1999; Pineda et al., 2000; Muthukumaraswamy and Johnson, 2004; Muthukumaraswamy and Singh, 2008; Oberman et al., 2008), and is thought to include premotor cortices (dorsal and ventral) and the inferior parietal cortex in which mirror neurons have also been measured in monkeys (Keysers and Gazzola, 2009; Caspers et al., 2010; Rizzolatti and Sinigaglia, 2010), with more recent evidence also pointing to an important role for the somatosensory cortex in the MNS (Keysers et al., 2010; Caspers et al., 2011). While no overall consensus exists as to the role of mirror neurons in social cognition (Hickok, 2009), one prominent hypothesis suggests that the observer's ability to embody the observed action as his or her own provides a neural scaffolding that facilitates behaviors and cognitive outcomes involved in social cognition, such as understanding actions, imitation, speech and language, theory of mind, social communication, and empathy (Rizzolatti and Craighero, 2004; Ferrari et al., 2009).

In the monkey premotor cortex, mirror neurons were also found to be sensitive to the acoustic correlates of actions, and the corresponding action sound by itself is sufficient to activate these premotor cells (Kohler et al., 2002; Keysers et al., 2003). Similarly, the premotor, posterior parietal and somatosensory cortices of humans show voxels that are active both while performing an action and listening to a similar action (Gazzola et al., 2006), and this activity is somatotopically organized, with more dorsal aspects of the premotor and parietal cortex more active during the execution and sound of hand actions, and more ventral aspects more active during the execution and sound of mouth actions. This somatotopical pattern allows classification of what action someone has performed by using the activity pattern while listening to actions (Etzel et al., 2008). Thus, by extension, the human MNS would appear to be multimodal, i.e., activated by motor, visual, auditory, as well as perhaps other sensory inputs associated with the action (Aglioti and Pazzaglia, 2010). Relatively few studies, however, have investigated the auditory properties of the human MNS, although it has been argued that non-action (environmental) and action-related sounds (those that are reproducible by the body) are likely processed by separate neural systems (Pizzamiglio et al., 2005). Non-action related sounds appear to involve the temporal poles, while action-related sounds appear to involve the same neural machinery as the visual MNS. Because increasing the exposure and proficiency with a given physical action provides for greater activation of auditory mirroring circuits (Ricciardi et al., 2009) and a perceptual-motor link that is rapidly established (Lahav et al., 2007), it has been proposed that these associations result from the Hebbian association between motor programs and what they sound like while we perform an action. Re-afference, input that results from the agent's movement, ensures that premotor neurons that cause the action will have firing that is temporally correlated with that of the auditory neurons that represent the re-afferent sound of the action (Keysers and Perrett, 2004). Perhaps one main difference between auditory and visual mirroring is that while visual aspects of mirroring appears to involve bilateral activity in left and right hemispheres, auditory aspects of mirroring has been reported to be primarily left-lateralized, particularly in the parietal cortex, including the posterior parietal and somatosensory cortex (Gazzola et al., 2006; Lahav et al., 2007). This is not true for environmental sounds, that do trigger robust right hemispheric activations as well (Gazzola et al., 2006). The left lateralization may reflect semantic associations of the sounds that have been previously established.

Mirroring activity cannot be directly recorded in humans except under special circumstances, (see Mukamel et al., 2010), but a number of recent studies have suggested that mirroring may be indirectly measured in the mu frequency band of the EEG (alpha: 8–13 Hz and beta: 15–25 Hz recorded over sensorimotor cortex) (Hari et al., 2000; Muthukumaraswamy et al., 2004; Oberman et al., 2005; Pineda, 2005). Sensorimotor neurons fire synchronously at rest, leading to high-amplitude mu oscillations, and asynchronously during self-movement and the observation of movement, leading to reduced amplitude of the mu band (called mu suppression or event related desynchronization-ERD) (Pineda, 2005). Mu suppression or ERD during action observation, in the absence of self-performed action, has been hypothesized to reflect the downstream modulation of sensorimotor neurons by premotor mirror neurons (Muthukumaraswamy et al., 2004; Oberman et al., 2005; Pineda, 2005). A recent combined EEG-fMRI study has explored the relationship between mu suppression (as measured through EEG) and blood oxygen level dependent (BOLD) activity in regions normally associated with the MNS (as measured using fMRI) during both action observation and action execution (Arnstein et al., 2011). The study found that mu suppression in the alpha band during both action observation and action execution went hand-in-hand with increases in BOLD activity in the dorsal premotor cortex, the inferior parietal lobe and the posterior aspects of the somatosensory cortex (BA2). A weaker association was also found between activity in the ventral premotor cortex and mu suppression. All of these regions are associated with the MNS and have strong cortico-cortico connections in the human and non-human brain with the primary sensorimotor region lining the central sulcus (BA4 and BA3) where the mu rhythm is thought to be generated (Shimazu et al., 2004). Therefore, it is plausible that activity in these MNS regions, during action observation and execution, could desynchronize activity around the central sulcus, and thereby cause the mu suppression in the EEG signal. Furthermore, results of several human mu suppression studies parallel primate single-cell recordings in terms of the object-directedness and sensitivity of the electrophysiology to action observation (Muthukumaraswamy et al., 2004). Consistent with this hypothesis, Keuken et al (Keuken et al., 2011) recently showed that using TMS to disrupt activity in the inferior frontal gyrus directly impacts the modulation of mu rhythms over sensorimotor cortex.

To date no investigations have examined the relationship between auditory aspects of mirroring and EEG mu rhythm suppression in humans in order to inform models of connectivity between these domains. One goal of this study was to test the hypothesis that action-related sounds are processed differently compared to non-action related sounds, as reflected in mu rhythm oscillations. We will specifically assess whether mu rhythm suppression reflects action or non-action related activity. In Studies 1 and 2 participants listened to sounds as well as performed actions while blindfolded that corresponded to those sounds. During the active listening portion of Study 1, participants made overt physical responses to oddball sounds. To assess responses to sounds alone, participants made covert responses in Study 2. In both studies, we predicted that representation of action-based sounds would elicit greater mu-suppression reflecting greater engagement of mirroring processes compared to environmental sounds. That is, we expected that action-related sounds (those interpreted vis-a-vis the observer's own bodily representation) would cause greater mu suppression compared to non-action related sounds.

MATERIALS AND METHODS

PARTICIPANTS

Twenty-eight healthy undergraduate students, including one older student (12 males and 16 females of varied ethnicities; mean age = 20.3 ± 6.2 years; range = 17–47 years) attending the University of California, San Diego (UCSD) participated in Study 1. In Study 2, a different group of twenty eight undergraduate students (13 males and 15 females; mean age = 20.4 ± 1.1 years; range = 18–23 years) participated. All participants were assumed to have normal hearing if they were able to identify the stimuli during an initial auditory identification task. Those who described themselves as left-handed on a self-report questionnaire were excluded from the study. All gave written informed consent prior to taking part and were compensated with course credit for their voluntary participation. The experiment was reviewed and approved by the UCSD Internal Review Board.

AUDITORY STIMULI

The auditory stimulus set was obtained from one of the co-authors (C.K.) who previously used it in an fMRI study (Gazzola et al., 2006) that investigated the human auditory MNS. The stimulus set consisted of three categories of sounds (see **Table 1**): Action (mouth- and hand-based sounds), Non-Action (environmental sounds), and Control or "Fuzzy" (phase-scrambled versions of both mouth and hand control sounds). There were five unique sounds per each category (25 total sounds with each sound presented for 4 s). The Action sounds (e.g., mouth: crunching candy and hand: ripping paper) were tangible sounds that could be easily reproduced by the listener. The Non-Action sounds were comprised of environmental sounds (e.g., howling wind or water dripping). Each control sound was based on one of the action sounds, and resulted from a reverse Fourier transform in which frequencies up to 125 Hz preserved their original phase and all frequencies above 125 Hz had their phase exchanged with that of another frequency. Accordingly, the control sounds were equivalent with respect to the bottom-up global frequency composition of the Action sounds, but were perceived as "fuzzy" because they were phase-scrambled and unrecognizable. For more information on how the sounds were developed see Gazzolla et al. (Gazzola et al., 2006).

Table 1 | Auditory stimuli used for Studies 1 and 2.

SOUND CATEGORY	DESCRIPTION
Mouth	Crunching a hard candy Kissing Gargling Crunching chips Finishing a beverage with a straw
Hand	Ripping a sheet of paper Unrolling scotch tape Zipping a zipper Opening a soda can Crushing a soda can
Environmental	Train passing by Howling wind Waves breaking on the shore Electric discharge Water dripping
Hand control (Fuzzy)	Crumple can Open can Zip Scotch Paper
Mouth control (Fuzzy)	Kiss Candy Chips Gargle Straw

GENERAL EXPERIMENTAL PROCEDURE

All participants took part in an auditory task first and a motor task second. The auditory task was always run before the motor task in order to avoid the possibility that the memory of executing the actions would bias perceptual brain activity. Participants initially completed a general screening questionnaire that enabled the experimenter to exclude individuals due to claustrophobia, prior experience, etc. Prior to EEG recording, participants took part in an Auditory Identification Task in which they were asked to listen attentively and identify the various auditory stimuli. Prior to the presentation of a sound, the experimenter announced the category to which the sound belonged (e.g., Hand Sound). If after three attempts, the participant incorrectly identified the sound, the experimenter would correctly identify the sound for the participant. The sound was played once more before moving on to the next sound to ensure participants now could identify the sound. Participants were not asked to identify nor discriminate control sounds. The experimenter played one of these control sounds and explained that they belonged in their own category of "fuzzy sounds" and did not need to be identified. Prior to the motor task, participants "practiced" performing the motor actions at least once following an experimenter's cue to make sure they followed the protocol.

EEG RECORDING

Participants were instructed not to consume caffeine nor use any hair products the day of the experiment. During EEG capping, they were seated in a comfortable recliner chair inside an acoustically- and electromagnetically-shielded chamber. After light abrasion of EEG electrode sites using NuPrep Gel, disk electrodes were applied using 10–20 conductive paste on the orbital bone below the left eye and the mastoid bone behind both ears. The eye electrode was used to monitor eye blinks and horizontal eye movements. The mastoid electrodes were computationally linked and used as reference electrodes. Seventeen electrodes embedded in a cap were positioned using the International 10–20 system at the following sites: F7, F8, F3, F4, FZ, C3, CZ, C4, P3, PZ, P4, T3, T4, T5, T6, O1, O2. Electrolytic gel was injected at each electrode site and the scalp lightly abraded with a thin wooden dowel to reduce the electrode-skin impedance to below 10 kΩ. The EEG data were recorded with a Neuroscan Synamps system (500 Hz sampling rate, 0.30–30 Hz bandpass filter). Participants were blindfolded and asked to keep their eyes closed during the various task conditions. A video monitoring system was used to ensure that participants remained still and that their hands were in resting position during EEG data collection.

AUDITORY TASK

Study 1

A trial consisting of a sequence of three pseudo-randomly selected sounds from the same category (e.g., Hand sound—Hand sound—Hand sound) was presented at an inter-stimulus interval (ISI) of 1 s. No individual sound appeared twice within the same trial. Sixty trials (twelve from each sound category) were randomized and presented (inter-trial interval or ITI of 3 s) through circumaural headphones (Sony MDR XD 100) using Presentation software (NeuroBehavioral Systems). An additional five randomly interspersed sequences contained "oddball" events. These sequences contained a final sound that was out-of-category (e.g., Mouth sound—Mouth sound—Hand sound). Participants were instructed to click a computer mouse placed under their right hand when detecting such an oddball event. This task was necessary to ensure that participants were *actively* listening to all the stimuli. Control sounds were presented as triplets but were not used as oddball events. While analyzed for accuracy as a behavioral task, these oddball event trials were excluded from further analysis in order to avoid motor contamination of the EEG data. After the task, participants were given the opportunity to take a short break prior to the start of the motor task.

Study 2 modifications to auditory task

In the second study, the ISI was increased to five seconds and the ITI to seven seconds to increase the amount of time participants had to process the individual sound stimuli. The type of response to oddball events also differed, with covert responses in Study 2 to avoid the effects of motor actions. Like Study 1, sequences with "oddball" events were randomly interspersed in between the normal trials. However, instead of actively using a mouse to indicate the oddball events, participants were asked to covertly count the total number of oddballs presented throughout the auditory task. At the end of the block of trials, subjects were asked for the total number of oddball events counted. This task was necessary to ensure that participants were *actively* listening to all the stimuli. Control sounds were not used as oddball events. While analyzed for accuracy as a behavioral task, these oddball event trials were excluded from further analysis in order to avoid any type of motor contamination of the EEG data. After the task, participants were given the opportunity to take a short break prior to the start of the motor task.

MOTOR TASK

In both Studies 1 and 2, participants were also asked to execute four actions associated with the sounds they heard. One was "zipping a zipper" (hand action) in which participants were provided a zippered jacket to put on prior to the start of the motor task. When cued, they were to move their hands from resting position on the armchair, zip the jacket up and down four times and return their hands to resting position. A second action, "ripping paper" (hand action) involved cueing the participant to move both hands from resting position on the armchair to the center where an experimenter would hand them a paper towel to rip. Participants would rip the paper towel three times, drop the scraps on the floor, and move their hands back to resting position. A third action, "sipping from a straw" (mouth action) involved cueing the participant by placing the straw to their lips and asking them to pretend drinking through the straw three times. The final action was "kissing" (mouth action) in which subjects were cued to make three kissing motions (i.e., purse and release their lips, thus making a smooching sound). During these actions, participants were blindfolded to prevent them from seeing their own actions, and circumaural headphones delivered white noise loud enough to prevent the participants from hearing the sound effects of their own actions. Experimenters used haptic cues [e.g., touching of hand] to prompt the participant to begin each action (the cues and actions were explained to the participant and practiced prior to EEG recording). Each of the four actions was performed twice, for a total of eight motor actions within a single block of trials. The order of the actions was determined through a random number generator, and was unique to each participant. In addition, the block of trials was repeated eight times for a total of 64 motor actions per subject. One experimenter delivered the haptic cues while a second confederate used a keyboard to send pulses via keyboard to the EEG computer demarcating the onset and offset of each action (see cues in **Table 2**).

DATA ANALYSIS

Eye blinks and movement artifacts were digitally identified in the EOG recording and removed. Other types of EEG artifacts were also automatically and manually removed prior to analysis. Data were only analyzed if sufficiently "clean" EEG, with no movement or eye blink artifacts, were present. Between 10 and 30% of the data were removed for individual participants. For each cleaned segment the integrated power in the 8–13 Hz mu range was computed using a Fast Fourier Transform. Data were segmented into epochs of 2 s beginning at the start of the segment. Fast Fourier Transforms were performed on the epoched data (1024 points or 2046 ms). A cosine window was used to control for artifacts resulting from data splicing.

Suppression of the 8–13 Hz band in both the auditory and motor tasks was computed as the ratio of power in response to Action sounds, Non-Action sounds, and motor movements, relative to control sounds. A ratio was used to control for variability in absolute power as a result of individual differences in scalp thickness and electrode impedance, as opposed to absolute differences in electrical activity. Since ratio data are inherently non-normal as a result of lower bounding, a log transform was used for statistical analyses. A log ratio of less than zero indicates suppression whereas a value of zero indicates no suppression and values greater than zero indicate enhancement.

Accuracy on the Auditory Oddball Task was calculated as hits plus correct rejections divided by total number of blocks. For EEG suppression, an omnibus ANOVA was first run followed by distinct ANOVAs for midline (Fz, Cz, Pz), frontal (F3, F4, F7, F8), centro-parietal (C3, C4, P3, P4), temporal (T3, T4, T5, T6), and occipital (O1, O2) sites. Stimulus type (mouth sound, hand

Table 2 | Four Actions Performed During the Motor Task (MT).

Motor action	Cue	Onset	Offset
Zipping a zipper	Pull on jacket	Move from resting position	Return to resting position
Ripping paper	Touch hand	Move from resting position	Return to resting position
Sipping through a straw	Put straw to lips	Cue	Finish third "sip"
Kissing	Touch cheek	Cue	Finish third "kiss"

sound, motor mouth, motor hand, environmental sounds) and electrodes were used as within-subject factors with Greenhouse-Geisser corrections applied to the degrees of freedom and only the corrected probability values reported. Partial Eta scores (h_p^2) are also reported. Pairwise comparisons were conducted using Tukey's Honest Significant Difference (HSD), while a Bonferroni correction was applied to correct for multiple comparisons.

RESULTS

Trial lengths were longer in Study 2 (7 s ITI) than in Study 1 (3 s ITI) to allow for more processing of the stimulus, and the type of response to oddball trials differed, with overt responses used in Study 1 and covert responses in Study 2. Nonetheless, no statistical differences were found between the studies and therefore only the combined results are reported.

AUDITORY IDENTIFICATION TASK

During the Auditory Identification Task, participants were able to identify sounds with a high degree of accuracy within three times of listening to a sound. The specific results for Hand, Mouth, and Environment sounds were 95, 98, and 93%, respectively. During the oddball trials, participants were able to correctly detect the oddball event with 97% accuracy.

EEG 8–13 Hz SUPPRESSION

There was a main effect of stimulus type across all electrodes, $F_{(4, 220)} = 63.2$, $p < 0.01$, $\eta_p^2 = 0.535$. Pairwise comparisons showed that all but audio hand vs. environmental sounds were highly significant ($p < 0.01$). There was also a main effect of electrodes, $F_{(16, 880)} = 7.9$, $p < 0.01$ and a stimulus type x electrode interaction, $F_{(64, 3520)} = 5.99$, $p < 0.01$.

Individual ANOVAs for subset of the electrodes (frontal, centro-parietal, midline, temporal, occipital) showed similar results as the omnibus ANOVA, as shown in **Figure 1** for centro-parietal sites. Likewise, frontal electrodes showed a main effect of stimulus type, $F_{(4, 220)} = 48.8$, $p < 0.01$, $\eta_p^2 = 0.470$. Pairwise comparisons for this subset of electrodes indicated significant differences for all comparisons except the audio hand vs. environmental sounds. There was a significant stimulus type x electrodes interaction, $F_{(12, 660)} = 3.29$, $p < 0.01$, with greater suppression over right (F4) compared to left (F3) anterior frontal sites (see **Figure 2**). This difference occurred primarily for hand sounds.

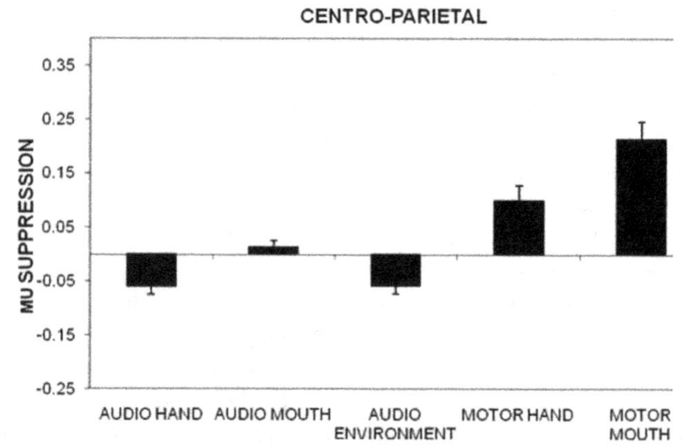

FIGURE 1 | Mu suppression over centro-parietal regions (C3, C4, P3, P4) in the action (hand, mouth) and non-action (environmental) auditory conditions as well as during the motor actions (hand, mouth). Mu suppression is determined as the log of the ratio between experimental condition and baseline condition. Error bars are standard error of the mean.

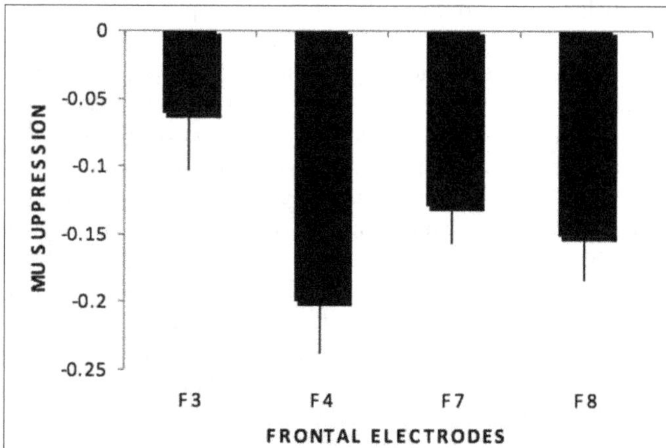

FIGURE 2 | Mu suppression across stimulus type at frontal regions (F3, F4, F7, F8) showing the stimulus type by electrode interaction in which greater mu suppression was recorded over right (F4) compared to left (F3) anterior frontal sites but not over more ventral anterior sites (F7, F8).

Centro-parietal electrodes exhibited a main effect of stimulus type, $F_{(4, 220)} = 31.6$, $p < 0.01$, $\eta_p^2 = 0.365$. Like the frontal electrodes, pairwise comparisons indicated significant differences for all comparisons except the audio hand vs. environmental sounds. There was also a main effect of electrodes, $F_{(3, 165)} = 3.08$, $p < 0.05$ with significantly more suppression over left (C3, P3) compared to right (C4, P4) hemisphere sites. A stimulus type x electrode interaction, $F_{(12, 660)} = 3.09$, $p < 0.05$ showed that in the audio hand and the environmental sounds conditions there was greater suppression compared to other conditions and more over left hemisphere for the audio hand condition and over the right hemisphere for environmental sounds (see **Figure 3**).

Midline electrodes showed a statistically significant main effect of stimulus type, $F_{(4, 220)} = 55.0$, $p < 0.01$, $\eta_p^2 = 0.500$, with all pairwise comparisons showing significant differences. A main effect of electrodes, $F_{(2, 110)} = 7.5$, $p < 0.01$, showed greater suppression occurring at the central (Cz) compared to frontal (Fz) and parietal (Pz) sites. There was also an interaction between stimulus type and electrodes, $F_{(8, 440)} = 9.5$, $p < 0.01$ with audio hand showing the greatest suppression.

Temporal electrodes exhibited a statistically significant main effect of stimulus type, $F_{(4, 220)} = 52.0$, $p < 0.01$, electrodes, $F_{(3, 165)} = 25.5$, $p < 0.01$, and an interaction between stimulus type and electrodes, $F_{(12, 660)} = 4.28$, $p < 0.01$.

Occipital electrodes showed a main effect of stimulus type, $F_{(4, 220)} = 42.1$, $p < 0.01$, with all audio sounds (hand, mouth, environmental) showing suppression compared to more positive responses during motor actions. There was also a main effect of electrodes, $F_{(1, 55)} = 15.2$ $p < 0.01$, such that greater suppression was seen over left (O1) compared to the right (O2) hemisphere.

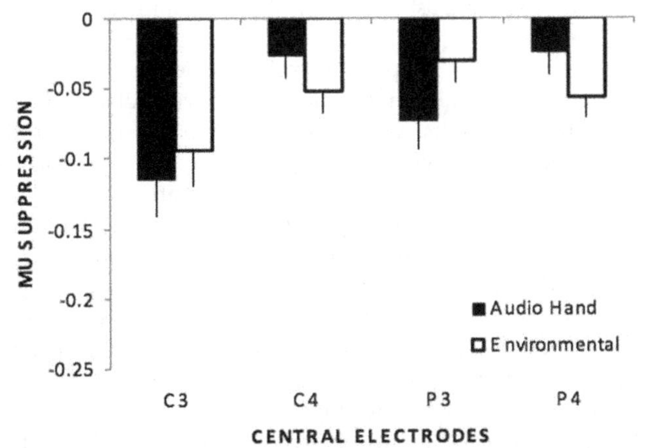

FIGURE 3 | Mu suppression over centro-parietal regions (C3, C4, P3, P4) showing that although no differences occurred between these sounds (audio hand vs. environmental), a stimulus type by electrode interaction showed that audio hand sounds exhibited greater suppression over left hemisphere sites (C3, P3) while environmental sounds exhibited greater suppression over right hemisphere sites (C4, P4).

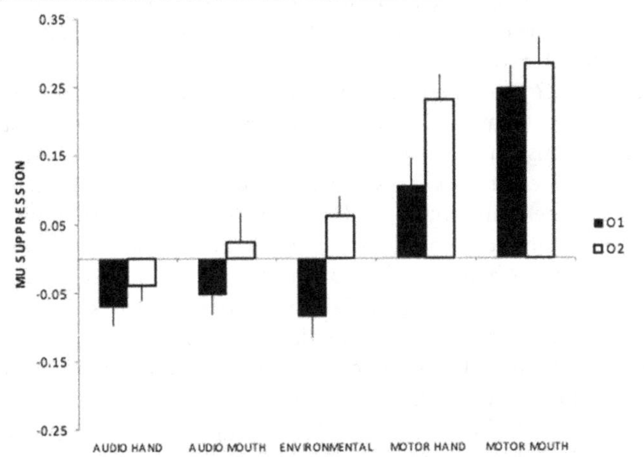

FIGURE 4 | Mu suppression over occipital regions (O1, O2) showing suppression over left (O1) while there was relative enhancement over right (O2) sites to environmental and motor actions.

Finally, there was an interaction between stimulus type x electrodes, $F_{(4,\ 220)} = 4.2$, $p < 0.01$ such that the greatest amplitude differences between left and right hemisphere sites occurred for environmental sounds (see **Figure 4**).

DISCUSSION

Results from this study show that EEG 8–13 Hz mu rhythms exhibit amplitude modulation not only during the performance of an action (synchronization) but also during hearing of action related sounds as well as non-action related sounds (desynchronization). Synchronization during action execution has been previously reported and while differences in the direction of modulation may reflect motor vs. mirroring processes, they may also involve increases in sensitivity to motivationally meaningful events (Pineda and Oberman, 2006). Differences in the spatial distribution of the mu suppression triggered by the action vs. the environmental sounds may reflect different neural sources, with action related sounds displaying a locus over left hemisphere in the anterior-posterior axis while non-action environmental sounds display primarily a right hemisphere locus.

A concurrent fMRI-EEG experiment (Arnstein et al., 2011) has shown that mu suppression during action observation and execution, as measured in the EEG over central electrodes (C3), directly correlated with BOLD increases in the dorsal premotor, and parietal cortex (posterior SI and adjacent posterior parietal lobe). Activity in the ventral premotor cortex was less correlated with mu suppression over C3. Because the exact same sound stimuli used here have been used previously in an experiment using fMRI (Gazzola et al., 2006), we can use the results of the fMRI-EEG study to link the results from the current EEG study and the past fMRI experiment. In particular, Gazzola et al. (2006) found that in the left hemisphere, the hand action sounds recruited the dorsal premotor and somatosensory cortex more than the environmental sounds [Figure S1 in Gazzola et al. (2006)], while the reverse was true for the right hemisphere. Here, we find the same lateralization pattern, with hand action sounds producing more mu suppression than environmental sounds over C3 (left) and the environmental sounds producing more mu suppression than the hand-action sounds over C4 (right). In addition, (Gazzola et al., 2006) found a somatotopic activation pattern, with hand action sounds and hand-action execution recruiting the dorsal premotor and mid-parietal cortex, while mouth action sounds and mouth action execution activated the ventral premotor cortex and the ventral-most parietal cortex. In the fMRI-EEG study, the dorsal but not the ventral premotor cortex, and the mid- rather than ventral parietal cortex reliably predicted mu suppression over C3. Accordingly, one would expect more mu suppression over C3 for the hand than mouth-actions. For the sounds, this was exactly what was found in the present experiment. For the action execution, mu suppression was not found for either of the action types, but the mu-power over C3 was lower for the hand than the mouth action execution. Accordingly, the two experiments using fMRI and EEG, respectively, find compatible results in terms of lateralization and somatotopical arrangement of the activation triggered using the same auditory stimuli.

These observations are also congruent with previous studies that have used different sounds but indicated that action sounds (those that are reproducible by the body) and non-action related sounds are processed by separate neural systems in the human brain (Pizzamiglio et al., 2005). More specifically Pizzamiglio et al. report that left posterior superior temporal and premotor areas appear to reflect action-related sounds, while bilateral areas in the temporal pole appear to respond to non-action related sounds. The present findings of a left hemisphere locus for action-related sounds underscore the fact that auditory aspects of mirroring, as reflected in the dynamics of the EEG mu rhythm, exhibits similar functional specialization inherent in processing auditory sounds with semantic meaning (Zahn et al., 2000). Furthermore, sounds associated with different effectors, e.g., hand compared to mouth action sounds, show distinct modulations of this rhythm. Hence, the data are consistent with the idea that biological sounds engage mirroring processes (both synchronization and desynchronization actions) in a manner similar to that which occurs during the observation and reproduction of motor actions (Pfurtscheller and Lopes da Silva, 1999; Neuper et al., 2006). The multi-sensory properties of the human MNS is thus assumed to help build a more accurate representation of sensorimotor activity from the visual, auditory, and other information embedded in the observation of other individuals. Whether these various aspects of the input are processed simultaneously or treated equally is left for future research.

Desynchronization or suppression of EEG rhythms has generally been interpreted as a correlate of an activated cortical area with increased excitability, while synchronization has been interpreted as a correlate of a deactivated cortical region (Pfurtscheller, 2001; Pineda, 2005). Mu rhythm oscillations in the present study were enhanced (meaning that the underlying neurons were less active and more synchronized) for mouth compared to hand stimuli, both while performing the movements in the Motor task and hearing the sounds in the Auditory task. In addition to fitting with the data of Gazzola et al. (Gazzola et al., 2006), using the same stimuli, the interpretation of these differences in mouth- and hand-related processing is also compatible with the findings of Pfurtscheller and Neuper (Pfurtscheller and Neuper, 1994) who reported that excitation of one sensorimotor area is typically accompanied by inhibition of a neighboring sensorimotor area as a result of lateral inhibitory connectivity. Consistent with this idea, mu rhythms recorded at central sites (C3, C4), which are located closer to the hand than mouth area in the motor strip, showed suppression to hand-related sounds and enhancement to mouth-related sounds. These center-surround effects, however, were asymmetrical since enhancements to mouth-related sounds were typically $>20\%$, while suppressions to hand-related sounds were typically $<10\%$. The basis for such an asymmetry is unclear although it appears consistent with greater suppression occurring to hand-related sounds at the C3 and C4 electrode sites. This difference cannot be attributed to task performance because no difference in counting of oddball control trials occurred for mouth- and hand-related sounds.

Participants understood and actively listened to the sounds as indicated by the results of the Auditory Identification Task and responses to the oddball events during the Auditory Task condition. The EEG findings are therefore not likely due to differences in perceptual or attentional factors but more consistent with the assumption that mirroring is reflected in the dynamics of the mu rhythm. That is, meaningful action sounds trigger greater mirroring as reflected in more mu suppression because they are embodied by the listener in order to understand them. This is supported by the different patterns of mu suppression to action (Mouth and Hand-based sounds) and non-action (Environmental) sounds. That is, greater suppression was recorded over the left hemisphere (especially over parietal areas) in response to action compared to non-action sounds but this is reversed over the right hemisphere. Thus, it is congruent with the idea that the mu rhythms (and the premotor to sensorimotor cortex connection) indexes auditory activity related to mirroring and that such a system exhibits lateralized processing as a function of the semantic associations with the sounds.

Studies 1 and 2 of the present work were designed to address the influence of motor preparation to report oddballs on the mu suppression results. We required participants in one study to make overt responses by clicking a mouse and in a separate study make covert responses by mentally counting the oddball trials. Both overt and covert responding requires motor planning. However, in one case it specifically involves an effector, such as the hand, while in the other it avoids such effector-based preparation. Since no significant differences occurred between the two studies, it suggests that EEG mu rhythms are either unaffected by the type of motor preparation or similar motor preparation occurs for both overt and covert responding.

When we observe another person moving, we only see the external consequences of their actions. To reproduce this action, we need instead to produce motor programs that produce a similar action. Clearly, the visual signals entering the eye during action observation are fundamentally different from the motor commands that need to be generated to perform a similar action. For one to map observed actions onto similar states in one self to understand or imitate the actions of others poses what has been called the correspondence problem in mirroring (Brass and Heyes, 2005). Specifically, how do observed movements actually map onto the observer's own motor system to enable everything from simple motor imitation to visceral discomfort upon seeing a queasy face? That is, how do we actually translate what we see into what we do (Brass and Heyes, 2005; Pineda, 2005)? In the visual domain, this correspondence problem is constrained by the fact that the observer can witness what body part the agent has used to perform the action. In the auditory domain, such information is lacking. When you hear the crunching of the soda can, it is impossible to know whether the left hand or the right was used. Perhaps it was the left or right foot used. Either is impossible to know with the given piece of sound information. Nevertheless, hand-action sounds and mouth-action sounds generated different patterns of mu suppression, which mirrors the relative amount of mu suppression during action execution, and previous fMRI studies have shown the existence of somatotopic brain activity (Gazzola et al., 2006) that allows classification as to which effector was used from sounds alone (Etzel et al., 2008). It has been proposed, that this somatotopy is the result of Hebbian learning: while we crush a coca-cola can with our right hand, we simultaneously perform the motor program, and hear (through what is called re-afference) the sound of this action. Through Hebbian learning, neurons in high-level auditory cortex that respond to the sound of this action then would enhance their synaptic connections with motor neurons in the parietal and premotor cortex that caused the action and with neurons in SI that sense the tactile consequences of performing such hand actions (Keysers and Perrett, 2004). Thereafter, listening to the sound would trigger, through these Hebbian associations, the motor programs corresponding to that action and the somatosensory representations of what such actions feel like. Because such motor programs and somatosensory fields are located more dorsal in the premotor, somatosensory and posterior parietal cortices than for mouth motor programs (Gazzola et al., 2006), the sound of such actions that we normally perform with our hands will trigger activity preferentially in these more dorsal regions in fMRI (Gazzola et al., 2006) and causing maximum mu suppression under C3 in the present study. While performing mouth actions like gurgling, we can hear and feel ourselves perform the action, and neurons in the high-level auditory cortex responding to the sound of actions we normally do with the mouth will wire together with the more ventrally located mouth motor and somatosensory representations in the premotor and parietal lobe. Accordingly, hearing such sounds will later trigger more ventral activity in the premotor and parietal lobe (Gazzola et al., 2006) and less mu suppression over C3. In support of the notion that brain activity in premotor and posterior parietal cortex is triggered by sounds as a result of Hebbian associations rather than inborn processes, Lahav et al. (Lahav et al., 2007) has shown that no premotor activity occurs to the sound of piano music in piano naïve listeners. However, a few hours of piano lessons, during which participants repeatedly experience the temporal contingencies between pressing piano keys and musical notes suffices to train new neural connections: after the training, piano music suddenly did trigger premotor activation in regions used to perform hand actions while listening to the learned piano melodies.

Environmental sounds such as the sound of a train passing are at first glance not considered body action-related, and it may seem odd that they should trigger any mu suppression at all. However, it is not unthinkable that they could be variably embodied, via Hebbian learning processes, in different individuals. Does John associate the sound of a train passing with the vibrations of his morning commute on the locomotive? Does Suzie associate the sound of a train passing with using her arm to move her electric train along the play tracks? The fact that such environmental sounds in the present study exhibit significant levels of mu suppression is consistent with this embodied argument for non-action stimuli. Nonetheless, much more research is needed to clarify these explanations.

CONCLUSION

The findings of this study provide support for a mirroring system in the human brain that responds to specific sounds, as well as greater understanding of the distinctions and similarities between processing the auditory and visual aspects of mirroring. The patterns of mu suppression across cortical regions to different categories of sounds and to effector-specific sounds suggest differential engagement of this mirroring system in the human brain when processing different category of sounds and may offer a potential set of signals to explore for the development of a passive brain computer interface. Clearly, future studies are needed to specifically investigate that possibility, as well as the effects of auditory and motor tasks on special populations, such as autistic individuals, which in turn could provide insight on the degree of importance of the auditory MNS in social interactions and language.

ACKNOWLEDGMENTS

We would like to thank Drs. Marta Kutas, Andrea Chiba, Inna Fishman, and Sarah Creel for their help and feedback throughout this project. We would also like to thank all those from the Cognitive Neuroscience Laboratory at UCSD for their logistical and moral support: Alan Kiang, Adrienne Moore, Max Keuken, Heather Pelton, Jia-Min Bai, Conny Soest, Dan Lotz, Nick Pojman, Alexy Andrade, Albert Anaya, and Alicia Trigeiro. We would like to thank Valeria Gazzola and Lisa-Aziz Zadeh for helping to record the original auditory stimuli.

FUNDING

Christian Keysers was supported by VIDI grant 452-04-305 of the Netherlands Science Foundation (N.W.O.) and ERC grant 312511 of the European Research Council.

REFERENCES

Aglioti, S. M., and Pazzaglia, M. (2010). Representing actions through their sound. *Exp. Brain Res.* 206, 141–151. doi: 10.1007/s00221-010-2344-x

Arnstein, D., Cui, F., Keysers, C., Maurits, N. M., and Gazzola, V. (2011). mu-suppression during action observation and execution correlates with BOLD in dorsal premotor, inferior parietal, and SI cortices. *J. Neurosci.* 31, 14243–14249. doi: 10.1523/JNEUROSCI.0963-11.2011

Brass, M., and Heyes, C. (2005). Imitation: is cognitive neuroscience solving the correspondence problem? *Trends Cogn. Sci.* 9, 489–495. doi: 10.1016/j.tics.2005.08.007

Buccino, G., Binkofski, F., and Riggio, L. (2004). The mirror neuron system and action recognition. *Brain Lang.* 89, 370–376. doi: 10.1016/S0093-934X(03)00356-0

Caspers, S., Eickhoff, S. B., Rick, T., von, K. A., Kuhlen, T., Huang, R., et al. (2011). Probabilistic fibre tract analysis of cytoarchitectonically defined human inferior parietal lobule areas reveals similarities to macaques. *Neuroimage* 58, 362–380. doi: 10.1016/j.neuroimage.2011.06.027

Caspers, S., Zilles, K., Laird, A. R., and Eickhoff, S. B. (2010). ALE meta-analysis of action observation and imitation in the human brain. *Neuroimage* 50, 1148–1167. doi: 10.1016/j.neuroimage.2009.12.112

Cochin, S., Barthelemy, C., Lejeune, B., Roux, S., and Martineau, J. (1998). Perception of motion and qEEG activity in human adults. *Electroencephalogr.Clin. Neurophysiol.* 107, 287–295. doi: 10.1016/S0013-4694(98)00071-6

Cochin, S., Barthelemy, C., Roux, S., and Martineau, J. (1999). Observation and execution of movement: similarities demonstrated by quantified electroencephalography. *Eur. J. Neurosci.* 11, 1839–1842. doi: 10.1046/j.1460-9568.1999.00598.x

di Pellegrino, G., Fadiga, L., Fogassi, L., Gallese, V., and Rizzolatti, G. (1992). Understanding motor events: a neurophysiological study. *Exp. Brain Res.* 91, 176–180. doi: 10.1007/BF00230027

Etzel, J. A., Gazzola, V., and Keysers, C. (2008). Testing simulation theory with cross-modal multivariate classification of fMRI data. *PLoS ONE* 3:e3690. doi: 10.1371/journal.pone.0003690

Fadiga, L., Buccino, G., Craighero, L., Fogassi, L., Gallese, V., and Pavesi, G. (1999). Corticospinal excitability is specifically modulated by motor imagery: a magnetic stimulation study. *Neuropsychologia* 37, 147–158. doi: 10.1016/S0028-3932(98)00089-X

Fadiga, L., Craighero, L., and Olivier, E. (2005). Human motor cortex excitability during the perception of others' action. *Curr. Opin. Neurobiol.* 15, 213–218. doi: 10.1016/j.conb.2005.03.013

Ferrari, P. F., Bonini, L., and Fogassi, L. (2009). From monkey mirror neurons to primate behaviours: possible "direct" and "indirect" pathways. *Philos. Trans. R. Soc. Lond. B Biol. Sci.* 364, 2311–2323. doi: 10.1098/rstb.2009.0062

Gazzola, V., Aziz-Zadeh, L., and Keysers, C. (2006). Empathy and the somatotopic auditory mirror system in humans. *Curr. Biol.* 16, 1824–1829. doi: 10.1016/j.cub.2006.07.072

Grezes, J., Armony, J. L., Rowe, J., and Passingham, R. E. (2003). Activations related to "mirror" and "canonical" neurones in the human brain: an fMRI study. *Neuroimage* 18, 928–937. doi: 10.1016/S1053-8119(03)00042-9

Hari, R., Levanen, S., and Raij, T. (2000). Timing of human cortical functions during cognition: role of MEG. *Trends Cogn. Sci.* 4, 455–462. doi: 10.1016/S1364-6613(00)01549-7

Hickok, G. (2009). Eight problems for the mirror neuron theory of action understanding in monkeys and humans. *J. Cogn. Neurosci.* 21, 1229–1243. doi: 10.1162/jocn.2009.21189

Iacoboni, M. and Dapretto, M. (2006). The mirror neuron system and the consequences of its dysfunction. *Nat. Rev. Neurosci.* 7, 942–951. doi: 10.1038/nrn2024

Iacoboni, M., Woods, R. P., Brass, M., Bekkering, H., Mazziotta, J. C., and Rizzolatti, G. (1999). Cortical mechanisms of human imitation. *Science* 286, 2526–2528. doi: 10.1126/science.286.5449.2526

Keuken, M. C., Hardie, A., Dorn, B. T., Dev, S., Paulus, M. P., Jonas, K. J., et al. (2011). The role of the left inferior frontal gyrus in social perception: an rTMS study. *Brain Res.* 1383, 196–205. doi: 10.1016/j.brainres.2011.01.073

Keysers, C., and Gazzola, V. (2009). Expanding the mirror: vicarious activity for actions, emotions, and sensations. *Curr. Opin. Neurobiol.* 19, 666–671. doi: 10.1016/j.conb.2009.10.006

Keysers, C., Kaas, J. H., and Gazzola, V. (2010). Somatosensation in social perception. *Nat. Rev. Neurosci.* 11, 417–428. doi: 10.1038/nrn2833

Keysers, C., Kohler, E., Umilta, M. A., Nanetti, L., Fogassi, L., and Gallese, V. (2003). Audiovisual mirror neurons and action recognition. *Exp. Brain Res.* 153, 628–636. doi: 10.1007/s00221-003-1603-5

Keysers, C., and Perrett, D. I. (2004). Demystifying social cognition: a Hebbian perspective. *Trends Cogn. Sci.* 8, 501–507. doi: 10.1016/j.tics.2004.09.005

Kohler, E., Keysers, C., Umilta, M. A., Fogassi, L., Gallese, V., and Rizzolatti, G. (2002). Hearing sounds, understanding actions: action representation in mirror neurons. *Science* 297, 846–848. doi: 10.1126/science.1070311

Lahav, A., Saltzman, E., and Schlaug, G. (2007). Action representation of sound: audiomotor recognition network while listening to newly acquired actions. *J. Neurosci.* 27, 308–314. doi: 10.1523/JNEUROSCI.4822-06.2007

Maeda, F., Kleiner-Fisman, G., and Pascual-Leone, A. (2002). Motor facilitation while observing hand actions: specificity of the effect and role of observer's orientation. *J. Neurophysiol.* 87, 1329–1335. doi: 10.1152/jn.00773.2000

Mukamel, R., Ekstrom, A. D., Kaplan, J., Iacoboni, M., and Fried, I. (2010). Single-neuron responses in humans during execution and observation of actions. *Curr. Biol.* 20, 1–7. doi: 10.1016/j.cub.2010.02.045

Muthukumaraswamy, S. D., and Johnson, B. W. (2004). Changes in rolandic mu rhythm during observation of a precision grip. *Psychophysiology* 41, 152–156. doi: 10.1046/j.1469-8986.2003.00129.x

Muthukumaraswamy, S. D., Johnson, B. W., and McNair, N. A. (2004). Mu rhythm modulation during observation of an object-directed grasp. *Brain Res. Cogn. Brain Res.* 19, 195–201. doi: 10.1016/j.cogbrainres.2003.12.001

Muthukumaraswamy, S. D., and Singh, K. D. (2008). Modulation of the human mirror neuron system during cognitive activity. *Psychophysiology* 45, 896–905. doi: 10.1111/j.1469-8986.2008.00711.x

Neuper, C., Wortz, M., and Pfurtscheller, G. (2006). ERD/ERS patterns reflecting sensorimotor activation and deactivation. *Prog. Brain Res.* 159, 211–222. doi: 10.1016/S0079-6123(06)59014-4

Oberman, L. M., Hubbard, E. M., McCleery, J. P., Altschuler, E. L., Ramachandran, V. S., and Pineda, J. A. (2005). EEG evidence for mirror neuron dysfunction in autism spectrum disorders. *Cogn. Brain Res.* 24, 190–198. doi: 10.1016/j.cogbrainres.2005.01.014

Oberman, L. M., Ramachandran, V. S., and Pineda, J. A. (2008). Modulation of mu suppression in children with autism spectrum disorders in response to familiar or unfamiliar stimuli: the mirror neuron hypothesis. *Neuropsychologia* 46, 1558–1565. doi: 10.1016/j.neuropsychologia.2008.01.010

Parsons, L. M., Fox, P. T., Downs, J. H., Glass, T., Hirsch, T. B., Martin, C. C., et al. (1995). Use of implicit motor imagery for visual shape discrimination as revealed by PET. *Nature* 375, 54–58. doi: 10.1038/375054a0

Pfurtscheller, G. (2001). Functional brain imaging based on ERD/ERS. *Vision Res.* 41, 1257–1260. doi: 10.1016/S0042-6989(00)00235-2

Pfurtscheller, G., and Lopes da Silva, F. H. (1999). Event-related EEG/MEG synchronization and desynchronization: basic principles. *Clin. Neurophysiol.* 110, 1842–1857. doi: 10.1016/S1388-2457(99)00141-8

Pfurtscheller, G., and Neuper, C. (1994). Event-related synchronization of mu rhythm in the EEG over the cortical hand area in man. *Neurosci. Lett.* 174, 93–96. doi: 10.1016/0304-3940(94)90127-9

Pineda, J. A. (2005). The functional significance of mu rhythms: translating "seeing" and "hearing" into "doing." *Brain Res. Brain Res. Rev.* 50, 57–68. doi: 10.1016/j.brainresrev.2005.04.005

Pineda, J. A., Allison, B. Z., and Vankov, A. (2000). The effects of self-movement, observation, and imagination on mu rhythms and readiness potentials (RP's): toward a brain-computer interface (BCI). *IEEE Trans. Rehabil. Eng.* 8, 219–222. doi: 10.1109/86.847822

Pineda, J. A., and Oberman, L. M. (2006). What goads cigarette smokers to smoke? neural adaptation and the mirror neuron system. *Brain Res.* 1121, 128–135. doi: 10.1016/j.brainres.2006.08.128

Pizzamiglio, L., Aprile, T., Spitoni, G., Pitzalis, S., Bates, E., D'Amico, S., et al. (2005). Separate neural systems for processing action- or non-action-related sounds. *Neuroimage* 24, 852–861. doi: 10.1016/j.neuroimage.2004.09.025

Ricciardi, E., Bonino, D., Sani, L., Vecchi, T., Guazzelli, M., Haxby, J. V., et al. (2009). Do we really need vision? how blind people "see" the actions of others. *J. Neurosci.* 29, 9719–9724. doi: 10.1523/JNEUROSCI.0274-09.2009

Rizzolatti, G., and Craighero, L. (2004). The mirror-neuron system. *Annu. Rev. Neurosci.* 27, 169–192. doi: 10.1146/annurev.neuro.27.070203.144230

Rizzolatti, G., and Sinigaglia, C. (2010). The functional role of the parieto-frontal mirror circuit: interpretations and misinterpretations. *Nat. Rev. Neurosci.* 11, 264–274. doi: 10.1038/nrn2805

Shimazu, H., Maier, M. A., Cerri, G., Kirkwood, P. A., and Lemon, R. N. (2004). Macaque ventral premotor cortex exerts powerful facilitation of motor cortex outputs to upper limb motoneurons. *J. Neurosci.* 24, 1200–1211. doi: 10.1523/JNEUROSCI.4731-03.2004

Zahn, R., Huber, W., Drews, E., Erberich, S., Krings, T., Willmes, K., et al. (2000). Hemispheric lateralization at different levels of human auditory word processing: a functional magnetic resonance imaging study. *Neurosci. Lett.* 287, 195–198. doi: 10.1016/S0304-3940(00)01160-5

9

EEG-based workload estimation across affective contexts

Christian Mühl[1]*, Camille Jeunet[1,2] and Fabien Lotte[1,3]

[1] *Institut National de Recherche en Informatique et en Automatique, Bordeaux Sud-Ouest, Talence, France*
[2] *Laboratoire Handicap et Système Nerveux, University of Bordeaux, Bordeaux, France*
[3] *Laboratoire Bordelais de Recherche en Informatique (LaBRI), Talence, France*

***Correspondence:**
Christian Mühl, Institut National de Recherche en Informatique et en Automatique, Bordeaux Sud-Ouest, 200, Rue de la Vieille Tour, 33405 Talence, France
e-mail: c.muehl@gmail.com*

Workload estimation from electroencephalographic signals (EEG) offers a highly sensitive tool to adapt the human–computer interaction to the user state. To create systems that reliably work in the complexity of the real world, a robustness against contextual changes (e.g., mood), has to be achieved. To study the resilience of state-of-the-art EEG-based workload classification against stress we devise a novel experimental protocol, in which we manipulated the affective context (stressful/non-stressful) while the participant solved a task with two workload levels. We recorded self-ratings, behavior, and physiology from 24 participants to validate the protocol. We test the capability of different, subject-specific workload classifiers using either frequency-domain, time-domain, or both feature varieties to generalize across contexts. We show that the classifiers are able to transfer between affective contexts, though performance suffers independent of the used feature domain. However, cross-context training is a simple and powerful remedy allowing the extraction of features in all studied feature varieties that are more resilient to task-unrelated variations in signal characteristics. Especially for frequency-domain features, across-context training is leading to a performance comparable to within-context training and testing. We discuss the significance of the result for neurophysiology-based workload detection in particular and for the construction of reliable passive brain–computer interfaces in general.

Keywords: workload, stress, brain–computer interface, classification, electroencephalography, passive brain computer interface

INTRODUCTION

The increasing complexity and autonomy of information systems rapidly approaches the limits of human capability. To avoid overload of the users in highly demanding situations, a dynamic and automatic adaptation of the system to the user state is necessary. Reliable knowledge about the user state, especially his workload, is a key requirement for a timely and adequate system adaptation (Erp et al., 2010). Examples are systems supporting air traffic control, pilots, as well as medical and emergency applications.

Conventional means of workload assessment, such as self-assessment and behavior, are intrusive or limited in their sensitivity, respectively (Erp et al., 2010). Physiological sensors, assessing for example the galvanic skin response (GSR) or elecrocardiographic activity (ECG), offer an unobtrusive and continuous measure that has been found sensitive to workload (Verwey and Veltman, 1984; Boucsein, 1992). In the last two decades, neurophysiological activity became popular as a modality for the measurement of mental states in general and of workload in specific. So-called "passive brain-computer interfaces" (pBCI, Zander and Kothe, 2011) are able to measure neuronal activity in terms of the electrophysiological activity of neuron populations as in the case of EEG or the oxygination of the cerebral blood flow as for functional near-infrared spectroscopy (fNIRS). Both approaches have been found informative regarding the detection of cognitive load (Brouwer et al., 2012; Solovey et al., 2012), and there is evidence for a partially superior sensitivity of neural measurements compared to other physiological sensors (Mathan et al., 2007) or self-report (Peck et al., 2013).

Most experiments on passive BCI use a very controlled approach, which naturally limits the range of real-world conditions they reflect. While this control is necessary to ensure the psychophysiological validity of the mental state detection, their results lack a certain ecological validity, they can not be generalized to other contexts. This might be one of the most impeding problems for the creations of passive BCI systems that work in the real world, since daily life is characterized by the variability of the conditions we function under. A prominent example are changes of affect while working, for example working under the pressure of an impending evaluation vs. work without pressure. A system that is supposed to work in such contexts needs to be calibrated and tested in them. Previous research in the domain of pBCI largely ignored the problem. To shed light on the interaction of mental state classification and change of affective context, we devised a protocol that recreates conditions of work, requiring different effort, during relaxed conditions and under psychosocial stress in a controlled environment. To study the resilience of a state-of-the art workload detection system to changes in affective context, we train subject-specific classifiers in either stressed or non-stressed context and test their performance within the same and in the other context.

In summary, the contributions of this paper for the study of the effect of affective context on workload classification are:

1. The creation and validation of a novel protocol to test interactions of workload classifier performance and affect[1].
2. The design and evaluation of a workload classifier generalizing across affective contexts.
3. Quantifying the impact across affective context generalization on classification performance, with and without across context-training.

Below, we will give the reader some background to neurophysiology-based detection of workload under varying (affective) user states and its potential interactions with stress responses. Then, we will introduce the employed approaches to manipulate the user's mental state, the used devices, and the applied signal processing and classification algorithms. We will then report the nature of the found effects, discuss their relevance, and conclude with the general consequences and limitations of the presented findings.

RELATED WORK

DETECTION OF WORKLOAD FROM NEUROPHYSIOLOGY

Mental workload can be defined as (perceived) relationship between the amount of mental processing capability and the amount required by the task (Hart and Staveland, 1988). The closer the requirements are to the actual capabilities, the higher is the (perceived) workload. Therefore, a general strategy for workload manipulation is the manipulation of task demand or difficulty (Gevins et al., 1998; Grimes et al., 2008; Brouwer et al., 2012), though alternative strategies, such as the manipulation of feedback or participant motivation (Fairclough and Roberts, 2011), exist.

Already in 1998, Gevins et al. (1998) showed that EEG is a viable source of information regarding the workload of a person, enabling 95% accuracy when using about 30 s of signal. However, there are many factors that can affect the performance of classification algorithms, such as the number of training data available, their distribution, their separability between classes, the data signal-to-noise ratio, the similarity (in terms of data distribution) of the training data and testing data, etc. (Duda et al., 2001). The estimation of these performances also depends on the number of testing data available (Müller-Putz et al., 2008), and the way they are estimated (cross-validation, independent test set). Finally, more BCI-specific factors affect the performances, such as whether the classification is subject-specific or subject-independent (see, e.g., Lotte et al., 2009), which subjects are used (there is a huge between-subject variability), whether the training and testing data are from the same session (e.g., same day) or not, etc. (Lotte et al., 2007). In this regard, Grimes et al. (2008) showed that a number of factors, such as the numbers of channels, amount of training data, or length of trials, have a strong influence on classification performance of workload classifiers. For example, reducing the length of the signal from 30 to 2 s reduces the classification performance on two workload levels from almost 92% to about 75%. Similar tradeoffs between optimal and practical signal processing settings are reported for channel number and training time. Another work, by Brouwer et al. (2012), studied in a similar setup the feasibility of different types of features (i.e., from the time- and frequency-domain, and combined) to differentiate workload levels, finding that the different feature types work comparably well with accuracies of about 85% after 30 s. Reducing the signal length to 2 s reduced the accuracy to about 65%. Zarjam et al. (2013) showed that workload manipulated by an arithmetic task can be classified with a performance of 83% for seven workload levels. Walter et al. (2013) tested the generalization of workload classifier from simple tasks, such as go/no-go, reading span, n-back tasks, to complex tasks involving diagram and algebra problems. While they were able to train well-performing classifiers for the simple tasks, reaching performances of about 96% for two classes on signals of a few seconds length, a cross-testing of a workload classifier trained on a simple task to a complex task did not succeed. However, since in both studies the order of workload levels was not randomized, a temporal trend present in the features could have biased the results toward a higher accuracy. Overall, these studies show that the workload level can be classified from neurophysiological activity. Indeed, it has also been suggested that neurophysiological information is more sensitive than information from other physiological signals (Mathan et al., 2007). Most importantly, these studies show that different factors, mainly methodological differences in workload induction, signal acquisition and processing, can have significant influences on the classification results.

However, to date there have only been few studies regarding the influence of the mental state changes during training and testing on the classifier performance. For active BCI, Reuderink and colleagues studied the influence of frustration on left and right hand movement classification during a computer game, using freezing screens and button malfunctions as induction tools (see Reuderink et al., 2013). The resulting loss of control (LOC) during "frustrating" episodes, surprisingly led to higher classification performance than during normal, relaxed game play (Reuderink et al., 2011). Zander and Jatzev (2012) induced LOC in a similar way during a simple behavioral task, the RLR paradigm, which resulted in lower classification performance. For passive BCI and specifically for workload level detection, only Roy et al. (2012) tested the impact of fatigue on EEG signal characteristics and workload classification performance. With increasing fatigue, the differentiating signal characteristics diminished and, consequently, the classification performance declined. This lack of research on interactions between passive BCI and changes in user state is problematic, since BCIs in general have been found susceptible to changes in task-unrelated mental states during classification, such as attention, fatigue or mood. Specifically, it is believed that variations in task-unrelated mental states are partially responsible for what is called non-stationarities of the signal, the change of its statistical properties over time, and thereby the source of one of the most notorious problems for BCI (Krusienski et al., 2011; van Erp et al., 2012).

In the next section, we will briefly introduce the concept of stress, which is another possible contextual factor influencing workload estimation that is occurring during daily life and work, and thus might be a relevant source of variance for workload detection devices.

[1]The validation of the administered stress-induction protocol was presented at the PhyCS 2014 conference (see Jeunet et al., 2014 for more details).

STRESS RESPONSES AND WORKLOAD

The psychophysiological concept of "stress," was introduced in 1936 by Selye (1936) to describe "the non-specific response of the body to any demand for change." In that sense, it is an organism's response to an environmental situation or stimulus perceived negatively—called a "stressor"—which can be real or imagined, that taxes the capacities of the subject, and thus has an impact on the body's homeostasis (that is to say that the constants of the internal environment are modified). To face the demand (i.e., to restore homeostasis), two brain circuitries can be activated during a "stress response cascade" (Sinha et al., 2003; Dickerson and Kemeny, 2004; Taniguchi et al., 2009): the sympatho-adrenomedullary axis (SAMa, also called the noradenergic circuitry) and the hypothalamus-pituitary gland-adrenal cortex axis (HPAa). On the one hand, the SAMa induces the release of noradrenaline which allows immediate physical reactions (such as increased heart rate and skin conductance, or auditory and visual exclusion phenomena) associated with a preparation for violent muscular action (Dickerson and Kemeny, 2004). On the other hand, the HPAa activation (which is lower) results in the releasing of cortisol the purpose of which is to redistribute energy in order to face the threat. Thus, more energy is allocated to the organs that need it most (brain and heart), while non-necessary organs for immediate survival (reproductive, immune and digestive systems) are inhibited. This stress response cascade ends when homeostasis is restored.

However, stress can be of different types, such as physical, psychological or psychosocial (Dickerson and Kemeny, 2004), each kind of stress being associated with a specific response. Indeed, physical stress, induced by extreme temperatures or physical pain for example, is associated with an increase of heart rate (Loggia et al., 2011), skin conductance (Boucsein, 1992; Buchanan et al., 2006) and subjective stress ratings but with only a weak cortisol response (Dickerson and Kemeny, 2004). These results suggest that this kind of stress induces an activation of the SAMa but only a weak activation of the HPAa. Psychological or mental stress, associated with difficult cognitive tasks, uncontrollability or negative emotions is associated with a weak release of cortisol (weak HPAa activation), but strong effects on heart rate and skin conductance (strong SAMa activation) (Boucsein, 1992; Reinhardt et al., 2012). Finally, psychosocial stress, triggered by a social evaluation threat (that is to say a situation in which the person's own estimated social value is likely to be degraded), and added to by a feeling of uncontrollability (in particular during the Trier Social Stress Task (TSST) Kirschbaum et al., 1993), has been shown to induce a strong activation of both the SAMa (Hellhammer and Schubert, 2012) and the HPAa (Dickerson and Kemeny, 2004).

Psychosocial stress and workload potentially can interact on physiological, neurophysiological and behavioral levels. Since workload can also be understood as the response to a particular type of psychological stressor, such as increased task demand, both concepts are associated with the activation of the sympathetic nervous system (see SAMa above). Furthermore, psychosocial stress and workload share also neurophysiological responses. From research in the neurosciences, and consistent with the notion of neural response systems, we know that stress has strong correlates in the EEG as well. One of the most prominent correlates of anxiety, as induced by psychosocial stress, is found in the alpha band, and specifically in brain asymmetry. Tops et al. (2006) proposed that cortisol administration (which simulates a stress situation) leads to a global decrease of cortical activity (except for the left frontal cortex in which activity is increased). However, other studies (Lewis et al., 2007; Hewig et al., 2008) showed that stress was associated with a higher activity in the right hemisphere, and that the right hemisphere activation was correlated with negative affect. For Crost et al. (2008), the explanation of these conflicting results would be that an association between EEG-asymmetry and personality characteristics, such as anxiousness, may only be observed in relevant situations to the personality dimensions of interest. For workload, on the other hand, we know that the alpha band plays a role in terms of increased sensory processing leading to decreased occipito-parietal alpha power (Gevins et al., 1998; Brouwer et al., 2012), as well as for frontal alpha asymmetry covarying with changes in engagement (Fairclough and Roberts, 2011). From a theoretical point of view, Eysenck and Derakshan (2011) suggested that increasing anxiety, for example due to psychosocial stress, has effects on different cognitive processes, leading to impaired processing efficiency and performance effectiveness. Specifically for workload-related processes, their "attentional control theory" suggests that anxiety impairs efficient function of inhibition and shifting mechanisms of the central executive, subsequently decreasing attentional control and increasing distraction effects of irrelevant stimuli. However, these deficits might not necessarily lead to decreases of performance if they are compensated by alternative strategies, such as enhanced effort.

Summarizing, increases in workload, as induced by higher task demand, can be subsumed under the concept of psychological stress and have been found to lead to increasing physiological and neurophysiological activity that has also been found responsive to anxiety as induced by psychosocial stress. Furthermore, cognitive theories propose links between anxiety and pre-attentional and attentional cognitive processes, which are expressed in behavior and physiology. Due to these possible interactions of workload and stress, it seems relevant to experimentally study the effect of stress on workload detection.

RESEARCH QUESTIONS

The work on the effects of potential contextual factors, such as moods or fatigue, on the stability of BCI performance, and the physiological and psychological links between stress and cognitive processes suggests that stress can be a relevant factor influencing the classification of workload levels. In more general, the findings of context-dependency of BCI performance make it seem imperative to explore the effect of factors, such as mood, on brain signals and classifier performance, to gain insight into the relevance of task-unrelated mental states on classifier performance, and to find ways to render classifiers robust against such changes. Specifically, for the development of reliable passive BCIs in the wild, those functioning robustly in private or work environments, the influence of contextual changes of mental states that are predominant in the context of application have to be explored. That is why we test the robustness of three workload classifiers, using features from either frequency-, time-, or both domains, to the influence of (psychosocial) stress. We let participants work under different levels of workload, while either under the impression of being observed and validated, or while being relaxed and free from this kind of pressure. We are interested in the effect of the contextual manipulation of stress on the classifier performance and in testing cross-context training as a simple and straightforward remedy to the problem. Thus, we address the following questions:

Q1: Can we induce stress and workload in a controlled manner? We validated stress and workload manipulation of our experimental protocol using participants' self-assessments, behavioral performance, and physiological indicators of sympathetic nervous system (SNS) activation (i.e., GSR, ECG). Stress is expected to increase perceived anxiety and SNS activity, while workload increase should be reflected in increased perceived arousal and mental effort, decreased performance, as well as increased SNS activity (Verwey and Veltman, 1984; Boucsein, 1992).

Q2: Can we train a workload classifier based on the data collected via this protocol? To ensure that we are using a state-of-the-art workload classifier, we trained the classifier on all data, irrespective of context, as done in conventional studies. We expect a performance of about 70% as shown by Grimes et al. (2008) and Brouwer et al. (2012) under similar conditions.

Q3: Does the classifier generalize across affective contexts, and if so, how well? To study the effect of different affective contexts on the classification performance, we compared the results from classifiers trained in either stressful or non-stressful context and applied it then to test data from the same ("within") or the other context ("across"). We expect a higher "within" compared to "across" performance to indicate the difficulty of the classifier to generalize.

Q4: Does training based on multiple context render the classifier resistant against changes in affective context,and if so, how resistant? To test if the training with combined data from both affective contexts is effecting the classifier's capability to generalize, we compare the performance depending on the training context ("single," that is training on only stress or non-stress context, or "combined," that is training over contexts) and expect higher performance for a classifier trained on data from the combined contexts.

MATERIALS AND METHODS

As mentioned before, we designed a protocol in which subjects had to do cognitive tasks involving two levels of mental workload, manipulated via task difficulty, while being exposed to two levels of psychosocial stress. We used the EEG signals collected with this protocol to design and assess a workload classifier across different stress conditions. This section describes in details the subjects involved, the protocol and the method to validate it, the EEG-based workload classifier used and the evaluations performed with it.

PARTICIPANTS

Twelve female and twelve male participants were recruited for our experiment. The participants were between 18 and 54 years old, with a mean age of 24.7 ± 7.9, and except four all were right-handed. Educations varied between high school degree and Ph.D., with a mean education of 3.1 ± 2.4 years after high school. To be admitted, people had to be at least 18 years, to speak the local language and to sign an informed consent. Furthermore, non-inclusion criteria were applied: bad vision, heart condition, neurological or psychological diseases, and affective troubles. Moreover, people were asked to select a time for the experiment in which they would feel alert. Finally, we asked them not to drink coffee and tea less than 2 h before the experiment.

MATERIAL

For our recordings, we used the following sensors: ElectroEncephaloGram (EEG, 28 active electrodes in a 10/20 system without T7, T8, Fp1, and Fp2), ElectroCardioGram (ECG, two active electrodes), facial ElectroMyoGram (EMG, two active electrodes), ElectroOculoGram (EOG, four active electrodes), breath belt (SleepSense), pulse (g.PULSEsensor), and a galvanic skin response sensor (g.GSRsensor). All sensors were connected and amplified with three synchronized g.USBAmp amplifiers (g.tec, Austria). The workload task was designed in the Presentation software (Neurobehavioral Systems, www.neurobs.com/presentation) and EEG signals were recorded and visually inspected with Open ViBE (Renard et al., 2010). **Figure 1** shows a participant sitting fully-wired in the experimental environment.

Subjects were first asked to sign an informed consent and to fill out three questionnaires: one assessing personal characteristics (such as gender, age and education) and form Y-A (anxiety state) and Y-B (anxiety trait) of the State-Trait Anxiety Inventory (STAI) (Spielberger et al., 1970) (see below for details). Then, all the sensors were installed and a 3 min baseline recorded. To avoid order effects, we counterbalanced the order of stress and relax condition (affective context) and 0-back and 2-back task (workload blocks), resulting in four scenarios (see **Figure 2A**). Each scenario was composed of 12 workload blocks in the stressful and 12 workload blocks in the relaxed context. The scenarios therefore begin with either relaxation or stress induction, and the workload blocks either start with the low workload (0-back) or high workload (2-back) condition. In each affective context, the subject performs, in alternating order, six times each workload condition (low/high) ($6 \times 2 \times 2 = 24$ min per block), with a short break after six tasks (i.e., after about 12 min). After each context was absolved, that is

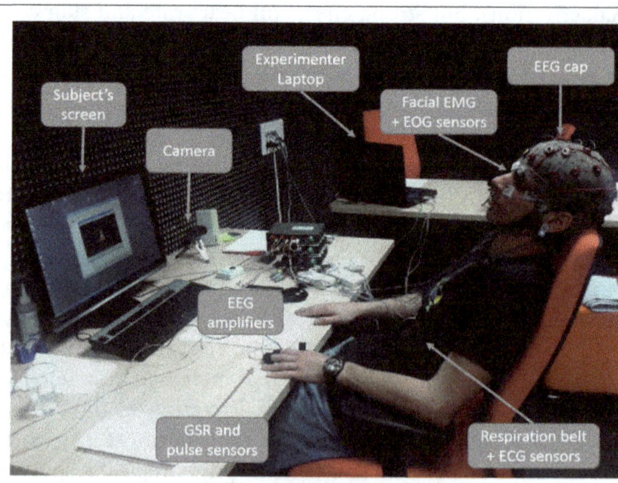

FIGURE 1 | A fully wired participant in the experimental environment during the relaxation induction period.

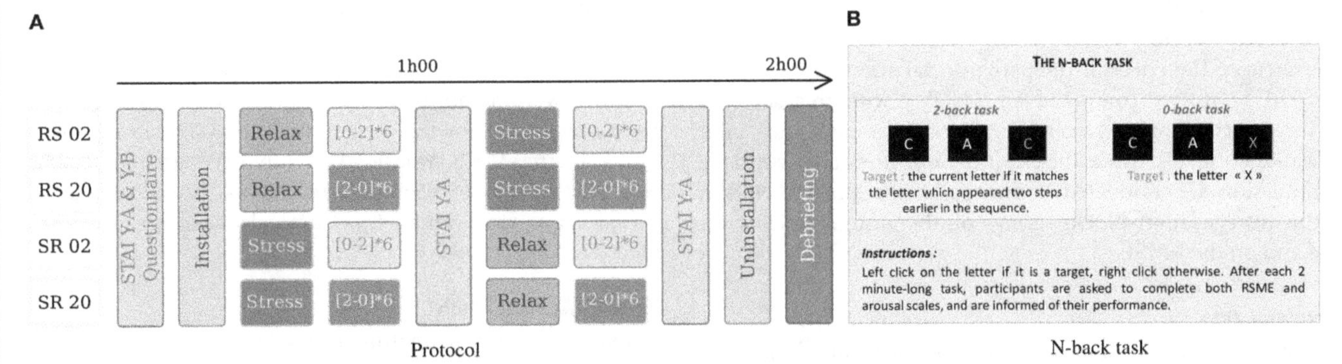

FIGURE 2 | The experimental protocol (A) with four scenarios, used for counterbalancing the order of conditions: the easy (0-back task) and difficult (2-back) workload tasks that follow the (R)elax and (S)tress induction procedures. "RS02" means that relaxation context is followed by stress context and that the interleaved workload blocks start with the 0-back condition. The N-back task **(B)** requires responses to target and non-target characters.

after the induction phase and the 12 workload blocks, the STAI form Y-A questionnaire was administered again to assess the anxiety state. Finally, the sensors were removed and the participant was debriefed about the aim of the experiment.

Stress and relaxation inductions

In order to manipulate stress, we used a stress-induction protocol based on the Trier Social Stress Task (TSST) (Kirschbaum et al., 1993) and a relaxation condition using a resting phase, music and/or videos. The stress-induction protocol is composed of three parts lasting together about 15 min and it requires the participation of three people, "the committee," who are presented as being body language experts. In the first part, a member of the committee asks the subject to prepare, during 5 min, a fake job interview for a position fitting the professional profile of the subject. During the second part, the committee asks the person to do this job interview and to speak about himself for 5 min. They tell the subject that he is filmed for a future behavioral analysis and take notes during the whole interview. The committee acts as being serious and neutral/unresponsive toward the subject. The third part is a 3 min long arithmetic task (the subject has to count from 2083 to 0 by steps of 13) and to begin again at any mistake or hesitation. At the end of this protocol, in order to keep the stress level high, the committee tells the subject he will be filmed during the workload tasks and that he will have to do another interview, which will be longer, and a self-evaluation based on the recorded film material after it. Furthermore, during the experiment, participants are receiving visual feedback about their performance in the workload tasks. During the stress condition, these feedbacks have been modified to display a performance 5–10% below their actual performance. Thereby, this protocol includes psychosocial stress and uncontrollability in order to maximize the chance to trigger a stress response for all the participants (Dickerson and Kemeny, 2004). On the other hand, the goal of the relaxation induction was to create a condition (referred to as "relax" condition) in which participants would be able to relax and thus execute the workload task without the influence of additional psychosocial and psychological stressors. To allow for an effective relaxation, participants were allowed to choose between resting in silence or select music/videos that would help them to feel calm (Krout, 2007). In order to measure the level of anxiety of the subjects and thereby to validate the stress/relax manipulation, the "State Trait Anxiety Inventory" (Spielberger et al., 1970) is used. It is composed of two scales of 20 propositions each: STAI form Y-A and STAI form Y-B. STAI form Y-A score measures anxiety state and is increased when the person currently experiences psychological stress. A college student (female/male) has a mean state anxiety index of 35/36, while values higher than 39/40 have been suggested to detect clinically significant symptoms (see Julian, 2011).

Workload tasks

We used the n-back task (Kirchner, 1958) as workload task (see **Figure 2B**), as it is easy to modify workload while keeping visual stimulation and behavioral motor requirements the same. Similar to Grimes et al. (2008) and Brouwer et al. (2012), we decided for a manipulation of task-difficulty to manipulate workload. Specifically, we used 0-back (low workload) and 2-back (high workload) varieties of the n-back task, which were presented in blocks of 2 min each. In both tasks, a stream of 60 white letters appears on a black background on the screen. Each letter is presented for 500 ms, followed by an inter-stimulus interval of 1500 ms. Among these letters, 25% are targets. In both tasks, when a letter appears, the subject is asked to perform a left mouse click if this is a target letter, and a right mouse click otherwise. For the 0-back task, the low workload condition, the target is the letter "X": each time an "X" appears, the subject has to do a left click, and in all the other cases he has to do a right click. For the 2-back task, the high workload condition, the subject has to do a left click if the letter that appears is the same as the one preceding the last letter. For example, if the sequence "C A C" appeared, the second "C" would be a target. At the end of each 2-min block, the subject has to report his level of arousal (on a scale from 1 to 9) (Bradley and Lang, 1994) and the perceived effort necessary to perform the task (Rating Scale of Mental Effort—RSME, Zijlstra, 1993). Finally, a screen with his performance during the block (see section 4.3.2) appears. As mentioned before, during the stressful condition, this displayed performance is lower than the actual performance to induce additional uncertainty.

PROTOCOL VALIDATION METHODS

Self-assessment data

To investigate the effect of the psychosocial stress induction on the STAI score, we computed an ANOVA with this score in the three factor-levels "baseline," "after relaxation," and "after stress induction." To assess the effect of both stress and workload manipulation, we conducted 2 (stress) × 2 (workload) ANOVAs for the averaged-over-blocks ratings on the arousal scale of the SAM and on the RMSE.

Behavioral data

To investigate the effects of the experimental manipulations on behavior, we calculated the performance per block based on the number of true positive (*TP*), true negative (*TN*), false negative (*FN*), and false positive (*FP*) responses resulting from the button presses within the n-back task (left click for targets, right click for non-targets) using the following equation: $Perf = \frac{(TP+TN)}{(TP+TN+FP+FN)}$. As for ratings, we analyzed the data in a 2 (stress) × 2 (workload) ANOVA.

Physiological data

Physiological responses were analyzed with respect to heart rate (HR) and galvanic skin response (GSR). Before applying statistical methods, the GSR data was pre-processed by extracting the mean GSR value (μS) for each block and then averaging these values over blocks as described above. The ECG signal was band-pass filtered between 5 and 200 Hz, applying a notch-filter 48–52 Hz to reduce power line noise, before mean HR for each of the blocks was extracted. As for the former analyses, we analyzed the data with a 2 (stress) × 2 (workload) ANOVA. We are reporting data as significant if $p < 0.05$ and as trend if $p < 0.1$. For all ANOVAs partial eta squared values ($\eta_p{}^2$) are calculated as a measure of effect size.

EEG SIGNAL PROCESSING

Our system aims at estimating the level of mental workload of the user from its EEG signals. To do so, we employed a machine learning approach based on state-of-the-art algorithms developed for Brain-Computer Interfaces (BCI) technologies (Lotte et al., 2007; Blankertz et al., 2008; Ang et al., 2012). This section describes the way EEG signals were preprocessed and segmented into trials, the machine learning algorithms used as well as the approach followed for the evaluating our method (see **Figure 3** for a schematic overview of these procedures).

EEG preprocessing and segmentation

We first cleaned signals from eye movements (EOG) contamination using the automatic method proposed in Schlögl et al. (2007). The EEG signals from each 2 min n-back task were

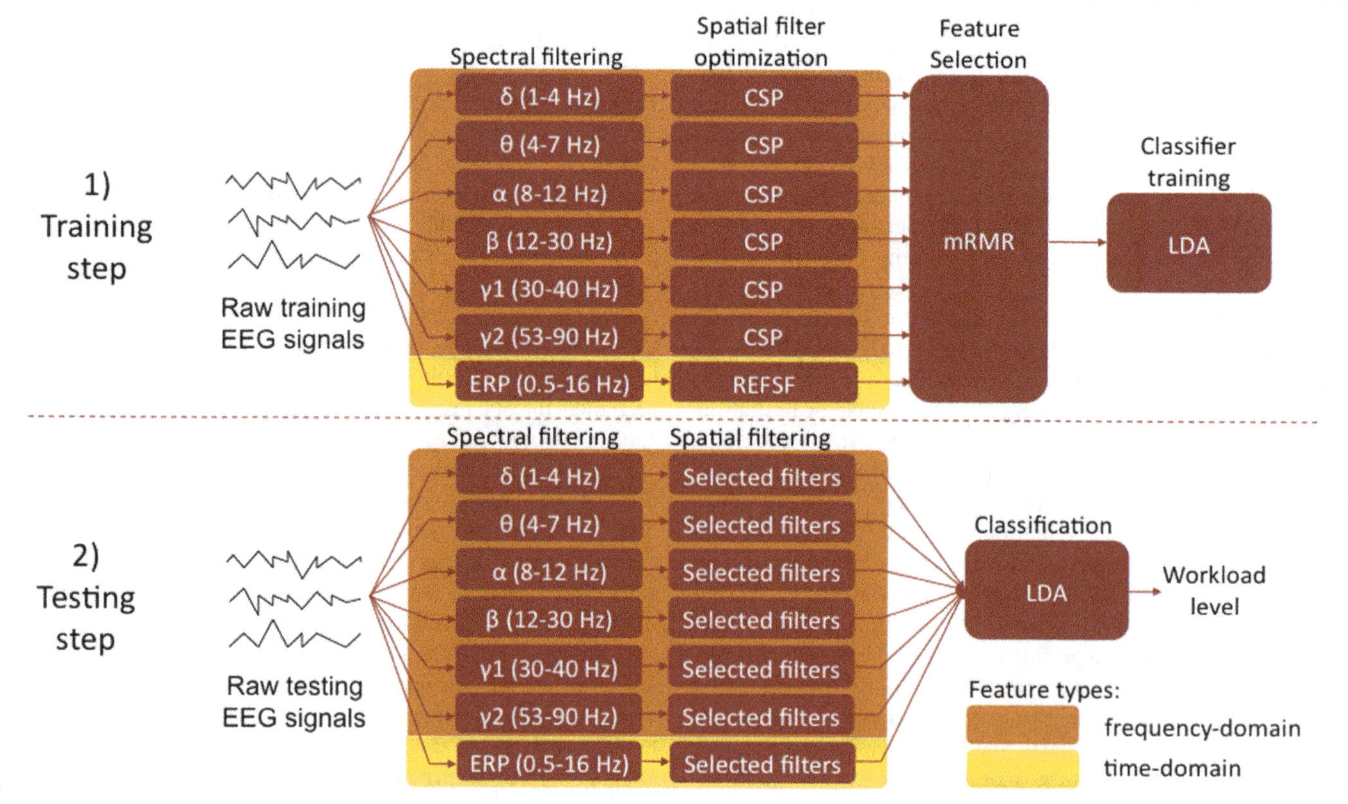

FIGURE 3 | Machine learning approach to workload level classification from EEG signals. Top: training set, aiming at identifying the relevant frequency bands (i.e., spectral filters) and channels (i.e., spatial filters), using the Filter Bank CSP and REFSF approach. **Bottom:** testing set, using the optimized spectral and spatial filter to estimate the workload level from an unknown EEG trial. (CSP, Common Spatial Patterns; REFSF, regularized Fisher spatial filter; mRMR, maximum Relevance Minimum Redundancy; LDA, Linear Discriminant Analysis).

then divided into 60 EEG trials, i.e., one EEG trial per letter appearance. More precisely, each EEG trial was defined as starting at a letter appearance onset and ending 2 s later, i.e., just before the next letter appearance. This resulted in 60 EEG trials per task, i.e., 720 trials per workload level (360 trials in the stressful condition, 360 in the non-stressful condition). Among them, trials corresponding to target letters were discarded in order to avoid confounding and interfering effects that may result from Event Related Potentials (ERP—notably a P300) likely to be triggered by target identification. This left 540 trials per workload levels (270 trials per psychosocial stress condition).

Machine Learning algorithms

In order to estimate workload levels from EEG signals, we investigated two different types of neurophysiological information: (1) oscillatory activity and (2) Event Related Potentials (ERP), both of which having been shown to be useful for such a task (Brouwer et al., 2012). We set up state-of-the-art signal processing pipelines in order to estimate workload using these two types of information, both individually and in combination (see **Figure 3**). They are described below:

Oscillatory activity. To classify low mental workload vs. high mental workload in EEG signals based on oscillatory activity, we used a variant of the Filter Bank Common Spatial Patterns (FBCSP) algorithm (Ang et al., 2012) in order to learn optimal spatial and spectral features, i.e., EEG frequency bands and channels. The FBCSP is one of the most efficient algorithms to extract spatio-spectral features from EEG signals. It was indeed the algorithm used by the winners of the last BCI competition on all EEG data sets (Ang et al., 2012; Tangermann et al., 2012), showing the superiority of this method over other approaches. The FBCSP-based approach we employed works as follows. The first step—the training step—consists in identifying the most relevant frequency bands (i.e., spectral filters) and EEG channels (i.e., spatial filters), using examples of EEG signals from the high and low workload conditions (see below for details on the definition of the training sets). To do so, we first filter each training EEG trial into multiple frequency bands using a bank of band-pass filters. Here we used band-pass filters in the following frequency bands, which correspond to classical EEG rhythms: δ (1–4 Hz), θ (4–8 Hz), α (8–12 Hz), β (12–30 Hz), γ (30–47 Hz), and high γ (53–90 Hz). Then for each of these bands, the band-pass filtered EEG trials are used to optimize spatial filters, i.e., linear combinations of the original EEG channels. These spatial filters are optimized using the Common Spatial Pattern (CSP) algorithm (Blankertz et al., 2008), which finds the optimal channel combination such that the power of the resulting spatially filtered signals is maximally discriminant between the two conditions (here, low and high workload). We optimize 12 (6 pairs) such CSP filters for each frequency band. Then, the power of the spectrally and spatially filtered EEG signals is used as features, resulting in each EEG trial being described by 72 features (12 CSP filters $\times$ 6 frequency bands). From these 72 features, the 18 most relevant ones are selected using the maximum Relevance Minimum Redundancy (mRMR) feature selection algorithm (Peng et al., 2005). This amounts to selecting the 18 most relevant pairs of spectral and spatial filters. Finally, the 18 selected power features are used to train a shrinkage Linear Discriminant Analysis (LDA) classifier (Blankertz et al., 2010; Lotte and Guan, 2010) to discriminate low workload EEG trials from high workload ones. This concludes the training step. For testing, i.e., to predict the workload level of a given EEG trial, the EEG signals are first filtered using the 18 selected pairs of spectral and spatial filters, then the power of the resulting signals is computing and given as input to the previously trained LDA classifier whose output indicates the workload level (high or low).

Event related potentials. To classifiy low mental workload vs. high mental workload in EEG signals based on ERP, we first band-pass filtered the signals between 0.5 and 16 Hz, and downsampled them to 36 Hz, to reduce the signal dimensionality. We only used the first second of EEG signals from each trial (i.e., the first second after letter presentation in the N-back task) to analyse ERP, i.e., 36 samples per channels. Then, based on these 1-second of EEG signals from the training set, we learned optimal spatial filters for the discrimination of ERP based on EEG samples, by using the Fisher Spatial Filters (FSF) proposed by Hoffmann et al. (2006). We extracted 6 such spatial filters, which resulted in 216 features (6 filters $\times$ 36 EEG samples per filter), using a regularization parameter $\lambda = 0.4$ for optimizing the FSF for all subjects. We finally selected 18 features (i.e., 18 EEG samples) out of these 216 initial ones, using mRMR feature selection. These 18 selected features were used to train a shrinkage LDA. For testing, the EEG signals were preprocessed in the same way (i.e., band-pass filtered in 0.5–16 Hz and downsampled to 36 Hz), spatially filtered using the 6 Fisher Spatial Filters optimized during training, and the 18 resulting selected features were used as input to the previously trained LDA classifier whose output indicates the workload level (high or low).

Combination of oscillatory activity and ERP. In order to combine both oscillatory activity and ERP information, we extracted 18 FBCSP features as described above and 18 ERP features, as described above as well, from each trial. These 36 features were concatenated into a single feature vector, which was used as input to a shrinkage LDA classifier.

Evaluation scheme

The performance of our workload-level estimator was assessed using sixfold stratified Cross-Validation (CV), separately for each subject. This means the data from each subject was divided into six parts, each part containing the same number of trials from each class (high/low workload). Five of these parts were used for training, i.e., to identify the relevant spectral and spatial filters, as well as to train the LDA classifier. The 6th part was used for testing the resulting workload-level estimator for that subject. This process was repeated six times, with each part used exactly once as the testing set. For three subjects we used only three- and fourfold CV due to missing blocks in the end of the recording. The performance, here the classification accuracy (i.e., rate of trials with correctly estimated workload-level), hence obtained on each testing part are then averaged to give a final performance of the workload-level estimator for that subject.

The goal of our work is to design a generic workload-level estimator, usable in practice, i.e., that can work across different affective contexts (here, different psychosocial stress levels). To do so, we performed different evaluations to estimate (1) the general performance of our system, independently of the affective context; (2) how it behaves *within* a given affective context; (3) how it behaves *across* different affective contexts, i.e., can a workload-level estimator calibrated on data from a given affective context (e.g., a relaxed condition) be used to estimate workload in another affective context (e.g., a stressful condition), (4) if effects of time can explain across-context classification performance loss, and (5) whether calibrating our system with data from different affective contexts makes the system better or worse, even if used in a single affective context. Different sub-parts of the data were thus used for training and testing within our CV scheme, in particular:

1. **General performance estimation:** This is the overall evaluation, in which we used all the data, from both affective contexts, i.e., with EEG trials from both the relaxed and the stressful conditions. Therefore, within each fold of the CV, 20 blocks (i.e., 900 trials) were available for training, and 4 blocks (i.e., 180 trials) were available for testing. The number of trials from each workload-level (high/low) and each psychosocial stress (relaxed/stressful) was balanced in both the training and testing set.
2. **Within affective context performance estimation:** This evaluation assessed the performance of our system when calibrated on a single affective context and tested on the same affective context. This is the evaluation generally performed in previous works, in which a single affective context is considered. Therefore, in each fold of the cross-validation, 10 blocks (i.e., 450 trials) were available for training, all coming from the relaxed (resp. stressful) condition, and 2 blocks (i.e., 90 trials) were available for testing, all coming as well from the relaxed (resp. stressful) condition. The number of trials from each workload-level was balanced in both the training and testing set.
3. **Across affective context performance estimation:** This evaluation assessed the performance of our system when calibrated on a given affective context and tested on a different affective context. This evaluation is usually ignored in current workload-level estimation works. Previous works indeed implicitly considered that the user was always in the same affective state, which is very unlikely in practice and can thus compromise the usability of the system. Therefore, in each fold of the cross-validation, 10 blocks (i.e., 450 trials) were available for training, all coming from the relaxed (resp. stressful) condition, and 2 blocks (i.e., 90 trials) were available for testing, all coming from the other affective context i.e., the stressful (resp. relaxed) condition. The number of trials from each workload-level was balanced in both the training and testing set.
4. **Investigation of time effects on classifier performance:** To rule out that a difference between within-context and across-context training is merely caused by the time passing between affective contexts, we devised an analysis similar to the above two analyses, but with first and second half of each context instead of relax and stress context. Therefore, we trained our classifiers on the data of 4 blocks and tested them on 2 blocks from either the same or the other half of the context. This was done in a threefold cross-validation scheme and resulted in two within and two across classification performance values (one from 1st half to second half, and one backwards) for each affective context. These were averaged over the affective contexts and yielded one value for the workload classification accuracy for within- and across-context (i.e., "half") per participant per half[2]. For a genuine effect of affective context instead of an effect of simply the time passing between both contexts, the "within vs. across halfs" performance loss for a classifier that was only trained on one half should be smaller compared to the loss between "within vs. across affective context" performance loss for a classifier that was only trained on one affective context.
5. **Calibration across affective context performance estimation:** When considering different affective contexts, an interesting question is whether using data from different contexts to calibrate the workload-level estimator will make it better or worse, notably as compared to the within affective context evaluation. Indeed, on the one hand, using data from different contexts can force the machine learning approach to identify workload indices that are invariant to the affective context, thus improving the system, but on the other hand it adds more noise and variability to the data, which can impede the machine learning process. Therefore, with this evaluation, in each fold of the cross-validation, 20 blocks were available for training, coming from both the relaxed and stressful condition, and 2 blocks were available for testing, coming from either the stressful or the relaxed condition (but not both). To ensure that the comparison of this approach with the within-context approach is fair, we had to use the same number of training trials for each approach. Indeed, using all the trials available in the 20 training blocks would mean using more training trials than in the within-context evaluation, which could result in higher performance simply due to a larger number of training trials. Therefore, for this last evaluation, we randomly selected 6 blocks from each context for training, from 4 of which all trials were used, while we selected every other trial from the remaining 2 blocks to keep the workload classes balanced within context. Further two blocks were selected from each context for testing. This procedure was repeated six times for a cross-validation comparable to the within-/across context evaluation.

RESULTS

In this section, we first present the validation analysis, suggesting that our protocol indeed induced different levels of workload and stress (Q1). Then the results of the EEG-based workload classification over, within, and across affective contexts are presented, showing that a state-of-the-art subject-specific workload

[2]For three subjects, the averaging only contained data from the stress context due to missing blocks in the 2nd half of the relax context.

classifier (Q2) has difficulty generalizing over affective contexts (Q3), but can be rendered less context-sensitive by calibration across affective contexts (Q4).

VALIDATION OF THE PROTOCOL

Subjective indicators

Each subject filled in three "STAI form Y-A" (state) questionnaires: one at the beginning ($STAI_{BL}$) of the experiment and one in the end of each affective context, that is after performing the n-back tasks under stress or relax condition (stress: $STAI_S$; relax: $STAI_R$) (see **Figure 4A**). Three data sets were excluded due to incompleteness. A repeated-measures ANOVA ($N = 21$) with the factor levels "baseline," "stress," and "relax" showed a significant difference of perceived anxiety between the conditions [$F_{(2, 20)} = 3.6225$, $p < 0.05$, $\eta_p{}^2 = 0.108$]. We conducted a *post hoc* analyses using paired t-tests with the hypothesis that subjectively perceived anxiety increases due to the stress induction procedure relative to baseline and relaxation condition. The results suggest that the stress-induction protocol indeed increases anxiety compared to baseline and relaxation condition, and keeps it significantly higher until measured in the end of the affective context (see **Figure 4A**): $STAI_S$ scores (mean $= 37.5 \pm 12.6$) are significantly higher [$t_{(20)} = 2.87$, $p = 0.01$] than $STAI_{BL}$ scores (mean $= 30.1 \pm 4.6$) and they are significantly higher [$t_{(20)} = 2.37$, $p = 0.028$] than $STAI_R$ scores (mean $= 32.2 \pm 8.6$). This increased anxiety seems mainly due to the interview and the apprehension of a final evaluation, rather than due to the n-back task as such: we found no difference between $STAI_R$ and $STAI_{BL}$ [$t_{(20)} = 1.27$, $p = 0.22$], that is when they performed the n-back tasks knowing that there would be no evaluation.

We furthermore asked the subjects after each block to rate their arousal on the respective scale of the Self-Assessment Maneken (see **Figure 4B**) and to rate the mental effort on the Rating Scale Mental Effort (see **Figure 4C**). Two data sets were excluded due to incompleteness. We submitted the data of each scale to a 2 (stress) × 2 (workload) repeated-measures ANOVA. Regarding the subjectively perceived arousal, we only found a main effect of the workload manipulation [$F_{(1, 21)} = 4.444$, $p = 0.047$, $\eta_p{}^2 = 0.175$] with higher perceived arousal for the 2-back task (mean $= 4.7 \pm 1.4$) compared to the 0-back task (mean $= 4.3 \pm 1.7$). Regarding the subjectively perceived workload, we only found a main effect of the workload manipulation [$F_{(1, 21)} = 63.216$, $p < 0.0001$, $\eta_p{}^2 = 0.751$] with higher perceived effort for the 2-back task (mean $= 48.1 \pm 11.5$) compared to the 0-back task (mean $= 28.6 \pm 12.9$).

Objective indicators

For the analysis of the objective indicator of behavioral performance, we logged all responses and computed the task accuracy for each task block (see **Figure 5A**). Two data sets were excluded due to incompleteness. We submitted the accuracy to a 2 (stress) × 2 (workload) repeated-measures ANOVA. As for the subjective indicators of perceived arousal and effort, we found a main effect of the workload manipulation [$F_{(1, 21)} = 65.251$, $p < 0.0001$, $\eta_p{}^2 = 0.757$] with higher accuracy for the simple 0-back task (mean $= 97.3 \pm 2.0$) compared to the hard 2-back task (mean $= 91.1 \pm 4.8$).

As a further objective indicator, we computed skin conductance level and heart rate. Four data sets were excluded due to incompleteness. For heart rate analysis a further data set was excluded due to malfunctioning sensors. We submitted the data of the physiological signals to a 2 (stress) × 2 (workload) repeated-measures ANOVA. For GSR (see **Figure 5B**), we found an increase of the skin conductance level [$F_{(1, 19)} = 4.4806$, $p = 0.048$, $\eta_p{}^2 = 0.191$], indicating higher sympathetic arousal during the stress condition (mean $= 3.83 \pm 2.05$) compared to the relax condition (mean $= 3.52 \pm 2.07$). Skin conductance level increased for high compared to low workload condition as well, however, not significantly. For HR (see **Figure 5C**), we found a trend toward an increase of the heart rate [$F_{(1, 18)} = 3.2123$, $p = 0.089$, $\eta_p{}^2 = 0.151$], indicating higher sympathetic arousal during the stress condition (mean $= 79.41 \pm 10.23$) compared to the relax condition (mean $= 78.30 \pm 10.08$). More importantly, we found a highly significant effect of the workload manipulation on

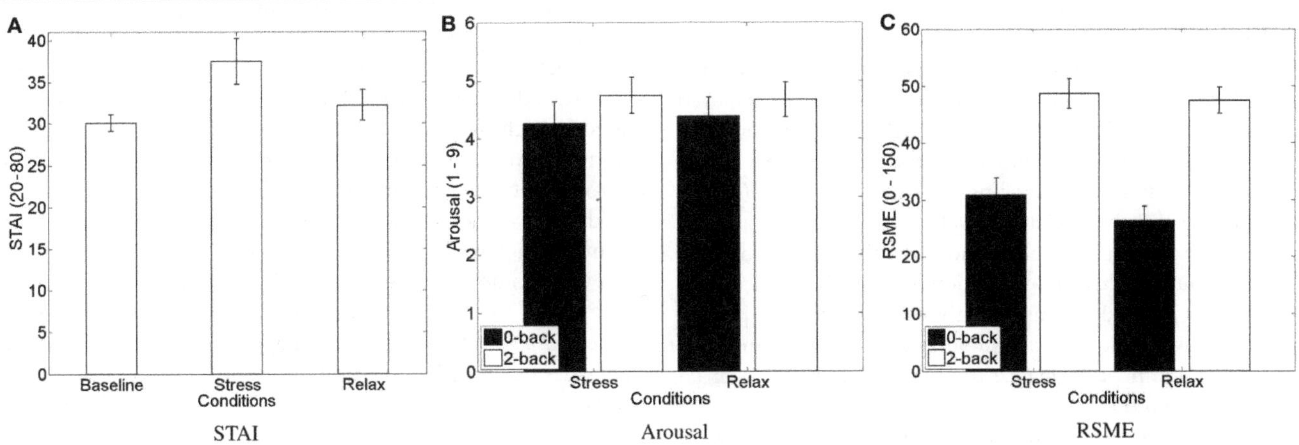

FIGURE 4 | Mean and standard error of mean of subjective stress level assessments. (A) STAI form Y-A scores, **(B)** SAM arousal scale, and **(C)** RSME. **(A)** Shows significant increase of perceived stress during the stressful condition compared to the baseline and the relax condition. **(B,C)** Show an increase of perceived arousal and mental effort for the 2-back compared to 0-back task.

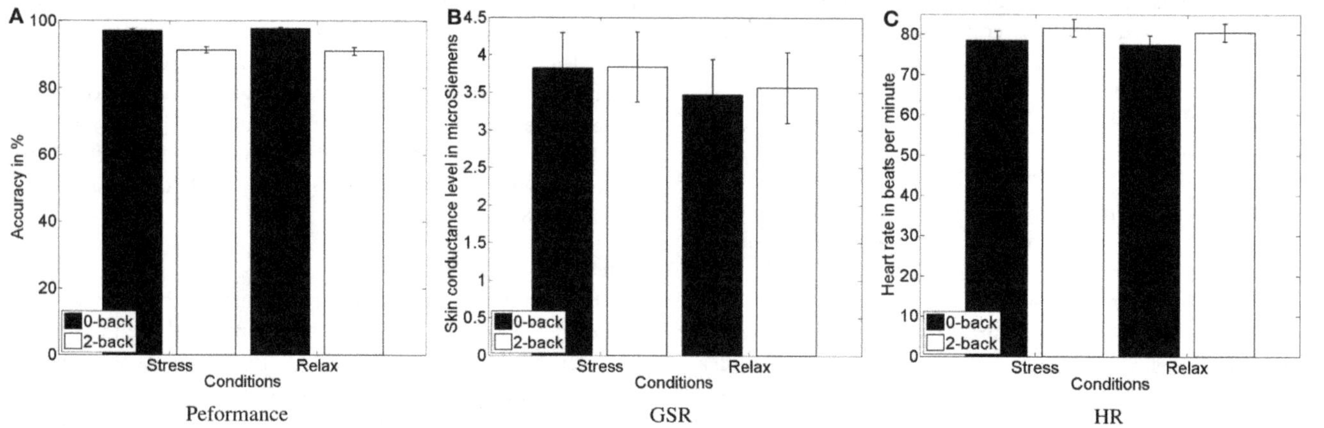

FIGURE 5 | Mean and standard error of the task performance (A), showing the decreased performance in high vs. low workload conditions, and of GSR response (B) and heart rate (C), indicating higher physiological activity in response to the psychosocial stress and workload manipulation, respectively.

HR [$F_{(1, 18)} = 36.1431$, $p < 0.0001$, $\eta_p{}^2 = 0.667$], with a higher HR for the more challenging 2-back task (mean $= 80.4 \pm 9.89$) compared with the relatively easy 0-back task (mean $= 77.27 \pm 10.19$).

In summary, we found evidence for the validity of the stress and workload induction (Q1) in both, the subjective (questionnaires) and objective (performance and physiological sensors) measures. This ensures that calibrating and evaluating a workload classifier on the EEG recorded with this protocol is meaningful.

CLASSIFICATION OF EEG

General performance estimation

In this section we report the general classification performance for a training on the whole data set, showing that our setup is state-of-the-art compared to similar studies hence positively answering question Q2. Specifically, we obtained performances similar to the best performances that were presented more recently with the n-back task paradigm and with 2 s short trials by Grimes et al. (2008) and Brouwer et al. (2012). The data of two participants was excluded due to incompleteness and of another one due to malfunctioning EEG sensors.

For the training and testing on the basis of all available data, those trials recorded during stress *and* relax context, we achieved an average classification accuracy of 76.1% when using only frequency-domain features, with performances between 58.7% and 95.4% (see **Figure 6**). According to Müller-Putz et al. (2008), we determined the above chance-level performance via a binomial test. For a two-class problem and given the number of 1080 trials used in our sixfold cross-validation scheme, the chance-level is at 53.1% for $p = 0.05$. Consequently, the classification performance was above chance for each subject, with a highly significant better-than-random performance for the average result over all subjects ($p \ll 0.0001$).

Subsequently, we tested the previously observed increase of performance for increasing decision intervals, that is when more data is available for testing (Grimes et al., 2008; Brouwer et al., 2012). A majority vote over the classifier decisions for all 45 relevant trials of a given block, using only frequency-domain features, leads to an accuracy of 96%, well over the 71% chance-level resulting from a binomial test on the basis of 24 decisions (one per block). For time-domain features, we observed an average accuracy of 74% for 2 s trials (of which only the first was used), and 96% for the judgement after 45 trials. For both feature varieties in combination, the 2-second accuracy was the highest with 80.4%, though the block-wise accuracy was only 94.4%. Since all accuracies are well over chance level the used classification schemes enable for a solid classification performance for all feature varieties with the combined frequency- and time-domain features performing best for short estimation intervals and separate feature varieties performing best for the long decision intervals.

From a scientific point of view it is necessary to know about the source of the classification performance: is the information of neural origin or is it derived from muscular activity that is known to contaminate higher frequency bands of the EEG (Goncharova et al., 2003)? Although this question is often eluded in previous works (Grimes et al., 2008), we tried to answer it by first computing the percentage of the features selected from each frequency band in the FBCSP algorithm. As **Figure 6** indicates, the majority (about 65%) of features selected with the mRMR feature selection algorithm employed came from lower frequency bands (i.e., delta, theta, alpha). However, the remaining 35% originated in high frequency bands, those over 12 Hz (beta, gamma, gamma2). To ensure that the classifier performance does rely on neuronal sources and not on muscle activity, we repeated the workload classifier evaluation excluding these potentially contaminated high frequency bands, both for training and testing. We achieved a somewhat lower, but again much better-than-random ($p \ll 0.0001$) classifier performance of 74.2%, with accuracies between 53.9% and 88.2%. This suggests that our workload classifier does rely mostly on neural information from low frequency bands.

Within- vs. across-context estimation

In this section we tested the generalization of the classifier to a different affective context (question Q3). To evaluate the effects of testing in dependence of training context, we conducted a 2 (training context: relax, stress) × 2 (testing context: same-as-training, different-from-training) repeated-measures ANOVA for each feature type. **Figures 7, 8** depict the average classifier performance when tested within and across affective context and the average loss of performance for the three used feature varieties (and the loss for the specific frequency bands), respectively.

The main effect found for the testing context when using frequency-domain features alone [$F_{(1,\ 20)} = 5.610$, $p = 0.028$, $\eta_p{}^2 = 0.219$] shows that the transfer from one context to another is problematic and results in a decrease of classifier performance (mean $= 69.4 \pm 9.7\%$) compared to testing on the same context as for the training (mean $= 72.4 \pm 9.4\%$). An exploratory analysis of the effect of context change on classifiers using only specific frequency bands revealed a significant contribution of the low frequency bands to the performance decline, while the less relevant high frequency bands were not or only minimally contributing (see **Figure 8**).

For time-domain features alone, the decrease of classifier performance for across context is as well significant, though stronger [$F_{(1,\ 20)} = 21.002, p < 0.001, \eta_p{}^2 = 0.512$], with a lower across-context classification performance (mean $= 69.1 \pm 5.5\%$) compared to within-context classification performance (mean $= 73.3 \pm 5.1\%$).

For frequency- and time-domain features combined, the decrease of classifier performance across-context (mean $= 73.2 \pm 8.8\%$) compared within-context (mean $= 77.3 \pm 7.9\%$) is as well marked [$F_{(1,\ 20)} = 12.104, p = 0.002, \eta_p{}^2 = 0.377$].

To rule out that the differences between within-context and across-context training were caused by the time passing between affective contexts, we divided each context into two parts (1st half,

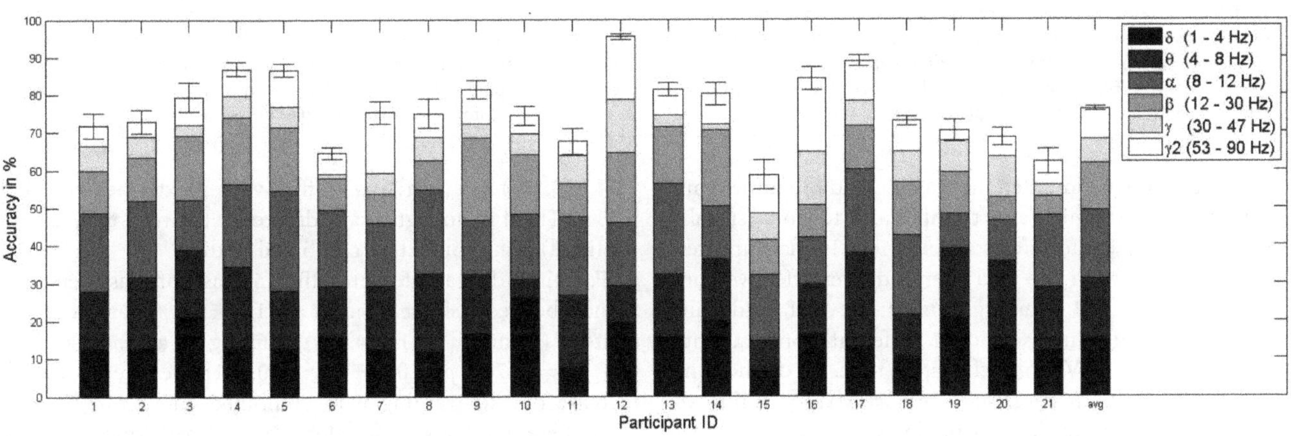

FIGURE 6 | Mean and standard error of the workload classification performance (sixfold cross-validation) per subject. The different colored subdivisions within each bar represent the percentage (total bar height = 100%) of features selected from a specific frequency band (delta, theta, alpha, beta, gamma, gamma2). For example, for subject 1 on average 9% of the features were chosen from the delta range. The last bar represents the mean classification accuracy over subjects and the average contribution from the frequency bands over subjects.

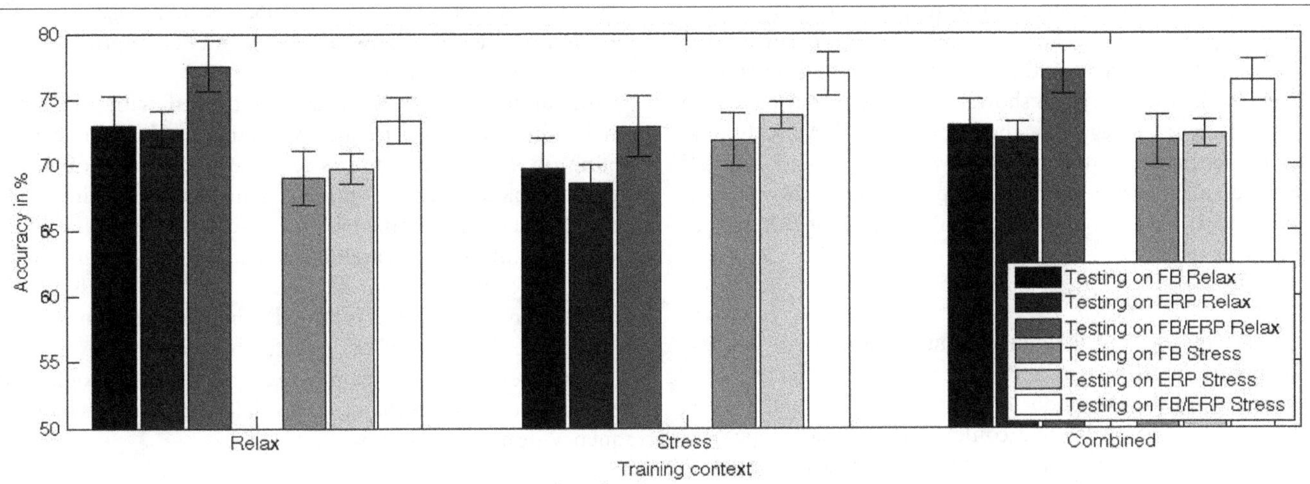

FIGURE 7 | Mean and standard error of the mean of the classification performance of a classifier trained in different training contexts (relax, stress, combined) and tested on data from relax and stress context. The differences between the testing performance for stress and relax context show an interaction between training and test factor: the difficulty of the classifier to generalize to another context. The higher performance for the combined training set relative to the training on data from a single context indicates a gain of the classifier in invariance and hence a protection against over-fitting.

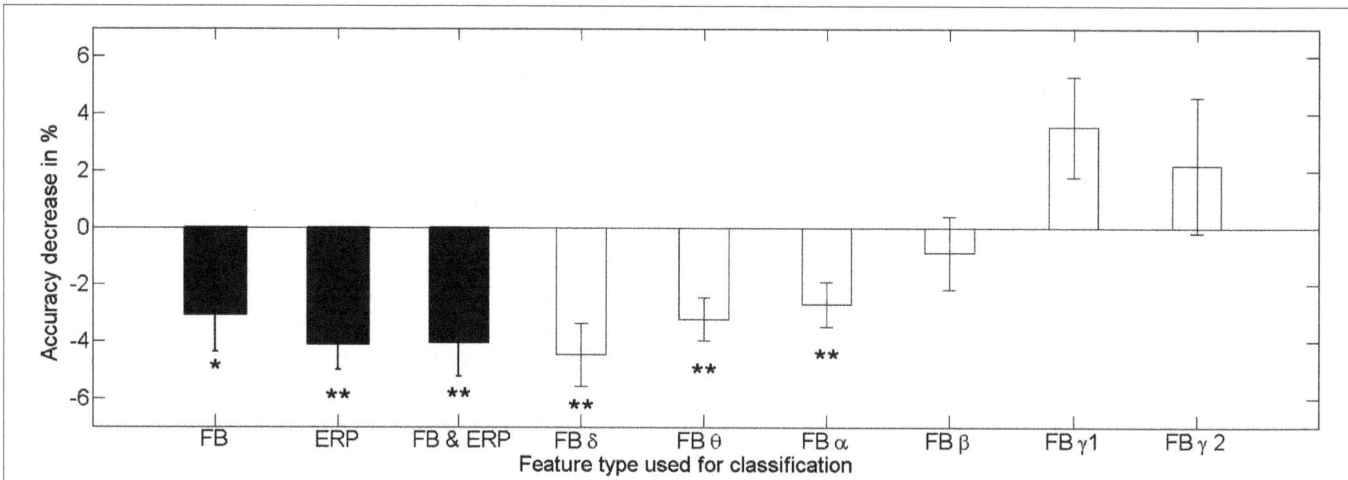

FIGURE 8 | Mean and standard error of the mean loss of the classification performance of a classifier trained and tested in different training contexts for the feature types from frequency-domain (FB), time-domain (ERP), both (FB and ERP), and for the individual frequency bands (FB $\alpha - \gamma 2$). The stars indicate the significance testing with the respective methods mentioned in the text ($^{*}p < 0.05$, $^{**}p < 0.01$). Only the low frequency bands show significant effects of performance detoriation in the phase of changing affective context, while the high frequency bands seem relatively stable against changes in context.

2nd half) and trained and tested the classifiers in the same manner as done for the within (e.g., training and test on 1st half) and across affective context (e.g., training on 1st half and test on 2nd half) tests. With the data averaged over affective contexts, we conducted a 2 (training context: 1st half, 2nd half) $\times$ 2 (testing context: same-as-training, different-from-training) repeated-measures ANOVA for each feature type. We did not find the pattern of performance loss that we observed for within vs. across affective context testing. Surprisingly, the only effect we found was a increase of performance for across vs. within context (half) testing for the frequency-domain only feature variety [$F_{(1,\ 20)} = 5.142, p < 0.04, \eta_p{}^2 = 0.204$] from 61.1% to 63.7%.

Summarizing, all feature varieties have been found susceptible to changes in affective context. For the frequency-domain features, only classifiers using the low frequency bands of delta, theta and alpha are significantly declining in performance when tested in an affective context different from the training context (see **Figure 8**). However, as we showed, these frequency bands are the most informative regarding the workload level. An additional test of the within vs. across effects between the 1st and 2nd half of the affective contexts on classifier performance showed that the time effect alone does not lead to a consistent decrease of performance.

Across-context calibration

To evaluate the use of a combined training context to increase the capability of the classifier to generalize over affective contexts (question Q4), we conducted a 2 (training context: average single, combined) $\times$ 2 (testing context: stress, relax) repeated-measures ANOVA for each feature type. The specific effects of across-context calibration in comparison to single context (stress and relax) calibration are depicted in **Figure 7**.

The main effect of the training context for frequency-domain features alone [$F_{(1,\ 20)} = 6.816,\ p = 0.017,\ \eta_p{}^2 = 0.254$] indicates a higher performance for training with combined (mean $=$ $72.4 \pm 9.5\%$) vs. with single affective context (mean $= 70.9 \pm 9.3\%$). There is no significant difference between testing on the (optimal) same context vs. combined testing.

For time-domain features the increase of classifier performance between single (mean $= 71.2 \pm 5.2\%$) and combined context (mean $= 72.1 \pm 4.9\%$) training is as well significant [$F_{(1,\ 20)} = 6.703, p = 0.017, \eta_p{}^2 = 0.251$]. Despite the observed increase due to training with combined data from both contexts, there is still a significant decrease of performance of about 1.2% relative to training and testing on the same context [$t_{(20)} = -3.526, p < 0.01$].

For frequency- and time-domain features combined, we observed an increase of classifier performance between single (mean $= 76.7 \pm 7.6\%$) and combined context training (mean $= 75.2 \pm 8.1\%$) with [$F_{(1,\ 20)} = 6.306, p = 0.021, \eta_p{}^2 = 0.240$]. There is no difference between testing on the (optimal) same context vs. combined testing.

Summarizing, for those classifiers trained with frequency-domain and combined frequency- and time-domain features, training on combined contexts leads to an increase of performance comparable with (optimal) same context training and testing. For classifiers trained with time-domain features only, we observe a significant increase of classification performance when training on combined context, but there is still a loss of performance compared to the (optimal) same context training and testing. Since the number of trials for both conditions are kept equal, this is evidence for a gain in resilience of the workload classifier against contextual changes, especially for classifiers based on frequency-domain features.

DISCUSSION

If we want to create passive brain-computer interfaces that work in the wild, we need to take the variability of such environments into account. To test how well a workload classifier would be able to cope with variability due to changes in affective context, we trained it on the data from a subject performing a task under the evaluative pressure of an impending interview, the same subject in a non-stressful setting, and from both contexts.

We validated the experimental protocol using subjective and objective indicators of the psychophysiological activation expected due to stress/relaxation induction and different workload levels. Though we did not see a significant difference in the perceived arousal measure (SAM), higher values for the STAI and increased sympathetic nervous system activity (as indicated by significant differences for GSR and a trend for HR) support a successful induction of anxiety in the stressful compared to the non-stressful condition. Higher perceived arousal and mental demand, higher sympathetic nervous system activity (as indexed by HR) as well as lower behavioral performance for high compared to low workload levels support the efficacy of the workload induction paradigm.

We showed that workload can be classified on the basis of 2 s of neurophysiological signals with an accuracy of 76.1%. This is comparable to previously reported results for such short intervals of data (Grimes et al., 2008; Brouwer et al., 2012). It was shown that the accuracy can be increased using decision-level fusion over the results of several trials (Brouwer et al., 2012) or simply by using longer signal epochs (Grimes et al., 2008), however, with the tradeoff of a less fine-grained, more discrete, and lagging measure of workload. We observed a similar increase of classifier performance to between 94.4% and 96% using a majority vote based on the classifier outcome of the relevant 45 trials of a given block.

While the source of information measured via EEG, neuronal or myographical, might seem of no immediate significance for an application on able-bodied users, it seems relevant to us to ensure that we indeed measure the neural activity implied by pBCI. In this regard, it is noteworthy that the distribution of relevant frequencies vary between subjects. While in general the majority of features (65%) is selected from low frequency bands (delta, theta, alpha), some subjects have a strong contribution of high frequencies (beta, gamma, gamma2) up to 50%. Since these higher frequency bands are notorious for their response to muscle activity in addition to neuronal information (Goncharova et al., 2003), we tested if the workload classification would suffer considerably when excluding them from the feature pool. The average performance did indeed decrease slightly to 74.2%. However, the highly significant above-chance performance over all subjects indicates an only marginal role of muscular activity in workload estimation[3]. This is in line with other studies that suggest a relevance of low frequency bands for workload (Jensen et al., 2002; Jensen and Tesche, 2002) and its estimation (Zarjam et al., 2013). Consequently, we showed that the trained classifier uses the neural correlates of workload to discern two workload levels with a performance equaling that reported in similar studies.

Regarding the classifier generalization to different affective contexts, we show that a classifier created in a non-stressful context can generalize to a stressful context and vice versa. However, the training context has a significant influence on the classification performance, with decreasing performance for cross-context classification (i.e., from 72.4% to 69.4% for frequency-domain features, from 73.3% to 69.1% for time-domain features, and from 77.3% to 73.2% for features from both domains). Interestingly, we found that a training which takes several relevant contexts into account enables the generalization of the classifier to a certain degree. Classifiers based on frequency-domain and on combined frequency- and time-domain features perform comparably well after training with data from both affective context (72.4% and 76.7%, respectively) as after being trained and tested within a specific context. Classifiers based on time-domain features profit as well from a training with data from both affective contexts (72.1%), but still show a declined performance relative to optimal, within-context training and testing.

The current study is limited in its generality by the use of a stress induction paradigm which manipulates affective context only once. We chose the TSST because it is a recognized standard of social stress induction and a powerful elicitor that allows to keep stimuli and task comparable during the workload session of stressful and non-stressful condition. However, since we have only two stress conditions and not several interleaved stress conditions, the stress manipulation is synonymous with a change in time, though with a counter-balanced order. Both affective contexts are separated by at least 10 min and we can not exclude that signal changes with time played a role for classifier performance. The analysis of effects of time within the affective contexts, however, did not reveal general performance decreases due to time passing and thus adds to the evidence of context-related performance loss. Similarly, the spread of training blocks over a larger time in combined compared to single testing contexts limits comparability of both performance measures. To ensure that our results hold for stress in specific, interleaved stress induction methods can be used, though a viable experiment length, reliability of stress induction, and comparability of stimuli and task need to be guaranteed.

Another limitation of the paradigm can result from a potential interaction of (psychosocial) stress and workload. For example, impaired cognitive processes or increased engagement in the face of evaluative pressure, could lead to differences in participant performance between affective contexts (Eysenck and Derakshan, 2011). Despite the lack of such interaction effects in our analysis, the possibility of participant's performance-related differences being reflected in brain activity is a general issue that needs to be considered, since such changes in brain activity would be only indirectly related to stress. Therefore, future research needs to identify the processes that are responsible for the signal variability in the face of psychosocial stress. On a related note, other stressors could be manipulated to identify the source of the performance decrease, for example in terms of impaired cognitive processes.

The result of our study suggests that classification performance for passive BCIs can be increased using not only a larger quantity of training data, but by introducing qualitative variations. Here, we varied the stress level of our participants during the task performance. This manipulation is comparable to the variation of the affective context of a task in real-world scenarios, for example task performance under pressure vs. normal task performance. Consequently, to create more reliable BCIs for

[3]Alternatively, the decrease might be due to the removal of relevant neural information represented in beta or gamma bands.

workload detection, robust against alterations in contextual conditions, such as affective factors (emotions, moods), the training data should include data collected under the relevant contextual conditions.

Zander and Jatzev (2012) found that certain metrics might enable the identification of phases of changed contexts and therefore identify phases were additional calibration might be necessary. One could then use transfer learning (Pan and Yang, 2010) or other re-calibration strategies to enable an adaptation of the transfer algorithm to the new context. However, the suggested metric specifically enables the detection of LOC, which is useful for the detection of perceived LOC and subsequent reliability decrease of active BCIs when environmental and internal factors of the user change. Passive BCIs are not directly related to a feeling of control since they do not enable nor aim at the intentional control of machines. Therefore, for passive BCI one needs other indicators of reliability.

Currently, several groups are investigating the cognitive, affective, and demographic factors that influence active BCI performance (see Lotte et al., 2013). We argue that a similar research program would allow to build more robust passive BCIs by (1) taking into account changes in relevant contextual factors (e.g., stress), (2) by exploring indicators of such changes or the subsequent loss of reliability, and (3) by the exploration of strategies to update the classifier in face of the loss of reliability due to contextual changes.

CONCLUSION

The current work has relevance for the development of passive brain-computer interfaces that are able to specifically classify one psychophysiological construct (e.g., workload), while being invariant to others (e.g., stress). We devised and validated a protocol to test the effect of stress on pBCI approaches. We showed that a classifier has trouble transfering from stressful training data to non-stressful test data and vice versa, indicating an influence of affective task context on the performance of a workload classifier. Moreover, we found that the classification profits from the training on a mix of the varied affective task contexts. Such classifiers perform comparably well to those trained and tested on the same affective context. More generally spoken, the results suggest that the classification performance is not only dependent on quantitative factors, such as the numbers of channels, amount of training data, or length of trials, but also on qualitative factors, such as the affective context. This underlines the need for studies that identify such contextual factors and that elucidate ways to deal with detrimental effects related to their influence. Future research and development of workload classification systems using physiological sensors needs to take the contextual factors into account to increase the generality and ecological validity of the system.

REFERENCES

Ang, K. K., Chin, Z. Y., Wang, C., Guan, C., and Zhang, H. (2012). Filter bank common spatial pattern algorithm on BCI competition IV datasets 2a and 2b. *Front. Neurosci.* 6:39. doi: 10.3389/fnins.2012.00039

Blankertz, B., Lemm, S., Treder, M., Haufe, S., and Müller, K.-R. (2010). Single-trial analysis and classification of ERP components—a tutorial. *Neuroimage* 56, 814–825. doi: 10.1016/j.neuroimage.2010.06.048

Blankertz, B., Tomioka, R., Lemm, S., Kawanabe, M., and Müller, K. R. (2008). Optimizing spatial filters for robust EEG single-trial analysis. *IEEE Signal Process. Mag.* 25, 41–56. doi: 10.1109/MSP.2008.4408441

Boucsein, W. (ed.). (1992). "Electrodermal Indices of Emotion and Stress, chapter 3," in *Electrodermal Activity* (New York, NY: Springer), 369–391.

Bradley, M. M., and Lang, P. J. (1994). Measuring emotion: the self-assessment Manikin and the semantic differential. *J. Behav. Ther. Exp. Psychiatry* 25, 49–59. doi: 10.1016/0005-7916(94)90063-9

Brouwer, A. M., Hogervorst, M. A., van Erp, J. B. F., Heffelaar, T., Zimmerman, P. H., and Oostenveld, R. (2012). Estimating workload using EEG spectral power and ERPs in the n-back task. *J. Neural Eng.* 9:045008. doi: 10.1088/1741-2560/9/4/045008

Buchanan, T. W., Etze, J. A., Adolphs, R., and Tranel, D. (2006). The influence of autonomic arousal and semantic relatedness on memory for emotional words. *Int. J. Psychophysiol.* 61, 23–26. doi: 10.1016/j.ijpsycho.2005.10.022

Crost, N. W., Pauls, C. A., and Wacker, J. (2008). Defensiveness and anxiety predict frontal EEG asymmetry only in specific situational contexts. *Biol. Psychol.* 78, 43–52. doi: 10.1016/j.biopsycho.2007.12.008

Dickerson, S. S., and Kemeny, M. E. (2004). Acute stressors and cortisol responses: a theoretical integration and synthesis of laboratory research. *Psychol. Bull.* 130, 355–391. doi: 10.1037/0033-2909.130.3.355

Duda, R. O., Hart, P. E., and Stork, D. G. (2001). *Pattern Recognition, 2nd Edn.* New York, NY: Wiley-Interscience

Erp, J. B. F., Veltman, H. J., and Grootjen, M. (2010). "Brain-Based indices for user system symbiosis, chapter 12" in *Brain-Computer Interfaces: Applying Our Minds to Human-Computer Interaction*, eds D. S. Tan and A. Nijholt (London: Springer), 201–219.

Eysenck, M. W., and Derakshan, N. (2011). New perspectives in attentional control theory. *Pers. Individ. Differ.* 50, 955–960. doi: 10.1016/j.paid.2010.08.019

Fairclough, S. H., and Roberts, J. S. (2011). Effects of performance feedback on cardiovascular reactivity and frontal EEG asymmetry. *Int. J. Psychophysiol.* 81, 291–298. doi: 10.1016/j.ijpsycho.2011.07.012

Gevins, A., Smith, M., Leong, H., McEvoy, L., Whitfield, S., Du, R., et al. (1998). Monitoring working memory load during computer-based tasks with EEG pattern recognition methods. *Hum. Factors* 40, 79–91. doi: 10.1518/001872098779480578

Goncharova, I., McFarland, D., Vaughan, T., and Wolpaw, J. (2003). EMG contamination of EEG: spectral and topographical characteristics. *Clin. Neurophysiol.* 114, 1580–1593. doi: 10.1016/S1388-2457(03)00093-2

Grimes, D., Tan, D. S., Hudson, S. E., Shenoy, P., and Rao, R. P. (2008). "Feasibility and pragmatics of classifying working memory load with an electroencephalograph," in *Proceedings of CHI 2008* (New York, NY: ACM Press), 835–844.

Hart, S. G., and Staveland, L. (1988). "Development of NASA-TLX (Task Load Index): results of empirical and theoretical research," in *Human Mental Workload* eds P. A. Hancock and N. Meshkati (Amsterdam: Elsevier), 139–183.

Hellhammer, J., and Schubert, M. (2012). The physiological response to trier social stress test relates to subjective measures of stress during but not before or after the test. *Psychoneuroendocrinology* 37, 119–124. doi: 10.1016/j.psyneuen.2011.05.012

Hewig, J., Schlotz, W., Gerhard, F., Breitenstein, C., Luerken, A., and Naumann, E. (2008). Associations of the cortisol awakening response (CAR) with cortical activation asymmetry during the course of an exam stress period. *Psychoneuroendocrinology* 33, 83–89. doi: 10.1016/j.psyneuen.2007.10.004

Hoffmann, U., Vesin, J., and Ebrahimi, T. (2006). "Spatial filters for the classification of event-related potentials," in *European Symposium on Artificial Neural Networks (ESANN 2006)* (Bruges).

Jensen, O., Gelfand, J., Kounios, J., and Lisman, J. E. (2002). Oscillations in the alpha band (9-12 Hz) increase with memory load during retention in a short-term memory task. *Cereb. Cortex* 12, 877–882. doi: 10.1093/cercor/12.8.877

Jensen, O., and Tesche, C. D. (2002). Frontal theta activity in humans increases with memory load in a working memory task. *Eur. J. Neurosci.* 15, 1395–1399. doi: 10.1046/j.1460-9568.2002.01975.x

Jeunet, C., Lotte, F., and Mühl, C. (2014). "Design and validation of a mental and social stress induction protocol towards load-invariant physiology-based stress detection," in *International Conference on Physiological Computing Systems* (Lisbon).

Julian, L. J. (2011). Measures of anxiety: state-trait anxiety inventory (STAI), beck anxiety inventory (BAI), and hospital anxiety and depression scale-anxiety (HADS-A). *Arthritis Care Res.* 63, S467–S472. doi: 10.1002/acr.20561

Kirchner, W. K. (1958). Age differences in short-term retention of rapidly changing information. *J. Exp. Psychol.* 55, 352–358. doi: 10.1037/h0043688

Kirschbaum, C., Pirke, K.-M., and Hellhammer, D. H. (1993). The "Trier Social Stress Test": a tool for investigating psychobiological stress responses in a laboratory setting. *Neuropsychobiology* 28, 76–81. doi: 10.1159/000119004

Krout, R. E. (2007). Music listening to facilitate relaxation and promote wellness: integrated aspects of our neurophysiological response to music. *Arts Psychother.* 34, 134–141. doi: 10.1016/j.aip.2006.11.001

Krusienski, D. J., Grosse-Wentrup, M., Galán, F., Coyle, D., Miller, K. J., Forney, E., et al. (2011). Critical issues in state-of-the-art brain–computer interface signal processing. *J. Neural Eng.* 8:25002. doi: 10.1088/1741-2560/8/2/025002

Lewis, R. S., Weekes, N. Y., and Wang, T. H. (2007). The effect of a naturalistic stressor on frontal EEG asymmetry, stress, and health. *Biol. Psychol.* 75, 224–239. doi: 10.1016/j.biopsycho.2007.03.004

Loggia, M. L., Juneau, M., and Bushnell, M. C. (2011). Autonomic responses to heat pain: heart rate, skin conductance, and their relation to verbal ratings and stimulus intensity. *Pain* 152, 592–598. doi: 10.1016/j.pain.2010.11.032

Lotte, F., Congedo, M., Lecuyer, A., Lamarche, F., and Arnaldi, B. (2007). A Review of classification algorithms for EEG-based brain-computer interfaces. *J. Neural Eng.* 4, R1–R13. doi: 10.1088/1741-2560/4/2/R01

Lotte, F., and Guan, C. (2010). "Learning from other subjects helps reducing brain-computer interface calibration time," in *International Conference on Audio, Speech and Signal Processing (ICASSP'2010)* (Dallas), 614–617. doi: 10.1109/ICASSP.2010.5495183

Lotte, F., Guan, C., and Ang, K. (2009). "Comparison of designs towards a subject-independent brain-computer interface based on motor imagery," in *International Conference of the IEEE Engineering in Medicine and Biology Society (EMBC) 2009* (Minneapolis), 4543–4546. doi: 10.1109/IEMBS.2009.5334126

Lotte, F., Larrue, F., and Mühl, C. (2013). Flaws in current human training protocols for spontaneous brain-computer interfaces: lessons learned from instructional design. *Front. Hum. Neurosci.* 7:568. doi: 10.3389/fnhum.2013.00568

Mathan, S., Feyereisen, T., and Whitlow, S. (2007). "WorkSense: exploring the feasibility of human factors assessment using electrophysiological sensors," in *Proceedings of ICACS* (Santa Monica).

Müller-Putz, G. R., Scherer, R., Brunner, C., Leeb, R., and Pfurtscheller, G. (2008). Better than random? A closer look on BCI results. *Int. J. Bioelectromagn.* 10, 52–55.

Pan, S. J., and Yang, Q. (2010). A survey on transfer learning. *IEEE Trans. Knowl. Data Eng.* 22, 1345–1359. doi: 10.1109/TKDE.2009.191

Peck, E. M. M., Yuksel, B. F., Ottley, A., Jacob, R. J., and Chang, R. (2013). "Using fNIRS brain sensing to evaluate information visualization interfaces," in *Proceedings of CHI 2013* (New York, NY: ACM Press), 473–482.

Peng, H., Long, F., and Ding, C. (2005). Feature selection based on mutual information: criteria of max-dependency, max-relevance, and min-redundancy. *IEEE Trans. Pattern Anal. Mach. Intell.* 27, 1226–1238. doi: 10.1109/TPAMI.2005.159

Reinhardt, T., Schmahl, C., Wüst, S., and Bohus, M. (2012). Salivary cortisol, heart rate, electrodermal activity and subjective stress responses to the Mannheim Multicomponent Stress Test (MMST). *Psychiatry Res.* 198, 106–111. doi: 10.1016/j.psychres.2011.12.009

Renard, Y., Lotte, F., Gibert, G., Congedo, M., Maby, E., Delannoy, V., et al. (2010). OpenViBE: an open-source software platform to design, test, and use brain-computer interfaces in real and virtual environments. *Presence Teleop. Virt.* 19, 35–53. doi: 10.1162/pres.19.1.35

Reuderink, B., Mühl, C., and Poel, M. (2013). Valence, arousal and dominance in the EEG during game play. *Int. J. Auton. Adapt. Commun. Syst.* 6:45. doi: 10.1504/IJAACS.2013.050691

Reuderink, B., Poel, M., and Nijholt, A. (2011). The impact of loss of control on movement BCIs. *IEEE Trans. Neural Syst. Rehab. Eng.* 19, 628–637. doi: 10.1109/TNSRE.2011.2166562

Roy, R., Bonnet, S., Charbonnier, S., and Campagne, A. (2012). "Time-on-task effect on workload level discriminability through electroencephalography," in *Proceedings of BIOMAG 2012* (Paris).

Schlögl, A., Keinrath, C., Zimmermann, D., Scherer, R., Leeb, R., and Pfurtscheller, G. (2007). A fully automated correction method of eog artifacts in eeg recordings. *Clin. Neurophysiol.* 118, 98–104. doi: 10.1016/j.clinph.2006.09.003

Selye, H. (1936). A syndrome produced by diverse nocuous agents. *Nature* 138:32. doi: 10.1038/138032a0

Sinha, R., Talih, M., Malison, R., Cooney, N., Anderson, G.-M., and Kreek, M.-J. (2003). Hypothalamic-pituitary-adrenal axis and sympatho-adreno-medullary responses during stress-induced and drug cue-induced cocaine craving states. *Psychopharmacology* 170, 62–72. doi: 10.1007/s00213-003-1525-8

Solovey, E., Schermerhorn, P., Scheutz, M., Sassaroli, A., Fantini, S., and Jacob, R. (2012). "Brainput: enhancing interactive systems with streaming fnirs brain input," in *Proceedings of CHI 2012* (Austin, TX), 2193–2202.

Spielberger, C. D., Gorsuch, R. L., and Lushene, R. E. (1970). *Manual for the State-Trait Anxiety Inventory.* Palo Alto, CA: Consulting Psychologists Press.

Tangermann, M., Müller, K. R., Aertsen, A., Birbaumer, N., Braun, C., Brunner, C., et al. (2012). Review of the BCI competition IV. *Front. Neurosci.* 6:55. doi: 10.3389/fnins.2012.00055

Taniguchi, K., Nishikawa, A., Sugino, T., Aoyagi, S., Sekimoto, M., Takiguchi, S., et al. (2009). *Method for Objectively Evaluating Psychological Stress Resulting When Humans Interact with Robots.* China: InTech.

Tops, M., van Peer, J. M., Wester, A. E., Wijers, A. A., and Korf, J. (2006). State-dependent regulation of cortical activity by cortisol: an EEG study. *Neurosci. Lett.* 404, 34–39. doi: 10.1016/j.neulet.2006.05.038

van Erp, J., Lotte, F., and Tangermann, M. (2012). Brain-computer interfaces: beyond medical applications. *IEEE Comput.* 45, 26–34. doi: 10.1109/MC.2012.107

Verwey, W. B., and Veltman, H. A. (1984). Detecting short periods of elevated workload : a comparison of nine workload assessment techniques. *J. Exp. Psychol. Appl.* 2, 270–285. doi: 10.1037/1076-898X.2.3.270

Walter, C., Rosenstiel, S. S., W., Gerjets, P., and Bogdan, M. (2013). "Using cross-task classification for classifying workload levels in complex learning tasks," in *Proceedings of ACII 2013* (Geneva), 876–881.

Zander, T., and Jatzev, S. (2012). Context-aware brain–computer interfaces: exploring the information space of user, technical system and environment. *J. Neural Eng.* 9:016003. doi: 10.1088/1741-2560/9/1/016003

Zander, T. O., and Kothe, C. (2011). Towards passive brain-computer interfaces: applying brain-computer interface technology to human-machine systems in general. *J. Neural Eng.* 8:025005. doi: 10.1088/1741-2560/8/2/025005

Zarjam, P., Epps, J., Chen, F., and Lovell, N. H. (2013). Estimating cognitive workload using wavelet entropy-based features during an arithmetic task. *Comput. Biol. Med.* 43, 2186–2195. doi: 10.1016/j.compbiomed.2013.08.021

Zijlstra, F. R. H. (1993). "*Efficiency in Work Behaviour: A Design Approach for Modern Tools*," Ph.D. thesis, Delft University of Technology.

10

Fusion of electroencephalographic dynamics and musical contents for estimating emotional responses in music listening

Yuan-Pin Lin[1,2]*, Yi-Hsuan Yang[3] and Tzyy-Ping Jung[1,2]

[1] Swartz Center for Computational Neuroscience, Institute for Neural Computation, University of California, San Diego, La Jolla, CA, USA
[2] Center for Advanced Neurological Engineering, Institute of Engineering in Medicine, University of California, San Diego, La Jolla, CA, USA
[3] Music and Audio Computing Lab, Research Center for IT Innovation, Academia Sinica, Taipei, Taiwan

Correspondence:
Yuan-Pin Lin, Swartz Center for Computational Neuroscience, Institute for Neural Computation, University of California, San Diego, 9500 Gilman Drive, Mail code 0559, La Jolla, CA 92093-0559, USA
e-mail: yplin@sccn.ucsd.edu

Electroencephalography (EEG)-based emotion classification during music listening has gained increasing attention nowadays due to its promise of potential applications such as musical affective brain-computer interface (ABCI), neuromarketing, music therapy, and implicit multimedia tagging and triggering. However, music is an ecologically valid and complex stimulus that conveys certain emotions to listeners through compositions of musical elements. Using solely EEG signals to distinguish emotions remained challenging. This study aimed to assess the applicability of a multimodal approach by leveraging the EEG dynamics and acoustic characteristics of musical contents for the classification of emotional valence and arousal. To this end, this study adopted machine-learning methods to systematically elucidate the roles of the EEG and music modalities in the emotion modeling. The empirical results suggested that when whole-head EEG signals were available, the inclusion of musical contents did not improve the classification performance. The obtained performance of 74~76% using solely EEG modality was statistically comparable to that using the multimodality approach. However, if EEG dynamics were only available from a small set of electrodes (likely the case in real-life applications), the music modality would play a complementary role and augment the EEG results from around 61–67% in valence classification and from around 58–67% in arousal classification. The musical timber appeared to replace less-discriminative EEG features and led to improvements in both valence and arousal classification, whereas musical loudness was contributed specifically to the arousal classification. The present study not only provided principles for constructing an EEG-based multimodal approach, but also revealed the fundamental insights into the interplay of the brain activity and musical contents in emotion modeling.

Keywords: EEG, emotion classification, affective brain-computer interface, music signal processing, music listening

INTRODUCTION

Through monitoring ongoing electrical brain activity, electroencephalography (EEG)-based brain-computer interfaces (BCIs) allow users to voluntarily translate their intentions into commands to communicate with or control external devices and environments, instead of using conventional communication channels, e.g., speech and muscles (Millan et al., 2010). Several types of EEG signatures are theoretically defined and empirically proved to be robust in actively and reactively actuating BCIs (Zander and Kothe, 2011), such as evoked potentials, event-related potential (ERP), and sensorimotor rhythms (Wolpaw et al., 2002). Nowadays, a new categorization called passive BCI was introduced (Zander and Kothe, 2011). It enables users to involuntarily interact with machines by means of implicit user states, e.g., emotion. Researches are attempting to augment BCI's ability with emotional awareness and intelligence in response to users' emotional states, so called affective brain-computer interfaces (ABCIs).

Emotion is a psycho-physiological process as well as a natural communication channel of human beings. Music is considered as an extraordinary mediator to evoke emotions and concurrently modulate underlying neurophysiological processes (Blood et al., 1999). Upon profound findings in musical emotions, using machine-learning methods to characterize spatio-spectral EEG dynamics associated with emotions has gained increasing attentions in the last decade, namely EEG-based emotion classification, due to its promise of potential applications such as musical ABCI (Makeig et al., 2011), neuromarketing (Lee et al., 2007), music therapy (Thaut et al., 2009), implicit multimedia tagging (Soleymani et al., 2012a; Koelstra and Patras, 2013) and triggering (Wu et al., 2008). Given diverse EEG patterns, the major efforts in the previous EEG-based emotion classification works (not limited to music stimuli) were to seek an optimal emotion-aware model by leveraging feature extraction, selection and classification methods (Ishino and Hagiwara, 2003; Takahashi, 2004; Chanel et al., 2009; Frantzidis et al., 2010; Lin et al., 2010b; Petrantonakis and Hadjileontiadis, 2010; Koelstra et al., 2012; Soleymani et al., 2012b). Despite many approaches and advances in EEG analysis in the past decade, how to precisely categorize EEG signals into distinct emotional states remains challenging.

Music is an ecologically valid and complex stimulus that conveys emotions to listeners through compositions of musical elements, such as mode, tempo and timber (Peretz et al., 1998; Schmithorst, 2005; Gomez and Danuser, 2007; Zatorre et al., 2007). Listeners would be able to more and less perceive and recognize the same emotions as the music expresses (Schmidt and Trainor, 2001; Juslin and Laukka, 2003). Analogous to the EEG domain, researchers in music signal processing field devoted to map acoustic characteristics of musical contents into emotion semantics labeled by human annotators, namely music emotion recognition (Yang and Chen, 2011, 2012). Most of previous works employed publicly available toolboxes, such as MIRToolbox (Lartillot and Toiviainen, 2007), Marsyas (Tzanetakis and Cook, 2002), and PsySound (Cabrera, 1999), to extract a wide variety of musical features and then used machine-learning algorithms to automatically learn the associations between extracted features and emotions expressed in music (Yang et al., 2008a; Aljanaki et al., 2013). The aforementioned evidence raises a natural question whether or not the acoustic characteristics of musical contents can further improve the EEG classification results.

Using EEG features in conjunction with other information sources recently shed light on this issue, for example peripheral biosignals (Chanel et al., 2009; Koelstra et al., 2012; Soleymani et al., 2012a), eye gaze (Soleymani et al., 2012a,b), musical structures (Koelstra et al., 2012), and facial expression (Koelstra and Patras, 2013) have been proposed. Particularly for the music study, Koelstra et al. (2012) reported that a multimodal approach, fusing decision outputs from EEG and music classifiers, marginally improved the classification performance over using solely EEG modality. It remained unclear whether or not the acoustic characteristics of musical contents effectively contribute to the emotion modeling.

This study attempted to examine the roles of EEG and music modalities in the multidiscipline emotion classification problem in music listening upon two posed hypotheses. The first hypothesis was that the EEG modality reflecting spatio-spectral brain activities of the whole brain about implicit emotion responses should dominate the multimodal approach for emotion classification, as compared to the music modality, in which the implicit emotions concerned the responses automatically induced by the stimulus itself (Gyurak et al., 2011). This study adopted machine-learning methods, i.e., feature extraction, selection, and classification, to systematically assess a composite feature space synchronizing EEG dynamics and musical characteristics in accordance to time scale. The relative contributions from EEG and music modalities then can be explored. Furthermore, one can imagine that the use of a high-density EEG montage over the whole head might be more difficult or impractical for real-life ABCI applications. The applicability of whole-head EEG dynamics (in the first hypothesis) might no longer hold if only few electrodes are available over a certain region or regions (Lin et al., 2010b). Thus, this study posed another hypothesis that the musical contents might complement less informative EEG dynamics for emotion classification and consequently improve over the EEG modality result. This study explored the minimal set of informative electrodes from multiple subjects for emotion classification. Such few electrodes mostly populated over the fronto-central regions were used to simulate the absence of whole-brain EEG dynamics. Exploring the validity of these two hypotheses might elucidate potential advantages and limitations in fusing EEG dynamics and musical contents for the emotion classification problem.

MATERIALS AND METHODS

EEG DATASET AND MUSIC EXCERPTS

This study adopted the Oscar movie soundtrack dataset (Lin et al., 2010b) to test the feasibility of using a multimodal approach for emotion classification. The EEG signals were collected from 26 healthy subjects who were undergraduate and graduate students (16 males, 10 females; age 24.40 ± 2.53) mostly from engineering-related colleges. The experiment protocol and EEG recording were approved by the Human Research Protections Program of National Taiwan University. The music-listening experiment targeted four emotion classes (joy, anger, sadness, and pleasure) in accordance to the two-dimensional circumplex emotion model composed of valence (positive-negative) and arousal (high-low) axes (Russell, 1980). Sixteen music excerpts from the soundtracks of Oscar winning movies were used to induce the targeted emotions. Each subject underwent a 4-block music experiment; each block contained four counterbalanced 30-s music trials corresponding to four targeted emotions. After music listening, the subjects labeled their felt emotions on a discrete scale, for example, joy (positive valence and high arousal), anger (negative valence and high arousal), sadness (negative valence and low arousal), and pleasure (positive valence and low arousal). In the experiment, a 32-channel Neuroscan EEG module placed according to the International 10–20 system (**Figure 1**) and referenced to the linked mastoids (algebraic average of left and right) was adopted to acquire EEG signals with a sampling rate of 500 Hz and a bandpass filter at 1–100 Hz. Subjects were asked to keep their eyes closed, remain seated, and minimize head/body movements. After the music experiment, each subject's data was consisted of 16 30-s EEG segments labeled by self-reported emotional states (joy, anger, sadness, or pleasure).

Referring to the recent works (Koelstra et al., 2012; Soleymani et al., 2012a,b; Koelstra and Patras, 2013), most of EEG-based classification tasks addressed and performed on the basis of emotional valence and arousal, e.g., categorizing EEG signals into positive or negative valence, instead of discrete emotion states. To make a direct comparison with the latest reports, this study addressed the binary emotion classification problem. The self-reported emotion labels of the Oscar movie soundtrack dataset were separately merged into the binary categories of valence and arousal. The valence scale comprised positive (joy and pleasure) and negative (anger and sadness) levels, whereas arousal scale contained high (joy and anger) and low (pleasure and sadness) levels. There were 16 pairs of 30-s EEG signals and music excerpts for each of 26 subjects available for analysis and comparison.

EEG FEATURE EXTRACTION

Previous neurophysiological studies documented EEG spectral changes either in distinct regions or between hemispheres (Davidson, 1992; Schmidt and Trainor, 2001; Aftanas et al., 2004; Sarlo et al., 2005; Sammler et al., 2007). Such evidence might in part facilitated the use of spectral dynamics within/between channels for the EEG-based emotion classification, e.g., spectra in individual channels and spectral asymmetry in left-right channel pairs (Lin et al., 2010b; Koelstra et al., 2012; Soleymani et al., 2012a; Koelstra and Patras, 2013). In the literature, the patterns of spectral differences along anterior and posterior brain regions have also been explored (Schmidt and Trainor, 2001; Sarlo et al., 2005). However, no study has attempted to address the feasibility of using spectral differences in fronto-posterior channel pairs in this domain. Prior to construct a multimodality approach, this study aimed to explore an optimal EEG features from different types, including the power spectral density in individual channels and the power spectral asymmetry in the left-right and fronto-posterior channels pairs.

For each of 16 30-s EEG trials, the short-time Fourier transform with non-overlapping 1-s Hamming window was applied to extract the power spectral density in five frequency bands, including delta (δ: 1–3 Hz), theta (θ: 4–7 Hz), alpha (α: 8–13 Hz), beta (β: 14–30 Hz), and gamma (γ: 31–50 Hz) over 30 channels (two reference channels were excluded). The band-specific power spectra of the individual channels formed a feature dimension of 150 (5 bands × 30 channels) and was labeled as PSD hereafter. To characterize the spectral-band asymmetry in respect of laterality (in left-right direction) and caudality (in fronto-posterior direction), this study defined two feature types namely DLAT and DCAU to separately extract the differential spectral asymmetry of 12 left-right and 12 fronto-posterior channel pairs from 30 individual channels, both forming a feature dimension of 60 (5 bands × 12 channel pairs). Furthermore, this study also named a feature type MESH by merging PSD, DLAT and DCAU, a dimension of 270, for comparison. **Table 1** summarizes the aforementioned four EEG feature types. It is noted that the feature vectors of each type were separately normalized to the range from 0 to 1.

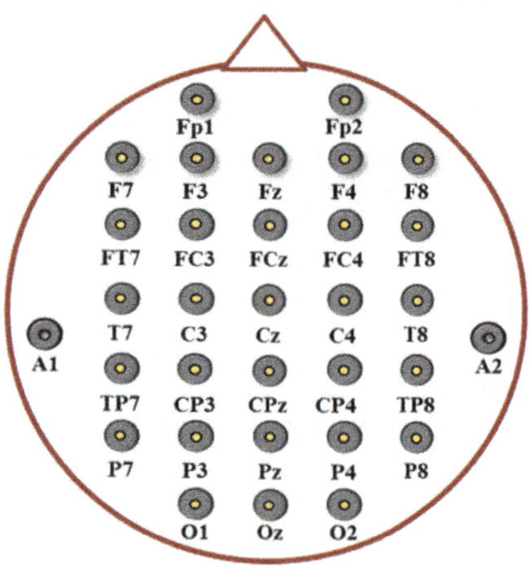

FIGURE 1 | Electrode placements of 32 channels according to the international 10–20 system.

MUSIC FEATURE EXTRACTION

Emotion expression in music is usually associated with different acoustic characteristics (Juslin, 2000; Gabrielsson and Lindström, 2010). This study employed commonly used music information retrieval toolboxes, i.e., MIRtoolbox (Lartillot and Toiviainen, 2007) and PsySound (Cabrera, 1999), to extract the acoustic features that represent various perceptual dimensions of music listening, including pitch, dissonance, loudness, and timber. The data samples of the musical features were aligned to the EEG features with one sample per second. The music feature types are summarized in **Table 2** and depicted as followings.

Pitch is the auditory attribute of sounds which can be ordered on a scale from low to high. The harmonic aspect of music can be described in terms of the relationship between two or more simultaneous pitches, whereas the melodic aspect is related to the temporal succession of pitches (Muller et al., 2011). This study used the MIRtoolbox to extract three major elements describing the pitch properties in music, including the key clarity, mode, and harmonic flux. The key clarity refers to the similarity (or key strength) that best describes one of the 24 musical keys, e.g., C major. Next, the musical mode represents the difference between the best major

Table 1 | A summary of EEG feature types.

Type	# Electrodes	# Features	Extracted features
DLAT	24	60	Five differential spectral band power (δ, θ, α, β, and γ) for 12 left-right electrode pairs: Fp1-Fp2, F7-F8, F3-F4, FT7-FT8, FC3-FC4, T7-T8, P7-P8, C3-C4, TP7-TP8, CP3-CP4, P3-P4, and O1-O2.
DCAU	24	60	Five differential spectral band power (δ, θ, α, β, and γ) for 12 fronto-posterior electrode pairs: Fp1-O1, Fp2-O2, F7-P7, F3-P3, Fz-Pz, F4-P4, F8-P8, FT7-TP7, FC3-CP3, FCz-CPz, FC4-CP4, and FT8-TP8.
PSD	30	150	Five spectral band power (δ, θ, α, β, and γ) for 30 electrodes: Fp1, Fp2, F7, F3, Fz, F4, F8, FT7, FC3, FCz, FC4, FT8, T7, C3, Cz, C4, T8, TP7, CP3, CPz, CP4, TP8, P7, P3, Pz, P4, P8, O1, Oz, and O2.
MESH	30	270	A combination of DLAT, DCAU, and PSD.

Table 2 | A summary of music feature types.

Type	# Features	Extracted features
Pitch	3	Key clarity, Mode, Harmonic flux
Dissonance	4	Tonal dissonance (HK,S), Spectral dissonance (HK, S)
Loudness	5	Loudness, Sharpness (Z, A), Timbral width, Volume
MFCC	13	MFCC coefficients (13 features)
MUSIC	25	A combination of Pitch, Dissonance, Loudness, and MFCC

key and the best minor key in key strength, which is often related to the sensation of valence in music (Gabrielsson and Lindström, 2010). The harmonic flux indicates a large difference in harmonic content between consecutive frames, such as chord changes, strong melody or bass line movement. This feature may be relevant as some psychology studies have found that large melodic intervals are perceived as more powerful (i.e., high-arousal) than small ones (Gabrielsson and Lindström, 2010).

Dissonance measures the harshness or roughness of the acoustic spectrum (Cabrera, 1999). The dissonance generally implies a combination of notes that sound harsh or unpleasant to people when played at the same time. Empirically, many musical pieces involve a balanced combination of consonance and dissonance sounds, e.g., the release of harmonic tension might create pleasure (Parncutt and Hair, 2011). Four elements describing the dissonance were calculated by the PsySound, including tonal dissonance (HK and S) and spectral dissonance (HK, S). The tonal and spectral dissonance measures the dissonance among tonal components and models the degree deviating from the noisiness of the sound, respectively. Note that HK and S are two methods forming the results in different scales.

Loudness is the perceptual intensity of sounds and depends primarily on the physical intensity as well as frequency and duration. This study employed the PsySound to derive five features depicting the human sensation of sound loudness across frequency, including loudness, sharpness (Z, A), timbral width, and volume. The loudness is an integral of the spectral distribution of loudness sensation. In general, loud music tends to be associated with high arousal and potency, whereas soft music relates to low arousal. Next, sharpness Z and A are two models distinctly characterizing the sharpness of the sound sensation in a scale from dull to sharp (Cabrera, 1999). The former model emphasizes high frequencies, whereas the later one is sensitive to the positive influence of loudness toward sharpness. The timbral width is defined as the flatness, i.e., width of the peak, of the loudness' spectral distribution, whereas the volume is derived based on the relative strength between total loudness and sharpness (Cabrera, 1999). The relationship between these two features and emotion processing is relatively less understood.

Timber that reflects the acoustic spectro-temporal characteristics is often considered as the quality of sound that makes a particular musical sound different from another. To model the timber, this study employed the MIRToolbox and computed the Mel-frequency cepstral coefficients (MFCC). MFCC characterizes the spectral shape of the sound by taking the coefficients of the discrete cosine transform of log-power spectra expressed on a non-linear perceptual-related Mel-frequency scale (Davis and Mermelstein, 1980). Typically, only the 10–20 lowest coefficients were retained for analysis (Muller et al., 2011). Referring to (Koelstra et al., 2012), this study only adopted the first 13 coefficients. The timber type was named as MFCC hereafter.

FUSION OF EEG AND MUSICAL FEATURES

Through using multidisciplinary signals, a multimodal approach can usually boost single modality results. Decision-level and feature-level fusions are two commonly used schemes to obtain the integration of multiple signal sources (Kittler et al., 1998; Sargin et al., 2007). The feature-level fusion works by concatenating features of different modalities and then feeding the composite feature vector to a classifier, whereas the decision-level fusion allows single modalities to process independently and then derive a final decision from multiple outputs. It is worth noting that since this study attempted to evaluate the relative contributions of EEG and music modalities, the feature-level fusion that synchronizes the features of different modalities along time more likely conforms to the objective. After applying a feature selection processing (described at the next section), this study defined a term, namely percent composition, to reveal the percentages of contributions of EEG and musical features to a multimodal feature composition. Prior to classification, each of the addressed EEG and musical features was independently normalized between 0 and 1, making features equally weighted to a classifier.

FEATURE SELECTION

Feature selection plays a chief role in solving classification problem. Given a plenty of raw features, the selection procedure is capable of extracting only a subset of task-relevant features while removing redundant/irrelevant ones. Feature reduction not only leads to computational efficiency, but also reduces the number of electrodes required in real-life applications (Lin et al., 2010b). This study employed an F-score index, a ratio of between- and within-class variations (Chen and Lin, 2006), to pinpoint the most emotion-relevant features/electrodes, which has been proven effective for the EEG-based emotion classification problem (Lin et al., 2010b). The F-score index of the ith feature is defined as following:

$$F(i) = \frac{\sum_{l=1}^{g} (\bar{x}_{l,i} - \bar{x}_i)^2}{\frac{1}{n_l}\sum_{l=1}^{g}\sum_{k=1}^{n_l} (\bar{x}_{k,l,i} - \bar{x}_{l,i})^2}$$

where $\bar{x}_i$ and $\bar{x}_{l,i}$ are the mean values of the ith feature for entire dataset and for class l ($l = 1 \sim g$, $g = 2$ for positive and negative classes in valence or high and low classes in arousal), respectively; $\bar{x}_{k,l,i}$ is the kth sample value of the ith feature for class l, and n_l is the number of samples in class l. The larger F-score value indicates higher discrimination power. It assumed that the features with highest F-score values account for the most emotion-tagged information and contribute more to emotion classification.

To test the first hypothesis, the F-score based feature selection was applied to each subject's EEG dataset separately to generate a subject-dependent EEG feature set. To test the second hypothesis, this study simulated the consequences of unavailability of whole-head EEG data. This study applied the F-score feature selection to explore the commonality of the informative EEG features from 26 subjects, i.e., subject-independent set. More specifically, an objective index, namely the level of feature independency (LFI), was defined as the number of subjects having the same informative features. After sorting and accumulating the F-score-sorted subject-dependent EEG features, the LFI-guided subject-independent EEG feature sets were then explored. The LFI value was empirically set and tested from 0.1 up to 0.6. Note that no informative features were commonly observed over 18 subjects (LFI = 0.7). The subject-independent EEG feature set with LFI = 0.6 was supposed to return a minimal set of electrodes to test the second hypothesis. It is also important to explore the common EEG patterns across subjects in emotion processing.

FEATURE CLASSIFICATION AND VALIDATION

Support vector machine (SVM) is a popular machine-learning algorithm that projects input data onto a higher dimensional feature space via a transfer kernel function, in which classification can be made more easily than in the original feature space. The iterative learning processing of an SVM eventually converges into optimal hyperplanes giving maximal margins between classes. This study used LIBSVM software (Chang and Lin, 2011) to build the SVM classifier and employed a radial basis function (RBF) kernel to non-linearly map the original data onto a higher dimensional space.

Regarding the classification validation, this study adopted a leave-trial-out (LTO) validation method to each individual's dataset to obtain the emotion classification results. The LTO validation provides a generalized performance by averaging classification results N times with each of N trials to be tested ($N = 16$ in this study). In each repetition, the SVM model was trained with 15 trials and then tested against the remaining trial. It is noted that prior to the LTO validation a grid-search procedure (Chang and Lin, 2011) was applied to the entire dataset to decide an optimal parameter pair (γ, C) for the size of the RBF kernel and the penalty of decision boundary from various pairs (γ: $2^{-1} \sim 2^3$, C: $2^{-4} \sim 2^1$), which corresponded to the best SVM training accuracy. The classification accuracy was defined by the ratio of correctly classified number of samples and the total number of samples. The averaged classification performance was obtained by averaging the classification results across 26 subjects. This study employed a paired t-test to access the statistical significance in classification performance between different feature types or modalities. As a baseline, the majority-voting accuracy defined by the majority class of the training data was also provided, i.e., random guessing. For example, given a training set consisted of positive (63%) and negative (37%) samples in the valence classification, the majority accuracy was 63% for assigning a new sample as positive valence. The significant difference of the obtained classification accuracy versus majority voting was tested using a one-sample t-test.

RESULTS

TESTING THE FIRST HYPOTHESIS: EEG DYNAMICS DOMINATED A MULTIMODAL APPROACH IN EMOTION CLASSIFICATION COMPARED TO MUSICAL CONTENTS

Figure 2 summarizes the valence and arousal classification results of the subject-dependent EEG feature types (DLAT, DCAU, PSD, and MESH). It is noted that the condition "without feature selection" shows the results using all the features, while the condition "with feature selection" shows the maximum accuracy through the add-one-feature-in procedure and the number of the features eventually used. In general, using different EEG feature types without the feature selection tended to have comparable results that were notably worse than majority voting. Using only informative features (with high F-score values), the classification accuracies for all the feature types were markedly improved ($p < 0.01$) upon the results without using feature selection, and were significantly better than the majority voting ($p < 0.01$). The MESH generated maximum accuracies of 76.08 ± 6.39% and 74.27 ± 4.82% for valence and arousal classification, respectively, which significantly outperformed other feature types ($p < 0.01$). The feature selection also considerably reduced the feature dimensionality from 270 to below 30. This was very likely attributed to the fact that the F-score feature selection effectively pruned the less informative features from the whole feature space, largely alleviating the interference caused by redundant/irrelevant features. Thus, the MESH was used to merge with musical contents to form a multimodal approach in the following sections.

Figure 3 summarizes the classification results using the subject-dependent EEG features (i.e., MESH), musical features (i.e., MUSIC), and subject-dependent multimodal approach. Note that the multimodal features were obtained by applying the F-score feature selection to the composite features of the MESH and MUSIC features. The multimodal approach obtained the maximum accuracies of 76.97 ± 6.18% and 76.25 ± 4.88% for valence and arousal classification, respectively. The results using musical features alone were around 65% and only significantly outperformed the majority voting for arousal classification but not for valence classification, which were all significantly worse than EEG and multimodality approaches ($p < 0.01$). The subject-dependent EEG features did not notably benefit from the inclusion of musical features. The classification performance using the multimodal features compared favorably ($p > 0.1$) to those using the EEG features.

Figure 4 further shows the percent composition of contributions of EEG and musical features to the subject-dependent multimodal approach. The composition was derived based on how many informative features led to the maximum classification accuracy. This result indicated that the EEG feature types, especially DLAT and DCAU, dominated the composition of multimodal features for valence and arousal classifications, while the musical features barely contributed. This might explain the marginal improvement using the multimodal approach versus the EEG-only modality.

In sum, the feature type MESH, consisted of the two-directional power asymmetry and individual power spectra across the whole scalp and frequency bands, better characterizing the

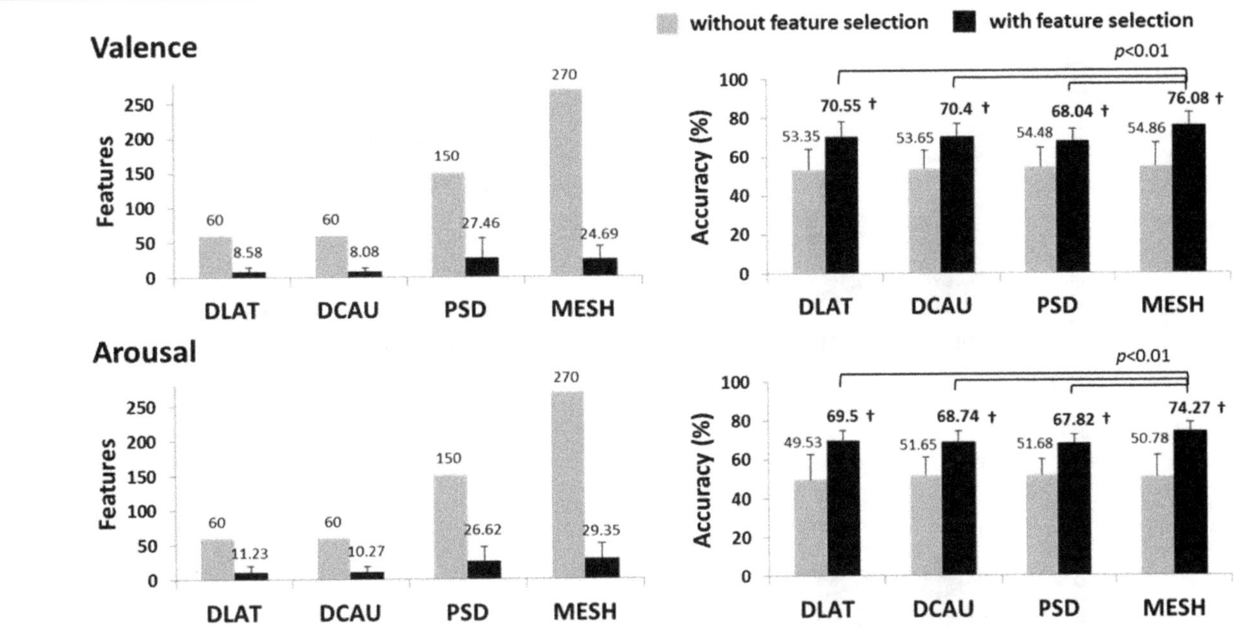

FIGURE 2 | The valence and arousal classification results using the subject-dependent EEG feature sets with/without the F-score based feature selection. The numbers above the bars represent the mean values of the results, whereas the numbers in bold indicate the accuracies significantly better ($p < 0.01$) than the majority voting accuracy (valence: ~63%, arousal: ~61%). †Indicates that the accuracy with feature selection significantly outperformed that without feature selection ($p < 0.01$).

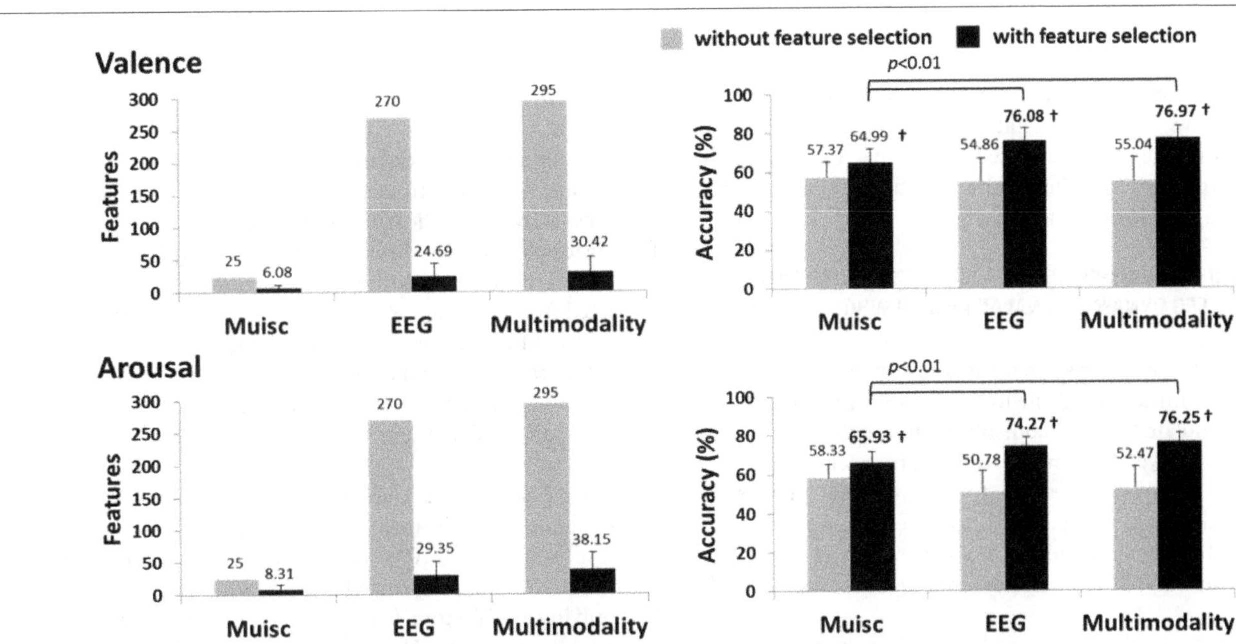

FIGURE 3 | The valence and arousal classification results using the subject-dependent multimodal approach with/without feature selection. The results of the subject-dependent EEG modality (feature type: MESH) and the music modality (feature type: MUSIC) are also provided for comparison. The numbers above the bars represent the mean values of the results, whereas the numbers in bold indicate the accuracies significantly better ($p < 0.01$) than the majority voting accuracy (valence: ~63%, arousal: ~61%). †Indicates that the accuracy with feature selection significantly outperformed that without feature selection ($p < 0.01$).

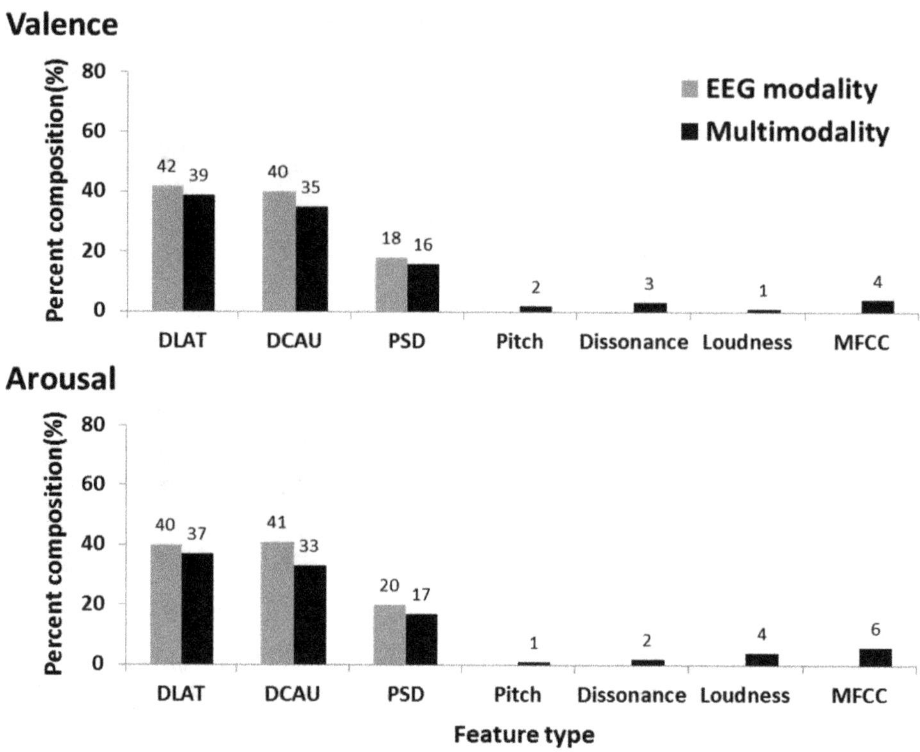

FIGURE 4 | The percent composition of contributions of EEG (DLAT, DCAU, and PSD) and musical (Pitch, Dissonance, Loudness, and MFCC) features to the subject-dependent multimodality. The composition of the subject-dependent EEG modality is also provided for comparison.

EEG dynamics about emotional responses than the musical features. The above empirical results proved the first hypothesis that the EEG modality that accessed spatio-spectral brain activity of the whole brain dominated the classification of emotional responses in the multimodal approach.

TESTING THE SECOND HYPOTHESIS: MUSICAL CONTENTS CAN COMPLEMENT EEG DYNAMICS UNAVAILABLE IN WHOLE-HEAD EEG RECORDINGS

To test the second hypothesis that musical contents can complement EEG dynamics unavailable in whole-head EEG recordings, this study simulated the circumstance of classifying emotion states based on fewer informative EEG features/electrodes. The LFI index (0.1~0.6) was defined to systematically reduce the whole-brain electrode montage (30) to different subsets of electrodes located at certain regions. Under such constrain, the relationship between the EEG dynamics and musical contents can be evaluated.

Figure 5 presents the valence and arousal classification results using the LFI-sorted subject-independent EEG features (i.e., MESH) with/without feature selection. Overall, the number of features can be seen to progressively reduce as the LFI value increased from 0.1 to 0.6. The number of electrodes required for the feature sets in turn was reduced. These feature sets, however, gave very limited estimations in emotional responses against the majority voting. The reason was attributed to the fact that the discriminative power of the subject-independent features with a compromise of a subject population might not be guaranteed to each of subjects. At LFI = 0.6, the required electrodes were dramatically reduced from the whole-scalp montage (30) to ten and seven electrodes for valence and arousal classification, respectively. As shown in **Figure 6**, most of the informative EEG features (listed in **Table 3**) were extracted from the fronto-central electrodes versus others. It is worth noting that the DLAT, extracted from left-right electrode pairs, dominated the composition of the EEG features, compared to others (DCAU and PSD). According to these results, the subject-independent EEG feature set (LFI = 0.6), which involved a low-density fronto-central montage, was adopted for emotion classification in the rest of the study.

Figure 7 shows the classification results using the subject-independent EEG features (i.e., MESH given LFI = 0.6), musical features (i.e., MUSIC), and subject-independent multimodal approach. Note that the sorted multimodal features were derived by applying the F-score feature selection to the composite feature vector of the MESH and MUSIC features. The multimodal approach resulted in the maximum accuracies of 66.93 ± 7.10% and 67.04 ± 5.78% for valence and arousal classification, respectively, following by the musical features and the EEG features. Most importantly, the multimodal approach outperformed the EEG-only features by around 6% for valence ($p < 0.05$) and 9% for arousal ($p < 0.01$) classification. There was no significant difference between the multimodal approach and the musical features ($p > 0.3$).

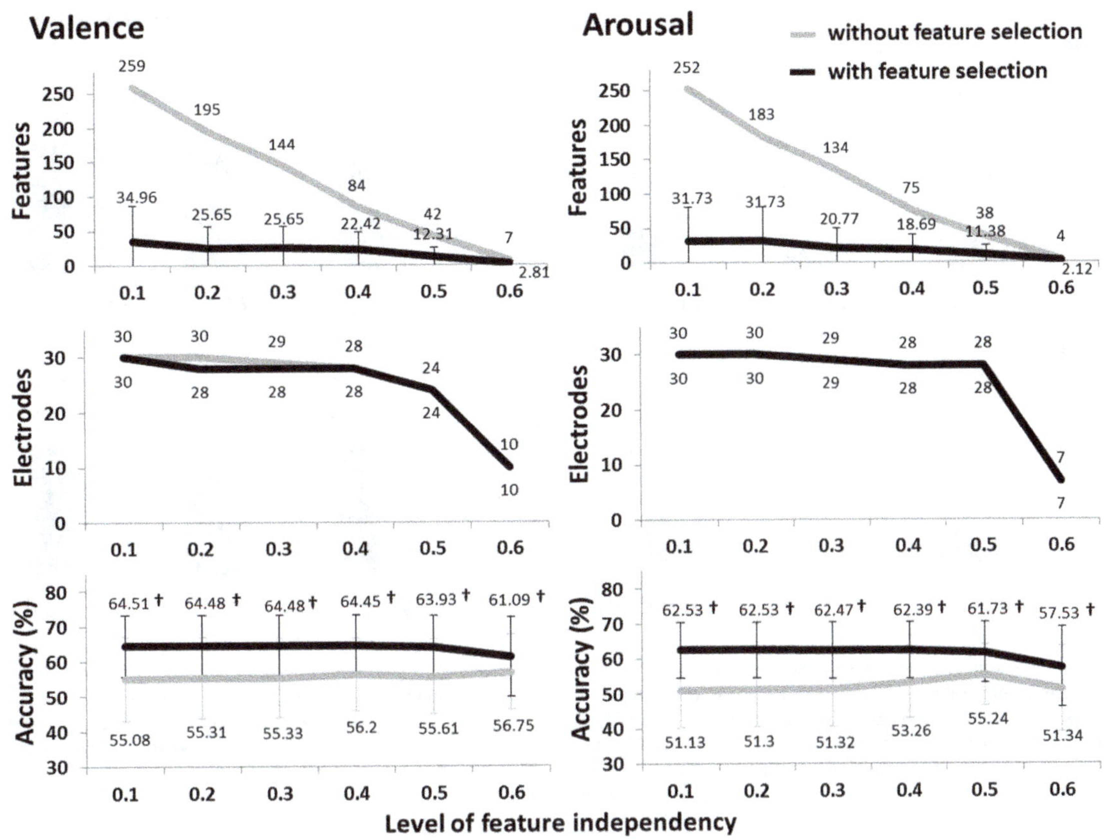

FIGURE 5 | The valence and arousal classification results of the subject-independent EEG features (type: MESH) in term of the average number of features, electrodes, and accuracies using with/without feature selection under the LFI criteria (0.1 ~ 0.6). The numbers near to the nodes represent the mean values of the results. [†]Indicates that the accuracy with feature selection significantly outperformed that without feature selection ($p < 0.01$), yet were comparable ($p > 0.1$) to majority voting accuracies (valence: ~63%, arousal: ~61%).

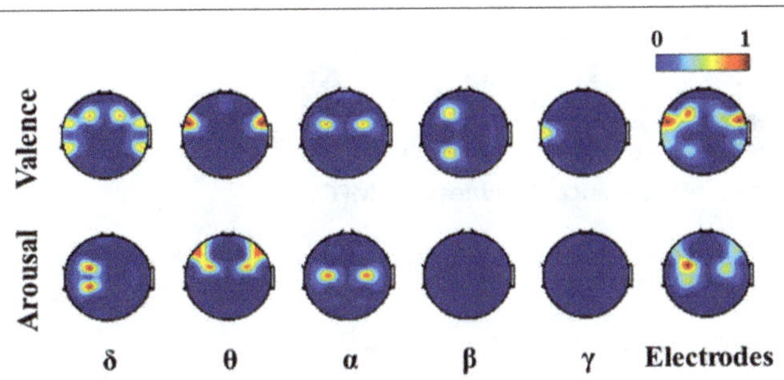

FIGURE 6 | The topographic mapping of informative EEG features consistently appeared in multiple subjects. The rightmost topography color-codes the importance of electrodes according to how frequent the electrodes were used to derive the corresponding features.

Table 3 | The informative EEG features that consistently appeared across multiple subjects.

Rank	Valence	Arousal
1	DLAT: FT7-FT8 (Theta)	DCAU: FC3-CP3 (Delta)
2	DLAT: FC3-FC4 (Alpha)	DLAT: C3-C4 (Alpha)
3	DLAT: F3-F4 (Delta)	DLAT: F7-F8 (Theta)
4	DLAT: FT7-FT8 (Delta)	DLAT: FC3-FC4 (Theta)
5	DLAT: TP7-TP8 (Delta)	
6	DCAU: F3-P3 (Beta)	
7	PSD: T7 (Gamma)	

Figure 8 shows the percent composition of contributions of EEG and musical features to the subject-independent multimodal features. As a baseline, the composition of the subject-independent EEG features is also provided. The comparative result showed the EEG and musical features performed complementarily in the multimodal approach. The musical features competed to the EEG features and replaced the ones with relatively low discriminative power, especially for arousal scale. This evidently explains the reason that the subject-independent multimodal approach leading to significant improvements upon the subject-independent EEG results. **Table 4** lists these informative musical features, which consistently appeared in above half of the subjects.

In sum, the EEG features extracted from a subset of brain regions was unable to effectively encompass the complex brain

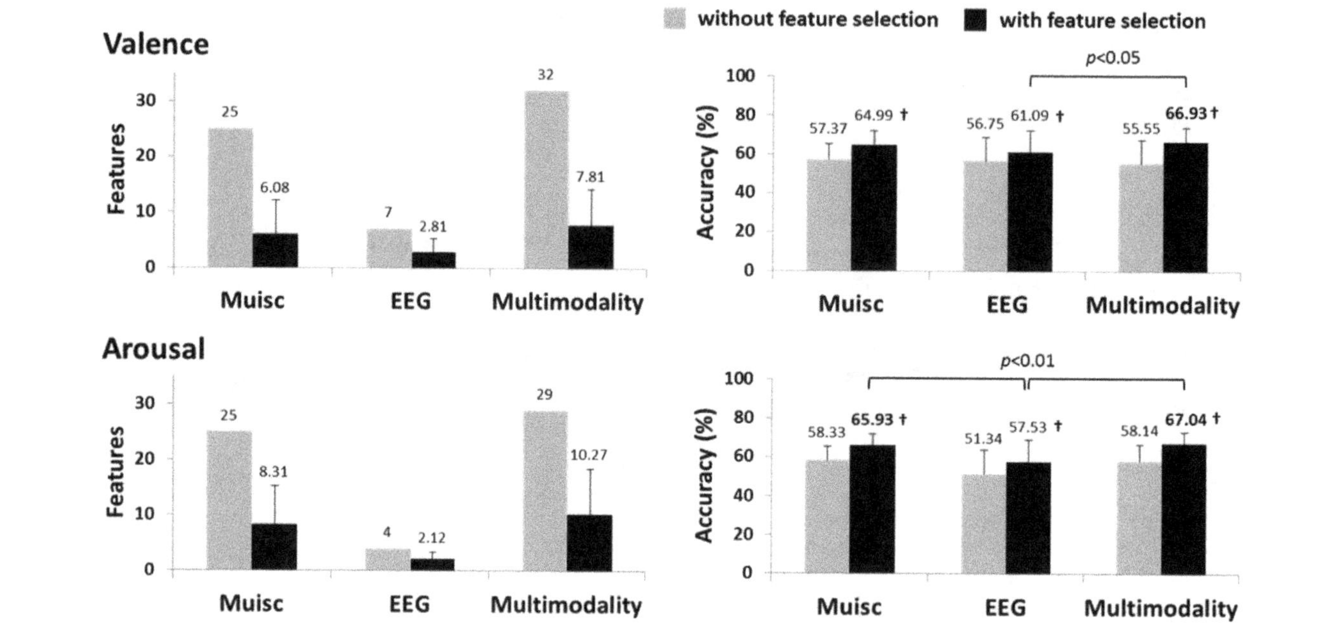

FIGURE 7 | The valence and arousal classification results using the subject-independent multimodal approach (LFI = 0.6) with/without feature selection. The results of the subject-independent EEG modality (feature type: MESH) and the music modality (feature type: MUSIC) are also provided for comparison. The numbers above the bars represent the mean values of the results, whereas the numbers in bold indicate the accuracies significantly better ($p < 0.02$) than the majority voting accuracy (valence: ~63%, arousal: ~61%). †indicates that the accuracy with feature selection significantly outperformed that without feature selection ($p < 0.01$).

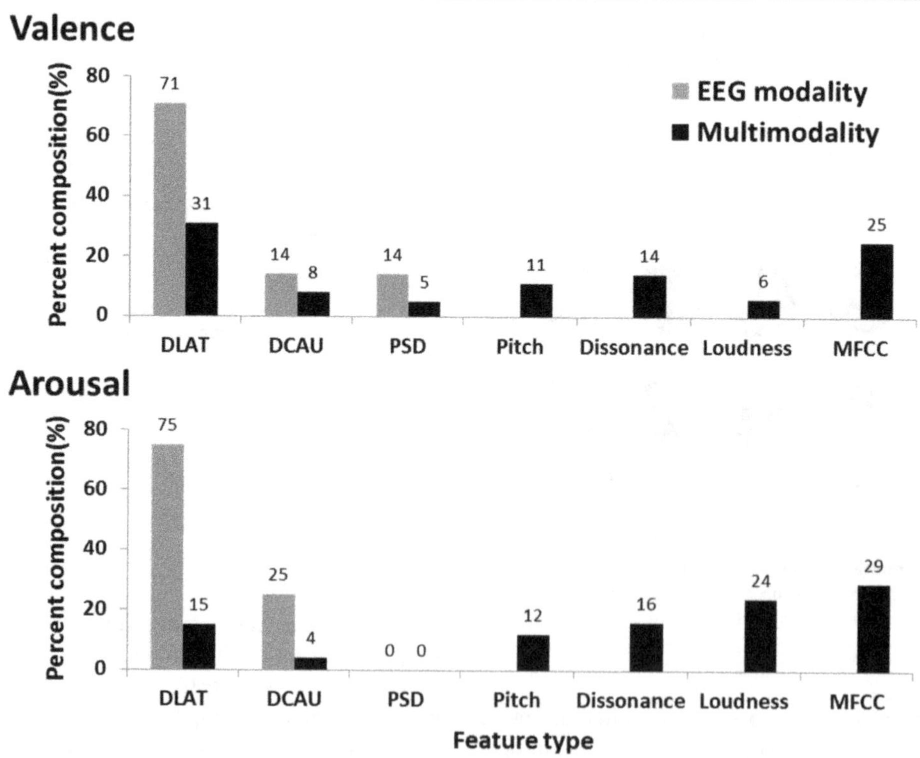

FIGURE 8 | The percent composition of contributions of EEG (DLAT, DCAU, and PSD) and musical (Pitch, Dissonance, Loudness, and MFCC) features to the subject-independent multimodality. The composition of the subject-independent EEG modality is also provided for comparison.

Table 4 | The informative musical features in the subject-independent multimodal approach.

Rank	Valence	Arousal
1	Dissonance: Spectral dissonance (S)	Loudness: Sharpness (Z)
2	Pitch: Mode	MFCC: 8th
3		Loudness: Sharpness (A)
4		Pitch: Harmonic flux

dynamics about emotions. The corresponding EEG features simply retuned the classification accuracy equivalent to random guessing. Under this circumstance, the EEG modality could benefit from the inclusion of the acoustic characteristics of musical contents. The aforementioned simulation result proved the second hypothesis that the musical contents can compensate for EEG dynamics unavailable in whole-head EEG recordings to improve the classification performance to some extent.

DISCUSSION

Music is an ecologically valid and complex stimulus that conveys emotions to listeners through musical composition. Using only EEG signals to classify music-induced emotional responses remained challenging. By exploiting the complementary nature of multidisciplinary modalities, the fusion of EEG and musical dynamics has been recently reported (Koelstra et al., 2012). However, it remains unclear when acoustic characteristics of musical contents effectively contribute to the modeling of emotional responses. To this end, this study adopted machine-learning methods, including feature extraction, selection and classification, to systematically assess a composite feature space by aligning EEG and musical features in time. The empirical results suggested that when EEG signals from the whole head were available, the inclusion of musical contents contributed little to the emotion classification model. On the contrary, if EEG dynamics only available from a small set of electrodes (likely the case in real-life BCI applications), the music modality tended to play a complementary role to enhance the EEG-based classification performance. To the best of our knowledge, no study has attempted to elucidate the roles of the EEG and music modalities in the emotion classification problem. The present study not only provided principles for building an EEG-based multimodal approach, but also revealed the fundamental insights into the interplay of the brain activity and musical contents in emotion modeling.

INDIVIDUAL VARIABILITY AND COMMONALITY OF THE EEG DYNAMICS FOR EMOTION CLASSIFICATION

Individual variability has been reported in emotion regulations (Gross and John, 2003). Such variability may introduce the disparity of informative EEG patterns across individuals or subgroups (Lin et al., 2010a, 2011). To estimate the emotional states, it is plausible to expect a subject-specific classification model that well learned from an individual would have an optimal classification accuracy (Lin et al., 2010b). In the present study, the comparison in valence and arousal classification using subject-dependent and -independent features addressed this issue. The classification performance using the LFI-guided subject-independent EEG features (c.f. **Figure 5**) was notably worse than that using the subject-dependent EEG set (c.f. **Figure 2**). The commonality of the valence- and arousal-specific EEG features/electrodes from multiple subjects was rather small. There were only seven and four informative EEG features consistently appeared in over 15 of 26 subjects for valence and arousal classification, respectively (c.f. **Table 3**). These results suggested that the individual variability substantially affected emotion classification, especially for arousal scale, and thereby posed a great challenge to learning a subject-independent emotion model using only the EEG signals.

However, it is worth noting that exploring a consensus set of emotion-relevant EEG activity from multiple subjects is of great important to normative emotion research. In this study, the electrodes placed over the fronto-central region were relatively discriminative for most of subjects (c.f. **Figure 6**), which was in line with the previous studies (Altenmuller et al., 2002; Lin et al., 2010a). Over the brain region, the lateralized power asymmetry (in the left-right direction) well characterized the changes of emotional states, which may be supported by the role of the frontal cortical lateralization in emotion processing (Altenmuller et al., 2002; Allen et al., 2004). Specifically, the frontal theta asymmetry (FT7-FT8) and the fronto-central alpha asymmetry (FC3-FC4) associated with the valence scale was in line with other studies (Davidson, 1992; Aftanas et al., 2001; Schmidt and Trainor, 2001), whereas the fronto-central theta asymmetry (F7-F8 and FC3-FC4) related to the arousal scale was supported by Aftanas et al. (2004). Furthermore, several informative spectral asymmetries in the delta band for both emotional valence and arousal partially conformed to the previous works (Lin et al., 2010a,b). Accordingly, the index of rhythmic lateralization presumably better differentiated the brain activity into emotional states and acted consistently for multiple subjects, compared to the caudality (power asymmetry in the fronto-posterior direction) and individual spectra.

THE ROLE OF EEG AND MUSIC MODALITIES IN EMOTION CLASSIFICATION

The empirical results of this study evidently suggested that the inclusion of the acoustic characteristics of musical contents did not guarantee to complement EEG dynamics in the emotion classification problem. One key factor is that whether or not the EEG signals can be extracted from the whole brain and across entire frequency bands to encompass the full emotion-modulated spatio-spectral dynamics.

The optimized subject-dependent results showed that the EEG modality with and without the inclusion of the music modality were comparable in the performance (c.f. **Figure 3**) and tended to dominate the feature composition in the multimodality model (c.f. **Figure 4**). This indicated that the musical content brought very limited or redundant discriminative power to the classification of emotional responses. The aforementioned individual variability might explain such results. The music modality that lacks of correlates of internal psychophysiological reactions might more and less introduce conflicts with the brain signals, i.e., EEG modality, in reflecting the felt emotional responses. It is true that the listeners might not actually perceive and experience the same emotion as music tried to express (Gabrielsson, 2002).

Accordingly, it is reasonable to conclude that if the informative EEG features can be obtained from the whole brain and entire frequency bands, the inclusion of musical contents barely contributed to the classification model. The multimodal approach might not be necessary.

However, in practical ABCI applications, an EEG cap with the whole-brain coverage might be impractical and unavailable in consumer-level headsets, e.g., the MindWave headset (NeuroSky, Inc.) and the Emotiv EPOC headset (Emotiv systems, Inc.). In this case, the EEG features measured by the electrodes sparsely placed at a certain brain region(s). The suboptimal EEG features returned very poor emotion classification performance (even lower than the random guessing, c.f. **Figure 7**). The music modality under this circumstance provided complementary information and replaced a set of EEG features with less discrimination power with the musical characteristics of timber and loudness (c.f. **Figure 8**). The musical dynamics tended to dominate the multimodal feature composition in the arousal scale as compared to valence. This phenomenon might be attributed to the fact that the music modality met a great challenge in modeling emotional valence (Macdorman et al., 2007; Yang et al., 2008b). This might also explain why the improvement in the classification performance was much noticeable in the arousal classification. Thus, the music modality was assumed to boost the EEG-based emotion classification performance if the EEG dynamics were substantially limited in certain brain regions.

INFORMATIVE MUSICAL CHARACTERISTIC FOR EMOTION CLASSIFICATION

By manipulating musical structures, conveying emotions in music is intuitively plausible (Peretz et al., 1998; Schmithorst, 2005; Gomez and Danuser, 2007; Zatorre et al., 2007). Several neurophysiological studies that devoted to the brain correlates in musical perception and emotion perception reported that some music-modulated brain activity were known to intervene in emotion processing (Blood et al., 1999; Tsang et al., 2001; Khalfa et al., 2005). It is reasonable to expect that there is a considerable amount of EEG rhythmicity that is not only engaged in emotion processing but also modulated by music perception. Thus, the acoustic characteristics of musical contents and EEG dynamics could somehow perform complementarily. As shown in **Table 4**, previous neurophysiological and music signal processing studies supported our findings. Several neurophysiological studies found that mode and consonance were relevant to the distinction of emotion valence (Tsang et al., 2001; Sammler et al., 2007), whereas the harmonics processing was very closely associated with emotional affect and intensity (Schmithorst, 2005). From musical signal processing aspect, Yang et al. (2008b) reported that the valence scale was better characterized by the dissonance and pitch-related features, whereas the arousal scale was better modeled by timber features. This was in line to the findings of spectral dissonance and mode for valence scale and a timber element (8th MFCC) for arousal scale. Aljanaki et al. (2013) recently also documented that the most important feature in the distinction of the arousal scale was the loudness, which supported our findings in arousal scale. It is encouraging that the consistent findings of the musical structures were conducted with different musical datasets.

COMPARING THE EMOTION CLASSIFICATION RESULTS WITH PREVIOUS WORKS

Recent works that adopted the EEG-based multimodal approach are described here. Koelstra et al. (2012) proposed to use a decision-level fusion scheme to construct a multimodal pipeline (EEG, peripheral biosignals, music) for emotional valence, arousal and liking classification while watching music videos. The classification performance using the EEG signals were marginally worse than that using musical features for valence (EEG: 58%, biosignals: 63%, music: 62%, majority: 59%) and arousal (EEG: 62%, biosignals: 57%, music: 65%, majority: 64%) classification. The fusion of EEG and musical features resulted in an optimal classification accuracy around 63% marginally outperformed EEG modality only for arousal classification. In the same year, Soleymani et al. (2012a) also adopted the decision-level approach and explored an optimal fusion pair among EEG signals, peripheral biosignals and eye gaze for affective recognition during video appreciation. The classification performance using the EEG-Gaze fusion was better than single modality results for valence (biosignals: 46%, EEG: 57%, gaze: 69%, fusion: 76%, random: 34%) and arousal (biosignals: 46%, EEG: 52%, gaze: 64%, fusion: 68%, random: 36%) classification. The authors later performed a following-up study (Soleymani et al., 2012b) to compare the schemes for fusing EEG and gaze modalities at feature and decision levels. The authors reported that the decision-level fusion returned better classification results compared to single modalities for valence (EEG: 50%, eye: 67%, decision: 69%, random: 33%) and arousal (EEG: 62%, eye: 71%, decision: 76%, random: 33%) classification, where the feature-level fusion (valence: 58%, arousal: 66%) just outperformed the EEG modality. A year later, Koelstra and Patras (2013) similarly assessed the feasibility of using the feature- and decision-based multimodality (EEG dynamics and facial expression characteristics). The authors documented that the feature-level fusion in general marginally improved the performance against single modalities for valence (EEG: 72%, face: 65%, fusion: 73%, majority: 62%) and arousal (EEG: 68%, face: 68%, fusion: 69%, majority: 62%) classification, whereas the fusion-level approach using an optimal weighting scheme led to more convincing improvement (valence: 74%, arousal: 72%). In the present study, the feature-level multimodal approach (EEG and musical features) was adopted to validate its feasibility of emotion classification in music listening. The empirical result showed that the subject-dependent multimodal approach marginally outperformed the single modalities for valence (EEG: 76%, music: 65%, fusion: 77%, majority: 63%) and arousal (EEG: 74%, music: 66%, fusion: 76%, majority: 61%) classification, whereas the subject-independent multimodal approach provided more convincing improvement for valence (EEG: 61%, fusion: 67%) and arousal (EEG: 58%, fusion: 67%) classifications.

It is worth mentioning that the comparison only based on classification accuracy might not be fair as a variety of factors might affect the classification results, such as but not limited to experimental conditions, stimulus types, multimodal sources, and signal processing steps. Thus, for a fair comparison in multimodality, this study summarized the differences between this and another related work (Koelstra et al., 2012) that also focused on the multimodality of EEG and musical dynamics. The obtained subject-dependent results of this study were evidently higher than theirs by at least 10%, whereas the subject-independent results of this study were marginally higher by around 3%, yet with fewer EEG features and electrodes. Despite the disparity in the selected musical features, the music modality results for emotional valence and arousal were comparable. Furthermore, compared to the studies using solely EEG modality (Koelstra et al., 2012; Soleymani et al., 2012a,b; Koelstra and Patras, 2013), the proposed subject-dependent EEG features (MESH) should be comparable to or even better than previous reports. Instead, the classification performance using the proposed subject-independent EEG set might only compare favorably to the study (Koelstra et al., 2012).

OUTPERFORMED EEG PATTERNS FOR EMOTION CLASSIFICATION

The MESH features in conjunction with the F-score feature selection produced a compact set of informative features and consequently optimized the classification performance, compared to others (DLAT, DCAU, and PSD) (c.f. **Figure 2**). The performance improvement might be attributed to the fact that emotion processing might accompany the EEG dynamics that varied distinctly within and between brain regions (Schmidt and Trainor, 2001; Aftanas et al., 2004; Sarlo et al., 2005; Sammler et al., 2007; Lin et al., 2010b). The MESH features that composed of two-directional power asymmetry (laterality and caudality) and individual spectra over the scalp allow seeking an optimal set for constructing a classification model for each individual. As referring to its feature composition (c.f. **Figure 4**), both DLAT and DCAU apparently dominated the EEG composition against the PSD. Specifically, the DLAT consistently appeared in multiple subjects (c.f. **Table 3**). These results suggested that the features depicting the directional spectral differences between brain regions might be of importance in the EEG-based emotion modeling.

THE CHOICE OF EEG ELECTRODE REFERENCE

The EEG signals analyzed in this study were recorded with the reference to the linked mastoids. The recorded potentials over the mastoids were conventionally believed to be neutral to the measured neural activities of interest, which were also adopted in previous music studies (Koelsch et al., 2007; Sammler et al., 2007). However, few reports demonstrated that the linked mastoids reference might introduce non-neutrality to the recorded EEG signals and distort the EEG spectra (Yao, 2001; Marzetti et al., 2007; Qin et al., 2010). Comparing the effects of different reference strategies on emotion classification is an important issue, but it is beyond the scope of this study. Interested readers can refer to the studies on reference techniques by Yao (2001), Marzetti et al. (2007), Qin et al. (2010).

FUTURE DIRECTION

Future efforts can be devoted to augment the multimodal classification performance as follows. First, data-driven approach, e.g., principal component analysis (Lin et al., 2009) and independent component analysis (Lin et al., 2010a), might be feasible to further elaborate the EEG spatio-spectral dynamics associated with implicit emotional responses. Second, advanced music signal processing techniques can be incorporated to extract other musical characteristics, e.g., rhythm. Lastly, the decision-level multimodal fusion has been reported to obtain convincing classification performance improvements over the feature-level fusion (Soleymani et al., 2012b; Koelstra and Patras, 2013). Following the explored EEG and musical features of this study, the fusion at the decision level can be further explored and compared.

REFERENCES

Aftanas, L., Varlamov, A., Pavlov, S., Makhnev, V., and Reva, N. (2001). Event-related synchronization and desynchronization during affective processing: emergence of valence-related time-dependent hemispheric asymmetries in theta and upper alpha band. *Int. J. Neurosci.* 110, 197–219. doi: 10.3109/00207450108986547

Aftanas, L. I., Reva, N. V., Varlamov, A. A., Pavlov, S. V., and Makhnev, V. P. (2004). Analysis of evoked EEG synchronization and desynchronization in conditions of emotional activation in humans: temporal and topographic characteristics. *Neurosci. Behav. Physiol.* 34, 859–867. doi: 10.1023/B:NEAB.0000038139.39812.eb

Aljanaki, A., Wiering, F., and Veltkamp, R. C. (2013). "MIRUtrecht participation in MediaEval 2013: emotion in music task," in *MediaEval Workshop*, Vol. 1043 (Barcelona).

Allen, J. J. B., Coan, J. A., and Nazarian, M. (2004). Issues and assumptions on the road from raw signals to metrics of frontal EEG asymmetry in emotion. *Biol. Psychol.* 67, 183–218. doi: 10.1016/j.biopsycho.2004.03.007

Altenmuller, E., Schurmann, K., Lim, V. K., and Parlitz, D. (2002). Hits to the left, flops to the right: different emotions during listening to music are reflected in cortical lateralisation patterns. *Neuropsychologia* 40, 2242–2256. doi: 10.1016/S0028-3932(02)00107-0

Blood, A. J., Zatorre, R. J., Bermudez, P., and Evans, A. C. (1999). Emotional responses to pleasant and unpleasant music correlate with activity in paralimbic brain regions. *Nat. Neurosci.* 2, 382–387. doi: 10.1038/7299

Cabrera, D. (1999). "Psysound: a computer program for psycho-acoustical analysis," in *Australian Acoustical Society Conference* (Melbourne, VIC), 47–54.

Chanel, G., Kierkels, J. J. M., Soleymani, M., and Pun, T. (2009). Short-term emotion assessment in a recall paradigm. *Int. J. Hum. Comput. Stud.* 67, 607–627. doi: 10.1016/j.ijhcs.2009.03.005

Chang, C.-C., and Lin, C.-J. (2011). LIBSVM: a library for support vector machines. *ACM Trans. Intell. Syst. Technol.* 2, 1–27. doi: 10.1145/1961189.1961199

Chen, Y. W., and Lin, C. J. (2006). "Combining SVMs with various feature selection strategies," in *Feature Extraction, Foundations and Applications*, eds I. Guyon, M. Nikravesh, S. Gunn, and L. A. Zadeh (Berlin; Heidelberg: Springer), 315–324.

Davidson, R. J. (1992). Anterior cerebral asymmetry and the nature of emotion. *Brain Cogn.* 20, 125–151. doi: 10.1016/0278-2626(92)90065-T

Davis, S. B., and Mermelstein, P. (1980). Comparison of parametric representations for monosyllabic word recognition in continuously spoken sentences. *IEEE Trans. Acoust. Speech Signal Process.* 28, 357–366. doi: 10.1109/TASSP.1980.1163420

Frantzidis, C. A., Bratsas, C., Papadelis, C. L., Konstantinidis, E., Pappas, C., and Bamidis, P. D. (2010). Toward emotion aware computing: an integrated approach using multichannel neurophysiological recordings and affective visual stimuli. *IEEE Trans. Inf. Technol. Biomed.* 14, 589–597. doi: 10.1109/TITB.2010.2041553

Gabrielsson, A. (2002). Emotion perceived and emotion felt: same or different? *Musicae Sci.* 5, 123–147. doi: 10.1177/10298649020050S105

Gabrielsson, A., and Lindström, E. (2010). "The role of structure in the musical expression of emotions," in *Handbook of Music and Emotion: Theory, Research, Applications*, ed P. N. Juslin (New York, NY: Oxford University Press), 367–400.

Gomez, P., and Danuser, B. (2007). Relationships between musical structure and psychophysiological measures of emotion. *Emotion* 7, 377–387. doi: 10.1037/1528-3542.7.2.377

Gross, J. J., and John, O. P. (2003). Individual differences in two emotion regulation processes: implications for affect, relationships, and well-being. *J. Pers. Soc. Psychol.* 85, 348–362. doi: 10.1037/0022-3514.85.2.348

Gyurak, A., Gross, J. J., and Etkin, A. (2011). Explicit and implicit emotion regulation: a dual-process framework. *Cogn. Emot.* 25, 400–412. doi: 10.1080/02699931.2010.544160

Ishino, K., and Hagiwara, M. (2003). "A feeling estimation system using a simple electroencephalograph," in *IEEE International Conference on Systems, Man and Cybernetics*, Vol. 4205, 4204–4209.

Juslin, P. N. (2000). Cue utilization in communication of emotion in music performance: relating performance to perception. *J. Exp. Psychol. Hum. Percept. Perform.* 26, 1797–1812. doi: 10.1037/0096-1523.26.6.1797

Juslin, P. N., and Laukka, P. (2003). Communication of emotions in vocal expression and music performance: different channels, same code? *Psychol. Bull.* 129, 770–814. doi: 10.1037/0033-2909.129.5.770

Khalfa, S., Schon, D., Anton, J. L., and Liegeois-Chauvel, C. (2005). Brain regions involved in the recognition of happiness and sadness in music. *Neuroreport* 16, 1981–1984. doi: 10.1097/00001756-200512190-00002

Kittler, J., Hatef, M., Duin, R. P. W., and Matas, J. (1998). On combining classifiers. *IEEE Trans. Pattern Anal. Mach. Intell.* 20, 226–239. doi: 10.1109/34.667881

Koelsch, S., Jentschke, S., Sammler, D., and Mietchen, D. (2007). Untangling syntactic and sensory processing: an ERP study of music perception. *Psychophysiology* 44, 476–490. doi: 10.1111/j.1469-8986.2007.00517.x

Koelstra, S., Muhl, C., Soleymani, M., Lee, J., Yazdani, A., Ebrahimi, T., et al. (2012). DEAP: a database for emotion analysis using physiological signals. *IEEE Trans. Affecti. Comput.* 3, 18–31. doi: 10.1109/T-AFFC.2011.15

Koelstra, S., and Patras, I. (2013). Fusion of facial expressions and EEG for implicit affective tagging. *Image Vis. Comput.* 31, 164–174. doi: 10.1016/j.imavis.2012.10.002

Lartillot, O., and Toiviainen, P. (2007). "A Matlab toolbox for musical Feature extraction from audio," in *International Conference on Digital Audio Effects*, 237–244.

Lee, N., Broderick, A. J., and Chamberlain, L. (2007). What is 'neuromarketing'? A discussion and agenda for future research. *Int. J. Psychophysiol.* 63, 199–204. doi: 10.1016/j.ijpsycho.2006.03.007

Lin, Y. P., Chen, J. H., Duann, J. R., Lin, C. T., and Jung, T. P. (2011). Generalizations of the subject-independent feature set for music-induced emotion recognition. *Conf. Proc. IEEE Eng. Med. Biol. Soc.* 2011, 6092–6095. doi: 10.1109/IEMBS.2011.6091505

Lin, Y. P., Duann, J. R., Chen, J. H., and Jung, T. P. (2010a). Electroencephalographic dynamics of musical emotion perception revealed by independent spectral components. *Neuroreport* 21, 410–415. doi: 10.1097/WNR.0b013e32833774de

Lin, Y. P., Jung, T. P., and Chen, J. H. (2009). EEG dynamics during music appreciation. *Conf. Proc. IEEE Eng. Med. Biol. Soc.* 2009, 5316–5319. doi: 10.1109/IEMBS.2009.5333524

Lin, Y. P., Wang, C. H., Jung, T. P., Wu, T. L., Jeng, S. K., Duann, J. R., et al. (2010b). EEG-based emotion recognition in music listening. *IEEE Trans. Biomed. Eng.* 57, 1798–1806. doi: 10.1109/TBME.2010.2048568

Macdorman, K. F., Ough, S., and Ho, C. C. (2007). Automatic emotion prediction of song excerpts: index construction, algorithm design, and empirical comparison. *J. New Music Res.* 36, 281–299. doi: 10.1080/09298210801927846

Makeig, S., Leslie, G., Mullen, T., Sarma, D., Bigdely-Shamlo, N., and Kothe, C. (2011). "First demonstration of a musical emotion BCI," in *Proceedings of the 4th International Conference on Affective Computing and Intelligent Interaction—*Volume Part II. (Memphis, TN: Springer-Verlag).

Marzetti, L., Nolte, G., Perrucci, M. G., Romani, G. L., and Del Gratta, C. (2007). The use of standardized infinity reference in EEG coherency studies. *Neuroimage* 36, 48–63. doi: 10.1016/j.neuroimage.2007.02.034

Millan, J. D., Rupp, R., Muller-Putz, G. R., Murray-Smith, R., Giugliemma, C., Tangermann, M., et al. (2010). Combining brain-computer interfaces and assistive technologies: state-of-the-art and challenges. *Front. Neurosci.* 4:161. doi: 10.3389/fnins.2010.00161

Muller, M., Ellis, D. P. W., Klapuri, A., and Richard, G. (2011). Signal processing for music analysis. *IEEE J. Sel. Top. Signal Process.* 5, 1088–1110. doi: 10.1109/JSTSP.2011.2112333

Parncutt, R., and Hair, G. (2011). Consonance and dissonance in music theory and psychology: disentangling dissonant dichotomies. *J. Interdiscipl. Music Stud.* 5, 119–166. doi: 10.4407/jims.2011.11.002

Peretz, I., Gagnon, L., and Bouchard, B. (1998). Music and emotion: perceptual determinants, immediacy, and isolation after brain damage. *Cognition* 68, 111–141. doi: 10.1016/S0010-0277(98)00043-2

Petrantonakis, P. C., and Hadjileontiadis, L. J. (2010). Emotion recognition from EEG using higher order crossings. *IEEE Trans. Inf. Technol. Biomed.* 14, 186–197. doi: 10.1109/TITB.2009.2034649

Qin, Y., Xu, P., and Yao, D. Z. (2010). A comparative study of different references for EEG default mode network: the use of the infinity reference. *Clin. Neurophysiol.* 121, 1981–1991. doi: 10.1016/j.clinph.2010.03.056

Russell, J. A. (1980). A circumplex model of affect. *J. Pers. Soc. Psychol.* 39, 18. doi: 10.1037/h0077714

Sammler, D., Grigutsch, M., Fritz, T., and Koelsch, S. (2007). Music and emotion: electrophysiological correlates of the processing of pleasant and unpleasant music. *Psychophysiology* 44, 293–304. doi: 10.1111/j.1469-8986.2007.00497.x

Sargin, M. E., Yemez, Y., Erzin, E., and Tekalp, A. M. (2007). Audiovisual synchronization and fusion using canonical correlation analysis. *IEEE Trans. Multimedia* 9, 1396–1403. doi: 10.1109/TMM.2007.906583

Sarlo, M., Buodo, G., Poli, S., and Palomba, D. (2005). Changes in EEG alpha power to different disgust elicitors: the specificity of mutilations. *Neurosci. Lett.* 382, 291–296. doi: 10.1016/j.neulet.2005.03.037

Schmidt, L. A., and Trainor, L. J. (2001). Frontal brain electrical activity (EEG) distinguishes valence and intensity of musical emotions. *Cogn. Emot.* 15, 487–500. doi: 10.1080/02699930126048

Schmithorst, V. J. (2005). Separate cortical networks involved in music perception: preliminary functional MRI evidence for modularity of music processing. *Neuroimage* 25, 444–451. doi: 10.1016/j.neuroimage.2004.12.006

Soleymani, M., Lichtenauer, J., Pun, T., and Pantic, M. (2012a). A multimodal database for affect recognition and implicit tagging. *IEEE Trans. Affect. Comput.* 3, 42–55. doi: 10.1109/T-AFFC.2011.25

Soleymani, M., Pantic, M., and Pun, T. (2012b). Multimodal emotion recognition in response to videos. *IEEE Trans. Affect. Computi.* 3, 211–223. doi: 10.1109/T-AFFC.2011.37

Takahashi, K. (2004). "Remarks on emotion recognition from multi-modal biopotential signals," in *IEEE International Conference on Industrial Technology* (Hammamet), 1138–1143.

Thaut, M. H., Gardiner, J. C., Holmberg, D., Horwitz, J., Kent, L., Andrews, G., et al. (2009). Neurologic music therapy improves executive function and emotional adjustment in traumatic brain injury rehabilitation. *Ann. N.Y. Acad. Sci.* 1169, 406–416. doi: 10.1111/j.1749-6632.2009.04585.x

Tsang, C. D., Trainor, L. J., Santesso, D. L., Tasker, S. L., and Schmidt, L. A. (2001). Frontal EEG responses as a function of affective musical features. *Biol. Found. Music* 930, 439–442. doi: 10.1111/j.1749-6632.2001.tb05764.x

Tzanetakis, G., and Cook, P. (2002). Musical genre classification of audio signals. *IEEE Trans. Speech Audio Process.* 10, 293–302. doi: 10.1109/TSA.2002.800560

Wolpaw, J. R., Birbaumer, N., McFarland, D. J., Pfurtscheller, G., and Vaughan, T. M. (2002). Brain-computer interfaces for communication and control. *Clin. Neurophysiol.* 113, 767–791. doi: 10.1016/S1388-2457(02)00057-3

Wu, T.-L., Wang, H.-K., Ho, C.-C., Lin, Y.-P., Hu, T.-T., Weng, M.-F., et al. (2008). "Interactive content presentation based on expressed emotion and physiological feedback," in *Proceedings of the 16th ACM International Conference on Multimedia* (Vancouver; British Columbia: ACM).

Yang, Y. H., and Chen, H. H. (2011). *Music Emotion Recognition.* Boca Raton, FL: CRC Press.

Yang, Y. H., and Chen, H. H. (2012). Machine recognition of music emotion: a review. *ACM Trans. Intell. Syst. Technol.* 3:40. doi: 10.1145/2168752.2168754

Yang, Y. H., Lin, Y. C., Cheng, H. T., Liao, I. B., Ho, Y. C., and Chen, H. H. (2008a). "Toward Multi-modal music emotion classification," in *Advances in Multimedia Information Processing—PCM 2008*, eds Y.-M. Huang, C. Xu, K.-S. Cheng, J.-F. Yang, M. N. S. Swamy, S. Li, and J.-W. Ding (Berlin; Heidelberg: Springer), 70–79. doi: 10.1007/978-3-540-89796-5_8

Yang, Y. H., Lin, Y. C., Su, Y. F., and Chen, H. H. (2008b). A regression approach to music emotion recognition. *IEEE Trans. Audio Speech Lang. Process.* 16, 448–457. doi: 10.1109/TASL.2007.911513

Yao, D. (2001). A method to standardize a reference of scalp EEG recordings to a point at infinity. *Physiol. Meas.* 22, 693. doi: 10.1088/0967-3334/22/4/305

Zander, T. O., and Kothe, C. (2011). Towards passive brain-computer interfaces: applying brain-computer interface technology to human-machine systems in general. *J. Neural Eng.* 8:025005. doi: 10.1088/1741-2560/8/2/025005

Zatorre, R. J., Chen, J. L., and Penhune, V. B. (2007). When the brain plays music: auditory-motor interactions in music perception and production. *Nat. Rev. Neurosci.* 8, 547–558. doi: 10.1038/nrn2152

11

A brain-computer interface for potential non-verbal facial communication based on EEG signals related to specific emotions

Koji Kashihara* *

Information Solution, Institute of Technology and Science, The University of Tokushima, Tokushima, Japan

***Correspondence:**
Koji Kashihara, Information Solution, Institute of Technology and Science, The University of Tokushima, 2-1 Minamijyousanjima, Tokushima 770-8506, Japan
e-mail: kashihara.koji@tokushima-u.ac.jp

Unlike assistive technology for verbal communication, the brain-machine or brain-computer interface (BMI/BCI) has not been established as a non-verbal communication tool for amyotrophic lateral sclerosis (ALS) patients. Face-to-face communication enables access to rich emotional information, but individuals suffering from neurological disorders, such as ALS and autism, may not express their emotions or communicate their negative feelings. Although emotions may be inferred by looking at facial expressions, emotional prediction for neutral faces necessitates advanced judgment. The process that underlies brain neuronal responses to neutral faces and causes emotional changes remains unknown. To address this problem, therefore, this study attempted to decode conditioned emotional reactions to neutral face stimuli. This direction was motivated by the assumption that if electroencephalogram (EEG) signals can be used to detect patients' emotional responses to specific inexpressive faces, the results could be incorporated into the design and development of BMI/BCI-based non-verbal communication tools. To these ends, this study investigated how a neutral face associated with a negative emotion modulates rapid central responses in face processing and then identified cortical activities. The conditioned neutral face-triggered event-related potentials that originated from the posterior temporal lobe statistically significantly changed during late face processing (600–700 ms) after stimulus, rather than in early face processing activities, such as P1 and N170 responses. Source localization revealed that the conditioned neutral faces increased activity in the right fusiform gyrus (FG). This study also developed an efficient method for detecting implicit negative emotional responses to specific faces by using EEG signals. A classification method based on a support vector machine enables the easy classification of neutral faces that trigger specific individual emotions. In accordance with this classification, a face on a computer morphs into a sad or displeased countenance. The proposed method could be incorporated as a part of non-verbal communication tools to enable emotional expression.

Keywords: neutral faces, source localization, aversive conditioning, face recognition, electroencephalogram, brain computer interfaces

INTRODUCTION

Unlike assistive technology for verbal communication, the brain-machine or brain-computer interface (BMI/BCI) has not been sufficiently established as a non-verbal communication tool for amyotrophic lateral sclerosis (ALS) patients (Nijboer et al., 2009; Tomik and Guiloff, 2010). Although face-to-face communication provides rich emotional information, late-stage ALS patients may experience difficulties in expressing their emotions because the disorder causes severe muscular paralysis (Iversen et al., 2008; Nijboer et al., 2009). Similarly, autistic individuals cannot adequately communicate negative feelings during non-verbal communication (Dalton et al., 2005). Emotions in these individuals will be easily predicted by looking at emotional facial expressions of visitors (e.g., positive feelings triggered by smiling faces and negative feelings stimulated by angry faces). However, people feel certain emotions even when observing an inexpressive face that is associated with an experience or socially relevant memory. Emotional prediction induced by inexpressive faces of visitors will necessitate advanced judgment underlain by various brain activities.

A crucial component of smooth communication is the ability to discern emotional states from facial expressions. Previous neuroimaging studies have implicated the fusiform gyrus (FG) and superior temporal sulcus (STS) as specifically involved in face processing activities (George et al., 1999; Leppänen and Nelson, 2009). This finding is supported by evidence that FG lesions in patients with prosopagnosia impair the ability to perceive facial configurations (Sergent and Signoret, 1992; Barton et al., 2002). The neural system for face perception is divided into a core system (the inferior occipital gyrus, lateral FG, and STS) for visual analysis and an extended system [intraparietal sulcus, amygdala (AMG), insula, etc.] for cognitive functioning in attention, mouth movement, facial expression or identity, and emotion (Haxby et al., 2000).

Healthy people easily respond to facial expressions that communicate happiness, sadness, and anger by using similar facial expressions. Although a patient with severe ALS cannot effectively form facial expressions, family members and carers could, to a certain extent, notice the patient's emotions from facial expressions in visitors. That is, the emotions in the patient will similarly correspond with the facial expressions at which he/she is looking (Keltner and Ekman, 2000). However, a more difficult requirement in coping with social situations is the ability to read an individual's emotional responses to neutral faces. In particular, a person may feel certain emotions when encountering neutral expressions that are associated with previous experiences. However, ALS or autistic individuals cannot directly express their emotions—a situation that diminishes their quality of life. For individuals who are unable to summon appropriate facial expressions during communication, desirable technologies are passive or affective BCIs (Nijboer et al., 2009; Zander et al., 2010) that enable the communication of specific emotions. Such technologies should facilitate real-time reception of and response to patients' emotions rather than be restricted to interpreting facial expressions.

Even a neutral face associated with previous information or memory (e.g., previously observed behavior and personal characteristics, familiar situations, etc.) can elicit various emotions (Todorov et al., 2007) and enhance brain activities (Kleinhans et al., 2007; Taylor et al., 2009). Experimental conditioning studies indicated that specific cues (e.g., angry or fearful faces) associated with negative feelings modulate AMG activity (Morris et al., 2001; Knight et al., 2009). Despite the progress made in research, however, a comprehensive conditioning study on inexpressive faces associated with negative emotions has not been conducted, with specific focus on the rapid neural dynamics (e.g., <1 s) in human cortex networks.

Although the effects of conditioned neutral faces remain unknown, previous studies on electromagnetic brain activity revealed significant electrical responses to faces at 100-ms (P1) and 170-ms (N170) latencies. P1 amplitudes in occipital regions are facilitated by visual stimuli, such as fearful faces (Pourtois et al., 2004). Specific N170 responses are characterized by posterior temporal negative deflection (Bentin et al., 1996; Eimer, 2000) and are slightly but more significantly enhanced in response to fearful faces than to other facial expressions (Batty and Taylor, 2003; Pegna et al., 2008). These face-specific amplitudes may therefore vary even when an individual looks at negatively conditioned inexpressive faces because of the modulation of emotional valances on the basis of individual experience.

Event-related potential (ERP) amplitudes for face stimuli have not been adequately elucidated. For example, some researchers showed that both famous and unfamiliar faces elicit identical amplitudes (Eimer, 2000; Schweinberger et al., 2002); they argue that late-period processing (e.g., 300–500 ms) is more important than early-period processing in the recognition of facial expressions or movements. By contrast, other studies revealed that familiar faces can enhance N170 amplitudes (Rossion et al., 1999; Caharel et al., 2002). In clarifying the reasons for the incongruence in results, a potentially promising approach is applying source localization to total channel responses to determine novel ways of explaining neuronal dynamics in the cortex, even under slightly differing EEG responses between experimental conditions.

Source localization supports the enhanced activation of the lateral FG at P1 and N170 latencies, such as the activation observed in the direct perception of facial expressions (Utama et al., 2009) and face processing during imaginary situations (Ganis and Schendan, 2008). Nevertheless, in the brain's neural response to inexpressive faces giving rise to negative emotions, definitive conclusions regarding the effects of source localization remain elusive. The primary purpose of this study, therefore, was to investigate the effects of aversively conditioned neutral faces on rapid central responses and evaluate the potential of electroencephalogram (EEG) signals as tools for detecting such responses. Source localization was performed to identify cortical activities. The emotions evoked by individual experience with a specific person may cause changes in physiological characteristics during rapid face processing.

If EEG signals can detect actual emotional responses to specific inexpressive faces, the results could be incorporated into the design and development of BMI/BCI-based non-verbal communication tools. Brain signals, such as EEG, magnetoencephalography (MEG), near-infrared spectroscopy, and electrocorticogram (ECoG) data, can be integrated with BMI/BCI functionality, thereby enabling the development of technologies that offer advantages to paralyzed patients (Lebedev and Nicolelis, 2006). In particular, ECoG or intracortical single-unit recordings show high spatial resolution and good signal-to-noise (S/N) ratio. Despite the advantage of this method, however, the invasive nature of the measurement may present technical difficulties and pose clinical risks (Leuthardt et al., 2004). By contrast, EEG or MEG signals can be non-invasively measured regardless of low spatial resolution and the presence of artificial noise (Gramfort et al., 2010). To improve poor S/N ratios, researchers have applied a wavelet transform with reasonable noise reduction to the single-trial classification of EEG signals (Tallon-Baudry et al., 1996; Hsu and Sun, 2009). EEG signals are also convenient for everyday measurement because EEG equipment is inexpensive and portable.

Because substantial changes in the EEG signals measured by scalp electrodes can be easily detected, extensive brain activity in the cortex (e.g., P300 responses) has been successfully employed in active BMI/BCI studies (Piccione et al., 2006; Mak et al., 2012). For non-verbal communication, the FG and STS regions are specifically involved in face processing (George et al., 1999; Hoffman and Haxby, 2000). For example, electrodes placed around posterior temporal regions can detect strong electrical responses to human faces, with the responses exhibiting 100-ms (P1) and 170-ms (N170) latencies (Bentin et al., 1996; Eimer, 2000). Especially for ALS patients who cannot freely move or speak, an important component of smooth communication is the ability to convey the emotions triggered by facial recognition to support persons. In this regard, therefore, real-time

BMI/BCI-based face recognition is a desirable next-generation application of EEG signals for the facilitation of non-verbal communication.

Support vector machines (SVMs) are useful and efficient methods for classifying biological signals (Lotte et al., 2007). However, a few problems are presented by parameter settings for SVMs that are directly linked to accuracy. To consider approaches to the use of BMI/BCIs with EEG signals, an essential requirement may be the abstraction of brain activity at functional frequencies under reduced artificial noise (Tallon-Baudry et al., 1996). Such issues are effectively addressed by time–frequency analyses (Kashihara et al., 2009), which could also elucidate the neural activities that are crucial for face processing. The time–frequency data for an SVM classifier enable the efficient extraction of meaningful changes in ERP responses. Accordingly, the second purpose of this study was to develop and evaluate an analytical method in which an SVM classifier evaluates negative emotional responses to inexpressive faces. The method was developed on the basis of time–course and time–frequency EEG data. A face morphing application triggered by the SVM classifier was also tested to determine its utility in non-verbal communication.

STUDY 1: EEG MEASUREMENT

Using EEG signals, this study investigated the effects of aversively conditioned neutral faces on rapid central responses. The emotions induced by individual experience with a specific person may modify the physiological characteristics that arise during face processing.

MATERIALS AND METHODS

Participants

A total of 22 right-handed healthy volunteers from Nagoya University were recruited for the study. The physiological responses of the 12 participants (6 males and 6 females; age: 27.0 ± 0.9 years) to conditioned neutral faces were examined. The remaining 10 participants (see Section Basic Study of Neutral Face Stimuli) were asked to take part in a basic experiment to evaluate the equality of the face stimuli used in this work. All the participants had normal or corrected-to-normal vision and had no history of serious medical problems. This study was approved by the ethics committee of our institute. Written informed consent was obtained from all the participants after they were provided an adequate description of the experiment.

Stimuli

Five inexpressive faces, as visual stimuli, were selected from the Japanese Female Facial Expression (JAFFE) database[1]. Thirty scenery images without artificial objects (e.g., skies, mountains, seas, etc.) were collected from free web sources. All the images were converted into grayscale bitmap images. The visual stimuli were presented on a 21-inch CRT monitor (640 × 640 pixels, with a resolution of 1024 × 768 pixels) that was positioned at the same height as the participants' eyes. The distance from the stimuli was set at 140 cm, indicating a visual angle within almost 5°. During the experiments, a loudspeaker was placed behind a participant and a 100-dB white noise burst was used as the auditory stimulus (Morris et al., 1998).

Procedure

After the sensors for the EEG measurement were attached onto the participants, they were asked to view a short series of images (10 trials) during the acclimation period. They were first asked to rate three face images, after which the two-phase experiment was initiated. The two phases were (1) aversive conditioning to a neutral face (*conditioning* phase) and (2) physiological measurement using the conditioned stimuli (*data acquisition* phase).

Conditioning phase. **Figure 1A** shows the experimental procedure adopted in the conditioning phase. A 500-ms "start" stimulus was followed by an interstimulus interval (ISI) between 800 and 1200 ms, after which one of the two faces selected from the dataset was presented onscreen for 1 s. A single neutral face (conditioned stimulus: CS+) was always followed by a 500-ms noise burst; the other face (CS−) was not paired with the noise burst. Fifty percent of all the face stimuli were of CS+ type (or CS−), and the image types were presented in random order. To evaluate the difference between the two faces, the participants were asked to press the left and right keys for the first and second faces, respectively. Intertrial interval (ITI) was varied between 5 and 6 s. This phase comprised 40 trials (20 trials under each stimulus condition). After all the trials were completed and the participants finished their 5-min rest period, the next phase was initiated.

Data acquisition phase. **Figure 1B** shows the experimental procedure used in the data acquisition phase. A 500-ms "start" stimulus was followed by an ISI jittered between 800 and 1200 ms.

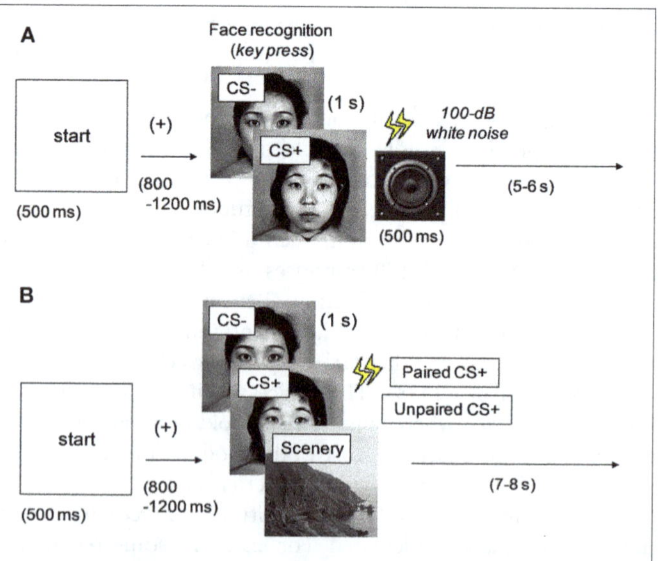

FIGURE 1 | Experimental procedures in the (A) conditioning and (B) data acquisition phases. One of the multiple images was presented at every trial. CS+, aversively conditioned face stimuli; CS−, unconditioned stimuli. All the faces were neutral; CS+ was followed by a noise burst in **(A)** (all) and **(B)** (50%).

[1]Lyons, M. J., Kamachi, M., and Gyoba, J. (1997). *Japanese Female Facial Expressions (JAFFE), Database of digital images.* Available online at: http://www.kasrl.org/jaffe_info.html

One of the two faces (CS+ and CS−) used in the conditioning phase or a scenery image (randomly selected from the dataset) was presented for 1 s. The images in the three types (unconditioned and conditioned neutral faces and scenery) were presented in random order. Half of the CS+ images were followed by a 500-ms noise burst (paired CS+), whereas the rest were presented without sound (unpaired CS+). This method was intended to efficiently maintain the effect of aversive or fear conditioning and was based on a procedure discussed in previous studies (Büchel et al., 1998; Morris et al., 2001). The CS− faces were always followed by silence, and the ITI was between 7 and 8 s.

This phase was initiated in three blocks, with each block involving 72 trials (24 trials for each image type). The rest period between the blocks was 5 min. To enable the participants to concentrate on the tasks, they were asked to press a key as quickly as possible when the cue stimulus of a railroad image was presented twice in a block. The participants were asked to refrain from body movements during the physiological measurement and to refrain from blinking during the image presentations. The face images (CS+, CS−, and a dummy) were also rated at the final period of the experiment.

Data acquisition

EEG recording. EEGs were recorded using EGI Inc.'s HydroCel Geodesic Sensor Net (65 channels) in accordance with the international 10-10 electrode system. The signals from an EEG amplifier (Net Amps 300) were sampled at 500 Hz with data acquisition software (Net Station ver. 4.2). The electrode impedances for all channels were kept below 50 kΩ, as recommended by EGI Inc. The EEG amplifier used in this study can record input with high electrode impedance, without the attachments causing scalp abrasions and without the need for a recording paste and gel. The recording net with electrodes uses a saline solution for the electrical conductor, thereby resulting in high electrode impedances. The high impedances are regulated by the amplifiers to guarantee recording accuracy (Ferree et al., 2001). The features of the EEG amplifier are also highly useful in EEG recordings for patients who cannot withstand lengthy setup procedures or painful scalp abrasions.

Rating of face stimuli. The participants were asked to rate neutral faces (0 = not at all, 1 = mild, 2 = moderate, 3 = strong, and 4 = extreme) to evaluate the changes in the emotions that arose [fear, anxiety, aversion, discomfort, anger, relief, favor, and pleasure in relation to social situations (Nesse, 2005)] before and after the experiment. Three images of neutral faces were randomly chosen from the database and presented onscreen; these images were the same as the CS+ and CS− faces and a dummy image that had not been presented in the previous experiments. The participants reported the emotions that they instantaneously experienced when they looked at the presented faces. In the final rating, the degree to which they experienced unpleasant feelings upon exposure to the noise burst (a five-point scale of 0–4) was confirmed by oral declaration.

Data analysis and statistics

All data are expressed as mean ± standard error. p-values less than 0.05 were considered statistically significant.

Event-related potentials. The average reference montage and a digital bandpass filter of 1–30 Hz were applied offline. For all the conditions, the EEG signals were segmented into epochs ranging from 100 ms before stimulus onset to 700 ms after stimulus onset. Baseline correction was performed by subtracting the mean of the 100-ms pre-stimulus interval from the data after stimulus onset. Trials in which ocular activity was greater than ±50 μV within a 50-ms period or movement artifacts with amplitudes exceeding ±200 μV were excluded from analysis. Although noise due to micromovements may contaminate EEG signals, sufficient signal averaging can eliminate as much of this noise as possible. After the trials were averaged in each condition, the grand average among the participants was calculated. Data on cue stimuli with key presses were excluded from the analysis. The regions of interest were the left (P7, P9, TP9) and right (P8, P10, TP10) posterior temporal regions that are correlated with face processing; the bilateral occipital electrodes (O1 and O2) that are related to attention in the primary visual cortex were used in the P1 analysis.

In the ERP responses at the posterior temporal regions, the maximum values between 60 and 120 ms and the minimum values between 100 and 200 ms were defined as P1 and N170 responses, respectively. For every amplitude in the early (P1 and N170) and late (average between 200 and 700 ms under a 100-ms analysis window) ERP components, repeated Two-Way ANOVA [two levels (left and right) in the bilateral recording sites; three levels (CS+, CS−, and scenery) in the presented images] was performed. In significant main effects, the Holm method was used for multiple comparisons.

Source localization. Standardized low-resolution electromagnetic tomography (sLORETA, the LORETA-KEY software package) was used for source localization, which has a possibility to estimate the local region from which cortical generators originate in each time window by solving the inverse problem (Pascual-Marqui, 2002). Because sLORETA analysis depends on noise levels (Grave de Peralta Menendez et al., 2009), the EEG data obtained after sufficient signal averaging were applied in the source localization. The solution space of sLORETA is restricted to 6239 voxels with a 5-mm^3 cortical gray matter.

The average of the post-stimulus period between 50 and 700 ms was compared with that of the baseline (100-ms pre-stimulus period) in each condition. The sLORETA images for the average of the ERP data in the P1 (60–120 ms), N170 (120–150 ms), and post-stimulus periods between 200 and 700 ms (100-ms time window without overlap: five windows) were then calculated to compare the difference between the CS+ and CS− conditions. The P1 and N170 periods that were analyzed were determined from the results on the ERP responses.

The statistical non-parametric map with smoothing and linear scaling (Nichols and Holmes, 2002) was used to estimate the significantly activated parts determined from the source localization between the CS+ and CS− conditions. Voxel-by-voxel t-tests of the LORETA images were performed. The significance threshold was based on a permutation test (6000 rounds). The corrected t-values were plotted onto a magnetic resonance imaging (MRI) template (Colin27 brain, T2-weighted images) with a color scale bar. As an experimental limitation, the correct location may have been slightly shifted because a standard brain template

(Colin27 brain) was used for each subject. All the *p*-values were one-tailed. Results are presented in the Montreal Neurological Institute coordinates with assigned Brodmann's area labels.

Rating of face stimuli. The first rating scores were subtracted from the final scores. A positive value indicates increased appeal and a negative value indicates the opposite. The extent to which the participants experienced unpleasant feelings upon exposure to the noise burst was calculated as the average across all the participants.

For the changes in rating scores before and after the conditioning experiment, repeated Two-Way ANOVA (three levels of CS+, CS−, and dummy images and eight levels of basic and social emotions) (Nesse, 2005) was carried out under the assumption of an equal-interval scale. For significant main effects, the Holm method was used for multiple comparisons.

RESULTS

ERP responses

Figure 2 shows the grand average of the ERP responses in the (**Figure 2A**) bilateral posterior temporal regions and (**Figure 2B**) two-dimensional topography at the focused latencies. At around 90 ms from face stimulus onset, the peak positive potential (P1) appeared, followed by a considerable negative potential (N170) at around 140 ms. Especially for late latency (600 ms in **Figure 2B**), the topographical maps of EEG activity changed across the image types.

ANOVA revealed the main effects of the image condition in the P1 [$F_{(2, 44)} = 4.15$, $p < 0.05$] and N170 amplitudes [$F_{(2, 44)} = 63.67$, $p < 0.01$] at the posterior temporal lobe. The N170 values for the face images were significantly ($p < 0.01$) greater than that for the scenery image in each hemisphere. However, these values did not significantly differ between CS+ and CS−. For the P1 amplitude at the occipital electrodes (O1 and O2), the main effects and interaction were statistically non-significant.

For the ERP responses between 200 and 700 ms (100-ms time window), ANOVA indicated that type of image exerted significant main effects: $p < 0.01$ in each period. For all the time windows, the average ERP values for the face images in each hemisphere were significantly lower than that for the scenery ($p < 0.01$). Especially in the period between 600 and 700 ms [$F_{(2, 44)} = 28.72$, significant main effect], the CS+ value in the right hemisphere decreased to a more significant extent than did the CS− value ($p < 0.05$).

Source localization

Table 1 shows the statistically significant regions among all the participants (baseline vs. post-stimulus response) in each experimental condition. In relation to the baseline, the significant areas localized by sLORETA ($p < 0.05$) were the bilateral FG, inferior temporal gyrus, and middle temporal gyrus for both the CS+ and CS− conditions. Especially in the CS+ condition, the right hemisphere exhibited stronger activity than did the left hemisphere. During the 600–700-ms latency, the right FG was more significantly activated under CS+ than under CS− (**Figure 3**; $p < 0.05$).

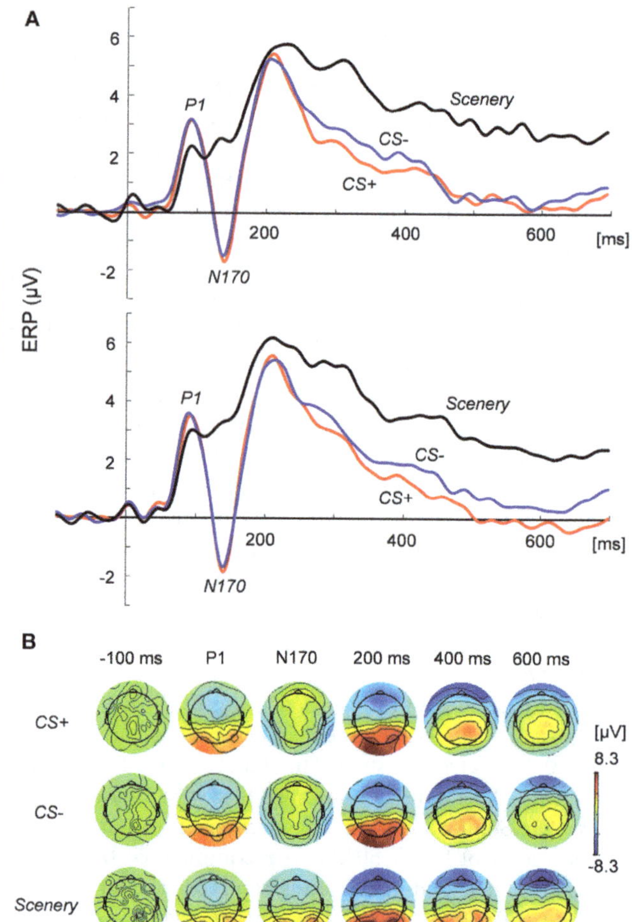

FIGURE 2 | ERP responses to and topography of the presented images. **(A)** ERP responses at the left (*top*) and right (*bottom*) posterior temporal regions under the CS+, CS−, and scenery conditions. **(B)** Two-dimensional topography of the presented images at P1, N170, and latencies of −100 (pre-stimulus), 200, 400, and 600 ms.

Rating of face stimuli

Figure 4 illustrates the affective changes found under the three face conditions. Overall, the rating scores for CS+ tended to reflect increased negative emotions and decreased positive emotions. ANOVA revealed the main effect of emotion [$F_{(7, 252)} = 6.17$, $p < 0.01$] and significant interaction [type of image × emotion, $F_{(14, 252)} = 4.54$, $p < 0.01$]. In the items showing a significant simple main effect, the CS+ and CS− conditions significantly differed in the rating scores for aversion ($p < 0.05$), discomfort ($p < 0.01$), relief ($p < 0.01$), and pleasure ($p < 0.05$). The changes in the scores for aversion ($p < 0.05$) and discomfort ($p < 0.05$) in the face under CS+ were significantly higher than those derived when the dummy was presented. The extent to which unpleasant feelings were experienced upon exposure to the noise burst was 3.0 ± 0.3 (75% of the max. score).

BASIC STUDY OF NEUTRAL FACE STIMULI

The same procedure as that applied in the data acquisition phase (see Section Procedure) was performed to evaluate the effect of

Table 1 | Brain areas of significant activity ($p < 0.05$) under the face image types in relation to the baseline.

Region	Side	MNI coordinates (mm)			*t*-value max	Voxels	BA
		x	*y*	*z*			
CS+ vs. BASELINE							
FG	Left	−55	−40	−30	9.5	5	20, 37
	Right	55	−40	−30	13.3	34	19, 20, 36, 37
ITG	Left	−55	−5	−40	10.2	5	20, 37
	Right	60	−35	−25	12.3	36	20, 37
MTG	Left	–	–	–	–	0	–
	Right	60	−45	−20	11.8	21	20, 21, 37, 38
CS− vs. BASELINE							
FG	Left	−55	−40	−30	16.7	44	19, 20, 36, 37
	Right	55	−40	−30	15.2	39	19, 20, 36, 37
ITG	Left	−55	−5	−40	17.2	50	20, 37
	Right	60	−35	−25	14.1	38	20, 37
MTG	Left	−60	−45	−20	15.5	31	20, 21, 37, 38
	Right	60	−45	−20	13.6	20	20, 21, 37, 38

CS+, conditioned stimulus; CS−, unconditioned stimulus. BA, Brodmann's areas; FG, fusiform gyrus; ITG, inferior temporal gyrus; MTG, middle temporal gyrus.

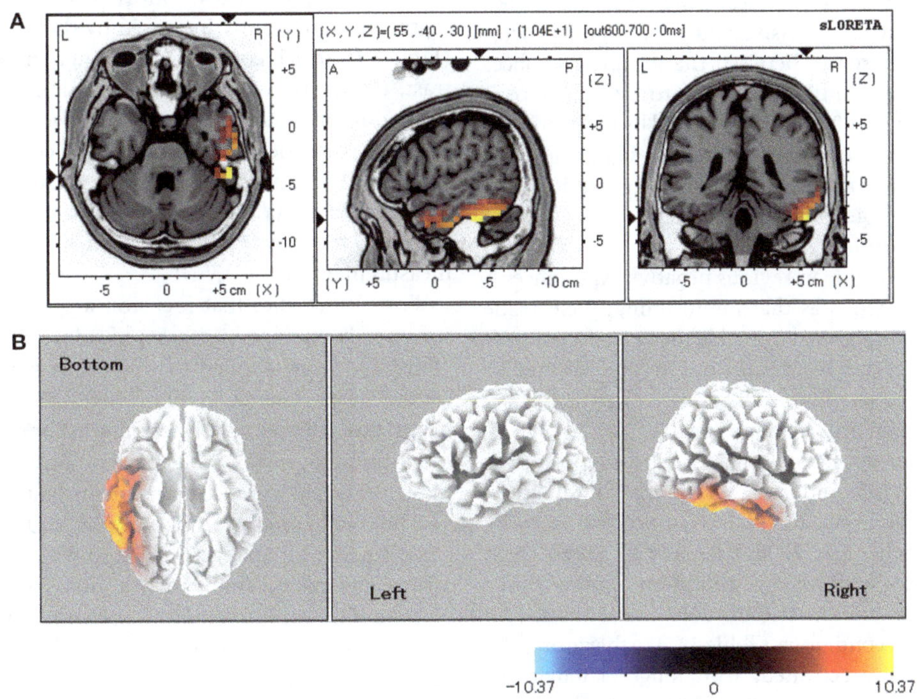

FIGURE 3 | sLORETA comparison of source localizations between the CS+ and CS− conditions. (A) MRI planes (Colin27 brain) in the axial, sagittal, and coronal views and **(B)** cortical maps from the bottom, left, and right sides of the average among the 600–700-ms latencies (CS+ vs. CS−). The statistically significant regions acquired from all the subjects were displayed on a standard brain template in **(A)**. The source estimation indicates the significant roles ($p < 0.05$ for all the subjects) of the right lateral fusiform gyrus.

neutral face stimuli under no condition (7 males and 3 females; age: 25.0 ± 0.7). The ITI was between 5 and 6 s because no aversive conditioning was applied. The parameters for the ERP responses (P1, N170, and latencies between 200 and 700 ms) and the significant source localization sites were statistically evaluated. The neutral faces exhibited no significant differences in terms of ERP response amplitudes and source estimation ($p > 0.05$), indicating equality across the image dataset.

DISCUSSION 1

Even for the inexpressive faces, aversive conditioning in which the noise burst was used induced a posteriori negative feelings.

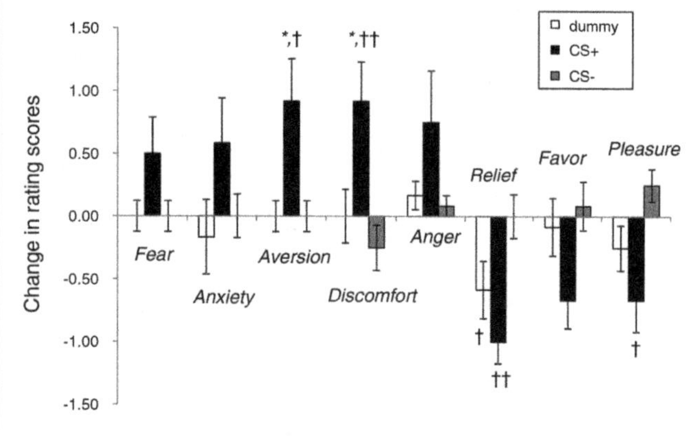

FIGURE 4 | Changes in the rating scores of emotional responses to neutral face stimuli before and after the conditioning experiments. $^{*}p < 0.05$ vs. a dummy; $^{\dagger\dagger}p < 0.01$, $^{\dagger}p < 0.05$ vs. CS−.

Although greater attention was paid to the faces than to the scenery, the CS+ and CS− conditions exhibited statistically non-significant differences in the N170 amplitudes in the posterior temporal regions and the P1 amplitudes at the O1 and O2 sites. This result indicates that an extensive and meaningful process of distinguishing the differences between the inexpressive faces would have worked, except in the early face processing. By contrast, the late ERP response (600–700 ms) evoked by the aversively conditioned neutral faces resulted in a statistically significant ERP component at the electrodes attached around the posterior temporal lobe; this result suggests the involvement of higher face recognition functions (Eimer, 2000) under situations wherein expressions are associated with a previous negative experience. A limitation of the experiment was that the meaningful electrode positions were carefully established to enable the detection of EEG responses. Nevertheless, other brain functions may be detected or missed, depending on region of interest. Severe ALS patients may also cause attenuated brain activity (Guo et al., 2010).

For facial expression or mental imagery, previous studies involving source estimation indicated that some brain areas, including the FG, are activated for early face processing at P1 and N170 (Ganis and Schendan, 2008; Utama et al., 2009). Even for the inexpressive faces with aversive conditioning, the source estimation in this study indicated continuous FG activation in both the CS+ and CS− conditions (**Table 1**). Furthermore, the right FG was significantly activated, with longer latencies of 600–700 ms under CS+ than under CS− (**Figure 3**). This result presumably reflects aversively conditioned responses to incoming noise burst.

The AMG is activated by short-term fear or aversive conditioning (Büchel et al., 1998; Morris et al., 2001; Knight et al., 2009), and viewing emotional faces effectively increases the connectivity between the AMG and FG (Leppänen and Nelson, 2009). The mental imaging of a face can also enhance FG activity (Ganis and Schendan, 2008). These findings suggest that recalling a conditioned face that reflects negative emotions similarly activates the FG and AMG. Because the results of the present study (**Table 1**, **Figure 3**) showed strong activation of the inferior temporal cortex (FG) rather than the STS, negative learning may have been performed via the inferior network for face recognition, through which the AMG and FG were accessed (Morris et al., 1998; Knight et al., 2009). The STS is generally activated by the recognition of gaze direction or facial expressions of emotion (Haxby et al., 2000). Because the visual targets (i.e., inexpressive faces) of the aversive conditioning in this study did not feature such dynamic movements, the STS activity may not have influenced conditioned facial perception and/or recognition.

The central responses were modulated primarily at the right sides of the FG; this modulation is related to the aversively conditioned neutral face stimuli. The activated area (**Table 1**) on the left-side FG (vs. the right side) under CS+ decreased to 1/7 (5 vs. 34 voxels), whereas the ratio under CS− (44 vs. 39 voxels) generally remained at around 1. This result presumably reflects the intensive recruitment of right-side neural functions in predicting impending danger. This finding is supported by previous studies in which the right-side FG activity in patients with prosopagnosia was dominant (Barton et al., 2002); this activity also dominated even during presentations of a fearful face to healthy participants (Pegna et al., 2008).

The aversion and discomfort reflected by the emotional ratings were significantly increased by the conditioned neutral face (**Figure 4**), which could trigger changes in brain activity. By contrast, the fearful emotion was non-significantly correlated with the conditioned neutral faces, which would have failed to induce the ERP responses (i.e., early face processing responses, such as P1 and N170) specific to typical fear stimuli (Batty and Taylor, 2003; Pegna et al., 2008). Note, however, that the participants in this study may have experienced unconscious fear during the EEG measurement.

For ERP studies that focus on a specific stimulus, sLORETA software is equipped with a procedure for baseline correction, which has been applied in numerous studies on source localization (e.g., Utama et al., 2009; Scharmüller et al., 2011). Nevertheless, baseline correction must be carefully used in source localization given the occurrence of local changes in each sensor location (http://www.electrical-neuroimaging.ch/faq.html).

The mathematical constraint in LORETA software is the smoothness of spatial activation, in which neighbor neurons are assumed to exhibit similar activations. From direct measurement on neural tissue, active states are characterized by a reduction in the synchrony of adjacent neurons (Cruikshank and Connors, 2008; Poulet and Petersen, 2008). Contrary to the LORETA hypothesis, sluggish states may be identified by the similarity in activity of neighbor neurons under a defined time window for source localization (Grave de Peralta Menendez and Andino, 2000).

The conditioned faces further emphasized activity in the right FG (i.e., face-selective cells) during late facial processing. The EEG equipment detected responses at the posterior temporal regions; these responses reflect activity in face-responsive neurons. Neutral stimuli other than faces would affect various brain areas with different EEG responses. Expert object recognition may stimulate the same face-selective cells (Tanaka and Curran, 2001), although such recognition is a rare response.

STUDY 2: APPLICATION OF A BRAIN-COMPUTER INTERFACE

Study 1 revealed that the posterior temporal lobe ERP responses to the aversively conditioned neutral faces significantly changed during late face processing. As previously stated, this study developed an efficient method for classifying implicit negative emotional responses to specific neutral faces by using EEG signals.

MATERIALS AND METHODS

Classification by SVM

The SVM classifier for determining a hyperplane that optimally separates samples from two classes with the largest margin (Cortes and Vapnik, 1995; Cristianini and Shawe-Taylor, 2000) was used in this study. An optimal SVM separating hyperplane is calculated by solving constrained optimization thus:

$$\min_{z,b,\xi}\left(\frac{1}{2}\|z\|^2 + C\sum_{i=1}^{l}\xi_i\right). \tag{1}$$

Equation (1) is subject to $y_i(z \cdot \phi(x_i) + b) + \xi_i \geq 1$ and $\xi_i \geq 0$ $(i = 1, \cdots, l)$, where l is the number of training vectors, $y_i \in \{-1, +1\}$ denotes the class label of the output, and $\|z\|^2 = z^T z$ represents the squared Euclidean norm. Weight parameter z determines the orientation of the separating hyperplane, b is a bias, ξ_i is the ith positive slack parameter, and ϕ shows a non-linear mapping function. Parameter C indicates the penalty term. With a large C, a high penalty is assigned to training errors. The two points closest to the hyperplane substantially affect the orientation, thereby resulting in a hyperplane that is close to other data points. With a small C, these points move inside the margin and the orientation of the hyperplane changes, thereby generating a large margin. To address this issue, a formulation of the SVM that uses the parameter $0 < \nu \leq 1$ can be applied. This parameter can regulate the fractions of support vectors and margin errors (ν-SVM).

The vector $\phi(x_i)$ that corresponds to a non-zero value is a support vector of the optimal hyperplane. A desirable approach is to use a small number of support vectors to complete a compact classifier. The optimal separating hyperplane is calculated as a decision surface of the form sgn:

$$f(x) = \text{sgn}\left(\sum_{i=1}^{L}\alpha_i y_i K(x_i, x) + b\right), \tag{2}$$

where $\text{sgn}(.) \in \{-1, +1\}$. K is the non-linear kernel function, and it projects samples to a high-dimension feature space via a non-linear mapping function. L is the number of support vectors. As the non-linear kernel, the radial basis function is defined as

$$K(x_i, x_j) = \exp\left(-\gamma\|x_i - x_j\|^2\right), \tag{3}$$

where the value of the kernel parameter γ determines the variance of the function.

Features for SVM

Figure 5A shows the diagram of the BCI based on the SVM classifier and face morphing application. Time–course and time–frequency data for the SVM classifier were extracted from the ERP responses to the face and scenery images.

(a) Time–course data: The time–course data that averaged between 600 and 700 ms at the right (P8, P10, TP10) posterior temporal regions were abstracted as the SVM features. These data correspond to the considerable change in the ERP responses to visual stimuli (**Figure 2A**).
(b) Time–frequency data: The time–frequency data obtained from the wavelet transform of raw data were regarded as the SVM features because raw signals can contaminate external noise. The EEG signals were convoluted by the complex Morlet wavelet (Tallon-Baudry et al., 1996; Kashihara et al., 2009) as follows:

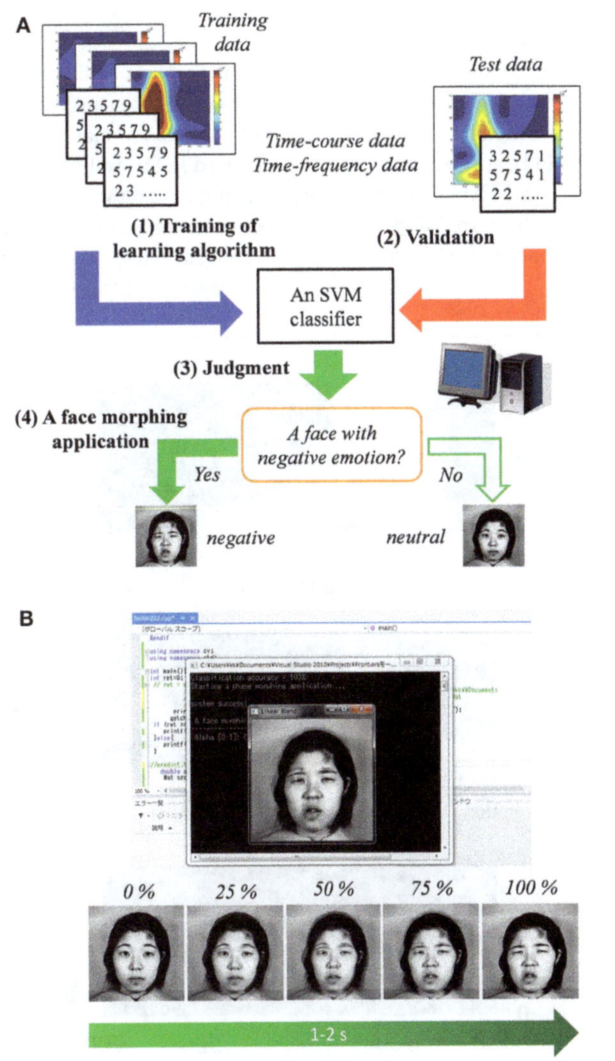

FIGURE 5 | (A) Diagram of the proposed method in which a support vector machine (SVM) classifier is used. **(B)** Illustration of the face morphing software triggered by the classifier's result.

$$w(t, f_0) = \exp\left(\frac{-t^2}{2\sigma_t^2}\right) \cdot \exp(2\pi f_0 it)/\sqrt{\sigma_t\sqrt{\pi}}. \quad (4)$$

The standard deviation of the time domain (σ_t) is inversely proportional to the standard deviation of the frequency domain $[\sigma_f = (2\pi\sigma_t)^{-1}]$. The effective number of oscillation cycles in the wavelet ($f_0/\sigma f$) was set at 6, with f_0 ranging from 4 to 12 Hz (i.e., theta and alpha bands) in increments of 0.1 Hz. After the subtraction of a linear trend, the continuous wavelet transform of a time series $[u(t)]$ was calculated as the convolution of a complex wavelet with $u(t)$: $\tilde{u}(t, f_0) = w(t, f_0) * u(t)$. The squared norm of the wavelet transform was calculated in a frequency band at around f_0. **Figure 6** shows examples of the wavelet transform in the ERP responses to the presented images. The power spectrum of the wavelet transform in the face stimulus indicated a characterized pattern, compared with that in the scenery stimulus.

VALIDATION OF THE SVM CLASSIFIER

Data and analysis

A 36-fold cross-validation among the three types of categorized data (unconditioned and conditioned neutral faces and scenery) was performed to evaluate the accuracy of the SVM classifier. The tested EEG data were the same as those used in Study 1 (12 participants). An SVM classifier trained by using 35 data was evaluated by using the remaining data (i.e., test data); this procedure was repeated, with modifications to the training and test data (a round robin for all the data: 36 rounds), to calculate classification accuracy. The independent parameter γ in Equation (3) was fixed at a constant value during this cross-validation ($\nu = 0.5$), thereby resulting in changes to the other parameters, such as the optimal objective value of the dual SVM problem and the bias term in the decision function. Here, the independent kernel parameter γ of Equation (3) was set as four types: 0.0001, 0.01, 1, and (number of features)$^{-1}$, and the accuracy of the cross-validation was computed for each kernel parameter. The tolerance of termination criterion for the SVM was set at ε^{-6}.

Classification results

Figure 7 shows the results of the 36-fold cross-validation regarding the performance of the SVM classifier in evaluating the negative emotional responses to inexpressive faces determined from the ERP responses. In both features, the SVM classifier exhibited an accuracy higher (80% at the maximum) than the chance level (i.e., 33% in each). Overall, the classification accuracies for the faces and scenery tended to be higher than those for the CS+ and CS− conditions. However, classification accuracy depended on the kernel parameter value. Compared with the time–course data of the SVM classifier, the wavelet-transform data showed stable accuracy in each category (e.g., almost 70% especially in the kernel parameter $\gamma = 0.01$ and 1), indicating the existence of the optimal parameter setting.

MORPHING APPLICATION

After the SVM classifier was trained by the above-mentioned training sample, the face morphing application (Microsoft

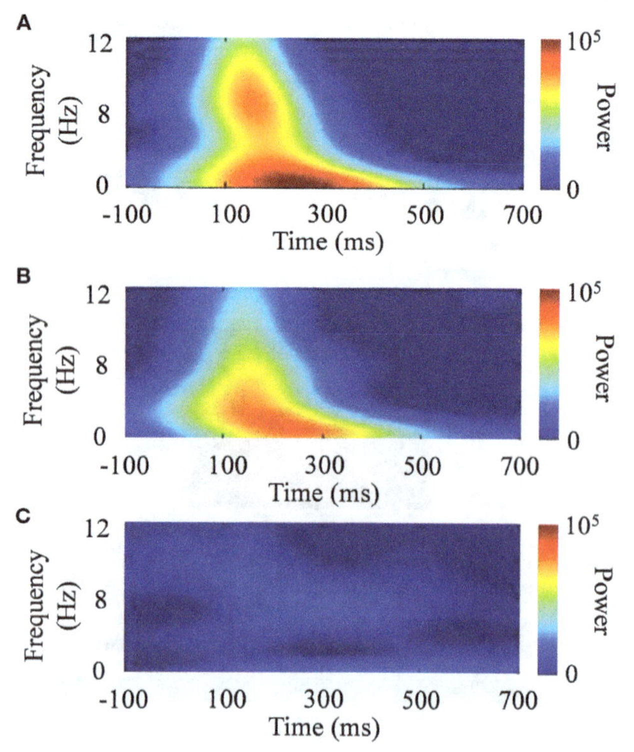

FIGURE 6 | Typical examples of time–frequency responses after the wavelet transform. **(A)** CS+, **(B)** CS−, and **(C)** scenery.

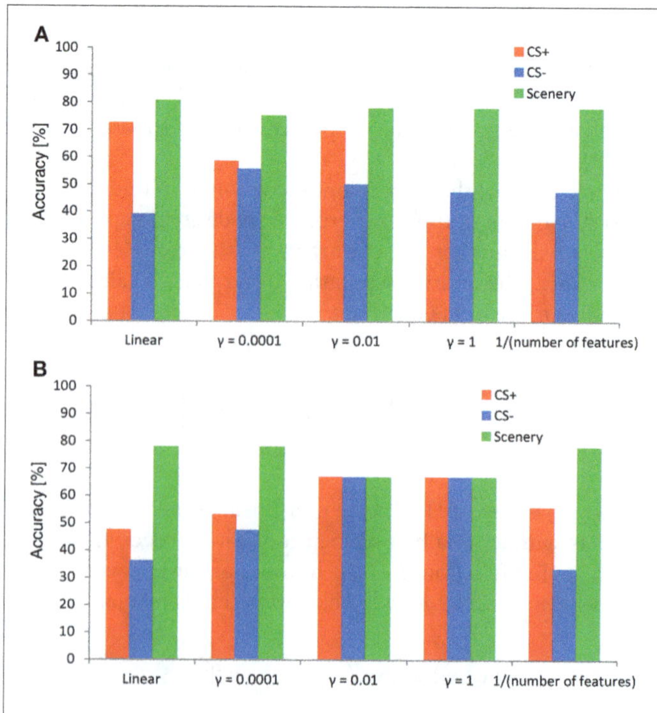

FIGURE 7 | Results of cross-validation using the SVM classifier. The SVM features **(A)** time–course and **(B)** time–frequency data.

Visual C++ 2012, OpenCV ver. 2.4, and LIBSVM ver. 3.17) was tested under the hypothesis of real-time data acquisition. When a neutral face associated with a negative emotion is predicted by the SVM classifier, the face morphing application is automatically triggered. As shown in **Figure 5B**, the target neutral face gradually (about 1–2 s) changed into a negative one (JAFFE database[1]). Therefore, individuals' emotions can be easily estimated using the proposed non-verbal communication tool.

DISCUSSION 2

In Study 2, the SVM classifier for non-verbal communication was evaluated by identifying the ERP responses to implicit emotional faces. For the control of mechanical or computer devices, active BMI/BCI studies have been based on the features of EEG data on various scalp regions (e.g., P300 responses) (Piccione et al., 2006; Mak et al., 2012). The present study especially focused on the activity of the posterior temporal lobe in relation to face processing; the SVM feature was used after the application of the wavelet transform. In the optimal range of the kernel parameter, the SVM classifier for the time–frequency domain showed stable accuracy (almost 70% in each category). Developing an auto-tuning method for appropriate parameter setting of the SVM classifier is an advantageous approach because of the individual differences of ERP responses. Thus, wavelet transform data will be effective for such a case. An accuracy higher than 60% will be regarded as a tentative indicator of a successful case for affective BCIs (Nijboer et al., 2009; Mak et al., 2011). A desirable future direction for BMI/BCI research is the development of small embedded systems for the everyday use of face morphing software that can reflect various emotions.

A critical safety problem arises when a patient experiences a severe accident as a malfunction occurs in active BCIs for basic motion (e.g., wheelchair, artificial arm, etc.). The proposed system is a device intended to enhance quality of life through emotional estimation. When a patient may possibly experience a negative emotion, the people around the patient (e.g., families, friends, and carers) can support him/her by paying particular attention to emotional estimation. If they recognize or predict the patient's negative emotions (e.g., 60 or 70% negative feeling, no perfect or maximum level for each emotion), the patient could live a full and humane life. Nevertheless, further studies on more accurate classifier methods are required. For example, a cascaded classifier may effectively increase classification accuracy.

Time–frequency analyses can identify the neural activities crucial for emotional face processing, but further modifications are required to obtain higher accuracy in SVM classification. This requirement may be satisfied with the direct image analysis (e.g., the bag of features scheme; Csurka et al., 2004) of contour maps in time–frequency data (Kashihara et al., 2011). Speeded-up robust features (SURF) and scale-invariant feature transform (SIFT) can effectively search for local information on object boundary (Bay et al., 2008). In the bag of features scheme, visual words are generated by the k-means algorithm to cluster the feature vectors of SIFT or SURF and create a visual vocabulary (Duda et al., 2001). Each image can be represented by a histogram of visual words. Therefore, the bag of features scheme may serve as a means of novel interpretation that determines the effective features of an SVM classifier and could extract meaningful changes in time–frequency data.

Several limitations constrain the practical application of the BCI approach adopted in this study. The specific brain region considered in the classification was limited to the right FG area identified by source localization from multiple electrodes attached onto a participant's scalp. Crucial issues for consideration are the separation of brain activities into multiple inputs and movement artifacts, which may influence the results of source localization. This study assumed application under a static measurement situation for patients and excluded active BCIs, such as moving artificial arms and wheelchairs. The next step, therefore, is to develop an accurate identifier that enables the practical application of BCIs and reduces noise; noise contamination of muscle or eye movements must be prevented through improvements in hardware, software, and algorithms.

To realize feature extraction from the frequency domain reducing external noise, data after the wavelet transform was used in machine learning (i.e., SVM); this application was implemented under the assumption that practical BCI analysis will be a component of future works. Experiment 2 was then performed to show the possibility of passive or affective BCI application for the detection of and response to high emotions. Therefore, the new techniques for wearable and hardware devices (robust to body movements) and efficient algorithms (e.g., signal filtering methods, including wavelet analysis) to eliminate external noise are desirable innovations for advancing the practical application of BCIs. In such application, accurate estimation from single trials can be factors for consideration.

The conditioned neutral facial stimuli (Experiment 1) were used to induce negative emotions based on previous experiences and to identify the specific brain area that is activated during such responses because dynamic EEG response has not been sufficiently clarified under such situations. As the next step, actual non-verbal communication should be evaluated by using real faces (families, friends, etc.) associated with patients' experiences and emotions.

Finally, the difficulty encountered in BCI training for autistic patients must be considered in the design and development of a practical system. EEG responses to facial stimuli and emotions may not require extensive training on scenarios such as those featuring active BCIs. Because posterior temporal regions are directly correlated with face processing primarily in the right FG, EEG responses might be measured in a straightforward manner, regardless of a specific training program.

CONCLUSION

Inexpressive faces associated with negative experiences induce aversive and unpleasant feelings. The ERP study and source localization revealed that the aversively conditioned neutral faces activated late face processing (600–700 ms), rather than early face processing (e.g., P1 and N170), in the right FG region. Further evaluations of emotionally conditioned faces would elucidate the complicated brain activities involved in social cognition. As a non-verbal communication tool for BMI/BCIs, the proposed SVM classifier has a possibility to enable the easy detection of inexpressive faces that trigger specific individual emotions. In accordance with this classification, a face on a computer morphs into an unpleasant look. In future studies, the proposed classification method, which uses EEG signals, could be integrated with non-verbal communication tools to enable the expression of other emotions. More accurate classifiers should also be investigated to realize the practical application of BMI/BCIs.

ACKNOWLEDGMENTS

This study was partially funded by a Grant-in-Aid for Scientific Research (C) from Japan Society for the Promotion of Science (KAKENHI, 25330171). The author would like to thank Nagoya University and JST for providing assistance during the EEG experiment.

REFERENCES

Barton, J. J., Press, D. Z., Keenan, J. P., and O'Connor, M. (2002). Lesions of the fusiform face area impair perception of facial configuration in prosopagnosia. *Neurology* 58, 71–78. doi: 10.1212/WNL.58.1.71

Batty, M., and Taylor, M. J. (2003). Early processing of the six basic facial emotional expressions. *Brain Res. Cogn. Brain Res.* 17, 613–620. doi: 10.1016/S0926-6410(03)00174-5

Bay, H., Ess, A., Tuytelaars, T., and Gool, L. V. (2008). Speeded-Up Robust Features (SURF). *Comput. Vis. Image Underst.* 110, 346–359. doi: 10.1016/j.cviu.2007.09.014

Bentin, S., Allison, T., Puce, A., Perez, E., and McCarthy, G. (1996). Electrophysiological studies of face perception in humans. *J. Cogn. Neurosci.* 8, 551–565. doi: 10.1162/jocn.1996.8.6.551

Büchel, C., Morris, J., Dolan, R. J., and Friston, K. J. (1998). Brain systems mediating aversive conditioning: an event-related fMRI study. *Neuron* 20, 947–957. doi: 10.1016/S0896-6273(00)80476-6

Caharel, S., Poiroux, S., Bernard, C., Thibaut, F., Lalonde, R., and Rebai, M. (2002). ERPs associated with familiarity and degree of familiarity during face recognition. *Int. J. Neurosci.* 112, 1499–1512. doi: 10.1080/00207450290158368

Cortes, C., and Vapnik, V. N. (1995). Support vector networks. *Mach. Learn.* 20, 273–297. doi: 10.1007/BF00994018

Cristianini, N., and Shawe-Taylor, J. (2000). *Introduction to Support Vector Machines and other Kernel-Based Learning Methods.* Cambridge: Cambridge University Press. doi: 10.1017/CBO9780511801389

Cruikshank, S. J., and Connors, B. W. (2008). Neuroscience: state-sanctioned synchrony. *Nature* 454, 839–840. doi: 10.1038/454839a

Csurka, G., Dance, C. R., Fan, L., Williamowski, J., and Bray, C. (2004). "Visual categorization with bags of keypoints," in *Proceedings of the IEEE Workshop on Statistical Learning in Computer Vision (SLCV'04)* (Prague), 1–16.

Dalton, K. M., Nacewicz, B. M., Johnstone, T., Schaefer, H. S., Gernsbacher, M. A., Goldsmith, H. H., et al. (2005). Gaze fixation and the neural circuitry of face processing in autism. *Nat. Neurosci.* 8, 519–526. doi: 10.1038/nn1421

Duda, R. O., Hart, P. E., and Stork, D. G. (2001). *Pattern Classification, 2nd Edn.* Singapore: John Wiley & Sons.

Eimer, M. (2000). The face-specific N170 component reflects late stages in the structural encoding of faces. *Neuroreport* 11, 2319–2324. doi: 10.1097/00001756-200007140-00050

Ferree, T. C., Luu, P., Russell, G. S., and Tucker, D. M. (2001). Scalp electrode impedance, infection risk, and EEG data quality. *Clin. Neurophysiol.* 112, 536–544. doi: 10.1016/S1388-2457(00)00533-2

Ganis, G., and Schendan, H. E. (2008). Visual mental imagery and perception produce opposite adaptation effects on early brain potentials. *Neuroimage* 42, 1714–1727. doi: 10.1016/j.neuroimage.2008.07.004

George, N., Dolan, R. J., Fink, G. R., Baylis, G. C., Russell, C., and Driver, J. (1999). Contrast polarity and face recognition in the human fusiform gyrus. *Nat. Neurosci.* 2, 574–580. doi: 10.1038/9230

Gramfort, A., Keriven, R., and Clerc, M. (2010). Graph-based variability estimation in single-trial event-related neural responses. *IEEE Trans. Biomed. Eng.* 57, 1051–1061. doi: 10.1109/TBME.2009.2037139

Grave de Peralta Menendez, R., and Andino, S. L. (2000). Discussing the capabilities of Laplacian Minimization. *Brain Topogr.* 13, 97–104. doi: 10.1023/A:1026603017734

Grave de Peralta Menendez, R., Hauk, O., and Gonzalez, S. L. (2009). The neuroelectromagnetic inverse problem and the zero dipole localization error. *Comput. Intell. Neurosci.* 2009:659247. doi: 10.1155/2009/659247

Guo, J., Gao, S., and Hong, B. (2010). An auditory brain-computer interface using active mental response. *IEEE Trans. Neural Syst. Rehabil. Eng.* 18, 230–235. doi: 10.1109/TNSRE.2010.2047604

Haxby, J. V., Hoffman, E. A., and Gobbini, M. I. (2000). The distributed human neural system for face perception. *Trends Cogn. Sci.* 4, 223–233. doi: 10.1016/S1364-6613(00)01482-0

Hoffman, E., and Haxby, J. (2000). Distinct representations of eye gaze and identity in the distributed human neural system for face perception. *Nat. Neurosci.* 3, 80–84. doi: 10.1038/71152

Hsu, W. Y., and Sun, Y. N. (2009). EEG-based motor imagery analysis using weighted wavelet transform features. *J. Neurosci. Methods* 176, 310–318. doi: 10.1016/j.jneumeth.2008.09.014

Iversen, I. H., Ghanayim, N., Kübler, A., Neumann, N., Birbaumer, N., and Kaiser, J. (2008). A brain-computer interface tool to assess cognitive functions in completely paralyzed patients with amyotrophic lateral sclerosis. *Clin. Neurophysiol.* 19, 2214–2223. doi: 10.1016/j.clinph.2008.07.001

Kashihara, K., Ito, M., and Fukumi, M. (2011). "An analytical method for face detection based on image patterns of EEG signals in the time-frequency domain. Workshop on Brain-Machine Interfaces," in *Proceedings of the 2011 IEEE International Conference on Systems, Man, and Cybernetics* (Anchorage), 25–29. doi: 10.1109/ICSMC.2011.6083637

Kashihara, K., Kawada, T., Sugimachi, M., and Sunagawa, K. (2009). Wavelet-based system identification of short-term dynamic characteristics of arterial baroreflex. *Ann. Biomed. Eng.* 37, 112–128. doi: 10.1007/s10439-008-9599-4

Keltner, D., and Ekman, P. (2000). "Facial expression of emotion," in *Handbook of Emotions, 2nd Edn.,* eds M. Lewis and J. M. Haviland-Jones. (New York, NY: Guilford Press), 236–249.

Kleinhans, N. M., Johnson, L. C., Mahurin, R., Richards, T., Stegbauer, K. C., Greenson, J., et al. (2007). Increased amygdala activation to neutral faces is associated with better face memory performance. *Neuroreport* 18, 987–991. doi: 10.1097/WNR.0b013e328165d189

Knight, D. C., Waters, N. S., and Bandettini, P. A. (2009). Neural substrates of explicit and implicit fear memory. *Neuroimage* 45, 208–214. doi: 10.1016/j.neuroimage.2008.11.015

Lebedev, M. A., and Nicolelis, M. A. (2006). Brain-machine interfaces: past, present and future. *Trends Neurosci.* 29, 536–546. doi: 10.1016/j.tins.2006.07.004

Leppänen, J. M., and Nelson, C. A. (2009). Tuning the developing brain to social signals of emotions. *Nat. Rev. Neurosci.* 10, 37–47. doi: 10.1038/nrn2554

Leuthardt, E. C., Schalk, G., Wolpaw, J. R., Ojemann, J. G., and Moran, D. W. (2004). A brain-computer interface using electrocorticographic signals in humans. *J. Neural Eng.* 1, 63–71. doi: 10.1088/1741-2560/1/2/001

Lotte, F., Congedo, M., Lécuyer, A., Lamarche, F., and Arnaldi, B. (2007). A review of classification algorithms for EEG-based brain-computer interfaces. *J. Neural Eng.* 4, R1–R13. doi: 10.1088/1741-2560/4/2/R01

Mak, J. N., Arbel, Y., Minett, J. W., McCane, L. M., Yuksel, B., Ryan, D., et al. (2011). Optimizing the P300-based brain-computer interface: current status, limitations and future directions. *J. Neural Eng.* 8:025003. doi: 10.1088/1741-2560/8/2/025003

Mak, J. N., McFarland, D. J., Vaughan, T. M., McCane, L. M., Tsui, P. Z., Zeitlin, D. J., et al. (2012). EEG correlates of P300-based brain-computer interface (BCI) performance in people with amyotrophic lateral sclerosis. *J. Neural Eng.* 9:026014. doi: 10.1088/1741-2560/9/2/026014

Morris, J. S., Öhman, A., and Dolan, R. J. (1998). Conscious and unconscious emotional learning in the human amygdala. *Nature* 393, 467–470. doi: 10.1038/30976

Morris, J. S., Büchel, C., and Dolan, R. J. (2001). Parallel neural responses in amygdala subregions and sensory cortex during implicit fear conditioning. *Neuroimage* 13, 1044–1052. doi: 10.1006/nimg.2000.0721

Nesse, R. M. (2005). Twelve crucial points about emotions, evolution and mental disorders. *Psychology Review* 11, 12–14. Available online at: http://www.hoddereducation.co.uk/Product?Product=9781471800962

Nichols, T. E., and Holmes, A. P. (2002). Nonparametric permutation tests for functional neuroimaging: a primer with examples. *Hum. Brain Mapp.* 15, 1–25. doi: 10.1002/hbm.1058

Nijboer, F., Carmien, S. P., Leon, E., Morin, F. O., Koene, R. A., and Hoffmann, U. (2009). "Affective brain-computer interfaces: Psychophysiological markers of emotion in healthy persons and in persons with amyotrophic lateral sclerosis," in *Affective Computing and Intelligent Interaction and Workshops, 2009. ACII 2009. 3rd International Conference on* (Amsterdam: IEEE), 1–11. doi: 10.1109/ACII.2009.5349479

Pascual-Marqui, R. D. (2002). Standardized low-resolution brain electromagnetic tomography (sLORETA): technical details. *Methods Find. Exp. Clin. Pharmacol.* 24(Suppl. D), 5–12.

Pegna, A. J., Landis, T., and Khateb, A. (2008). Electrophysiological evidence for early non-conscious processing of fearful facial expressions. *Int. J. Psychophysiol.* 70, 127–136. doi: 10.1016/j.ijpsycho.2008.08.007

Piccione, F., Giorgi, F., Tonin, P., Priftis, K., Giove, S., Silvoni, S., et al. (2006). P300-based brain computer interface: reliability and performance in healthy and paralysed participants. *Clin. Neurophysiol.* 117, 531–537. doi: 10.1016/j.clinph.2005.07.024

Poulet, J. F., and Petersen, C. C. (2008). Internal brain state regulates membrane potential synchrony in barrel cortex of behaving mice. *Nature* 454, 881–885. doi: 10.1038/nature07150

Pourtois, G., Grandjean, D., Sander, D., and Vuilleumier, P. (2004). Electrophysiological correlates of rapid spatial orienting towards fearful faces. *Cereb. Cortex* 14, 619–633. doi: 10.1093/cercor/bhh023

Rossion, B., Campanella, S., Gomez, C. M., Delinte, A., Debatisse, D., Liard, L., et al. (1999). Task modulation of brain activity related to familiar and unfamiliar face processing: an ERP study. *Clin. Neurophysiol.* 110, 449–462. doi: 10.1016/S1388-2457(98)00037-6

Scharmüller, W., Leutgeb, V., Schäfer, A., Köchel, A., and Schienle, A. (2011). Source localization of late electrocortical positivity during symptom provocation in spider phobia: an sLORETA study. *Brain Res.* 1397, 10–18. doi: 10.1016/j.brainres.2011.04.018

Schweinberger, S. R., Pickering, E. C., Jentzsch, I., Burton, A. M., and Kaufmann, J. M. (2002). Event-related brain potential evidence for a response of inferior temporal cortex to familiar face repetitions. *Cogn. Brain Res.* 14, 398–409. doi: 10.1016/S0926-6410(02)00142-8

Sergent, J., and Signoret, J. (1992). Varieties of functional deficits in prosopagnosia. *Cereb. Cortex* 2, 375–388. doi: 10.1093/cercor/2.5.375

Tallon-Baudry, C., Bertrand, O., Delpuech, C., and Pernier, J. (1996). Stimulus-specificity of phase-locked and non phase-locked 40-Hz visual responses in human. *J. Neurosci.* 16, 4240–4249.

Tanaka, J. W., and Curran, T. (2001). A neural basis for expert object recognition. *Psychol. Sci.* 12, 43–47. doi: 10.1111/1467-9280.00308

Taylor, M. J., Arsalidou, M., Bayless, S. J., Morris, D., Evans, J. W., and Barbeau, E. J. (2009). Neural correlates of personally familiar faces: parents, partner and own faces. *Hum. Brain Mapp.* 30, 2008–2020. doi: 10.1002/hbm.20646

Todorov, A., Gobbini, M. I., Evans, K. K., and Haxby, J. V. (2007). Spontaneous retrieval of affective person knowledge in face perception. *Neuropsychologia* 45, 163–173. doi: 10.1016/j.neuropsychologia.2006.04.018

Tomik, B., and Guiloff, R. J. (2010). Dysarthria in amyotrophic lateral sclerosis: a review. *Amyotroph. Lateral Scler.* 11, 4–15. doi: 10.3109/17482960802379004

Utama, N. P., Takemoto, A., Koike, Y., and Nakamura, K. (2009). Phased processing of facial emotion: an ERP study. *Neurosci. Res.* 64, 30–40. doi: 10.1016/j.neures.2009.01.009

Zander, T. O., Kothe, C., Jatzev, S., and Gaertner, M. (2010). "Enhancing human-computer interaction with input from active and passive brain-computer interfaces," in *Brain Computer Interfaces* (London: Springer), 181–199. doi: 10.1007/978-1-84996-272-8_11

12

What we can and cannot (yet) do with functional near infrared spectroscopy

Megan Strait* and Matthias Scheutz

Human-Robot Interaction Laboratory, Department of Computer Science, Tufts University, Medford, MA, USA

***Correspondence:**
Megan Strait, Human-Robot Interaction Laboratory, Department of Computer Science, Tufts University, 200 Boston Avenue, Medford, MA, 02155, USA
e-mail: megan.strait@tufts.edu

Functional near infrared spectroscopy (NIRS) is a relatively new technique complimentary to EEG for the development of brain-computer interfaces (BCIs). NIRS-based systems for detecting various cognitive and affective states such as mental and emotional stress have already been demonstrated in a range of adaptive human–computer interaction (HCI) applications. However, before NIRS-BCIs can be used reliably in realistic HCI settings, substantial challenges concerning signal processing and modeling must be addressed. Although many of those challenges have been identified previously, the solutions to overcome them remain scant. In this paper, we first review what can be currently done with NIRS, specifically, NIRS-based approaches to measuring cognitive and affective user states as well as demonstrations of passive NIRS-BCIs. We then discuss some of the primary challenges these systems would face if deployed in more realistic settings, including detection latencies and motion artifacts. Lastly, we investigate the effects of some of these challenges on signal reliability via a quantitative comparison of three NIRS models. The hope is that this paper will actively engage researchers to facilitate the advancement of NIRS as a more robust and useful tool to the BCI community.

Keywords: functional near infrared spectroscopy, brain–computer interfaces, human–computer interaction, reliability, signal processing

1. INTRODUCTION

The primary aim of human–computer interaction (HCI) research is to develop methods and tools to facilitate effective interaction between people and with computer systems. While current modes of interaction mainly rely on tactile communication, there is a growing body of research on using brain-based sensors as an additional information channel (e.g., Tan and Nijholt, 2010; Zander and Kothe, 2011; Strait et al., 2014a). Socially-aware systems that can *capture and respond to* changes in anxiety, attention, arousal, and other user states have been found to be more effective in engaging people (e.g., Szafir and Mutlu, 2012). Hence, research on neurophysiological signals has been gaining the attention of researchers in human–computer interaction in recent years (e.g., Bainbridge et al., 2012; Frey et al., 2014; Strait and Scheutz, 2014).

Amongst this work, electroencephalography (EEG) is the most widely used technology in HCI, as it provides high temporal resolution and has general success in measuring a wide array of user states such as workload, attention, fatigue, and affect (Frey et al., 2014). However, EEG has limited spatial resolution, thus constraining its applicability for measuring region-specific brain activity. Conversely, high spatial resolution can be achieved using fMRI, but at a cost to both participant mobility and temporal resolution (e.g., Canning and Scheutz, 2013; Frey et al., 2014). Hence, functional near infrared spectroscopy (NIRS; also referred to as fNIRS or fNIR) is a promising alternative, achieving some middle ground in spatial and temporal resolution as well as mobility between the EEG and fMRI technologies (e.g., Villringer et al., 1993; Hoshi, 2011).

Within the human–computer interaction community, NIRS has been primarily used in two ways: (1) for *evaluating* human–machine interactions (e.g., Hirshfield et al., 2009a, 2011a), and more recently, (2) as additional input *to adapt* user interfaces and computer systems based on the user's cognitive state (e.g., Solovey et al., 2012), which is generally referred to as a *passive* brain–computer interface (Zander and Kothe, 2011).

While there are a growing number of EEG-based brain–computer interfaces (BCIs) (e.g., George and Lecuyer, 2010), the development of NIRS-based BCIs has generally lagged behind (e.g., see **Table 1** vs. Frey et al., 2014). Moreover, as a consequence of the NIRS literature being dispersed across many publication outlets in HCI, neuroimaging, and brain–computer interface communities (and furthermore, of inconsistencies in results within and between these fields), the efficacy of NIRS-BCIs in realistic human–robot interactions (Canning and Scheutz, 2013) and HCI settings (Strait et al., 2013b) is relatively unknown and unexplored.

To date, NIRS has been shown to be quite successful in measuring a number of cognitive and affective states (e.g., Cutini et al., 2012) in highly controlled laboratory settings. Yet, substantial challenges persist concerning signal processing for more realistic settings, many of which have already been identified (e.g., Hoshi, 2003, 2007; Plichta et al., 2007; Cutini et al., 2011; Hoshi, 2011; Krusienski et al., 2011; Kirilina et al., 2012; Canning and Scheutz, 2013; Hu et al., 2013; Strait et al., 2013b, 2014b). And while these challenges are not necessarily unique to NIRS, (e.g., see the limitations of using functional magnetic resonance imaging Cacioppo et al., 2003; Logothetis, 2008 and EEG Lotte, 2011; Ohara et al.,

Table 1 | Resources for and applications of recent NIRS-based systems.

Reference(s)	Topic
Brigadoi et al., 2014	Comparison of motion correction techniques
Cutini et al., 2012; Canning and Scheutz, 2013	Review of NIRS for human–robot interaction
Cui et al., 2011	Comparison of NIRS and fMRI across multiple cognitive tasks
Hoshi, 2007, 2011	Review of the utility and limitations of NIRS
Oriheula-Espina et al., 2010	Taxonomy of influential factors in the reliability of NIRS
Scholkmann et al., 2014	Review of CW-NIRS instrumentation and signal processing
Tak and Ye, 2014	Review of statistical methods of analysis of NIRS data
Aoki et al., 2011, 2013	Negative mood during working memory tasks
Gupta et al., 2013	Correlates of quality of experience
Heger et al., 2013	Continuous decoding of valence and arousal
Hirshfield et al., 2011b	Frustration and surprise in human–computer interactions
Kawaguchi et al., 2011	Engagement in human–robot interaction
Luu and Chau, 2009	Single-trial decoding of preference
Peck et al., 2013	Online decoding of preference
Strait et al., 2013a	Correlates of moral decision-making
Strait and Scheutz, 2014	Discomfort in human–robot interactions
Tupak et al., 2014	Correlates of emotion regulation
Ayaz et al., 2010	Sliding-window motion artifact rejection
Ayaz et al., 2012	Workload assessment using n-back and air traffic control tasks
Coffey et al., 2012	Comparison of NIRS and EEG for measuring workload
Cui et al., 2010a	Simple signal noise reduction based on hemoglobin dynamics
Cui et al., 2010b	Speeded response detection of motor activity
Cutini et al., 2011	Probe placement method for multichannel NIRS
Derosiere et al., 2013	Review of NIRS for ergonomics
Fekete et al., 2011	Package for NIRS signal processing and statistical analysis
Ferrari and Quaresima, 2012	Review of NIRS general history and applications
Girouard et al., 2010	Review of NIRS for human–computer interaction
Herff et al., 2013a	Single-trial quantification of workload
Hirshfield et al., 2009b	Assessment of syntactic workload
Hu et al., 2013	Reduction of inter-trial variability using resting-state connectivity
Izzetoglu et al., 2010	Motion artifact cancelation using Kalman filtering
Kirilina et al., 2012	Method for separation of superficial and cortical signals
Lloyd-Fox et al., 2010	Review of the utility and limitations of NIRS for use with infants
Lu et al., 2010	Assessment of resting-state connectivity

(Continued)

Table 1 | Continued

Reference(s)	Topic
Molvi and Dumont, 2012	Wavelet-based motion artifact removal
Power et al., 2012	Intersession consistency of single-trial classification of workload
Robertson et al., 2010	Comparison of motion correction techniques
Sassaroli et al., 2009	Discrimination of mental workload levels
Scarpa et al., 2013	Reference method for improving reliability of event-related NIRS
Scholkmann et al., 2010	Motion artifact correction using spline interpolation
Schudlo and Chau, 2014	Online differentiation of workload and rest
Solovey et al., 2011	Discrimination of cognitive multitasking states
Strait et al., 2013b	Limitations/reliability of NIRS in realistic settings
Tanaka et al., 2012	Comparison of task-related component analysis for fMRI and NIRS
Tsuzuki and Dan, 2014	Method for identification of cortical sampling location
Virtanen et al., 2011	Accelerometer-based method for motion artifact correction
Ye et al., 2009	Package for NIRS signal processing and statistical analysis

In red: useful reviews of NIRS instrumentation and applications. In blue: NIRS-based investigations of neural signals that reflect affective states in particular.

2011; Brouwer et al., 2013; Frey et al., 2014), we are still lacking adequate solutions to overcome them.

Hence, the goals of this paper are the following: to provide (1) a review of what can be currently done with NIRS-BCIs for measuring cognitive and affective user states relevant to HCI, (2) a discussion of the effects of naturalistic and unconstrained interaction settings of HCI on signal reliability, and (3) a quantitative comparison of the performance of three modeling approaches in these more realistic settings. We first start with a review of the technology, including an overview of current NIRS-based systems and their limitations. We then identify and evaluate some of the challenges for model reliability, and conclude with a discussion of directions for future research to overcome those challenges.

2. FUNCTIONAL NEAR INFRARED SPECTROSCOPY

Functional near infrared spectroscopy is a neuroimaging technique (similar to fMRI) for measuring changes in blood-oxygenation (Hoshi, 2011). Due to the differences in absorptivity between oxygenated and deoxygenated hemoglobin and the transparency of biological tissue to light in the 700–1000 nm range, NIRS is able to capture the hemodynamic changes via the coupling of infrared light emission and detection (Hoshi, 2011). Change in hemoglobin concentration following a precipitating stimulus is referred to as the hemodynamic response (HDR) and can be used to make inferences about functional areas of the brain. Unlike EEG, however, most NIRS-based studies find the onset of the response lags behind the triggering events by at least 1–2 s (e.g., Cui et al., 2011), which then peaks

4–8 s after the stimulus onset and then dips back down over the course of several more seconds as homeostasis is reestablished (e.g., Matthews and Pearlmutter, 2008; Hoshi, 2011). For detailed reviews of hemodynamics and NIRS instrumentation, see for example: Lloyd-Fox et al. (2010); Hoshi (2011); Ferrari and Quaresima (2012); Scholkmann et al. (2014).

2.1. USING NIRS TO MEASURE COGNITIVE STATES

Within the field of HCI, discrimination of workload-based states is the predominant application of NIRS (e.g., Nozawa, 2010; Hirshfield et al., 2011a; Ayaz et al., 2012; Coffey et al., 2012; Herff et al., 2013a,b; Schudlo and Chau, 2014). There are also a growing number of affect-related studies using NIRS, with the primary focus on the detection of negatively-valenced and high-arousal states (e.g., Tupak et al., 2014). **Table 1** shows a number of relevant NIRS-related publications and a summary of their topics. Additionally, there are several comprehensive reviews of the utility and limitations of NIRS in general (Hoshi, 2011; Cutini et al., 2012; Brigadoi et al., 2014; Tak and Ye, 2014) and for human–robot interaction (Canning and Scheutz, 2013) in particular.

Although this set of measureable states (i.e., workload, negative affect) is a subset of that which is achieved using EEG (i.e., workload, attention, vigilance, fatigue, error recognition, affect, engagement, flow, and immersion; see Frey et al., 2014), NIRS may serve as a complimentary or alternative modality. Specifically, while some comparisons of EEG versus NIRS for workload detection found that NIRS is less effective across a population (i.e., better-than-chance classifications were observed for only 50% of participants using NIRS versus 80% of participants using EEG) (Coffey et al., 2012), NIRS has also been found to achieve better overall discrimination of two levels of workload compared to EEG (Hirshfield et al., 2009a). Hence, a combination of the two (both NIRS and EEG) may be more appropriate for general deployment in workload-related activities.

Moreover, as the prefrontal cortex shows functional coupling in response to emotionally-charged tasks (e.g., Strait et al., 2013a), NIRS may be of greater utility (than EEG) for the detection such localized affect-related brain activity. For instance, recent EEG-based studies have shown recognition rates of only mid-50% for two-way classification (Frey et al., 2014) which is substantially less than what has been achieved in similar paradigms using NIRS which show recognition rates of mid to high 60% (Heger et al., 2013). Although recent EEG-based research shows successful recognition rates of 85–90% for arousal and valenced-states (Liu et al., 2011), artifacts arising from the electrical activity of facial muscles were not controlled for in this work. Given such artifacts are both inherent to emotion induction paradigms and have been shown to have significant effects on frontal EEG channels (e.g., Heger et al., 2011), it is unlikely the above results are reliably detecting brain activity (versus EMG activity of facial muscles). Hence, NIRS may be a useful alternative for measuring affect-related activity. In particular, for NIRS-based affect-related studies (e.g., Aoki et al., 2011, 2013; Hirshfield et al., 2011a; Strait et al., 2013a; Strait and Scheutz, 2014; Tupak et al., 2014), the results are highly consistent across the various efforts and moreover, across a diverse set of contexts (i.e., threat, working memory tasks, moral decision-making, human-robot interactions) in which detection rates significantly better than chance have been achieved. However, as this body of work—similar to Liu et al. (2011)—relies on frontally-situated probes that are proximal to primary facial muscles, the measurements might still reflect some degree of EMG artifacts rather brain activity alone.

Furthermore, as the majority of these studies have been conducted in offline settings, affect detection may still be premature for passive NIRS-BCIs. There exist but a few attempts (moreover, with mixed results) at single-trial and online decoding of affective states (specifically Luu and Chau, 2009; Heger et al., 2013; Peck et al., 2013). Regarding the detection of user preferences (e.g., affinity versus aversion), Luu and Chau originally showed an average classification accuracy of 80% in decoding users' preferences between two possible drinks in a single-trial NIRS paradigm (Luu and Chau, 2009). However, after an issue with the original methodology was identified (Dominguez, 2009), reanalysis yielded an average classification accuracy of 54% (Chau and Damouras, 2009) which was not significantly better than chance. Similarly, in an online classification paradigm, Peck and colleagues investigated preference decoding as a means of providing implicit ratings of movies (Peck et al., 2013). However, comparison of the NIRS-based recommendations (recommendations based on classification of the users' NIRS data) versus random movie recommendations did not show any significant difference. Despite the unsuccessful approaches to decoding of preference states, the work of Heger and colleagues suggests that offline experimentation on the detection of certain affective states may indeed extend to more realistic settings. In Heger et al. (2013), they showed three affect classes (high valence, high arousal, and high valence/arousal) could be reliably (63–69% average classification accuracies) discriminated from neutral for an eight-subject sample in an asynchronous classification paradigm. However, their recognition of high-valenced versus high-arousal states did not perform significantly better than chance (average accuracy of 53%), thus suggesting the granularity of passive NIRS-BCIs for affect recognition is limited.

2.2. EXEMPLARS OF NIRS-BCIs

While investigation into NIRS-based detection of affect is growing, on the forefront of state-of-the-art NIRS-BCIs is the development of NIRS as a passive input modality (referred to here as "NIRS-pBCI") based on workload-related user states. **Table 2** shows a detailed summary of known demonstrations of NIRS-pBCIs. Aside from the couple aforementioned attempts at online affect detection (Heger et al., 2013; Peck et al., 2013), these systems are primarily based on the decoding of workload-related states (i.e., Matsuyama et al., 2009; Solovey, 2012; Solovey et al., 2012; Girouard et al., 2013; Afergan et al., 2014; Schudlo and Chau, 2014). Here we discuss three such systems in detail regarding their approaches to the online decoding of cognitive states as well as their current limitations.

2.2.1. Reference channel/thresholding

Matsuyama and colleagues created a simple, proof-of-concept NIRS-pBCI based on the detection of workload-related

Table 2 | Current passive NIRS-BCI systems (listed by first author).

References	Model	Latency (s)	Classes	Accuracy (%)	*N*
Girouard et al., 2013	Workload	30	2	82	9
Heger et al., 2013	Affect	5	2	68	8
Matsuyama et al., 2009	Workload	9	2	NA	9
Peck et al., 2013	Affect	25	5	27	14
Schudlo and Chau, 2014	Workload	20	2	77	10
Solovey et al., 2012	Workload	40	2	68	3

Model refers to the type of state information of interest, latency is the delay imposed by the signal processing on onset detection, and N indicates the population sample size.

hemodynamic changes (Matsuyama et al., 2009). Their study was a preliminary attempt at using passive monitoring of users' cognitive state to adapt a robot's behavior. Using a 35-channel NIRS instrument, they measured participants' prefrontal cortex while they solved arithmetic problems. As a proof-of-concept of NIRS-based robot adaptivity, they developed their NIRS-pBCI to send a primitive motion command to a robot when it detected changes in hemoglobin associated with the arithmetic problem solving (i.e., when an increase in oxygenated hemoglobin was observed corresponding to the participant actively working on a arithmetic problem). They used a simple combination of thresholding and reference channel for noise subtraction to detect task-evoked changes in oxy-hemoglobin. Specifically, to avoid noise from widespread brain activity, they computed the difference between two regions—a target region and a reference region (F7-F4, coordinates according to the International 10–20 placement system). Then, using a single threshold (max F7-F4 difference in oxy-hemoglobin), their NIRS-pBCI would cause the robot to move whenever this threshold was surpassed. While there exist many sound BCIs for the direct control of robotic systems (e.g., Canning and Scheutz, 2013), their NIRS-BCI system was not intended to use workload-related activity to directly control a robot. Rather, it served as an effective demonstration that a NIRS-based BCI can passively monitor a person's cognitive workload to initiate behavioral changes in a robot. However, this work also exposed a particular shortcoming of NIRS that is an obstacle for its effectiveness in more realistic scenarios, namely that of onset detection latency (Canning and Scheutz, 2013). Specifically, using their approach to workload monitoring, the time between a participant beginning the arithmetic problem and the transmission of the motor control signal ranged from just few seconds to over 15 s (Matsuyama et al., 2009). As task-related hemodynamic changes in oxygenated hemoglobin occur over several seconds (Coyle et al., 2007), this delay was (and is) somewhat unavoidable due to the inherent hemodynamics; however, recent work has demonstrated vast reductions in temporal delays to onset detection (Cui et al., 2010b), which suggests improvement may be possible.

2.2.2. Temporal dynamics

Similar to Matsuyama et al. (2009), we previously participated in the development of a passive NIRS-BCI aimed at adapting a robot's behavior based on a person's detected multitasking state (Solovey et al., 2012). A two-probe NIRS instrument (with four sources per probe) was used to image participants' prefrontal cortex, while they worked with two simulated robots on a human-robot team task. Here we designed a naive SVM (support vector machine) classification model based on gross temporal dynamics, built by the Sequential Minimal Optimization (SMO) algorithm available in the Weka (Waikato Environment for Knowledge Analysis[1]) library (Hall et al., 2009) and trained using data collected while participants performed a variant of the n-back task. Specifically, the SVM was trained on feature vectors containing every measure of amplitude of both oxy- and deoxy-hemoglobin over the course of a 40 s period of n-back performance. That is, for a device with a sampling rate of 6.25 Hz and a task period of 40 s, a single training example was a vector of 40 s $\times$ 6.25 cycles/second $\times$ 2 signals (oxy and deoxy) $\times$ 2 probes $\times$ 4 sources/probe, or 4000 features. This naive approach was a first attempt at capturing temporal patterns over the full time course of a person performing the n-back task. The n-back task, rather than human–robot team task, was used for training in order to avoid potential variations implicit in the team task, but we expected participants to show similar patterns in their NIRS data across both tasks as both induced similar levels of subjectively reported mental stress.

In the human–robot team task, we hypothesized that adapting the level of a robot's autonomy would lead to better task performance and better perceptions of teamwork. Thus, while participants performed the team task, classifications of their mental workload dynamically adapted the autonomy of one of the robots according to the participant's multitasking state. An initial evaluation (Solovey, 2012; Solovey et al., 2012) showed successful task completion was significantly moderated by adaptivity: the dynamic adaptivity of the robot's autonomy improved task performance (82% of participants successfully completed the team task versus a baseline performance rate of 45%). This system was thus a substantial extension of Matsuyama et al. (2009), as it was the first NIRS-BCI to demonstrate effective improvements on a *realistic* task. However, in a recent series of reinvestigations (Strait et al., 2014b) of this system's classification performance, the average classification accuracy on an alternative dataset (of mental arithmetic) was only 54.5% ($SD = 14.3\%$) suggesting limited generalizability of the system's signal processing. Additionally, this NIRS-pBCI was found effective (statistically better than chance) for only 10 of 40 participants in this alternative dataset (Strait et al., 2014b), which suggested limited utility for a more realistic population sample (i.e., when $N = 40$ versus $N = 3$ in the initial evaluation). This finding was consistent with one recent investigation (Coffey et al., 2012) which showed better-than-chance NIRS-based classifications for only 5 out of 10 participants on a workload task, but not with another recent investigation (Hirshfield et al., 2009a), which showed the reverse. Hence it remains to-date unclear whether one modality or the other (EEG versus NIRS) is better for measuring workload-related signals, if either, or if it is largely a function of the signal processing methods employed.

[1]The Weka Java libarary contains a collection of common tools for data processing, classification, visualization, and other common analyses for data mining. For more information, see Hall et al. (2009).

2.2.3. Combination temporal/spatiotemporal dynamics

Schudlo and Chau (2014) also developed an online NIRS–BCI which was driven by a mental arithmetic; however, unlike previous NIRS-pBCIs, their system also accommodated an unconstrained rest state. That is, while previous examples of NIRS-pBCIs have been demonstrated to function in online settings (e.g., Matsuyama et al., 2009; Solovey et al., 2012; Girouard et al., 2013), they all employ a synchronous training paradigm, which does not clearly allow the user to remain in an unconstrained resting state for an unfixed length of time. Given this gap in the NIRS-pBCI literature, Schudlo and Chau investigated whether prefrontal activity corresponding to mental arithmetic and unconstrained rest could be differentiated online at a practical accuracy for more realistic BCI use. Here the prefrontal cortex was sampled (using a nine-channel spectrometer) while participants selected letters from an on-screen scanning keyboard via intentionally controlled brain activity (mental arithmetic). To classify the hemodynamic activity, a combination of temporal features (extracted from the NIRS signals) and spatiotemporal features (extracted from dynamic NIRS topograms) were used in a majority vote combination of multiple linear classifiers. The online classification results showed an average accuracy of 77.4% ($SD = 10.5\%$), with 8 of the 10 participants showing accuracies significantly above chance. Considering previous results showing significant detection accuracies in less than half of participants (Coffey et al., 2012; Strait et al., 2014b), the findings of Schudlo and Chau's work are particularly promising, and suggest that mental workload, using a more complex classification approach, may indeed be effective at driving a passive NIRS-BCI.

2.3. CONSIDERATIONS

The previous section detailed three examples of state-of-the-art passive NIRS-BCIs, which intended to serve both as proof-of-concept demonstrations of NIRS being successfully utilized as a passive input to a computer system, as well as of the challenges to achieving more robust NIRS-pBCIs. While there are numerous factors that contribute to the reliability and robustness of a NIRS-based system (e.g., Oriheula-Espina et al., 2010), we highlight some of the more pressing of these considerations, as well as the differences in signal processing that may contribute to decrements to signal reliability in moving from offline NIRS-based systems to online, passive BCIs.

In the standard, *offline* approaches to signal processing of NIRS data, the signals are short (3–60 s) and heavily filtered *post hoc* (with roughly the following measures)—*detrending* (removal of low frequency signal artifacts and drift), *smoothing* (removal of systemic artifacts such as cardiac pulsations, respiration, and Mayer waves), *motion correction* (reduction of motion artifacts), and *data reduction* (removal of noisy or corrupt trials; averaging over repetitions of a task and/or truncation of the signal to reduce temporal variation; using summary statistics, e.g., area-under-the-curve, percent signal change to represent the overall hemodynamic response) (see Cui et al., 2010a; Oriheula-Espina et al., 2010; Hoshi, 2011; Brigadoi et al., 2014; Scholkmann et al., 2014; Tak and Ye, 2014). Such processing can result in dramatic reductions of signal noise, however, in online, passive settings, signal processing faces substantial challenges (Canning and Scheutz, 2013; Schudlo and Chau, 2014), three of which we detail here.

2.3.1. Onset latency

In moving from offline to fully online, unconstrained, real-time analysis, NIRS-pBCIs suffer a loss in signal processing as well as task information which may result in increased signal noise, and hence, increased unreliability. Specifically, while offline paradigms have known onsets and offsets of the task stimulus, such an oracle is lost in an online, asynchronous scenario. That is, the difficulty in offline processing is primarily to identify whether a trial contains a significant change in hemodynamic activity in response to a particular stimulus. Whereas, in passive (online) systems, not only must we identify whether the signal contains a significant hemodynamic response, but also where such a response begins and terminates. While these fundamental differences in offline versus online protocols is not a new consideration for the signal processing or EEG communities (e.g., Lotte, 2011), they underscore a necessary consideration when transitioning from proof-of-concept (offline) systems to robust online, passive systems that has yet to receive much discussion regarding NIRS-based BCIs. For instance, while both Girouard and colleagues (Solovey, 2012; Girouard et al., 2013) as well as Schudlo and Chau (Schudlo and Chau, 2014) achieved accuracies that were relatively high for online classification of NIRS data with their NIRS-pBCIs, their systems implicitly required delays in the detection of task-related onsets of 20–40 s. Such delays limit the execution of passive NIRS-based adaptivity to only after a significant amount of time has elapsed.

2.3.2. Participant mobility

In addition to the loss of onset/offset oracles, signal noise is also problematic for passive BCI systems. In particular, unrestricted participant mobility can cause motion artifacts which degrade the NIRS signals (e.g., Canning and Scheutz, 2013). These artifacts can be caused by movement of the sensors on the skin, facial expressions, and head orientation (Matthews and Pearlmutter, 2008; Robertson et al., 2010). As techniques for online, asynchronous filtering are limited (e.g., Ayaz et al., 2010; Cui et al., 2010a), other attempts at combating motion artifacts include restricting participant mobility (e.g., using chin rests and mechanical supports, Coyle et al., 2007), which are not particularly suited for *realistic* HCI settings and furthermore, such restrictions on participant mobility significantly reduce the value gained in using NIRS over fMRI. There are, however, a growing number of proposals for real-time motion artifact correction in natural environments, such as the adjustment of the signal based on statistical associations between oxy- and deoxy-hemoglobin values (Cui et al., 2010a), the use of linear quadratic estimation (Izzetoglu et al., 2010), and the use of complimentary physiological measures (Falk et al., 2011).

2.3.3. Task-unrelated activity

Lastly, task-unrelated activity such as resting-state fluctuations (Hoshi, 2011; Hu et al., 2013) or whole brain activity (Matsuyama et al., 2009) can degrade the signal quality. That is, separating task-related from unrelated cortical activity and signal noise can be difficult in some cases (e.g., Kirilina et al., 2012). For example, to separate task-related activity from unrelated whole brain activity, a reference channel outside the cortical region of interest has been used as a method to subtract out the task-unrelated activity (Matsuyama et al., 2009; Lu et al., 2010; Scarpa et al., 2013). This method, however, is impractical when multiple channels are not available (e.g., as was the case in Solovey et al., 2012) and moreover, assuming the reference is neutral (that the activity at the reference region is unrelated to the task-evoked activity), it relies on the quality of the channel placements, which is in itself a challenge for NIRS (Plichta et al., 2007). However, there are a couple of recent proposals for improving the identification of sampling region using probabilistic registration methods of probe placement based on a reference-MRI database (Tsuzuki and Dan, 2014), as well as for separating superficial from cortical signals (Kirilina et al., 2012) and for using resting-state connectivity for reducing inter-trial variability (Hu et al., 2013).

3. INVESTIGATION

To empirically investigate some of the aforementioned challenges to signal reliability, we collated a large NIRS dataset which we used in the construction of three basic models. The dataset contains (1) 18 training samples of resting versus workload-induced states, during which participant mobility was restricted; (2) 18 training samples (rest versus workload) where mobility was *unrestricted*; and (3) one testing sample of a more realistic task paradigm (i.e., prolonged rest and task periods similar to the human–robot team task in Solovey et al., 2012). Here, we first compare the performance of three basic NIRS models (using 10-fold cross-validation) when trained on data with and without participant movement. Following, we then look at the relative model performances when applied to the more realistic testing sample.

3.1. DATASET

To compare the relative performance of three modeling approaches, as well as the effects of unrestricted participant mobility on model performance, we obtained the dataset from Strait et al. (2013b) for further analysis. The dataset contains 40 Tufts University students and staff (18 male; ages 18–45, $M = 23.4$, $S = 5.8$), sampling prefrontal hemodynamic activity (recorded bilaterally using a two-channel ISS OxiplexTS, with a temporal resolution of 6.25 Hz) while participants performed a workload-inducing arithmetic task. All participants were healthy, right-handed, with normal or corrected-to-normal vision, and reported no known history of neurological or psychiatric disorder. To secure the NIRS probes to the participant's forehead, we used a fitted black cap. To minimize signal noise due to ambient light, the room lights were turned off during the recording periods and all stimuli were presented via white text on a black background. Each participant performed two blocks of the workload task (each block comprised of nine trials of arithmetic, nine trials of rest)—one block with their motion restricted (using a zero-gravity chair and verbal instructions to remain motionless) and one with their motion unrestricted (using a simple office chair and verbal instructions to sit naturally). While the trials were each separated by a 30 s fixation cross, here we refer to trial as a sampling period comprised of the participant performing the task or resting only. That is, the trials contained measurements sampled while the participant was actively performing the task or (exclusive) resting.

3.1.1. Signal processing

Prior to analysis, the dataset was first converted using the modified Beer-Lambert Law (MBLL), which yielded a measure of Hb (deoxygenated) and HbO (oxygenated hemoglobin) at each time point for each of two sensors positioned over the left and right prefrontal cortex (PFC), respectively, for a total of four time-series signals (left Hb, HbO; right Hb, HbO). We then detrended the signals by subtracting out the signal obtained from a low-pass filter (1st degree Savitsky-Golay with a cut-frequency of 0.01 Hz) and smoothed the resulting signals using another low-pass FIR filter (1st degree Savitsky-Golay with a cut-frequency of 0.15 Hz) to reduce the effects of systemic physiological artifacts (namely, cardiac pulsations and respiration). Lastly, we applied a correlation-based signal correction (Cui et al., 2010a) to reduce the effects of motion artifacts. Although all signal processing was applied *post hoc* and offline, online implementations of similar filters have been suggested to be equally effective (Cui et al., 2010a,b).

3.1.2. Modeling

We constructed our models using the nine arithmetic and nine rest training trials (measured under restricted mobility conditions) based on three relatively successful approaches to classifying NIRS data: (1) the reference channel/threshholding approach described in Matsuyama et al. (2009), and the slightly more complex SVM-based approaches of (2) Cui et al. (2010b) and (3) Solovey et al. (2012). Here we implemented the reference channel/thresholding approach put forth by Matsuyama et al. (2009), such that we calculated the difference in oxy-hemoglobin between the two sensors placed bilaterally on the PFC (left PFC—right PFC). This roughly corresponds to the probe placement used in Matsuyama et al. (2009), with the probe measuring the left PFC placed more anterior and medial to the F7 region of interest. To classify the rest versus workload states, this model compares each time point in the left-right oxy-hemoglobin difference against a single baseline value (the average of the max differences during the observed in the resting trials). If the difference at the current time point exceeds the baseline value, the system classifies it as task-evoked activation. To compare more sophisted approaches, we implemented a simple SVM model based on Cui et al. (2010b) which uses four features—the amplitude of left and right oxy/deoxy—and again performs a classification of each timepoint. While this approach is still relatively simple, it capitalizes on the correlations between oxy/deoxy hemodynamics, as well as possible left/right synchronies. Lastly, we compared both approaches with the results of the model described in Solovey (2012) and Solovey et al. (2012), which uses the entire time course of a training sample (see Strait et al., 2014b for details).

3.2. RESULTS

The results of the cross-validation are shown in **Table 3**, where accuracy refers to the overall recognition rate of both classes (rest and task). The results of the Matsuyama thresholding model (Matsuyama et al., 2009) are depicted in the first column section (average time to onset detection, M_{on}, and average classification accuracy, $M_{acc(1)}$). The middle column section depicts the results of the simple SVM model (Cui et al., 2010b), and the rightmost column section depicts the results of the more complex SVM model[2] (Solovey et al., 2012). Using the thresholding approach, we found an average task detection latency of 12.6 (±7.6) s across participants ($N = 40$), with individual averages

[2]The model based on Solovey et al. (2012) and results of its cross-validation are also described in Strait et al. (2014b). However, all additional analyses and discussion presented here of its performance are novel.

Table 3 | Relative model performances in nine-fold cross-validation.

Subject	M_{on}	SD	$M_{acc(1)}$	SD	t_{obs}	$M_{acc(2)}$	SD	t_{obs}	$M_{acc(3)}$	SD	t_{obs}
1	12.2	8.2	49.2	30.6	−0.07	58.4	19.2	1.37	48.9	11.5	−0.30
2	11.6	8.6	47.4	30.6	−0.25	**64.7**	21.1	2.19	37.5	13.8	−2.86
3	5.3	6.2	60.6	28.0	1.13	**70.1**	12.4	5.11	52.4	16.5	0.46
4	5.5	3.6	**70.6**	16.8	3.68	**75.2**	12.7	6.31	46.2	12.6	−0.95
5	12.9	10.6	50.1	31.4	0.00	57.8	19.9	1.24	52.8	15.2	0.58
6	9.8	7.0	47.3	26.2	−0.31	57.0	17.8	1.24	54.2	16.9	0.78
7	11.3	7.8	44.6	22.5	−0.71	**74.2**	25.4	3.01	**65.6**	10.0	4.93
8	15.3	10.7	44.1	37.2	−0.47	**67.8**	13.6	4.14	53.8	16.6	0.72
9	7.0	4.1	59.3	15.7	1.77	53.8	17.6	0.68	60.4	18.8	1.74
10	9.0	6.8	54.3	26.5	0.48	**73.1**	14.3	5.11	**67.0**	10.8	4.97
11	17.6	6.6	22.5	16.5	−4.99	**68.6**	16.8	3.49	**60.8**	16.3	2.09
12	3.1	2.6	**84.9**	10.1	10.42	**83.5**	10.2	10.37	**57.3**	11.6	1.99
13	10.3	4.5	52.0	22.0	0.27	61.7	20.6	1.79	**63.9**	14.9	2.95
14	8.5	5.8	**68.5**	19.6	2.82	47.4	16.6	−0.49	55.6	14.2	1.24
15	9.6	8.5	50.4	31.0	0.03	51.6	21.2	0.23	**73.6**	11.0	6.78
16	11.2	7.9	49.0	23.7	−0.12	55.1	16.9	0.95	**75.7**	9.0	9.03
17	13.0	7.8	49.4	24.8	−0.07	**68.0**	17.6	3.24	61.1	23.7	1.48
18	10.1	8.1	55.7	30.4	0.56	51.9	17.2	0.34	40.5	7.4	−4.91
19	15.9	8.3	44.0	27.2	−0.66	46.1	13.9	−0.88	46.2	13.3	−0.90
20	8.0	6.3	51.1	26.0	0.12	50.0	18.4	0.00	43.1	11.2	−1.94
21	4.6	3.7	**72.9**	26.7	2.56	45.0	21.5	−0.73	52.1	14.0	0.47
22	20.3	11.8	17.1	24.0	−4.12	53.2	16.5	0.61	50.0	15.7	−0.02
23	12.5	10.5	38.8	31.4	−1.06	48.4	13.9	−0.33	**65.3**	17.2	2.81
24	13.8	6.2	46.7	20.1	−0.49	55.2	11.9	1.38	47.2	12.2	−0.72
25	22.7	8.9	23.7	29.1	−2.70	**67.4**	7.8	7.03	53.1	16.5	0.59
26	18.6	11.0	25.8	28.2	−2.57	48.4	13.3	−0.35	43.7	21.6	−0.92
27	9.0	5.4	58.2	14.8	1.65	**62.8**	18.0	2.26	57.6	16.5	1.45
28	21.8	8.4	21.2	26.5	−3.26	**66.4**	9.2	5.64	34.0	9.3	−5.44
29	9.0	8.2	51.1	24.7	0.14	56.4	21.2	0.94	48.6	14.1	−0.31
30	15.4	7.4	46.6	26.7	−0.37	**61.4**	16.2	2.23	**62.1**	9.8	3.90
31	17.9	9.5	35.1	34.5	−1.29	**75.6**	9.0	9.03	54.2	10.8	1.22
32	27.5	5.3	8.2	17.8	−7.03	**65.9**	12.8	3.94	51.4	14.0	0.31
33	18.5	11.5	28.3	32.0	−2.03	**66.9**	14.0	3.83	**71.2**	18.1	3.70
34	4.2	2.0	**64.8**	22.2	1.99	**59.6**	11.9	2.55	56.6	13.6	1.53
35	9.6	7.0	56.9	24.5	0.84	51.6	18.9	0.27	52.8	14.2	0.62
36	11.5	8.1	55.4	26.3	0.61	**66.3**	7.9	6.55	45.8	18.8	−0.70
37	14.8	11.0	44.6	32.0	−0.50	**67.7**	18.3	3.05	59.0	17.3	1.65
38	25.3	8.4	5.6	9.8	−13.6	**58.9**	8.9	3.17	52.1	14.2	0.46
39	7.1	5.8	61.7	25.2	1.39	52.5	19.3	0.40	56.2	17.8	1.10
40	13.1	12.7	47.8	36.5	−0.18	53.8	18.6	0.64	54.9	13.0	1.19
Overall	12.6 s	7.6	46.6%	17.2		**60.5%**	15.8		**54.5%**	14.3	

The Matsuyama approach is shown in the left column section (with both onset latency and classification accuracy shown). Middle shows the model based on Cui et al. and far right, the Solovey et al. model. In red: rates that are significantly above chance (right-tailed t-test, $t_{crit}(8) = 1.8595$).

ranging from 3.1 to 27.5 s (see **Table 3**, left). However, the recognition rate of this model did not perform better than chance ($M = 46.6\%$, $SD = 17.2\%$). Whereas, both the more complex SVM models performed significantly above chance recognition levels (simple SVM: $M = 60.5\%$, $SD = 15.8\%$, $p < 0.0001$ and complex SVM: $M = 54.5\%$, $SD = 14.3\%$, $p = 0.0037$). However, between these two SVMs, the more simple approach of the two (Cui et al., 2010b) performed significantly better both in terms of classification accuracy ($p = 0.0035$) and across the subject population (with 20/40 participants showing significant recognition rates) versus the more complex approach (with 10/40 showing significant rates).

To examine the effects of (semi) unrestricted participant mobility, we next re-constructed each of the three models using the motion-*unrestricted* set of training samples (again nine of each rest and arithmetic trials). Using nine-fold cross-validation of these samples, we found neither the thresholding nor simple SVM approaches were significantly affected in terms of classification accuracy ($M = 45.2\%$, $SD = 18.2\%$, $p = 0.5459$; and $M = 60.4\%$, $SD = 15.4\%$, $p = 0.8850$, respectively), nor in onset latency for the thresholding approach ($M = 13.7$ s, $SD = 5.7$ s, $p = 0.1446$). However, the performance of the more complex SVM model was significantly degraded, with an average classification accuracy of 25.3% ($SD = 7.3\%$, $p < 0.0001$).

To investigate the relative performances of each of these three models in a more realistic task paradigm, we tested each of the classification approaches (using the models trained on the motion-*restricted* training samples) on the testing sample (3.5 min rest, 3.5 min arithmetic, 3.5 min post-arithmetic rest). Here we observed a significant reduction in classification accuracy for the simple SVM model ($M = 54.6\%$, $SD = 14.4\%$, $t_{obs} = 1.74$), but not the complex SVM ($M = 48.5\%$, $SD = 15.1\%$, $t_{obs} = 0.67$). However, the simple SVM still performed significantly above chance ($t_{obs} = 2.02$, $t_{crit}(39) = 1.68$). There was not any significant change in accuracy for the thresholding model ($M = 43.9\%$, $SD = 10.5\%$, $t_{obs} = 0.84$).

3.3. DISCUSSION

3.3.1. Model performance

In comparison to Matsuyama et al. (2009), the simple reference channel/thresholding combination approach on the dataset used here showed onset latencies substantially slower ($M = 12.6$ s, $SD = 7.6$ s) than theirs ($M = 9.1$ s, $SD = 4.3$ s). This increase in delay and variability may be in part due to a different and larger sample population, as well as the placement of the probes (the positioning used here was inexact and slightly more anterior and medial in comparison to Matsuyama et al., 2009). Hence, the measured activity by the channel used for reference may not have been entirely distinct from the target region-of-interest. In any case, our results confirm a temporal limitation for workload-based state detection, at least when using a minimal (two-probe) NIRS instrument. That is, a fair onset detection delay (9–13 s) will be encountered using this method (see **Figure 1**). However, more problematic for this method is the classification accuracy: which failed to perform any better than chance overall. While this naive detection approach may work appropriately for contexts in which the duration of the passive adaptivity is not important, for contexts in which it is (e.g., if a robot should only act autonomously while a person is multitasking or mentally stressed), this may not serve as the best model. Similarly, a model that is very complex also may not be the best approach. Specifically, the more simplistic SVM model significantly outperforms the more complex SVM, both in terms of overall accuracy (60.5% versus 54.5%) and within the population (effective for 20 participants versus only 10 using the complex SVM). As SVMs are known to produce poor performance on highly-dimensional data with few training samples (Cortes and Vapnik, 1995), this difference in performance here between the two SVMs might be attributable to the availability of only 18 training samples total in combination with the complex SVM (which employs 4000 features in its model of workload-based activity) versus the simple SVM (which makes use of only four features). For instance, Power and colleagues showed a nearly 15% improvement in classification accuracy in

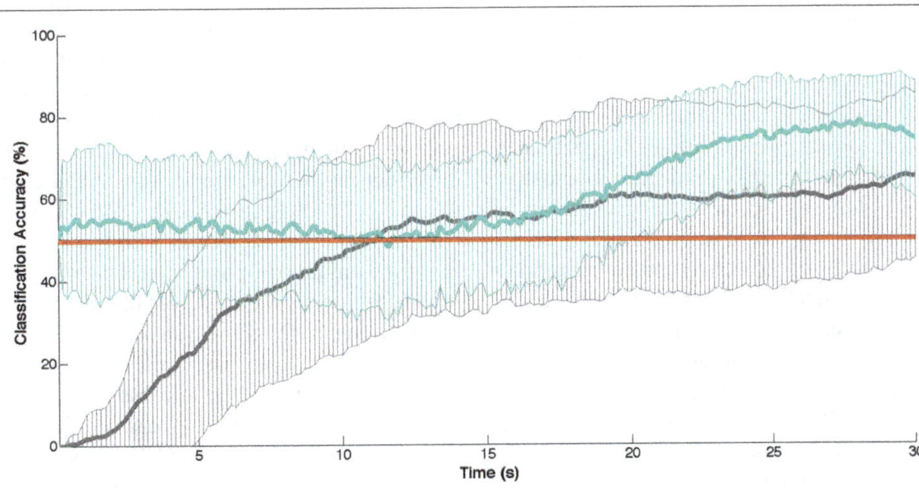

FIGURE 1 | Cross-validation results: mean classification accuracy (±*SD*) at each time point of the training task (30 s) with chance-level accuracies indicated in red. In gray: the thresholding approach (Matsuyama et al., 2009). In blue: the naive SVM approach (Cui et al., 2010b).

using 80 versus 10 training samples (Power et al., 2012). Thus, given more training samples, we might expect the complex SVM approach to show better recognition rates.

3.3.2. Model performance subject to movement

When we next re-trained our models using the training samples with semi (participants were still tethered within range of the NIRS device) unrestricted participant mobility, we found neither the thresholding nor simple SVM approaches were significantly affected. However, the performance of the more complex SVM model was significantly degraded, with an average classification accuracy of 25.3% ($SD = 7.3\%$, $p < 0.0001$). This difference in effects may be due to the difference in approach, where the more simplistic approaches of Matsuyama et al. (2009) and Cui et al. (2010b) classify the NIRS signal at every time point versus the more complex model which classifies a sizable window of the data. Hence, while a motion artifact may significantly degrade the overall measurement sample (thus resulting in lower accuracy of the complex SVM), an individual timepoint may not be so influenced. Potential influences on these models, however, may have been obscured in part by the filtering methods (namely, the correlation-based signal correction to attenuate movement artifacts). Hence it is worth further consideration when developing a NIRS-BCI, as to what signal processing is necessary depending on the context in which it will be used (i.e., if participants will be moving). Lastly, we looked at model performance given a more realistic task paradigm. Here we observed a significant reduction in overall classification accuracy for the simple SVM model, but not for the complex SVM or thresholding model. While the performance of the simple SVM was still statistically significantly above chance, passive adaptivity of a system based on this model would be unlikely to have any serious effects (and thus would be considerably difficult to measure in terms of behavior enhancements of the user).

3.3.3. Limitations

In this section, we systematically investigated three recently-proposed models of NIRS data and their performances when subject to certain factors of more realistic HCI settings (namely participant motion and semi-undefined task durations). While this evaluation serves to highlight the challenges of these factors to achieving more robust NIRS-based systems, there are also a number of limitations to the interpretation of results. In particular, all three modeling approaches performed significantly worse than prior work, with the thresholding approach showing a substantial increase in onset latency and the two SVMs a substantial decrease in accuracy (roughly 15% and 13%, respectively) than the models on which they were based. It is likely that these differences are at least in part due to the sample size, as the sample population used in this study is meaningfully larger than all prior work ($N = 7$ in Matsuyama et al. and $N = 3$ in both Cui et al. and Solovey et al.). It is also likely that they are attributable partially to differences in the task (e.g., numeric versus the alphameric n-back task used in Solovey et al.), region of measurement (prefrontal cortex versus motor cortex measured in Cui et al.), and placement of probes (the 10–20 system was used in Matsuyama et al., but no standardized coordinates were used in this investigation). Hence, it is impossible to speculate as to whether the above effects would be observed in exact replications of prior work. However, these limitations in themselves raise an important consideration regarding NIRS-based research: specifically, whether underpowered studies generalize over larger populations and whether the methods for signal processing and modeling generalize across functional regions of the brain and over a variety of tasks.

4. CONCLUSIONS

The aim of this paper was to provide (1) an overview of what we can do with NIRS-BCIs for measuring cognitive and affective user states, (2) a discussion of the effects of naturalistic and unconstrained interaction settings of HCI on signal reliability, and (3) a quantitative comparison of the performance of three recent modeling approaches in these more realistic settings. Specifically, we described two primary cognitive and affective states (mental workload and negative affect) measureable with NIRS, as well as two modes of use (evaluatory and passive). Additionally, we emphasized the distinction of offline versus online (real-time) signal processing for NIRS-based BCIs. The prototypical application of NIRS as an evaluation tool is as an offline *post hoc* analysis of a signal recorded during some stimulus. However, the usage of NIRS as a passive BCI (involving the online processing of hemodynamic data) has emerged, and with it, a number of challenges have followed.

We discussed some of those key challenges (participant mobility, more naturalistic interaction) and investigated their effects with a comparative analysis of three recently-proposed modeling techniques. The results of our investigation highlight several considerations, including detection latencies (the temporal delay between a precipitating stimulus and the detection of the stimulus-evoked hemodynamic changes), performance of the model in more naturalistic contexts (i.e., when participant mobility is unrestricted), and the generalizability of current training paradigms (i.e., offline, time-restricted) to the asynchronous, online paradigms of more realistic settings (e.g., Brouwer et al., 2013). The results also underscore several additional considerations, namely efficacy of a NIRS-BCI across a population (i.e., whether the signal processing and modeling approach effective for the whole population or only a small proportion) and task/region-specificity of a technique. While these challenges are not particularly new to the field, or to BCI in general, both the review of the literature and the empirical evaluation highlight the dependencies between performance, signal processing, and experimental context. Research efforts on all these fronts are mutually complementary and necessary to the advancement of NIRS as a tool for human–computer interaction.

NIRS-based systems have already been used in a range of applications, such as the quantification of mental workload and differentiation of aroused/valenced states; however, substantial challenges remain to be addressed before NIRS can become a practical and robust tool for passive BCIs. The challenges emphasized here concern detection latency, signal processing, as well as better understanding of hemodynamic changes over undefined task durations. While there are numerous challenges that have been raised previously (both in NIRS and EEG research), they remain to-date unaddressed. It is thus our hope that this survey and dataset will facilitate researchers to actively engage in NIRS-related research that will help overcome current challenges and make NIRS a more robust and useful tool to the BCI community.

ACKNOWLEDGMENT

This material is based upon work supported by the National Science Foundation under Grant No. ISS-1065154.

REFERENCES

Afergan, D., Peck, E., Solovey, E., Jenkins, A., Hincks, S., Chang, R., et al. (2014). "Dynamic difficulty using brain metrics of workload," in *CHI*. New York, NY: ACM.

Aoki, R., Sato, H., Katura, T., Matsuda, R., and Koizumi, H. (2013). Correlation between prefrontal cortex activity during working memory tasks and natural mood independent of personality effects: an optical topography study. *Psychiatry Res. Neuroimag.* 212, 79–87. doi: 10.1016/j.pscychresns.2012.10.009

Aoki, R., Sato, H., Katura, T., Utsugi, K., Koizumi, H., Matsuda, R., et al. (2011). Relationship of negative mood with prefrontal cortex activity during working memory tasks: an optical topography study. *Neurosci. Res.* 70, 189–196. doi: 10.1016/j.neures.2011.02.011

Ayaz, H., Izzetoglu, M., Shewokis, P., and Onaral, B. (2010). Sliding-window motion artifact rejection for functional near-infrared spectroscopy. *Conf. Proc. IEEE Eng. Med. Biol. Soc.* 2010, 6567–6570. doi: 10.1109/IEMBS.2010.5627113

Ayaz, H., Shewokis, P., Bunce, S., Izzetoglu, K., Willems, B., and Onaral, B. (2012). Optical brain monitoring for operator training and mental workload assessment. *Neuroimage* 59, 36–47. doi: 10.1016/j.neuroimage.2011.06.023

Bainbridge, W. A., Nozawa, S., Ueda, R., Okada, K., and Inaba, M. (2012). A methodological outline and utility assessment of sensor-based biosignal measurement in human-robot interaction. *Int. J. Soc. Rob.* 4, 303–316. doi: 10.1007/s12369-012-0146-y

Brigadoi, S., Ceccherini, L., Cutini, S., Scarpa, F., Scatturin, P., Selb, J., et al. (2014). Motion artifacts in functional near-infrared spectroscopy: a comparison of motion correction techniques applied to real cognitive data. *Neuroimage* 85, 181–191. doi: 10.1016/j.neuroimage.2013.04.082

Brouwer, A.-M., van Erp, J., Heylen, D., Jensen, O., and Poel, M. (2013). "Effortless passive BCIs for healthy users," in *HCII*, (Berlin, Heidelberg: Springer), 615–622.

Cacioppo, J., Berntson, G., Lorig, T., Norris, C., Rickett, E., and Nushbaum, H. (2003). Just because you're imaging the brain doesn't mean you can stop using your head: a primer and set of first principles. *J. Personality Soc. Psychol.* 85, 650–661. doi: 10.1037/0022-3514.85.4.650

Canning, C., and Scheutz, M. (2013). Function near-infrared spectroscopy in human-robot interaction. *J. Hum. Rob. Interact.* 2, 62–84. doi: 10.5898/jhri.v2i3.144

Chau, T., and Damouras, S. (2009). Reply to 'on the risk of extracting relevant information from random data.' *J. Neural Eng.* 6, 058002. doi: 10.1088/1741-2560/6/5/058002

Coffey, E., Brouwer, A.-M., and van Erp, J. (2012). "Measuring workload using a combination of electroencephalography and near infrared spectroscopy," in *HFES*. doi: 10.1177/1071181312561367

Cortes, C., and Vapnik, V. (1995). Support-vector networks. *Mach. Learn.* 20, 273–297.

Coyle, S., Ward, T., and Markham, C. (2007). Brain-computer interface using a simplified functional near-infrared spectroscopy system. *J. Neural Eng.* 4, 219. doi: 10.1088/1741-2560/4/3/007

Cui, X., Bray, S., Bryant, D., Glover, G., and Reiss, A. (2011). A quantitative comparison of nirs and fmri across multiple cognitive tasks. *Neuroimage* 54, 2808–2821. doi: 10.1016/j.neuroimage.2010.10.069

Cui, X., Bray, S., and Reiss, A. (2010a). Functional near infrared spectroscopy (NIRS) signal improvement based on negative correlation between oxygenated and deoxygenated hemoglobin dynamics. *Neuroimage* 49, 3039–3046. doi: 10.1016/j.neuroimage.2009.11.050

Cui, X., Bray, S., and Reiss, A. (2010b). Speeded near infrared spectroscopy (NIRS) response detection. *PLoS ONE* 5:e15474. doi: 10.1371/journal.pone.0015474

Cutini, S., Moro, S., and Bisconti, S. (2012). Functional near infrared optical imaging in cognitive neuroscience: an introductory review. *J. Near Infrared Spectrosc.* 20, 75–92. doi: 10.1255/jnirs.969

Cutini, S., Scatturin, P., and Zorzi, M. (2011). A new method based on ICBM152 head surface for probe placement in multichannel fNIRS. *Neuroimage* 54, 919–927. doi: 10.1016/j.neuroimage.2010.09.030

Derosiere, G., Mandrick, K., Dray, G., Ward, T., and Perrey, S. (2013). NIRS-measured prefrontal cortex activity in neuroergonomics: strengths and weaknesses. *Front. Hum. Neurosci.* 7:583. doi: 10.3389/fnhum.2013.00583

Dominguez, L. (2009). On the risk of extracting relevant information from random data. *J. Neural Eng.* 6, 058001. doi: 10.1088/1741-2560/6/5/058001

Falk, T., Guirgis, M., Power, S., and Chau, T. (2011). Taking nirs-bcis outside the lab: achieving robustness against environment noise. *Neural Syst. Rehabil. Eng.* 19, 136–146. doi: 10.1109/TNSRE.2010.2078516

Fekete, T., Rubin, D., Carlson, J., and Mujica-Parodi, L. (2011). The NIRS analysis package: noise reduction and statistical inference. *PLoS ONE* 6:e24322. doi: 10.1371/journal.pone.0024322

Ferrari, M., and Quaresima, V. (2012). A brief review on the history of human functional near-infrared spectroscopy (fNIRS) development and fields of application. *Neuroimage* 63, 921–935. doi: 10.1016/j.neuroimage.2012.03.049

Frey, J., Mühl, C., Lotte, F., and Hachet, M. (2014). "Review of the use of electroencephalography as an evaluation method for human-computer interaction," in *International Conference on Physiological Computing Systems (PhyCS)*. (Lisbon).

George, L., and Lecuyer, A. (2010). "An overview of research on 'passive' brain-computer interfaces for implicit human-computer interaction in *International Conference on Applied Bionics and Biomechanics*. (Venice).

Girouard, A., Solovey, E., Hirshfield, L., Peck, E., Chauncey, K., Sassaroli, A., et al. (2010). "From brain signals to adaptive interfaces: using fNIRS in HCI," in *Brain-Computer Interfaces*, eds D. S. Tan and A. Nijholt (New York, NY: Springer), 221–237.

Girouard, A., Solovey, E., and Jacob, R. (2013). Designing a passive brain computer interface using real time classification of functional near-infrared spectroscopy. *Int. J. Auton. Adapt. Commun. Syst.* 6, 26–44. doi: 10.1504/IJAACS.2013.050689

Gupta, R., Laghari, K., Arndt, S., Schleicher, R., Moller, S., O'Shaughnessy, D., et al. (2013). "Using fNIRS to characterize human perception of TTS system quality, comprehension, and fluency: preliminary findings," in *International Workshop on Perceptual Quality of Systems (PQS)*.

Hall, M., Frank, E., Holmes, G., Pfahringer, B., Reutemann, P., and Witten, I. (2009). The WEKA data mining software: an update. *ACM SIGKDD Explor. Newslett.* 11, 10–18. doi: 10.1145/1656274.1656278

Heger, D., Mutter, R., Herff, C., Putze, F., and Schultz, T. (2013). "Continuous recognition of affective states by functional near infrared spectroscopy signals," in *Affective Computing and Intelligent Interaction (ACII)*. doi: 10.1109/ACII.2013.156

Heger, D., Putze, F., and Schultz, T. (2011). "Online recognition of facial actions for natural EEG-based BCI applications," in *Affective Computing and Intelligent Interaction (ACII)*. (Berlin, Heidelberg: Springer-Verlag), 436–446.

Herff, C., Heger, D., Fortmann, O., Hennrich, J., Putze, F., and Schultz, T. (2013a). Mental workload during n-back task—quantified in the prefrontal cortex using fNIRS. *Front. Hum. Neurosci.* 7:935. doi: 10.3389/fnhum.2013.00935

Herff, C., Heger, D., Putze, F., Hennrich, J., Fortmann, O., and Schultz, T. (2013b). Classification of mental tasks in the prefrontal cortex using fNIRS. *Conf. Proc. IEEE Eng. Med. Biol. Soc.* 2013, 2160–2163. doi: 10.1109/EMBC.2013.6609962

Hirshfield, L., Chauncey, K., Gulotta, R., Girouard, A., Solovey, E., Jacob, R., et al. (2009a). "Combining electroencephalograph and functional near infrared spectroscopy to explore users' mental workload," in *HCII*, (Heidelberg: Springer-Verlag Berlin), 239–247.

Hirshfield, L., Solovey, E., Girouard, A., Kebinger, J., Jacob, R., Sassaroli, A., et al. (2009b). "Brain measurement for usability testing and adaptive interfaces: an example of syntactic workload with functional near infrared spectroscopy," in *CHI*, (New York, NY: ACM), 2185–2194.

Hirshfield, L., Gulotta, R., Hirshfield, S., Hincks, S., Russell, M., Ward, R., et al. (2011a). "This is your brain on interfaces: enhancing usability testing with functional near-infrared spectroscopy," in *CHI*, (New York, NY: ACM), 373–382.

Hirshfield, L., Hirshfield, S., Hincks, S., Russell, M., Ward, R., and Williams, T. (2011b). "Trust in human-computer interactions as measured by frustration, surprise, and workload," in *Foundations of Augmented Cognition* (Orlando, FL), 507–516.

Hoshi, Y. (2003). Functional near-infrared optical imaging: utility and limitations in human brain mapping. *Psychophysiology* 40, 511–520. doi: 10.1111/1469-8986.00053

Hoshi, Y. (2007). Functional near-infrared spectroscopy: current status and future prospects. *J. Biomed. Opt.* 12:062106. doi: 10.1117/1.2804911

Hoshi, Y. (2011). Towards the next generation of near-infrared spectroscopy. *Philos. Trans. R. Soc. A Math. Phys. Eng. Sci.* 369, 4425–4439. doi: 10.1098/rsta.2011.0262

Hu, X., Hong, K., and Ge, S. (2013). Reduction of trial-to-trial variability in functional near-infrared spectroscopy signals by accounting for resting-state functional connectivity. *J. Biomed. Opt.* 18:17003. doi: 10.1117/1.JBO.18.1.017003

Izzetoglu, M., Chitrapu, P., Bunce, S., and Onaral, B. (2010). Motion artifact cancellation in NIR spectroscopy using discrete kalman filtering. *Biomed. Eng. Online* 9, 16. doi: 10.1186/1475-925X-9-16

Kawaguchi, Y., Wada, K., Okamoto, M., Tsujii, T., Shibata, T., and Sakatani, K. (2011). "Investigation of brain activity after interaction with seal robot measured by fnirs," in *Robot and Human Interactive Communication*, 308–313. doi: 10.1109/ROMAN.2012.6343812

Kirilina, E., Jelzow, A., Heine, A., Niessing, M., Wabnitz, H., Bruhl, R., et al. (2012). The physiological origin of task-evoked systemic artifacts in functional near infrared spectroscopy. *Neuroimage* 61, 70–81. doi: 10.1016/j.neuroimage.2012.02.074

Krusienski, D., Grosse-Wentrup, M., Galan, F., Coyle, D., Miller, K., Forney, E., et al. (2011). Critical issues in state-of-the-art brain-computer interface signal processing. *J. Neural Eng.* 8:025002. doi: 10.1088/1741-2560/8/2/025002

Liu, Y., Sourina, O., and Nguyen, M. (2011). "Real-time EEG-based emotion recognition and its applications," in *Transactions on Computational Science XII*, eds M. L. Gavrilova, C. J. Kenneth Tan, A, Sourin, and O, Sourina (Berlin: Springer), 256–277. doi: 10.1007/978-3-642-22336-5_13

Lloyd-Fox, S., Blasi, A., and Elwell, C. (2010). Illuminating the developing brain: the past, present and future of functional near infrared spectroscopy. *Neurosci. Biobehav. Rev.* 34, 269–284. doi: 10.1016/j.neubiorev.2009.07.008

Logothetis, N. (2008). What we can do and what we cannot do with fMRI. *Nature* 453, 869–878. doi: 10.1038/nature06976

Lotte, F. (2011). "Brain-computer interfaces for 3d games: hype or hope?" in *Foundations of Digital Games* (New York, NY: ACM), 325–327. doi: 10.1145/2159365.2159427

Lu, C., Zhang, Y., Biswal, B., Zang, Y., Peng, D., and Zhu, C. (2010). Use of fNIRS to assess resting state functional connectivity. *J. Neurosci. Methods* 186, 242–249. doi: 10.1016/j.jneumeth.2009.11.010

Luu, S., and Chau, T. (2009). Decoding subjective preference from single-trial near-infrared spectroscopy signals. *J. Neural Eng.* 6, 016003. doi: 10.1088/1741-2560/6/1/016003

Matsuyama, H., Asama, H., and Otake, M. (2009). "Design of differential near-infrared spectroscopy based brain machine interface," in *Robot and Human Interactive Communication*, 775–780. doi: 10.1109/ROMAN.2009.5326215

Matthews, F., and Pearlmutter, B. (2008). Hemodynamics for brain-computer interfaces. *Signal Process.* 25, 87–94. doi: 10.1109/MSP.2008.4408445

Molvi, B., and Dumont, G. (2012). Wavelet-based motion artifact removal for functional near-infrared spectroscopy. *Physiol. Meas.* 33, 259. doi: 10.1088/0967-3334/33/2/259

Nozawa, T. (2010). Autonomous adaptive agent with intrinsic motivation for sustainable hai. *J. Intell. Learn. Syst. Appl.* 2, 167–178. doi: 10.4236/jilsa.2010.24020

Ohara, K., Sellen, A., and Harper, R. (2011). "Embodiment in brain-computer interaction," in *CHI*. doi: 10.1145/1978942.1978994

Oriheula-Espina, F., Leff, D., James, D., Darzi, A., and Yang, G. (2010). Quality control and assurance in functional near infrared spectroscopy (fNIRS) experimentation. *Phys. Med. Biol.* 55, 3701–3724. doi: 10.1088/0031-9155/55/13/009

Peck, E., Afergan, D., and Jacob, R. (2013). "Brain sensing as input to information filtering systems," in *4th Augmented Human International Conference, AH'13*, (Stuttgart, Germany) 142–149.

Plichta, M., Herrmann, M., Baehne, C., Ehlis, A., Richter, M., Pauli, P., et al. (2007). Event-related functional near-infrared spectroscopy (fNIRS) based on craniocerebral correlations: reproducibility of activation? *Hum. Brain Mapp.* 28, 733–741. doi: 10.1002/hbm.20303

Power, S., Kushki, A., and Chau, T. (2012). Intersession consistency of single-trial classification of prefrontal response to mental arithmetic and no-control state by NIRS. *PLoS ONE* 7:e37791. doi: 10.1371/journal.pone.0037791

Robertson, F. C., Douglas, T. S., and Meintjes, E. M. (2010). Motion artifact removal for functional near infrared spectroscopy: a comparison of methods. *IEEE Trans. Biomed. Eng.* 57, 1377–1387. doi: 10.1109/TBME.2009.2038667

Sassaroli, A., Zheng, F., Hirshfield, L., Coutts, M., Girouard, A., Solovey, E., et al. (2009). "Application of near-infrared spectroscopy for discrimination of mental workloads," *SPIE*. doi: 10.1117/12.807737

Scarpa, F., Brigadoi, S., Cutini, S., Scatturin, P., Zorzi, M., Dell'Acqua, R., et al. (2013). A reference-channel based methodology to improve estimation of event related hemodynamic response from fNIRS measurements. *Neuroimage.* 72, 106–119. doi: 10.1016/j.neuroimage.2013.01.021

Scholkmann, F., Kleiser, S., Metz, A., Zimmermann, R., Pavi, J., Wolf, U., et al. (2014). A review on continuous wave functional near-infrared spectroscopy and imaging instrumentation and methodology. *Neuroimage* 85, 6–27. doi: 10.1016/j.neuroimage.2013.05.004

Scholkmann, F., Spichtig, S., Muehlemann, T., and Wolf, M. (2010). How to detect and reduce movement artifacts in near-infrared imaging using moving standard deviation and spline interpolation. *Physiol. Meas.* 31, 649–662. doi: 10.1088/0967-3334/31/5/004

Schudlo, L., and Chau, T. (2014). Dynamic topographical pattern classification of multichannel prefrontal NIRS signals: online differentiation of mental arithmetic and rest. *J. Neural Eng.* 11:016003. doi: 10.1088/1741-2560/11/1/016003

Solovey, E., Lalooses, F., Chauncey, K., Weaver, D., Parasi, M., Scheutz, M., et al. (2011). "Sensing cognitive multitasking for a brain-based adaptive user interface," in *Conference on Human Factors in Computing Systems (CHI)*, 383–392. doi: 10.1145/1978942.1978997

Solovey, E., Schermerhorn, P., Scheutz, M., Sassaroli, A., Fantini, S., and Jacob, R. (2012). "Brainput: enhancing interactive systems with streaming fNIRS brain input," in *CHI*, (New York, NY: ACM), 2193–2202. doi: 10.1145/2207676.2208372

Solovey, E. T. (2012). *Real-Time fNIRS Brain Input for Enhancing Interactive Systems*. PhD thesis, Tufts University.

Strait, M., Briggs, G., and Scheutz, M. (2013a). "Some correlates of agency ascription and emotional value and their effects on decision- making," in *Conference on Affective Computing and Intelligent Interaction (ACII)*, (Washington, DC), 505–510. doi: 10.1109/ACII.2013.89

Strait, M., Canning, C., and Scheutz, M. (2013b). "Limitations of NIRS-based BCI for realistic applications in human-computer interaction," in *BCI Meeting*, (Monterey, CA), 6–7.

Strait, M., Canning, C., and Scheutz, M. (2014a). "Let me tell you! investigating the effects of robot communication strategies in advice- giving situations based on robot appearance, interaction modality and distance," in *Human-Robot Interaction (HRI)*, (New York, NY: ACM). doi: 10.1145/2559636.2559670

Strait, M., Canning, C., and Scheutz, S. (2014b). "Reliability of NIRS-Based BCIs: a placebo-controlled replication and reanalysis of Brainput," in *Human Factors in Computing (CHI), Extended Abstracts*. doi: 10.1145/2559206.2578866

Strait, M., and Scheutz, M. (2014). "Using near infrared spectroscopy to index temporal changes in affect in realistic human–robot interactions," in *Physiological Computing Systems (PhyCS), Special Session on Affect Recogntion from Physiological Data for Social Robots.*

Szafir, D., and Mutlu, B. (2012). "Pay attention! designing adaptive agents that monitor and improve user engagement," in *Conference on Human Factors in Computing Systems (CHI)*, (New York, NY: ACM), 11–20. doi: 10.1145/2207676.2207679

Tak, S., and Ye, J. (2014). Statistical analysis of fNIRS data: a comprehensive review. *Neuroimage* 85, 92–103. doi: 10.1016/j.neuroimage.2013.06.016

Tan, D., and Nijholt, A., editors (2010). *Brain-Computer Interfaces: Applying Our Minds to Human-Computer Interaction*. London: Springer. doi: 10.1007/978-1-84996-272-8

Tanaka, H., Katura, T., and Sato, H. (2012). Task-related component analysis for functional neuroimaging and application to near-infrared spectroscopy data. *Neuroimage* 64, 308–327. doi: 10.1016/j.neuroimage.2012.08.044

Tsuzuki, D., and Dan, I. (2014). Spatial registration for functional near-infrared spectroscopy: from channel position on the scalp to cortical location in individual and group analyses. *Neuroimage* 85, 92–103. doi: 10.1016/j.neuroimage.2013.07.025

Tupak, S., Dresler, T., Guhn, A., Ehlis, A., Fallgatter, A., Pauli, P., et al. (2014). Implicit emotion regulation in the presence of threat: neural and autonomic correlates. *Neuroimage* 85, 372–379. doi: 10.1016/j.neuroimage.2013.09.066

Villringer, A., Planck, J., Hock, C., Schleinkofer, L., and Dirnagl, U. (1993). Near infrared spectroscopy (NIRS): a new tool to study hemodynamic changes during activation of brain function in human adults. *Neurosci. Lett.* 154, 101–104. doi: 10.1016/0304-3940(93)90181-J

Virtanen, J., Noponen, T., Kotilahti, K., Virtanen, J., and Ilmoniemi, R. (2011). Accelerometer-based method for correcting signal baseline changes caused by motion artifacts in medical near-infrared spectroscopy. *J. Biomed. Opt.* 16, 087005. doi: 10.1117/1.3606576

Ye, J., Tak, S., Jang, K., Jung, J., and Jang, J. (2009). NIRS-SPM: statistical parametric mapping for near-infrared spectroscopy. *Neuroimage* 44, 428–447. doi: 10.1016/j.neuroimage.2008.08.036

Zander, T., and Kothe, C. (2011). Towards passive brain-computer interfaces: applying brain-computer interface technology to human-machine systems in general. *J. Neural Eng.* 8, 025005. doi: 10.1088/1741-2560/8/2/025005

13

A new paradigm to induce mental stress: the Sing-a-Song Stress Test (SSST)

Anne-Marie Brouwer* and Maarten A. Hogervorst

TNO, Perceptual and Cognitive Systems, Soesterberg, Netherlands

Correspondence:
Anne-Marie Brouwer, TNO, Perceptual and Cognitive Systems, PO Box 23, Kampweg 5, 3769 ZG Soesterberg, Netherlands
e-mail: anne-marie.brouwer@tno.nl

We here introduce a new experimental paradigm to induce mental stress in a quick and easy way while adhering to ethical standards and controlling for potential confounds resulting from sensory input and body movements. In our Sing-a-Song Stress Test, participants are presented with neutral messages on a screen, interleaved with 1-min time intervals. The final message is that the participant should sing a song aloud after the interval has elapsed. Participants sit still during the whole procedure. We found that heart rate and skin conductance during the 1-min intervals following the sing-a-song stress message are substantially higher than during intervals following neutral messages. The order of magnitude of the rise is comparable to that achieved by the Trier Social Stress Test. Skin conductance increase correlates positively with experienced stress level as reported by participants. We also simulated stress detection in real time. When using both skin conductance and heart rate, stress is detected for 18 out of 20 participants, approximately 10 s after onset of the sing-a-song message. In conclusion, the Sing-a-Song Stress Test provides a quick, easy, controlled and potent way to induce mental stress and could be helpful in studies ranging from examining physiological effects of mental stress to evaluating interventions to reduce stress.

Keywords: stress, arousal, paradigm, heart rate, skin conductance

INTRODUCTION

When studying physiological effects of sudden arousing and negative emotional events, it is desirable to induce a considerable amount of emotional stress in an easy, controlled and efficient manner, while respecting ethical standards with regard to experimental participants. A range of protocols in this direction has been described in the literature. Kreibig (2010) lists experimental paradigms of 134 studies on effects of emotion on autonomic nervous system activity. With respect to the negative emotions fear and anxiety, paradigms that have been used include watching film clips (Eisenberg et al., 1988), viewing pictures from the standardized International Affective Picture System (IAPS) by Lang et al. (2005) (Ritz et al., 2005), listening to sounds from the standardized International Affective Digitized Sound system (IADS) by Bradley and Lang (2007) (Brouwer et al., 2013), listening to music (Krumhansl, 1997), expecting an electrical shock (Bloom and Trautt, 1977), mental imagery (Van Diest et al., 2006), negative events in a gaming context (Brouwer et al., 2011), recall of personal emotional events and directed facial expression (Ekman et al., 1983). The paradigm that has become the worldwide standard for inducing psychological stress is the Trier Social Stress Test (TSST—Kirschbaum et al., 1993). In this paradigm, participants are asked to take over the role of a job applicant. They are informed that they will be giving a speech to a "selection committee" consisting of three people, and that their speech performance will be video and audio recorded for analysis. At the start of the procedure, participants get to see the business-like equipped test room with the committee, wearing white coats. During a stress anticipation interval of 10 min, participants prepare a speech that should convince the selection committee that they are the perfect candidate for a job. Participants are provided with paper and pencil to help them prepare. Following the stress anticipation interval, they deliver their speech standing in front of the selection committee. The members of the committee respond in a standardized, non-emphatic way. After 5 min of free speech, the participant is instructed to perform a serial subtraction task aloud, having to start over again on each mistake. In a later version, the paradigm has been adapted slightly to involve two to three people in the selection committee and only 3 min of preparation time (Kudielka et al., 2007).

The TSST is considered the best available paradigm to reliably elicit strong neuroendocrine stress responses (Dickerson and Kemeny, 2004). Responses of the sympathetic nervous system are also strong in comparison to other paradigms. Heart rate increases in the order of 17 bpm (Kirschbaum et al., 1993; 20 bpm in a TSST for groups: von Dawans et al., 2011) when comparing a baseline measurement to a measurement taken at the end of the 10-min preparation interval. In a public speaking task that is comparable to the TSST but that made use of a virtual rather than a real audience (Westenberg et al., 2009), heart rate increased with about 10 bpm and skin conductance increased with approximately 2 μS. In their TSST review paper, Kudielka et al. (2007) mention a heart rate increase of 15–25 to the psychosocial stressor. It is unclear though which heart rate values are compared to arrive at this estimate. It probably involves heart rate during performance of the task, which is arguably the time that the most stress is experienced but which is also confounded by standing and talking such that part of the increase in heart rate is likely due to physical activity. As a rough comparison to physiological effects found using the TSST, viewing arousing pictures with negative valence usually elicits short rises in skin conductance of at most a few tenths of μS (Codispoti et al., 2001; Codispoti and De Cesarei, 2007) while heart rate decelerates for about one or at most a few bpm (Codispoti and De Cesarei, 2007; Brouwer et al., 2013).

The stress elicited by the TSST is multi-facetted. Participants perform cognitive tasks while preparing and delivering a speech, they are standing upright and talking, but the element that is considered to be mainly responsible for at least the strong neuroendocrine stress responses is social-evaluative threat (Dickerson and Kemeny, 2004). Social-evaluative threat occurs when an important aspect of the self-identity is, or could be negatively judged by others.

While the TSST elicits reliable stress responses and is a well-studied paradigm, it is a relatively complicated procedure geared to examining neuroendocrine responses. We present an easy, short and effective stress-inducing paradigm that is geared toward examining stress responses controlled by the sympathetic nervous system such as skin conductance and heart rate. These stress responses typically occur faster than neuroendocrine responses. However, they can also be strongly affected by posture or body movements such as speech, so it is important to keep these constant across stress levels. In our paradigm, participants are presented with neutral messages on a screen, interleaved with 1-min time intervals. The final message is that the participant should sing a song aloud after the interval has elapsed. Participants sit still during the whole procedure. Skin conductance and heart rate are compared between time intervals that follow neutral messages and the one that follows presentation of sing-a-song "stress" message. In contrast to the TSST and a number of other stress inducing paradigms, both body movements and sensory input are kept constant while only mental stress is varied. This ensures that effects of the stress message on skin conductance and heart rate can only be attributed to psychological processes, and are not caused or partly caused by an increase in visual input or by the fact that the individual starts moving or talking.

In accordance to the stress inducing potency of social-evaluative threat, earlier studies indicate that anticipating and watching oneself singing with an audience, does indeed elicit emotional stress. In a study by Harris (2001) participants sang "Star Spangled Banner" while being recorded on video. After singing, there was a 10-min break followed by a 6-min relaxation period during which physiological baseline measures were taken. Then, the participant watched the video tape together with the experimenter and two confederates. No instructions were given to the participants on how to behave during this viewing interval. During the first minute of the viewing interval, heart rate was 4.5 (first study) or 3 (second study) bpm higher than during the baseline measurement. Changes in heart rate were significantly correlated with subjective ratings of feeling calm ($r = -0.43$) and feeling embarrassed ($r = 0.38$). Hofmann et al. (2006) investigated autonomic correlates of social anxiety and embarrassment in shy and non-shy individuals. They informed their participants upon arrival in the lab that they would be asked to give a speech and to sing in front of a video camera. Their results indicated that anticipating singing results in a stronger increase of heart rate (compared to an eyes-closed baseline) than either anticipating giving a speech or watching videos of the performance together with confederates. Average heart rate increase was 11 bpm, and skin conductance increased with approximately 4 μS.

The main aim of the present study was to examine the potency of our Sing-a-Song Stress Test to elicit stress-related increases in heart rate and skin conductance. On the one hand, we expected the test to be effective given relatively strong effects of previous studies on social evaluative threat and singing, on the other hand, effect sizes may have been expected to be small since we excluded effects of confounds that possibly contributed to effects in other studies. We checked whether eventual increases could be detected by a change detection algorithm on the level of an individual participant, simulating an online stress detection algorithm in a situation that a participant is sitting still. Ultimately, we are interested in online and real-life detection of sudden stress based on physiological signals—if possible without attaching sensors to the body. Wieringa et al. (2005) showed that it is possible to recover heart rate from no-contact recorded images. Poh et al. (2010) described a robust algorithm to determine heart rate from varying color of a face as recorded by a camera. A similar algorithm has been exploited in Vital Signs Camera technology by Philips. To compare the performance of this technology to heart rate as measured using traditional electrocardiography (ECG), we measured heart rate using ECG and a camera simultaneously. A previous experiment indicated that heart rate based on camera images is very similar to heart rate extracted from ECG when averaging across 2 min intervals (Hogervorst et al., 2013).

MATERIALS AND METHODS

PARTICIPANTS

Twenty-five participants (15 female, 10 male) took part in the experiment. They were between 19 and 50 years old with a mean age of 30 and a standard deviation of 11 years. None of them suffered from a heart disease or took drugs that affect heart rate, as verified through a questionnaire. Participants received a monetary reward to make up for their travel and time. The study is in accordance with the Declaration of Helsinki and has been approved of by the local ethics committee. All participants signed an informed consent form prior to taking part in the experiment.

MATERIALS

Stimuli

We selected nine phrases that were approximately of the same length and structure as the 10th sentence which was the following (translated into English): "Task: start singing a song aloud when the counter reaches zero. Keep sitting still until that moment." Since we did not want the other nine phrases to elicit stress, we picked neutral phrases from the Dutch Wikipedia site about vacuum cleaners. A translated example is "Phrase: the first vacuum cleaner was constructed by Sweep Company. This was in 1907 and the device was called hoover."

ECG and skin conductance

To record ECG, we used self-adhesive Kendall Neonatal ECG electrodes (TYCO healthcare, Neustadt, Germany). The ECG channel electrode was placed at the sixth left intercostal space (midclavicular line); the reference electrode was placed at the first right intercostal space (midclavicular line); the ECG ground electrode was placed at the sixth right intercostal space (midclavicular line). Recording frequency was 256 Hz. To record skin conductance, we used the g.GSRsensor2 from G.tec Medical engineering (G.tec GmbH, Schiedlberg, Austria). Electrodes were applied to the fingertips of the index finger and the middle finger. Physiological data was processed by a G.tec USB Biosignal amplifier.

Vital Signs camera

Heart rate was also determined using a camera and Philips Vital Signs camera software. The camera was an IDS UI-2220SE-C-HQ (uEye SE) 12-bit color camera, recording raw RGB-video, 8-bit per channel at 20 Hz and 768 × 576 pixels. The Vital Signs camera software requires the user to initially indicate a skin location by drawing a rectangle around a suitable face region as displayed on a monitor. This region is then automatically tracked. The Vital Signs camera software derives a measure of heart rate from subtle variations in skin color. Each measure is based on a window of 25.6 s and the resulting heart frequency is reported with a resolution of 0.039 Hz or 2.34 bmp at an output frequency of 20 Hz.

PROCEDURE

Participants were not given any instructions prior to the study e.g., with respect to eating and drinking or physical activity prior to coming into the lab. The participant, as well as two confederate "participants" (one male and one female), were picked up by the experimental leader from the waiting area. In the experimental room, the experimental leader explained that they would be sitting in turn behind the monitor while heart rate and skin conductance are monitored and they are filmed by a camera. The task description was to sit as still as possible and silently read the messages that appear on the monitor, interchanged by a counter counting down from 60 to 0 s. They were told that one of the messages could entail a task that they then needed to carry out after the subsequent counter reached 0. Participants were not told that the experiment was about stress or involved singing. Subsequently, the participant and the confederates filled out the informed consent form as well as a questionnaire with general questions about age, use of cigarettes, coffee and alcohol, physical activity and cardiovascular health. The experimental leader then appointed the real participant as the one to start, seated him or her behind the monitor and then attached the physiological sensors. The monitor was in between the participant and the confederates, who were sitting on chairs facing a wall such that the angle between their gaze and that of the participant was 90 degrees. After the experiment, participants were asked whether they had believed that the confederates were experimental participants. They were also asked to indicate the stress they experienced during the minute before singing on a scale of 1 (not stressed at all) to 10 (extremely stressed). The experimental room did not have windows to the outside. Lighting was constant office lighting.

ANALYSIS

ECG and skin conductance

The ECG signal was filtered by the g-tec amplifier with a 0.5–100 Hz band pass filter, and afterwards by a 2.5 Hz high-pass 2-sided Butterworth filter. R wave to R wave interval (RRI, the interval between successive heart beats) was extracted from this signal. Outliers resulting from the RRI derivation were determined by calculating differences from a moving median as calculated over 30 samples. Values outside the 5–95% quantile range were removed. For each participant, we then determined the mean RRI of each of the 1-min count-down intervals (blocks), and mean RRI was converted to HR (bpm). Also, mean skin conductance level was calculated over the 1-min blocks.

Statistical analysis

In order to test whether heart rate and skin conductance show a sudden increase after presentation of the sing-a-song sentence, we performed paired *t*-tests on values of heart rate and skin conductance averaged over the 1-min blocks after offset of the 9th (vacuum cleaner) message and the 10th (sing-a-song) message, for each participant. Correlations are computed between subjective stress ratings and differences in heart rate between the 9th and the 10th block as well as between subjective stress ratings and differences in skin conductance between the 9th and the 10th block. Positive values indicate higher values in the 10th than in the 9th block.

Stress detector

By designing a set of stress detectors based on detecting changes in state, we wanted to get an impression to what extent the onset of the sing-a-song message could be detected for a single individual and in real time. Note that it was not our goal to design the most optimal detector. Performance of these detectors can thus be considered to be the lower bound to performance under the circumstances tested.

Basic change detection algorithm

The "normal" state of the signal was described by calculating the average and standard deviation of the signal during blocks 1–9 of the experiment, for each of the participants separately. Next, a normalized signal, akin to the *z*-score, was computed by subtracting the mean signal and dividing this difference by the standard deviation. A threshold was set above which a signal was considered to be deviating from normal, therewith signaling a change of state. Here, a change was assumed to correspond to the onset of stress. For each of the types of signals (as used in different detector types as described below) a suitable threshold was chosen, such that a change in physiological state was most often detected in block 10 and least often in other blocks (false alarms).

Detector types

Detectors were designed that made use of the various types of information available. Two detectors were based on heart rate only: one was based on heart rate derived from the ECG signal and one on heart rate derived from the camera data. The stress detection threshold for these detectors was set to a value of 4.

For skin conductance we used two different types of detectors. One detector used the raw signal with a threshold value of 6. Another detector used a filtered version of skin conductance. Filtering was done by subtracting the mean over the interval starting at 33 s and ending 3 s before the current moment from the mean over the last 3 s. This filter acts as an edge detector and eliminates slow variations in the skin conductance. The filtered signal was used as signal input to the basic change detection algorithm. We used a threshold value of 6 for this skin conductance edge detector (i.e., the same as for the skin conductance detector based on the raw signal). The skin conductance edge detector turned out to perform better than the detector based on the raw signal due to the existence of slow variations in the skin conductance level.

Finally, a detector was constructed in which the skin conductance edge output and ECG heart rate were combined. Both signals were converted to a normalized z-score before they were combined by calculating the square root over the sum of squares and dividing by the square root of 2: $z = \text{sqrt}(x^2 + y^2)/\text{sqrt}(2)$ (where x is the z-score of the skin conductance signal, y is the z-score of heart rate, and z is the combined z-score). In correspondence with the individual thresholds (6 and 4) the threshold for the combined signal was set to 5.

RESULTS

GENERAL

All 25 participants started singing. Three participants accidentally started to sing too early, that is, before the counter had reached zero. After the experiment had ended, four participants stated that they had doubted that the confederates were real participants. None of them was a participant who started singing early. The data of the three early singing participants are excluded from further analyses to prevent confounding the mental stress interval with body movements.

HEART RATE RESPONSE

Heart rate responses to the presentation of the sing-a-song sentence were generally very strong as indicated by the data of an example participant in **Figure 1A**. For every participant, heart rate was on average higher in the 10th than in the 9th block. **Figure 2A** indicates the heart rate for each of the 10 blocks averaged across participants. A paired t-test indicates a significant difference between the 9th and the 10th block ($t_{21} = 6.21$, $p < 0.001$, mean difference: 15.3 bpm, Cohen's d: 1.63, paired t-tests comparing the 10th block to all other blocks resulted in p-values < 0.001 as well).

SKIN CONDUCTANCE RESPONSE

Like heart rate responses, skin conductance responses to the presentation of the sing-a-song sentence were generally very strong. Data of an example participant is presented in **Figure 1B**. For two of the participants, skin conductance recording failed. For all of the 20 remaining participants, skin conductance was on average higher in the 10th than in the 9th block. **Figure 2B** indicates the average skin conductance in the different blocks. A paired t-test indicates a significant difference between the 9th and the 10th block [$t_{(19)} = 5.37$, $p < 0.001$, mean difference: 10.9 μS, Cohen's d: 0.81, paired t-tests comparing the 10th block to all other blocks resulted in p-values < 0.001 as well].

SUBJECTIVE RATINGS

The subjective rating of experienced stress was missing for one out of 22 participants. Ratings vary from 2 to 10 with a mean of 6.4 and a standard deviation of 2.1. As indicated in **Figure 3A**, subjective ratings correlated with skin conductance response (i.e., the difference in mean skin conductance level between the 9th and the 10th block: $r = 0.50$, $p = 0.03$). We did not find a significant correlation between subjective ratings and heart rate response (**Figure 3B**; $r = 0.26$, $p = 0.26$).

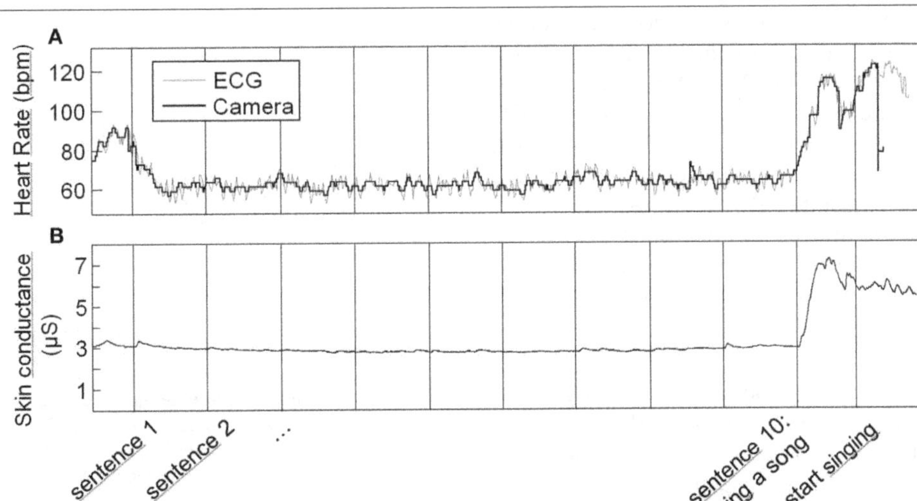

FIGURE 1 | Heart rate (A) and skin conductance (B) of an example participant across the whole experiment. Vertical lines indicate the sentence onsets except for the very last one that corresponds to singing onset. Heart rate depicted by the gray line is heart rate derived from ECG; heart rate depicted by the black line is heart rate derived from the camera.

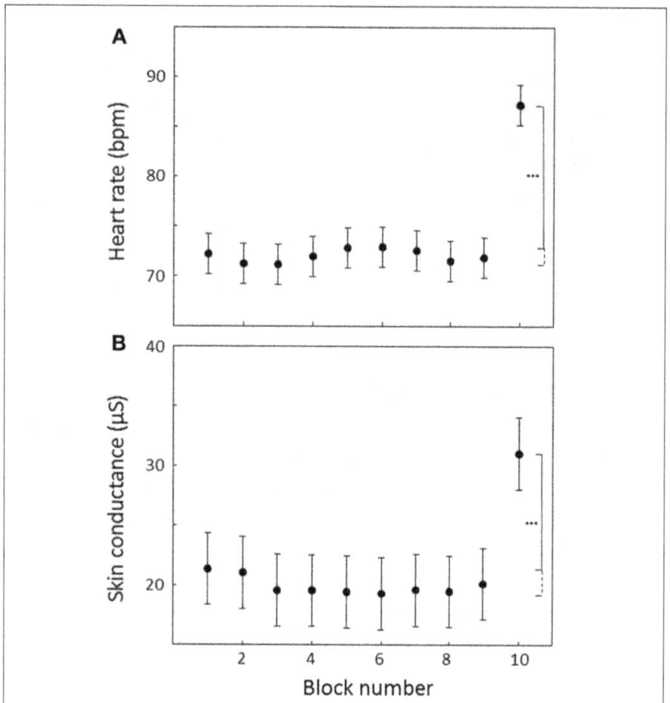

FIGURE 2 | Heart rate (A) and skin conductance (B) averaged across 1-min count-down blocks across all subjects. Block 10 is the count-down block following the sing-a-song sentence. Error bars indicate standard errors of the mean. Stars indicate that heart rate and skin conductance are significantly higher in block 10 compared to all other blocks at an alpha level of 0.001.

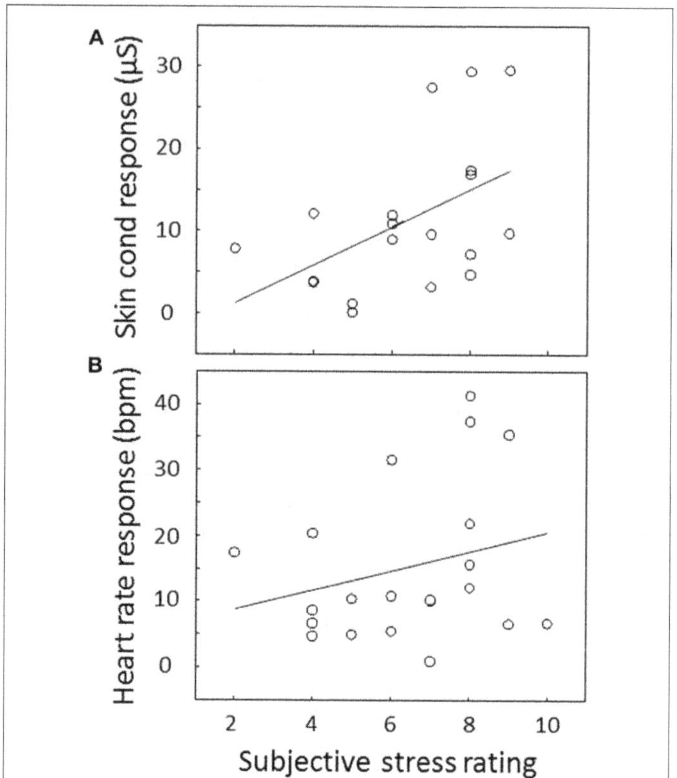

FIGURE 3 | Association between subjective stress and (A) skin conductance and (B) heart rate response. Responses are determined by the difference in average skin conductance level or heart rate between the 9th and the 10th block and plotted against subjective stress rating for each participant. The correlation between subjective stress and skin conductance response was significant; the correlation between subjective stress and heart rate response was not. The plotted lines are linear regression lines.

VITAL SIGNS CAMERA SYSTEM

There is a strong correspondence between heart rate as determined by the Vital Signs camera system and ECG. The example data in **Figure 1A** show that while the high frequency heart rate variability cannot be closely followed due to limited resolution, the heart rate as given by the camera system nicely follows the ECG data. The scatter plot presented in **Figure 4** represents average heart rate values for each of the 25 participants and each 1-min block as based on the camera and ECG. On average, ECG indicates a heart rate that is 0.55 bpm faster ($SD = 2.22$) than the Vital Signs Camera system. The median indicates a 0.25 bpm faster heart rate. The mean absolute difference is 0.92 bpm ($SD = 2.09$). The median absolute difference is 0.38 bpm. 77% of the heart rate values as measured by the camera is within 1 bpm difference from ECG; 90% is within 2 bpm difference.

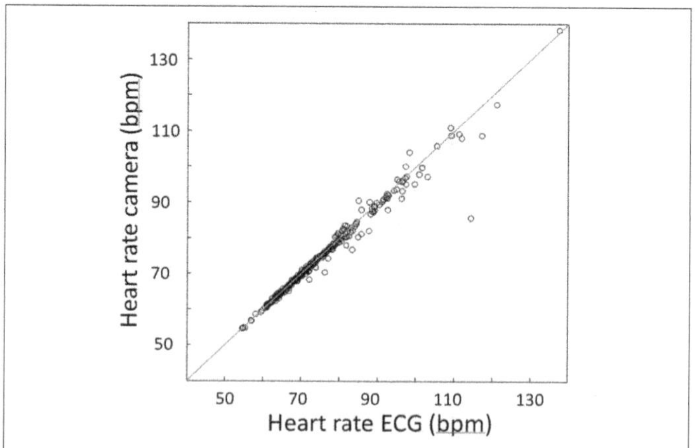

FIGURE 4 | Association between heart rate as determined by the camera and heart rate as determined by ECG. The diagonal line is the unity line. Each symbol represents the average heart rate as derived from ECG and the camera for one 1-min block for one participant.

STRESS DETECTOR

Table 1 shows the results of the various stress detectors for 20 participants since data of the three participants that started to sing early and the data of the two participants with failed skin conductance recording were excluded. Shown are the number of participants for which a state change was detected in block 10 ("Detections") and the total number of detected state changes during blocks 1–9 (false alarms: "FAs") over all participants. The false alarms often occurred at the start of the experiment and seemed at least partly be due to signal recording artifacts. When false alarms occurring during the first 20 s of the experiment were not counted, this resulted in a 60% reduction of false alarms as indicated in the table. The last two columns show the mean and median detection times (DTs), indicating the time between the

Table 1 | Threshold settings and results for the different stress detectors.

Detector	Threshold	Detections	FAs	FAs after 20 s	Mean *DT*	Median *DT*
Skin conductance raw	6	15 (75%)	0	0	15.3	6.8
Skin conductance edge	6	17 (85%)	7	2	7.7	6.7
Heart rate camera	4	16 (80%)	13	7	23.3	26.0
Heart rate ECG	4	17 (85%)	3	1	24.3	22.1
Heart rate ECG + skin conductance edge	5	18 (90%)	2	0	11.1	8.1

"Detections" are the number (and %) of participants out of 20 for which stress was detected in the 10th block. "FAs" are the total number of false alarms ("stress detections" in block 1–9). "FAs after 20 s" represents the same but after excluding the first 20 s of block 1. "Mean DT" and "Median DT" (detection time in s) indicate when stress was detected relative to the onset of the sing-a-song sentence.

start of block 10 and detection. For determining detection times, we only used blocks in which a state change was detected. These detection times are quite short, especially considering that the participant and his/her physiological system need some time to react to the stimulus.

Of the single sensor detectors the skin conductance edge detector performs best, detecting a change in the 10th block for 85% of the participants. The detector that uses the raw skin conductance signal shows the lowest detection performance (75% of the participants) indicating that preprocessing is required to compensate for the slow variations in the raw signal.

The detector that uses heart rate as derived from ECG seems to perform better than the one based on the camera in terms of the number of detections and the number of false alarms. Whereas both signals are largely the same, the resolution of the camera signal is limited resulting in more noise.

The detector that uses a combination of heart rate (from ECG) and filtered skin conductance performs best, with a detection rate of 90% (18 out of 20 subjects) and only two false alarms that were both found during the first 20 s of the experiment. The missed detections by the 5 different detectors originate from 8 participants, labeled "A" through "H" in **Table 2**. This table shows the overlap of participants with missed detections across the different detectors. For one of the participants ("A"), none of the detectors detected a state change in block 10. It is possible that this participant simply did not experience stress. Participants B and C did not show a detectable skin conductance response to the stress message while heart rate did show a response. The converse is true for participants D and E. More noisy variants of skin conductance (i.e., the raw data version) and heart rate (i.e., the camera version) resulted in below detection effects for three participants for one or the other signal (participant F, G, and H).

Table 2 | Participants without detected stress response for at least one detector.

Detector	Participant							
	A	B	C	D	E	F	G	H
Skin conductance raw	×	×	×			×	×	
Skin conductance edge	×	×	×					
Heart rate camera	×			×	×			×
Heart rate ECG	×			×	×			
Heart rate ECG + skin conductance edge	×		×					

*The missed detections per detector equal the number of detections as presented in **Table 1** subtracted from 20 (the number of included participants).*

DISCUSSION

THE SING-A-SONG STRESS TEST

The Sing-a-Song Stress Test proved to be an effective way to induce stress: rises in heart rate and skin conductance across 1 min, or even a fraction thereof, were in the same order as those elicited by the TSST viewed over 10 min. Rises in heart rate and skin conductance responses were an order of magnitude larger than those generally reported to be elicited by perceptual stimuli. Most subjective stress ratings reflected moderate to strong experienced stress, and individual subjective ratings correlated with rises in skin conductance. The same trend was observed for heart rate. As opposed to the TSST, our paradigm features a sudden stressor with known onset which makes it suitable to investigate physiological responses in short time windows. This paradigm also offers a clear within-subject baseline that controls for sensory input and body movement, and that is close in time to the stress interval (i.e., the 9th "neutral" count-down block as compared to the 10th "stress" count-down block). Since the paradigm only involves a passive audience of two confederates who are, during the experiment, not directly in the line of sight of the participant, possible effects of confederates behaving differently toward different participants are minimized. The limited role of the confederates would also potentially enable the use of different confederates within one project. The Sing-a-Song Stress procedure is short, with a complete experiment lasting about 11 min. The only equipment that is needed is a computer and a screen presenting messages at fixed time intervals. The limited number and role of the confederates, the short procedure and the fact that no special equipment is needed make the paradigm low-cost. Since participants do not move and are in front of a monitor rather than in front of a real-life audience, the test could in principle be applied in an MRI scanner (as also addressed in Quaedflieg et al., 2013). Stress induction paradigms, such as the Sing-a-Song Stress Test, can be useful in a range of stress-related studies (Kudielka et al., 2007). Examples include validating stress response sensitivity of physiological sensors or signal processing algorithms, evaluating interventions to reduce stress or examining the association between personality characteristics and stress responses.

LIMITATIONS OF THE PARADIGM, POSSIBLE IMPROVEMENTS AND FUTURE EXPERIMENTS

The instruction of singing after the 10th count-down interval was not followed by three out of 25 participants. They started singing earlier than that and we had to exclude these data to prevent confounding the mental stress interval with body movements. If we had included data of these participants, mean heart rate increase would still have been 15.3 bpm (as is the average hart rate increase without these participants), while the skin conductance increase would on average have been larger (12.6 μS rather than 10.9 μS). This stronger response would both be consistent with an effect of movement or a different kind of breathing, and of early singers being more stressed than the other participants which would arguably be consistent with the fact that they were not able to follow the instruction.

The Sing-a-Song Stress Test induces stress by asking participants to sing a song after a designated interval is over. While physiological effects can only be due to mental processes, we do not know exactly which mental processes contribute to the observed effects, similar to the TSST. Both the TSST and the Sing-a-Song Stress Test involve mental workload besides social anxiety and (anticipated) embarrassment. The cognitive task of our participants was arguably easier than preparing a speech, but they did need to choose a song to sing. Increasing workload (therewith probably also increasing stress) has been found to be associated with increasing heart rate and skin conductance. In an experiment that varied workload while keeping perceptual input and movement constant, heart rate was about 4 bpm higher and skin conductance level about 1.5 μS higher in a quite difficult high workload condition compared to a very easy, low workload condition (Brouwer et al., 2014). While it may be impossible to completely disentangle mental processes such as workload and more emotion-related stress for all individuals, as well as to properly equate the strengths of these processes, it seems that in general effects of workload on physiology are less strong than effects of emotional stress (Harris, 2001; Hofmann et al., 2006). Future experiments using the Sing-a-Song Stress Test could dissociate workload and emotional stress to some extent by telling participants which well-known song they are supposed to sing or by replacing the neutral messages by neutral mental tasks. Also, overall mental stress may be increased by increasing the workload aspect of the task (e.g., "sing a song that is about a city and that none of the participants before you have sung").

Stress responses when repeating the paradigm in the same individual could reveal to what extent there is habituation. If stress can be repeatedly induced, this would increase the value of the test for fMRI studies. For the TSST and other stress protocols, habituation of the neuroendocrine processes has been reported but the sympathetic nervous system has been found to respond more uniformly to repeated exposure to psychosocial challenge (Kudielka et al., 2007).

Future studies that may help to further improve the paradigm include examining the effect of the number of confederates (with a minimum of zero—where the experimental leader is the only audience available) as well as the effect of the role they play. Now we had confederates waiting in the waiting area and fill out forms so as to make the participants believe that they were really fellow participants, but this may not be necessary. Four of the 25 participants indicated after the experiment that they had doubted that the confederates were real participants. While obviously, this number of participants is too low to allow firm statements on the possible effect of believing the scenario, these four participants did not show a trend to weaker physiological or subjective stress responses. Another way of improving the paradigm could be to reduce the number of neutral messages. **Figure 2** shows that there is not much heart rate and skin conductance variation over the first nine blocks suggesting that e.g., four rather than nine blocks may be sufficient. Finally, future experiments should include a baseline subjective stress rating before the experiment starts, and not only after the stress interval. While the time of baseline would be different than the physiological baseline at block 9, taking the difference between the baseline and the subjective rating about experienced stress in block 10 would remove the effect of differences between participants in rating own subjective stress in general. This difference measure would probably comprise a more sensitive subjective stress measure that is expected to correlate better with skin conductance and heart rate responses.

DETECTING SUDDEN INCREASE IN STRESS: APPLICATIONS

This study provides a clear and well-controlled example of the strong effects of mental stress on heart rate and skin conductance. We implemented simple algorithms that could be used in real time to identify a sudden increase in stress within an individual and showed that this was also possible, be it to a lesser extent, using only a camera based heart detection system. This may enable potential applications. Examples are the evaluation of interventions (e.g., scents) that reduce the stress inducing quality of certain stimuli (e.g., a dentist drill) or supporting a therapist when administering anxiety-evoking stimuli in exposure therapy (Popovic et al., 2006). Applications of stress detectors would be particularly valuable in cases where individuals cannot or do not want to express the stress they experience. This could be the case in patients who cannot express themselves effectively due to physical or mental limitations. Stress detectors may help to clarify how they experience certain medical treatments and how they can be modified to elicit less stress in general or in a particular individual. In the safety domain, stress detectors (from a distance) may be one way to increase the chances of picking the appropriate individuals from a waiting line for search by looking at responses to stimuli like the appearance of a drugs sniffing dog. Of course, many of these situations do involve potential effects of movement that we here carefully excluded. These effects will give rise to false alarms. False alarm rates could be reduced by taking into account concurrent measurements of movements. It may also be necessary to limit application of such a stress monitor to situations where there are very little movements. Regardless, in any application the presence of false alarms should be dealt with, e.g., by treating the system as one of several (fallible) stress indicators, or, in the case of evaluating interventions, by looking at the mean of large data sets. Not discussed here, but essential when designing applications around mental stress detection are privacy concerns.

CONCLUSIONS

By making use of the relatively strong effects of social evaluative threat on physiological measures of stress, we designed a new experimental paradigm to induce stress at a clearly specified moment in time in an easy and effective way. The effects of heart rate and skin conductance turned out to be strong and detectable on the level of an individual participant. We hope that the Sing-a-Song Stress Test will facilitate standardized studies on mental stress that are controlled for sensory and movement confounds.

ACKNOWLEDGMENTS

Thanks to Manje Brinkhuis for running the experiment, and members of the project team Wouter Vos and Marc Menkhorst. Financially enabled by the Netherlands Ministry of Safety and Justice within the programme "Innovatie Maatschappelijke Veiligheid" initiated by the Center "Innovatie en Veiligheid," Utrecht. Additional support came from the BrainGain Smart Mix Programme of the Netherlands Ministry of Economic Affairs and the Netherlands Ministry of Education, Culture and Science.

REFERENCES

Bloom, L. J., and Trautt, G. M. (1977). Finger pulse volume as a measure of anxiety: further evaluation. *Psychophysiology* 14, 541–544. doi: 10.1111/j.1469-8986.1977.tb01195.x

Bradley, M. M., and Lang, P. J. (2007). "*The International Affective Digitized Sounds (2nd Edn. IADS-2): Affective Ratings of Sounds and Instruction Manual. Technical Report B-3.* Gainesville, Fl: University of Florida.

Brouwer, A.-M., Hogervorst, M. A., Holewijn, M., and van Erp, J. B. F. (2014). Evidence for effects of task difficulty but not learning on neurophysiological variables associated with effort. *Int. J. Psychophysiol.* 93, 242–252. doi: 10.1016/j.ijpsycho.2014.05.004

Brouwer, A.-M., Neerincx, M. A., Kallen, V. L., van der Leer, L., and ten Brinke, M. (2011). EEG alpha asymmetry, heart rate variability and cortisol in response to virtual reality induced stress. *J. Cyberther. Rehabil.* 4, 21–34.

Brouwer, A.-M., van Wouwe, N., Muehl, C., van Erp, J. B. F., and Toet, A. (2013). Perceiving blocks of emotional pictures and sounds: effects on physiological variables. *Front. Hum. Neurosci.* 7:295. doi: 10.3389/fnhum.2013.00295

Codispoti, M., Bradley, M. M., and Lang, P. J. (2001). Affective reactions to briefly presented pictures. *Psychophysiology* 38, 474–478. doi: 10.1111/1469-8986.3830474

Codispoti, M., and De Cesarei, A. (2007). Arousal and attention: picture size and emotional reactions. *Psychophysiology* 44, 680–686. doi: 10.1111/j.1469-8986.2007.00545.x

Dickerson, S. S., and Kemeny, M. E. (2004). Acute stressors and cortisol responses: a theoretical integration and synthesis of laboratory research. *Psychol. Bull.* 130, 355–391. doi: 10.1037/0033-2909.130.3.355

Eisenberg, N., Fabes, R. A., Bustamante, D., Mathy, R. M., Miller, P. A., and Lindholm, E. (1988). Differentiation of vicariously induced emotional reactions in children. *Dev. Psychol.* 24, 237–246. doi: 10.1037/0012-1649.24.2.237

Ekman, P., Levenson, R. W., and Friesen, W. V. (1983). Autonomic nervous system activity distinguish between emotions. *Science* 221, 1208–1210. doi: 10.1126/science.6612338

Harris, C. R. (2001). Cardiovascular responses of embarrassment and effects of emotional suppression in a social setting. *J. Pers. Soc. Psychol.* 81, 886–897. doi: 10.1037/0022-3514.81.5.886

Hofmann, S. G., Moscovitch, D. A., and Kim, H. J. (2006). Autonomic correlates of social anxiety and embarrassment in shy and non-shy individuals. *Int. J. Psychophysiol.* 61, 134–142. doi: 10.1016/j.ijpsycho.2005.09.003

Hogervorst, M. A., Brouwer, A.-M., and Vos, W. (2013). "Physiological correlates of stress in individuals about to undergo eye laser surgery,"in *2013 Humaine Association Conference on Affective Computing and Intelligent Interaction* (Washington, DC: IEEE Computer Society), 473–478.

Kirschbaum, C., Pirke, K. M., and Hellhammer, D. H. (1993). The "Trier Social Stress Test"—a tool for investigating psychobiological stress responses in a laboratory setting. *Neuropsychobiology* 28, 76–81. doi: 10.1159/000119004

Kreibig, S. D. (2010). Autonomic nervous system activity in emotion: a review. *Biol. Psychol.* 84, 394–421. doi: 10.1016/j.biopsycho.2010.03.010

Krumhansl, C. L. (1997). An exploratory study of musical emotions and psychophysiology. *Can. J. Exp. Psychol.* 51, 336–353. doi: 10.1037/1196-1961.51.4.336

Kudielka, B. M., Hellhammer, D. H., and Kirschbaum, C. (2007). "Ten years of research with the Trier Social Stress Test—revisited," in *Social Neuroscience: Integrating Biological and Psychological Explanations of Social Behavior*, eds E. Harmon-Jones and P. Winkielman (New York, NY: Guilford Press), 56–83.

Lang, P. J., Bradley, M. M., and Cuthbert, B. N. (2005). *International Affective Picture System (IAPS): Affective ratings of Pictures and Instruction Manual. Technical Report.* Gainesville, Fl: University of Florida

Poh, M.-Z., McDuff, D. J., and Picard, R. W. (2010). Non-contact, automated cardiac pulse measurements using video imaging and blind source separation. *Opt. Express* 18, 10762–10774. doi: 10.1364/OE.18.010762

Popovic, S., Slamic, M., and Cosic, K. (2006). "Scenario self-adaptation in virtual reality exposure therapy for posttraumatic stress disorder," in *Novel Approaches to the Diagnosis and Treatment of Posttraumatic Stress Disorder*, ed M. J. Roy (Amsterdam: IOS Press), 135–147.

Quaedflieg, C. W. E. M., Meyer, T., and Smeets, T. (2013). The imaging Maastricht Acute Stress Test (iMAST): a neuroimaging compatible psychophysiological stressor. *Psychophysiology* 50, 758–766. doi: 10.1111/psyp.12058

Ritz, T., Thöns, M., Fahrenkrug, S., and Dahme, B. (2005). Airways, respiration, and respiratory sinus arrhythmia during picture viewing. *Psychophysiology* 42, 568–578.

Van Diest, I., Thayer, J. F., Vandeputte, B., Van de Woestijne, K. P., and Van den Bergh, O. (2006). Anxiety and respiratory variability. *Physiol. Behav.* 89, 189–195. doi: 10.1016/j.physbeh.2006.05.041

von Dawans, B., Kirschbaum, C., and Heinrichs, M. (2011). The Trier Social Stress Test for Groups (TSST-G): a new research tool for controlled simultaneous social stress exposure in a group format. *Psychoneuroendocrinology* 36, 514–522. doi: 10.1016/j.psyneuen.2010.08.004

Westenberg, P. M., Bokhorst, C. L., Miers, A. C., Sumter, S. R., Kallen, V. L., Van Pelt, J., et al. (2009). A prepared speech in front of a pre-recorded audience: subjective, physiological, and neuroendocrine responses to the leiden public speaking task. *Biol. Psychol.* 82, 116–124. doi: 10.1016/j.biopsycho.2009.06.005

Wieringa, F. P., Mastik, F., and van der Steen, A. F. (2005). Contactless multiple wavelength photoplethysmographic imaging: a first step toward "SpO2 camera" technology. *Ann. Biomed. Eng.* 33, 1034–1041. doi: 10.1007/s10439-005-5763-2

14

GASICA: generic automated stress induction and control application design of an application for controlling the stress state

Benny van der Vijgh[1,2]*, Robbert J. Beun[1], Maarten van Rood[1,2] and Peter Werkhoven[1]

[1] *Buys Ballot Laboratory, Department of Information and Computing Sciences, Utrecht University, Utrecht, Netherlands*
[2] *Department of Neurology and Neurosurgery, University Medical Center Utrecht, Utrecht, Netherlands*

***Correspondence:**
Benny van der Vijgh, Department of Neurology and Neurosurgery, University Medical Center Utrecht, Universiteitsweg 100, Utrecht 3584 CG, Netherlands
e-mail: b.h.vandervijgh@umcutrecht.nl

In a multitude of research and therapy paradigms it is relevant to know, and desirably to control, the stress state of a patient or participant. Examples include research paradigms in which the stress state is the dependent or independent variable, or therapy paradigms where this state indicates the boundaries of the therapy. To our knowledge, no application currently exists that focuses specifically on the automated control of the stress state while at the same time being generic enough to be used in various therapy and research purposes. Therefore, we introduce GASICA, an application aimed at the automated control of the stress state in a multitude of therapy and research paradigms. The application consists of three components: a digital stressor game, a set of measurement devices, and a feedback model. These three components form a closed loop (called a *biocybernetic loop* by Pope et al. (1995) and Fairclough (2009) that continuously presents an acute psychological stressor, measures several physiological responses to this stressor, and adjusts the stressor intensity based on these measurements by means of the feedback model, hereby aiming to control the stress state. In this manner GASICA presents multidimensional and ecological valid stressors, whilst continuously in control of the form and intensity of the presented stressors, aiming at the automated control of the stress state. Furthermore, the application is designed as a modular open-source application to easily implement different therapy and research tasks using a high-level programming interface and configuration file, and allows for the addition of (existing) measurement equipment, making it usable for various paradigms.

Keywords: GASICA, stress state, stress state control, psychological stressor, physiological response, feedback model, stressor game

INTRODUCTION

For various cognitive and affective (neuroscience) research and therapy purposes, information on the internal stress state of patients and participants and, desirably, exerting control over this stress state, is important. For instance, during exposure therapy it is of importance to have information concerning the internal stress state of a patient, and, based on the inclination of the therapist, either control this stress state to keep psychological responses to the exposed stimuli within certain boundaries, or leave the state as is, and use the received information to determine which states are optimal for a specific therapy. The same holds for various cognitive and affective research, e.g., memory and risk-taking research, where the stress state of a participant can act as a confounding factor during the research.

Currently, to our knowledge, no application exists that focuses specifically on the automated control of the stress state while at the same time being generic enough to be used in various therapy and research purposes. There exist tasks that allow to adjust the presented stressor intensity, for example the Montreal Imaging Stress Task (MIST, Dedovic et al., 2005). However, this adjustment cannot be done real-time: the intensity can only be set at the start of the task, hereby not allowing control over the stress state during the therapy or research paradigm. Therefore, we propose a new application in this paper, dubbed GASICA: *Generic Automated Stress Induction and Control Application.* This application is aimed at automated control of the internal stress state in various therapy and research paradigms by online and continuous monitoring of the stress state.

The stress state generally refers to the current state of stress present in the subject (i.e., a patient or participant). However, over the years, stress research has produced a myriad of definitions for the concept of stress, expressing a wide variety of views on the matter. This variety has emerged due to several reasons, such as the multidisciplinary nature of stress research and the developing view on stress in the past decades.

Our definition of stress is based on the definition by Newport and Nemeroff (2002) where stress is defined as any challenge to homeostasis of an individual that requires an adaptive response of that individual. In order to use this definition in the construct of GASICA, we use it in the following form: "*Stress is the state resulting from the ensemble of responses that are aimed at (facilitating) restoration and/or maintenance of (psychological) homeostasis to internal or external stimuli that present (perceived) challenges to this (psychological) homeostasis.*"

To be more specific, the stimulus presenting the challenge to (psychological) homeostasis will be referred to as the *stressor*, and the response to this challenge referred to as the *stress response*. In par with the interactional approach on stress (Jones and Bright, 2001), we furthermore identify variables influencing the relation between the stressor and stress response, referred to as *intervening variables*.

Stressors, stress responses and intervening variables can be divided into different categories. With regard to stressors, two of the categorizations that are often made and that are relevant to our application, are the division of stressors in *physical* and *psychological* stressors, and in *acute* and *chronic* stressors (see, amongst others, Jones and Bright, 2001; Dickerson and Kemeny, 2004). Physical stressors are in general defined as metabolically demanding stressors, such as physical exercise or a cold pressor task, where the hand of a subject is cooled down. Psychological stressors are in most cases defined as non-metabolically demanding stressors, for example as used in the Trier Social Stress Test, in which a subject is asked to perform a public speech task and mental arithmetic (Kirschbaum et al., 1993). The division between acute and chronic stressors refers to the length a stressor is presented. The precise boundary between these categories varies in the literature, although a consensus can be discerned on the stressor lengths on the ends of the spectrum: stressors that are presented within the realm of minutes are regarded as acute stressors and stressors that are present for weeks or longer will be regarded as chronic.

The stress response can also be divided into different categories. An often-made categorization is the distinction between *physiological*, *psychological* and *behavioral* stress responses (see, amongst others, Jones and Bright, 2001; Lovallo, 2005). Physiological stress responses can include, among others, alterations in heart rate (variability), cerebral activity, and electrodermal activity, while psychological responses typically include alterations in affect and cognition, and behavioral responses include alterations of the exhibited behavior.

Intervening variables have been divided into a broad array of different categories in the literature, depending on the aim of the categorization made. However, there are several categories that are prevalent throughout this literature. These categorizations include, amongst others, *individual difference variables*, including variables such as age, gender and personality type, and *environmental variables*, including variables such as the surrounding temperature.

Within the stressor and stress response categories we introduce a further distinction between *type* and *form*. This distinction will aid us in the further design and description of GASICA. We define within this context stressor types to refer to the manifestation of a stressor, i.e., the concrete entity that produces the stressor: for example a public speaking task, a mathematical task, or a digital game producing a stressor. Stressor form will refer to the kind of stressor(s) that is or are presented through this stressor type, for example workload, social-evaluative threat (the possibility of being negatively judged by others), or frustration.

Analogous we introduce the term stress response type to refer to the manifestation of physiological stress response(s), such as heart rate responses (e.g., an elevated heart rate), or cortisol responses (e.g., an increased cortisol level in the blood). Stress response form refers to the kind of physiological response system the response type is originating from, e.g., stress responses of the form *sympathetic* are originating from the sympathetic nervous system (responsible for the electrodermal stress response type), and *hemodynamic* responses are responses of the hemodynamic response system (responsible for changes in blood pressure).

The difference between the concepts stress and *arousal* remains an interesting point of discussion in the breadth of the stress research community. To our knowledge there is currently no consensus on how to separate the two. Of the different views that are currently present on this matter, we concur with the view expressed by Day and Walker (2007), in that the difference between these two concepts needs to be sought rather in a top-down characterization of qualitative appraisal, opposed to a bottom-up characterization of physiological responses. Based on this thought Day and Walker propose three ways in which stress differs from arousal. The first way is that stress differs from arousal in terms of the qualitative appraisal that precedes it. The second is that stress is only elicited by aversive challenges. And the third is that there is a difference in the resulting physiological state between stress and arousal, which the authors state based on, amongst others, memory research. However, the authors indicate that the exact differences between these physiological states are currently not elucidated.

In GASICA we will utilize an *acute psychological* stressor (i.e., a stressor that falls both in the psychological stressor category and the acute stressor category) and we will measure *physiological* stress responses (i.e., stress responses in physiological signals). An *acute* stressor is used since, for practical reasons, a stressor cannot be presented for days or weeks within the application, as this will not be suitable for most therapy and research paradigms. Furthermore, a *psychological* stressor is used, as this allows for more flexibility than a physical stressor. This because the adjustment of physical entities, e.g., changing the temperature of water, is more cumbersome and less flexible than the adjustment of a psychological stressor, allowing a more generic application. A *physiological* stress response is used as an indication of the internal stress state as this category of stress response is the best objectively measurable and quantifiable of the three different stress response categories. Therefore, in the context of our application, we further refine our definition of the stress state, defining it as the current overall stress response in spontaneously generated (neuro)physiological signals, i.e., the current sum of different (neuro)physiological stress response types.

In order to achieve the aim of automated controlling of the stress state, it is essential to control the stressor intensity *causing* the current stress state. Therefore, our proposed application consists of three components, depicted in **Figure 1**:

(1) A stressor, allowing to induce stress responses.

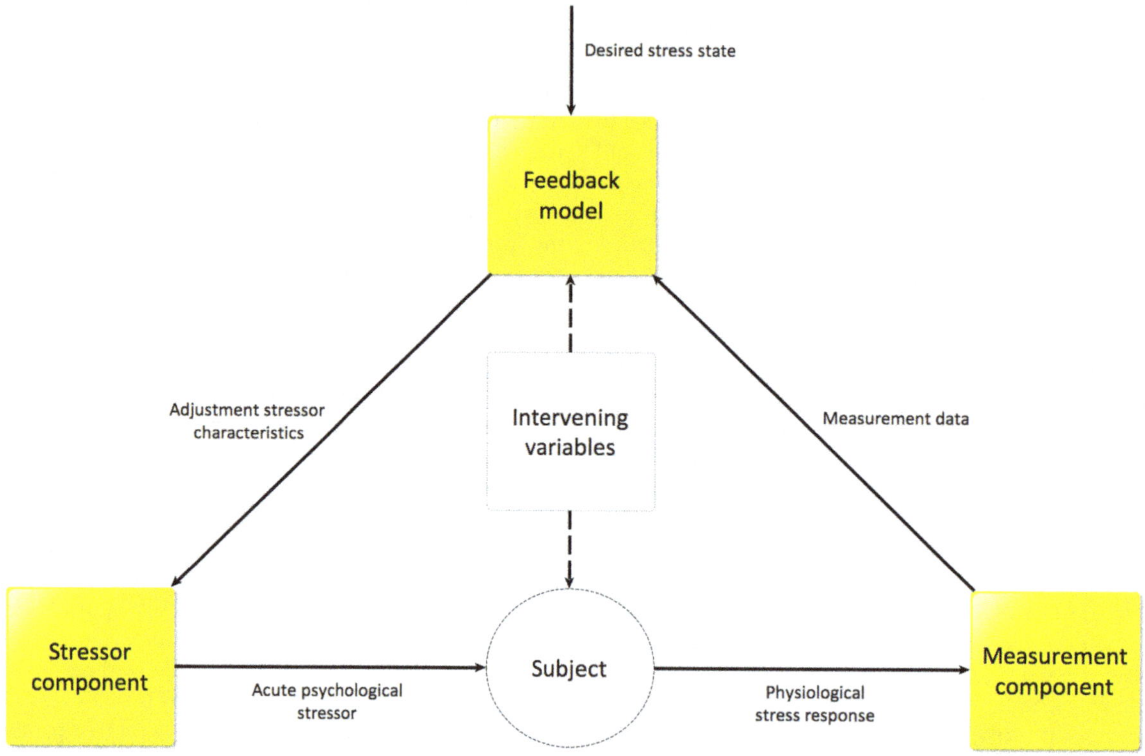

FIGURE 1 | Schematic overview of GASICA.

(2) Set of measurement devices, allowing for continuous and online measurement of several (neuro)physiological signals.
(3) Feedback model that derives the current internal stress state of the human subject based on the measured (neuro)physiological signals and adjusts the stressor characteristics based on this derived state and the desired stress state in the current paradigm.

In this paper, we will describe the design of GASICA by discussing each of the three separate components in detail in the upcoming sections.

GASICA

In this section we will further design the different components in our application (i.e., the stressor component, measurement component and the feedback model) using a top-down approach. In this design process we aim to maximize the diagnosticity, sensitivity, and reliability of GASICA, i.e., we aim to maximize the extent to which we are able to measure different levels psychological stress across inter- and intra-individual differences (for a detailed treatment of these concepts, see Fairclough, 2009). As the category of the utilized stressor and stress response are already determined, we will first determine the form and type of the utilized stressor and stress responses, using requirements formulated based on our aim to continuously measure and exert control over the stress state in various research and therapy paradigms. Subsequently we will determine the characteristics of the different components using a recent meta-analysis we conducted (van der Vijgh et al., 2015) as guideline. Finally we will determine the instantiations and/or implementations of the components, using sets of requirements and the meta-analysis as guidelines. This process is described in the following sections for the different components separately.

COMPONENT 1: STRESSOR

Stressor type

For the first component, the stressor, we utilize an acute psychological stressor. To determine the *type* of acute psychological stressor best suited for use in our application we formulated four requirements:

(1) Multidimensionality
The stressor should allow for presentation of multiple stressor forms (e.g., workload, emotion induction, and frustration) to make it suitable for multiple therapy and research designs.
(2) Adjustability
In order to allow for presenting different stressor intensities, the stressor characteristics should be adjustable, in a way that results in different stressor intensities. Furthermore, through this adjustment it should also be possible to adjust the stressor form presented.
(3) Real-time
The adjustment of the stressor characteristics should be possible in real-time, in order to respond to changing stress states. In this context, real-time refers to the realm of seconds,

so that the application can adjust the stressor within a couple of seconds when needed.

(4) Continuity
To allow continuous control over the stressor that is presented, it should be possible to both present and adjust the stressor continuously for a prolonged period of time.

When we look at acute psychological stressors to match against these requirements, we find a plethora of different stressor types. In an influential meta-analysis by Dickerson and Kemeny acute psychological stressors were subdivided in four mutually exclusive types: public speaking and verbal interaction tasks, cognitive tasks, emotion induction procedures, and noise exposure tasks (Dickerson and Kemeny, 2004).

Public speaking and verbal interaction tasks refer to tasks in which subjects have to verbally interact with other human subjects, such as in interviews or through public speaking. The stressor intensities of these tasks are hard to adjust, especially in real-time, and the tasks present a mostly one-dimensional stressor form, being mostly social stress (social-evaluative threat).

Cognitive tasks are tasks such as arithmetic tasks, the Stroop task, vigilance-reaction time tasks, and analytical tasks, e.g., puzzles. These kind of tasks are, especially when presented digitally, well adjustable, also in real-time, and can be presented continuously. However, these tasks also present a mostly one-dimensional stressor form, being workload.

Emotion inducement tasks are tasks that present emotion-eliciting material that elicit a negative affective state, such as the viewing of aversive pictures or film. These tasks are by definition one-dimensional in the sense that these only induce emotion as stressor form.

Noise exposure tasks exist of the presentation of loud noises. These kinds of tasks are also by nature one-dimensional.

Another widely used type of acute psychological stressor not discussed in this analysis consists of a combination of the latter three stressor types, hereby alleviating the limitation of one-dimensionality pertaining to the individual stressor types: a *digital stressor game*, i.e., a digital game producing a stressor. In a recent meta-analysis 5448 articles were found when using search phrases to find studies utilizing this type of stressor[1] , indicating the widespread use of this type of stressor (van der Vijgh et al., 2015). We adhere to the definition of a game used in this analysis: a game is defined as a type of play activity conducted in the context of a pretended reality, in which the player(s) try to achieve at least one arbitrary, nontrivial goal by acting in accordance with rules (Adams, 2010). Key elements in games are players, (inter)action, environment, goals, and rules. In a game, players interact with entities in the environment or with other players in accordance with a set of rules in order to achieve a set goal. In the case a player controls a specific entity, this entity is referred to as the avatar. Game characteristics are characteristics of any (part of) of the key elements or the game as a whole, such as the game type, the presence of game music or time pressure, or the amount of aversive stimuli present in the digital game.

As in digital games many, or even all, of the key elements are taken over by computer technology, this provides possibilities that allow to *adjust* the stressor intensity, in *real-time*, by adjusting the game characteristics of the digital game stressor. Also, by adjusting these game characteristics, it is possible to present *multi-dimensional* stressor forms, *continuously*, satisfying our requirements. Even more, a (digital) game provides a *narrative*, the pretended reality in which the goal that is set is tried to be achieved. This narrative provides possibilities to conceal the adjustments made to the stressor characteristics and changes between stressor forms from the subject by presenting these adjustments as part of the narrative. The presence of a narrative also provides a way to incorporate different research and therapy paradigms in the application, as it allows to create a specific narrative for each specific paradigm. Given these properties (adjustable, real-time, continuity, multidimensional, and a narrative), a digital game stressor is selected as the stressor type in our application.

Characteristics

In order to present different stressor intensities using this type of stressor, it is essential to have insight in which digital game characteristics elicit physiological stress responses, i.e., alter the stress state, and to what degree. Additionally, the effects of adjustments of these characteristics on the stress state should be predictable.

In the same meta-analysis by van der Vijgh et al. (2015), the relation between digital game characteristics and physiological stress responses is analyzed. Using meta-regression, this analysis identified four stressor game characteristics, presenting different stressor forms, that significantly moderated the physiological stress responses in a predictable and consistent manner. This indicates that these characteristics can be used to elicit stress responses and that adjustments of these characteristics are expected to result in predictable changes of the stress state. These four characteristics will therefore be instantiated in the digital game:

(1) Aversive stimuli
The first game characteristic identified is the presence and intensity of *aversive stimuli* in the digital game, such as the visual or auditory presentation of scenes of violence, blood, or gore. Aversive stimuli have been found to elicit physiological stress responses both inside as well as outside a digital game context. Outside the context of a game, the presentation of aversive stimuli such as in a picture rating task (Stegeren et al., 2008), passive viewing of aversive pictures (Sokhadze, 2007) or film viewing containing aversive stimuli (Miller et al., 1995) has been found to induce physiological stress responses such as alterations in heart rate, electrodermal activity and frontal EEG activity. Within the context of a game aversive stimuli can, for example, include the presence of violence, blood and gore (Hebert et al., 2005), and torture (Tafalla, 2007), also inducing physiological stress responses (Carnagey et al., 2007). This characteristic presents a stressor

[1]The search phrases used were *game AND physiolog** and *stress* AND game*, where *AND* indicates a logical conjunction and the asterisk ("*") indicates a wildcard, i.e., any combination of characters. The search was performed in Pubmed, Scopus, PsycInfo, and the IEEE Xplore Digital Library.

of the form emotion induction, as it induces a negative affect.

(2) Realism
This characteristic concerns the amount of *realism* presented in the digital game. This refers to the degree to which a subject will identify the presented stimuli as realistic. This characteristic does not present a separate stressor form in itself, but rather heightens the immersion, resulting in heightened physiological stress responses. Several studies have found the amount of realism in digital games to be related to resulting physiological stress responses. For example, Ivory and Kalyanaraman (2007) found that more technologically advanced, although otherwise comparable, digital games elicited higher electrodermal stress responses and Barlett and Rodeheffer (2009) showed that more realistic digital games significantly heighten the heart rate stress response.

(3) Game music
Game music refers to whether or not music is presented in the game. A recent overview provided by Sokhadze (2007) makes clear that although there are inconsistent results to be found, music has the potential to elicit physiological stress responses. Examples include work by Nyklicek et al. (1997), who found significant differences in both cardiovascular and respiratory variables in response to different fragments of music and white noise. Other physiological stress responses, such as in skin temperature, have also been found by, amongst others, McFarland (1985), who found that music with different valence and arousal (subjectively determined) have different effects on skin temperature. Game music induces emotion, the same stressor form as aversive stimuli.

(4) Game type
This characteristic concerns the *game type*, the type of digital game. Examples of different game types include action, adventure, strategy and management, role playing games (RPG), simulation or board and card games (Ritterfeld et al., 2009). In the meta-analysis, it was found that puzzle games induce the highest physiological stress responses. Game type in itself does not present a stressor form, as it acts as a container characteristic: the characteristics that are contained within a specific game type are responsible for the resulting stressor form.

Besides these four characteristics, several other game characteristics were identified in this meta-analysis to be related to physiological stress responses, but were not used in the meta-regression because these could not be objectively qualified or were not reported sufficiently in the included studies. As we aim to design an application that can be applied in various therapy and research paradigms, we aim to include as many different game characteristics as possible, allowing a wider range of stressor forms to be presented and thereby providing greater flexibility for use in more paradigms. Therefore, we screened these characteristics that were excluded from the meta-regression to see if these were fit to use in our stressor. Of these additional characteristics, three digital game characteristics are selected to be incorporated in the digital game, based on the property of these three characteristics to be adjustable during execution of the application, bringing the total of game characteristics used in our digital game stressor to seven:

(5) Time pressure
Time pressure refers to the presence of limited time before a certain goal has to be achieved. Studies utilizing time pressure paradigms (Wahlstrom et al., 2002) have consistently been found to elicit physiological stress responses. The stressor form time pressure presents is workload, as it increases the demand placed on the subject.

(6) Sound level
Sound level concerns the sound level at which auditory stimuli are presented during the game. This characteristic presents a stressor of the form noise induction and it has been shown that high sound levels, mostly studied at 75 dB and above, elicit physiological stress responses (Smith et al., 1997; Selander et al., 2009).

(7) Disabling of input
Disabling of input refers to the disabling of the control the subject has in the game making it harder to achieve the goals set, resulting in frustration and physiological stress responses (Reuderink et al., 2009).

In **Table 1** an overview is given of the seven included stressor game characteristics and the stressor forms these present.

Game design

The stressor game is designed around the seven selected game characteristics, aiming to provide a narrative through which the game characteristics can be adjusted as part of the narrative, reducing the possibility of subjects noticing the adjustments as being part of the stress state control method.

The game is designed as a 3D puzzle game because the same meta-analysis (van der Vijgh et al., 2015) indicated that this game type elicited the highest stress response of the analyzed game types. The narrative provided is that an adolescent boy or girl (i.e., the avatar, the entity that is controlled by the subject, gender is not made explicit) has to find notes that are scattered across the house and garden of his or her uncle, an inventor and scientist, who needs these notes within a given amount of time in order to finish his work. The boy/girl sets out to find these notes wearing one of the latest inventions by this uncle, a heavy suit that should help the subject to find these notes, outfitted with a radio and head up display that can present auditory and visual stimuli to the wearer. However, this suit turns out not to work as expected, malfunctioning from time to time, resulting in, for example, the possible presentation of images or sounds, and the restriction of movement. This suit allows the game characteristics to be altered as needed without the subject registering this as a conscious adaptation of the game, as these alterations are presented as malfunctions of the suit the subject is wearing. Furthermore, the narrative serves to heighten immersion and reduce boredom and annoyance by motivating the subject to keep participating in the current paradigm. The stressor game is designed to exclude fast-paced motor action or complicated cognitive tasks in order

Table 1 | Overview of stressor game characteristics, with presented stressor form, instantiation within the stressor game, the way the instantiations fit in the narrative and how these are adjusted in order to control the stress state.

Stressor game characteristic	Stressor form	Instantiation of characteristic	Narrative	Adjustment
Aversive stimuli	Emotion induction	IAPS and IADS	Malfunctioning of suit: unwanted presentation of pictures and sounds.	Absence/Presence of pictures and sounds, and selection of pictures and sounds of different values of new scale.
Realism	Not applicable	Point of view	Malfunctioning of suit: point of view is adjusted.	Point of view is either first or third person.
Game music	Emotion induction	Music samples	Malfunctioning of suit: unwanted presentation of music.	Absence/Presence of music, and selection of samples of different values of new scale.
Game type	Not applicable	Not applicable	Not applicable	Not applicable
Time pressure	Workload	Countdown	Uncle needs next notes quickly.	Absence/Presence of countdown and starting number.
Sound level	Noise induction	Sound level auditory stimuli	Malfunctioning of suit: volume built-in radio is adjusted.	Different sound levels.
Disabling input	Frustration	Disabling input	Malfunctioning of suit: movement is restricted.	Absence/Presence of disabling of input: if disabled, which key is disabled.

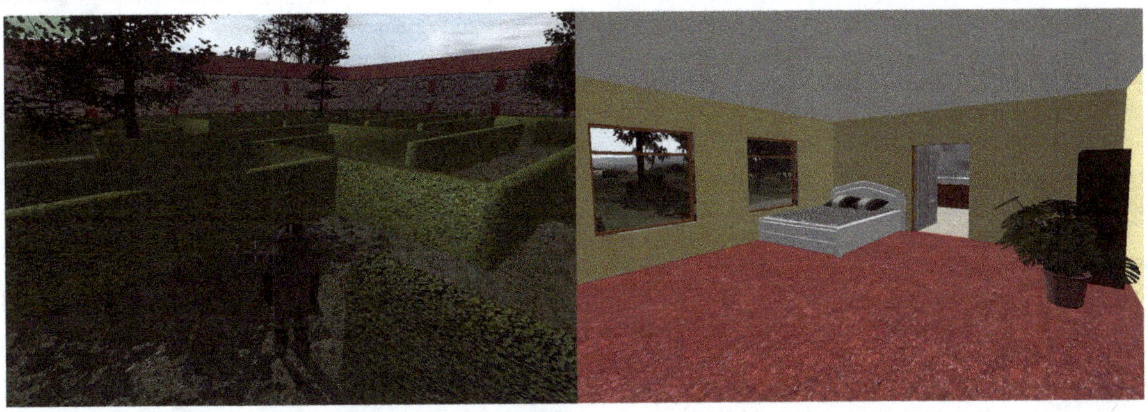

FIGURE 2 | Impression of condition 1 and 2 in the stressor game, respectively.

to prevent uncontrolled elements of the stressor to induce physiological reactions. Furthermore, the setting of the game does not include political or ideological content, to prevent unwanted side-effects, nor fast-paced visual or auditory sequences (e.g., no flashing lights) to prevent uncontrolled stress responses and to make sure the digital game can be utilized in multiple paradigms.

Within the game there are two separate conditions: a *fitting* and *manipulation* condition. The fitting condition serves to fit an individual feedback model for each subject. This condition consists of a maze (the garden of the uncle) that presents a homogeneous environment that is suited for the fitting of the feedback model (for more details, see Section Fitting). To prevent unwanted stressor effects of getting lost in the maze we placed trees as landmarks to help subjects find their way. The manipulation condition serves to utilize the fitted feedback model to control the stress state and to present tasks or therapy elements (for more details, see Section Overview). This condition is placed inside the house of the uncle. Impressions of both conditions are given in **Figure 2**.

Instantiations of characteristics

Within this design, the seven selected stressor game characteristics are instantiated in order to control the stress state. We chose instantiations that allowed changes to the characteristics to be immediately noticeable. An overview of the instantiations and how these fit in the narrative of the stressor game is given in **Table 1**.

Aversive stimuli are presented using the International Affective Picture System (IAPS) (Lang et al., 1988) and the International Affective Digitize Sounds (IADS) (Bradley and Lang, 1999), standard sets containing over 1000 pictures and 167 sounds respectively. These sets are scored on valence, arousal and dominance by subjects in an on-going sequence of studies, currently containing the scoring from over 18 separate studies. By summing the scores on inversed dominance, valence, and arousal, we derived a new scale in which a low value corresponded with images and sounds scored as unhappy, arousing and being controlled and higher values corresponded with images scored as happy, non-arousing and being in control. Pictures are presented full screen to achieve maximal effect, the subject is explained that this is displayed on the display incorporated in the suit, and sounds are presented over the built-in radio, both are malfunctions of the suit.

Realism is altered through changing the point of view to either 1st or 3rd person view, i.e., the view the subject has in the stressor game is either through the eyes of the avatar or from above, just beyond the avatar, having view of the complete avatar. Altering this view has been found by Dahlquist et al. (2010) to alter presence: in 1st person view a greater sense of presence was reported. This adjustment is also presented as a malfunction of the suit.

As game music has been found to induce different responses, it is hard to determine how to instantiate this characteristic. Based on the review provided by Sokhadze (2007) we used the results from the study by Nyklicek et al. (1997) as a basis, as this study was found to be the most comprehensive study, and having clear significant results. These results indicate the possibility to elicit different emotional states (recognized based on physiological responses), utilizing music excerpts that are characterized by valence and arousal dimensions. Based on these findings we chose to use a standard set of music excerpts, scored on several dimensions, including valence, and arousal, by 116 subjects (Eerola and Vuoskoski, 2011). We derived a new scale by summing the values for valence, tension, and energy. In this scale low values correspond to negatively valenced, tensed, and energetic music, and high values correspond to positively valenced, relaxed, and calm music. Music is presented over the built-in radio, in the narrative of the game this is explained as a malfunction of the suit.

The game type will not be altered during the execution of the game, and is set as a puzzle game. This is because changes in the game type has also consequences for the narrative and game design, which is undesirable.

Time pressure will be applied through a countdown presented to the subject indicating that he or she needs to find the next note before the timer reaches zero. This timer can be turned on or off and can start at any given number of seconds. Within the narrative of the game the time pressure is applied through the uncle announcing over the radio that he needs new notes quickly.

Sound level is adjusted by presenting the auditory stimuli in different intensities, this is presented as a malfunction of the radio in the suit.

Disabling input is induced by (partially) disabling control by disabling the keys needed to control the game. In the narrative of the game this is also a malfunction of the suit the subject is wearing.

Each of the stressor characteristics instantiations can be presented either *transient* or *state-wise*, as can be determined by the experimenter or therapist. This refers to the duration an adjustment of the instantiation is present: either for a set duration (that can be determined by the experimenter or therapist) or constantly, until it is adjusted again.

An additional strength of the included stressor game characteristics and the respective instantiations is that these present stressor forms have a high degree of ecological validity. This is due to fact that these stressors have a high correlation with stressors found in real life. Exemplars are the real-life depictions of aversive visual and auditory stimuli of the IAPS and IADS that are used, and the presentation of time pressure on task-completion, as presented through the countdown in the stressor game.

Implementation

In order to implement the stressor game we aimed to utilize a software environment which fulfilled three requirements:

(1) Data exchange
It must be possible to both import and export information into and from the environment during execution. Import is needed to receive information from the feedback model, in order to receive which game characteristics will be adjusted in what way. Export is needed to send markers to the measurement component or any additional hardware.

(2) Characteristic implementation
All of the selected game characteristics instantiations must be implementable in the environment. For example, the environment must allow for a high level of realism in order to be able to vary the amount of realism presented.

(3) Real-time adjustment
The implemented game characteristic instantiations must be real-time adjustable.

(4) High-level programming interface
In order to make the application suitable for different therapy and research paradigms, it is needed to have a high-level programming interface that allows to easily implement the needed research or therapy tasks within the application.

Based on these requirements the software environment Virtual BattleSpace 2 (VBS2) by Bohemia Interactive was selected (Simulations, 2011). This is a 3D simulation environment that allows for complete control over the simulation to adjust the relevant game characteristics and fulfill the above requirements. The subjects control the stressor game with the four directional keys of a standard alphanumeric keyboard.

COMPONENT 2: MEASUREMENT

Stress response types

In the measurement component we include a multitude of physiological stress response types, both to provide information suited for a variety of research and therapy paradigms as well as to gain as much information as possible regarding the current stress state. In order to determine which types and corresponding measurements are suitable for inclusion we drafted six requirements, the first three concerning the stress response types, the latter three concerning the corresponding measurements, given below:

(1) Responsivity
The stress response type should respond to the selected stressor game characteristics.

(2) Response consistency
In order to succeed in achieving the intended effect in the measured stress response upon adaptations of the stressor, the response must be consistent within a subject to a (digital game) stressor (adaptation), both quantitatively and temporally. This entails the response should have a consistent sign (either increasing or decreasing) between repeated presentations of an identical stressor game characteristic, and this response must occur within the same time span between repeated presentations. This consistency is only required for identical circumstances. For example the response is not

required to be consistent between cases where in one of the cases the stress response type is already at a physiological possible maximum or minimum.

(3) Low response latency
In order to be able to measure the effect of stressor characteristic adjustment and allow for any subsequent adjustments, the stress response must emerge after such an adjustment with the least amount of delay as possible. In practice, this requires the latency to be within the realm of seconds, in order to reliably determine the effect of a presented stressor.

(4) Measurement continuity
The measurement must be applicable continuously in order to keep continuous track of the stress state and the effects of stressor adjustments.

(5) Measurement inertion
In order to reliably relate the stress responses to adjustments in the stressor game, the measurement must be applicable without inducing an additional stress response or disturbing the experiment or therapy.

(6) Measurement fMRI compatibility
In order to allow usage of the application in additional research and therapy paradigms, the measurement must be applicable inside a MRI scanner, without disturbing (f)MRI imaging, allowing the use of the application in combination with this technique.

We compiled a list of all stress response types and corresponding measurements encountered in the meta-analysis on digital game characteristics utilized in the previous section (van der Vijgh et al., 2015), as this provides an exhaustive overview of the kind of measurements performed with stressor games in the past 36 years. We reviewed these types and measurements to match these against the above requirements. The results hereof are given in **Table 2**, using the same numbering of the requirements as above. **Table 2** contains 13 stress response types and corresponding measurements that meet all requirements. Although we aim for a multitude of measurements, including all these stress response types will require six different measurement devices[2] , which presents practical problems and is not expected to provide additional information concerning the overlap in the different stress response types and forms. Therefore, to reduce the number of needed measurement devices, we look at the stress response *form* the different stress response types have.

The types are either of the cardiac response form (measured using ECG and ICG), hemodynamic response form (measured with blood pressure monitor and photophlesmograph), stress responses stemming from sympathetic activation (measured using electrodes), and the neural stress form, measured using electroencephalography (EEG). In order to reduce the number of needed measurement devices, we chose one measurement from each stressor form by selecting the measurement of the stress response types with the highest mean effect. These mean effect sizes[3] are taken from the meta-analysis in which these stress response types were analyzed (van der Vijgh et al., 2015). For the different stress response forms and measurement combinations, these effect sizes are given in **Table 3**. Given this approach, we select to measure heart rate and heart rate variability (using ECG), systolic and diastolic blood pressure (using a blood pressure monitor), the electrodermal stress response type (electrodes) and the neural response using EEG.

Implementation

In order to implement the measurement component we aimed to utilize hardware and software that fulfilled three requirements:

(1) fMRI compatible
One of the requirements on the stress response types is that is possible to perform the measurement within a fMRI environment. Therefore, this requirement is extended to the hardware and software of the implementation as well.

(2) Continuous
We selected the stress response types amongst other things on the possibility to measure these continuously, therefore the hardware used to perform the measurement of these types also needs to be able to measure continuously.

(3) Broad spectrum
In order to make the application suitable for multiple research and therapy paradigms we select hardware and software that is easily extendable with measurement equipment for additional stress response types or the measurement of other dependent physiological variables, such as the use of EEG.

We were not able to find a manufacturer that provided interconnected equipment that fulfilled all our requirements and also measured all selected stress response types at the same time. We selected the system that fulfilled all three requirements and was able to measure the most stress response types at the same time. This is the fMRI-compatible equipment by Biopac Systems Inc. that allows continuous measurement of all our selected stressor types, except EEG. This results in the use of heart rate (variability), blood pressure and electrodermal activity measurements in the measurement component. The base station of this equipment, the *MP150*, allows easy extension with additional equipment through a plug-and-play interface which allows the plugging in of additional equipment by the same manufacturer, that is automatically recognized by the accompanying software, *Acqknowledge*. This ensures easy extension of the utilized stressor types, making the application suited for additional paradigms.

For the measurement of heart rate and variability with ECG we use the ECG 100C MRI amplifier with disposable electrodes in a lead-II type ECG. For the measurement of the electrodermal

[2]Heart rate and heart rate variability are measured using electrocardiography (ECG); systolic, diastolic and mean blood pressure are measured using a blood pressure monitor; electrodermal response is measured using electrodes on the skin; cardiac output, pre ejection period, cardiac index, left ventricular ejection time and vascular rigidity index are measured using impedance cardiography (ICG); digital blood volume pulse is measured using a photophlesmograph; and neural spectral power or event-related potentials are measured using electroencephalography (EEG).

[3]These mean effect sizes represent the difference between baseline measurements and measurements during digital stressor presentation.

Table 2 | Overview of stress response types and corresponding measurements matched against requirements for detemining the utilized stress response types in the measurement component.

Stress response type/Measure	1. Responsitivity	2. Response consistency	3. Low response latency	4. Measurement continuity	5. Measurement inertion	6. fMRI compatibility	Comment
Heart rate (HR)	+	+	+	+	+	+	
Diastolic blood pressure (DBP)	+	+	+	+	+	+	
Systolic blood pressure (SBP)	+	+	+	+	+	+	
Forearm blood flow (FBF)	+	+	+	−	+	+	4: Time needed to inflate cuff does not allow for continuous measurement.
Respiration rate (RR)	−	−	+	+	+	+	1/2: Voluntary control over RR interferes with responsitivity and response consistency.
Forearm vascular resistance (FVR)	+	+	+	−	+	+	4: Time needed to inflate cuff does not allow for continuous measurement.
Cardiac output (CO)	+	+	+	+	+	+	
Digital blood volume pulse (DBVP)	+	+	+	+	+	+	
Electrodermal activity (EDA)	+	+	+	+	+	+	
Total peripheral resistance (TPR)	−	+	+	+	+	+	1: No significant responses found in this response type.
Cortisol	+	+	−	+	+	+	3: Response peak around 20 min.
Pre ejection period (PEP)	+	+	+	+	+	+	
Respiratory sinus arrhythmia (RSA)	+	−	+	+	+	+	2: Voluntary control over respiration influences RSA.
Oxygen consumption (VO_2)	+	+	+	+	−	+	5: Requires cap, acting as stressor itself.
CO_2 Production VCO_2	+	+	+	+	−	+	5: Requires cap, acting as stressor itself.
Epinephrine (E)	−	+	+	−	+	+	1: No significant responses found in this response type. 4: Determining measure after measurement takes time.
Norepinephrine (NE)	−	+	+	−	+	+	1: No significant responses found in this response type. 4: Determining measure after measurement takes time.
Plasma renin activity (PRA)	−	+	+	−	+	+	1: No significant responses found in this response type. 4: Determining measure after measurement takes time.
Stroke volume (SV)	−	+	+	+	+	+	1: No significant responses found in this response type.
Tidal volume (TV)	−	−	+	+	−	+	1/2: Voluntary control interferes with responsitivity and response consistency. 5: Requires cap, acting as stressor itself.
Muscle activity	−	−	+	+	+	+	1/2: Inconsistency and lessened responsitivity due to (semi-) voluntary movements.
α-Amylase	−	+	+	−	+	+	1: No significant responses found in this response type. 4: Determining measure after measurement takes time.
Cardiac index (CI)	+	+	+	+	+	+	
Heather index (HI)	−	+	+	+	+	+	1: No significant responses found in this response type.
Heart rate variability (HRV)	+	+	+/−	+	+	+	3: Although HRV has a low response latency, in practice HRV measures in the frequency and phase domain require data in the realm of minutes to be determined, rendering a too high latency in practice. Time-domain measures do meet all requirements.
Left ventricular ejection time (LVET)	+	+	+	+	+	+	
Mean (Arterial) blood pressure (MAP/MBP)	+	+	+	+	+	+	
Mean systolic ejection time (MSER)	−	+	+	+	+	−	1: No significant responses found in this response type.
Pulse transit time (PTT)	−	+	+	+	+	+	1: No significant responses found in this response type.
Perceived/subjective stress	+	+	+	−	−	+	4/5: Cannot be measured continuously without disturbing experiment as it requires introspection.

(Continued)

Table 2 | Continued

Stress response type/Measure	1. Responsitivity	2. Response consistency	3. Low response latency	4. Measurement continuity	5. Measurement inertion	6. fMRI compatibility	Comment
Stroke volume index (SVI)	−	+	+	+	+	+	1: No significant responses found in this response type.
Total systemic resistance (TSR)	−	+	+	+	+	+	1: No significant responses found in this response type.
Vascular rigidity index (VRI)	+	+	+	+	+	+	
Activity/Electro- encephalography (EEG)	+	+	+	+	+	+	

A plus sign (+) indicates that the requirement of the respective column is met, a minus sign (−) indicates this requirement is not met. In the latter case, the comment column indicates why this is the case. Rows corresponding to stress response types and measurements that meet all requirements are given in gray.

Table 3 | Overview of stress response types fulfilling all requirements.

Stress response form	Stress response type	Measurement	Mean effect size
Cardiac	HR, HRV (time-domain)	ECG	0.73
Cardiac	CO, PEP, CI, LVET, VRI, MAP	ICG	0.59
Hemodynamic	SBP, DBP	Blood pressure monitor	0.93
Hemodynamic	DBVP	Photophlesmograph	0.84
Sympathetic	EDA	Electrodes	0.27
Neural	Event-related potentials (ERP), spectral power measures	EEG	Not available

Gray rows indicate selected types and forms for use in application.

response we use two disposable electrodes on the hand or foot connected to an EDA 100C MRI amplifier. For measuring systolic and diastolic blood pressure we use a small pressure pad on the thumb or elbow that detects these measures using continuous pressure, allowing for continuous measurement, connected to an HLT-100C amplifier. This method utilizes an additional software package for extraction of the systolic and diastolic blood pressure from the raw blood pressure signal, *Caretaker*, which transfers the measurement data to the *Acqknowledge* software.

COMPONENT 3: FEEDBACK MODEL

The feedback model serves to select the optimal adjustment of the stressor game characteristics, i.e., the adjustment that minimizes the difference between the current stress state and the desired stress state. To this end, it models the relations between the size of the stress response types selected in the previous section and the stressor game characteristics adjustments chosen in the preceding section. These relations are expressed in rules that are fitted for each individual subject during the fitting condition of the application. It is important to realize here that the formulas presented in this section can be used to calculate values to a precision that does not necessarily reflect the same precision of the entities these are presenting, i.e., the provided formulas and resulting values in this section should be seen as an approximation of the respective entities these present.

Stress state

In correspondence with our definition of the stress state as the ensemble of responses to internal or external stimuli that present (perceived) challenges to the (psychological) homeostasis, the stress state in the feedback model is expressed as the weighted summation of stress responses in the selected stress response types (i.e., heart rate, heart rate variability, blood pressure, and electrodermal response). In order to estimate this stress state, we calculate the *physiological activity state.* This latter state is derived by calculating the activity for each stress response type separately, expressed in the standardized mean difference effect between the baseline and stress response values, denoted as Hedges' g (Hedges, 1981). The formula for the size of the activity of a given stress response type expressed in g is given by:

$$g = \frac{\mu_{\text{stress response}} - \mu_{\text{baseline}}}{\sigma_{\text{baseline}}}$$

Here μ_{baseline} refers to the mean value of the specific stress response type (e.g., heart rate) during a baseline measure. This baseline measure is a measure of the physiological activity state of the subject in rest, before the start of the respective paradigm. This measure needs to be performed shortly before the application is used, while the subject is instructed to relax in the same position as he or she will be in when using the application. Furthermore, the $\mu_{\text{stress response}}$ and σ_{baseline} refer to the mean current physiological activity of a given type and the standard deviation of the corresponding baseline measurement values. In this manner, the sign of the resulting g will be positive when the physiological activity is higher compared to the corresponding baseline measurement, with the value indicating the change from baseline expressed in standard deviations. The physiological activity state, calculated as the weighted summation of these stress response types is given by:

$$p_c = \sum (g_i * w_i) \,/\, \sum w_i$$

Here p_c stands for the current physiological activity state, summing over all g_i, the current size of the respective stress response types, multiplied by w_i, representing the respective weights assigned to these types. These weights are introduced to allow specific stress response types to have more influence on the physiological activity state than other response types, by assigning the respective weight of this response type a higher value than other weights. This can be desirable in certain therapy or research paradigms in which specific stress response types are more informative for the aim of the paradigm than others. By default the weights are all initialized to the value of 1, resulting in all stress response types having the same influence on the physiological activity state. The state is normalized by dividing it by the summation of all weights. In this manner the normalized weights sum up to one, resulting in a physiological activity state p_c that is expressed in the weighted average standard deviations change from baseline, making interpretation more intuitive. Calculating p_c in this manner allows to combine multiple stress response types, takes personal variance in physiological signals of individual subjects into account and makes sure that the physiological activity state value is close to 0 at the beginning of each experiment, by using the baseline measurements.

We use this physiological activity state to estimate the current stress state s_c. Based on the current stress state estimated in this manner and the given desired stress state s_d, the feedback model selects a stressor characteristic adjustment that is predicted to result in a stress state that is closest to the desired stress state. In order to determine this adaptation, the feedback model utilizes *rules* that model the relation between stressor characteristic instantiations and the different stress response types.

Rules

For every stressor characteristic instantiation, the feedback model contains exactly one rule that models the relation between all the available adjustments of the instantiation and the corresponding responses in the different stress response types. For example, for the stressor characteristic "game music" the feedback model contains a rule that predicts the response for each of the different stress response types (i.e., heart rate (variability), blood pressure and the electrodermal response) for each of the possible adjustments, i.e., for each music sample that can be presented.

Two kinds of rules are contained in the feedback model: *discrete* and *continuous* rules. The discrete rule is used for modeling relations concerning stressor game characteristics that are instantiated in discrete levels, such as realism, which is instantiated by adjusting the point of view to either the first or the third person view, i.e., two levels. This kind of rule is represented as a matrix $\boldsymbol{D}_{ij}$, with the rows representing the change in the size of the respective response types, and the columns representing the transitions between levels of the stressor game characteristic instantiation. There are i rows, equal to the amount of stress response types, and j columns, equal to the number of 2-permutations of the set of levels of the stressor game characteristic [i.e., P(*amount of levels*, 2)], representing all the possible transitions from one level of a given characteristic to another. In this manner the element D_{ij} refers to the predicted change in response type i, i.e., $\Delta\ g_i$, when the stressor game characteristic transition is applied that belongs to column j. For example, the rule for transitions of the realism characteristic instantiation would consist of a four by two matrix, with the four rows presenting the changes in size of the different stress response types and the two columns representing the two possible transitions: from first to third point of view, and vice versa. Within this presentation, the predicted change in the current stress state, i.e., $\widehat{\Delta s_c}$, when applying transition j on the stressor game characteristic presented by discrete rule r_d, is therefore equal to the weighted summation (using the weights corresponding to the respective stress response types) of the elements in column j in matrix $\boldsymbol{D}$:

$$r_d(j) = \widehat{\Delta s_c} \quad with\ \widehat{\Delta s_c} = \sum\nolimits_i (\mathbf{D}_{ij} * w_i)$$

The continuous rule is used for modeling relations of stressor characteristics that are instantiated in a continuous manner, such as aversive stimuli, which is instantiated by using sounds and pictures from the IAPS and IADS using a continuous scale. This kind of rule consists of a simple linear regression model for each response type, in which the respective predicted response sizes are regressed on the continuous measure of the stressor characteristic. This entails that the predicted change in the current stress state, $\widehat{\Delta s_c}$, when applying an adjustment with value x of the continuous measure of the stressor game characteristic instantiation presented by the rule r_c, is equal to the weighted summation of the predicted changes in stress response type sizes, Δg_i. These changes are equal to the value predicted by the fitted regression model:

$$r_c(x) = \widehat{\Delta s_c} \qquad with\ \widehat{\Delta s_c} = \sum \left(\widehat{\Delta g_i} * w_i / \sum w_i\right)$$
$$with\ \widehat{\Delta g_i} = \beta_0 + \beta_1 \cdot x$$

In the example of the instantiation of aversive stimuli in the form of pictures from the IAPS, the desired change in the current stress state can be inserted, resulting in a value for x that corresponds to the value of the scale used for aversive pictures that is predicted to result in this desired change of stress state. Subsequently, the picture with the value closest to x is selected to be used as stressor game characteristic adjustment.

In order to select the stressor characteristic adjustment that is predicted to result in the stress state that is closest to the desired stress state, the feedback model will inspect the predicted stress state change of all rules when applied on the current stress state. Subsequently it will select the rule that results in the stress state that is closest to the desired stress state s_d and apply this rule, i.e., stressor characteristic adjustment, to the stressor game. This entails that one rule is executed at a time. When we consider all possible rules r with all possible input values x or j as a set R, this selection process is given by:

$$\min_{r(x \vee j) \in R} \{ s_d - (s_c + r(x \vee j))\}$$

In cases where two or more rules would result in identical predicted stress states that are both the closest to the desired stress state, the feedback model selects the rule that has the largest effect on the stress response type that has the value the farthest away from the desired stress state. This is applied to prevent flooring and ceiling effects of stress response types.

Fitting

In order to derive the rules of the feedback model for each individual subject, the subject is presented with a predetermined sequence of stressor characteristic adjustments in the fitting condition, i.e., the condition where the subject searches for notes in the maze in the garden. This sequence can be specified by the therapist or researcher, allowing to determine which rules will be used and therefore included in the feedback model and how many times and which specific adjustment will be presented.

The response to the adjustments are calculated by using the measurements x seconds before the adjustment as a baseline and the measurements y seconds after the adjustment as response, after which g is calculated for each stress response type as described in section Stress state. The values of x and y can be chosen by the therapist or researcher in order to allow for specific intervals of measurement suited for the specific stress response types being used. Because we only adjust one stressor characteristic at a time and keep all other variables that we identified as being relevant to the response constant, and do so in a homogeneous environment (the maze looks virtually the same at any given time), we take the measured response as representing the expected change in the stress response types after applying this specific adjustment. Although we aim to control all relevant variables and solely adjust the characteristic of interest, we would recommend therapists or researcher creating a sequence of adjustments to use multiple presentations of a specific adjustment, resulting in multiple-trial measurements in the fitting condition. In this manner, any remaining effect of variation in non-controlled variables on the measured response will be reduced.

The measured sizes of the response types to these stressor characteristics are used to fit the feedback model rules. For the discrete rules, this entails creating a matrix of the possible transitions between the levels together with the measured responses. The continuous rules are derived by constructing a simple regression model using least squares regression estimation (LSRE), with the measured responses as data to fit the regression model.

Intervening variables

Intervening variables, i.e., variables influencing the relation between the stressor and stress response, can intervene with the stress state that is predicted by a rule executed by the feedback model. In these cases, the feedback model cannot reliably predict, and therefore not control, the stress state. Currently, the feedback model controls for two kinds of intervening variables.

First, the model controls for intervening variables of the individual difference variables category, such as gender and age, by fitting an individual feedback model for every subject separately.

Second, the feedback model aims to reduce intervening flooring and ceiling effects of stress response types by selecting rules that have the largest effect on the stress response type that has the value the farthest away from the desired stress state.

Implementation

The feedback model is implemented in Python (van Rossum, 1995), as this language provides classes for interaction with the measurement component software *Acqknowledge* and is a high-level programming language, allowing easier adaptation in the future when this is needed for a given paradigm.

OVERVIEW

In **Figure 3** the schematic overview GASICA from **Figure 1** is revisited, and elaborated with the outcomes of the top-down design process of the different components as described in the previous sections. In this figure the constant loop performed in GASICA is depicted. In this loop the digital stressor game presents various stressor forms such as emotion induction, workload and frustration to the subject (**Table 1**) through the adjustment of (instantiations of) stressor game characteristics, e.g., the adjustment of time pressure through the presentation of a countdown. Simultaneously, five different physiological stress response types (i.e., heart rate, heart rate variability, diastolic, and systolic blood pressure, and electrodermal response) of different forms (respectively cardiac, hemodynamic, and sympathetic) are measured (**Table 3**). These measurements are relayed to the feedback model, which determines the current stress state and selects a rule (resulting in a adjustment of an instantiation of a game characteristic) that will minimize the difference between the desired stress state and the predicted current stress state after applying the rule. This rule is then applied in the stressor component, resulting in an adjustment of the game characteristic instantiations, hereby closing the loop that will run continuously. Because this loop runs continuously, any changes in the current stress state that are not a consequence of the adjustment of stressor characteristics (e.g., spontaneous drifts or influences of non-controlled variables) are constantly measured and corrected for. A narrative is used in the stressor game to prevent subjects to identify adjustments as part of the therapy or research intervention: the subject has to find notes wearing a heavy suit that contains a radio and display, and which malfunctions from time to time, resulting in for example, the presentation of images, sounds, and the restriction of movement. Intervening variables are taken into account by the feedback model in two ways, most prominently by constructing an individual feedback model for each subject.

Important to realize here is that GASICA utilizes single stressor characteristic adjustments to alter the stress state. However, the envisioned workings of GASICA do not rely on the expectation that single adjustments will result in the exact responses as found during the fitting condition. Because we *continuously* alter different characteristics, we get an ensemble of stressor manipulations that together have more power to alter the stress state toward the desired stress state. In other words, it is not the case that each specific, relatively mild, stressor is expected to elicit the exact response measured during the fitting, but rather the ensemble of all stressor characteristics that are continously presented

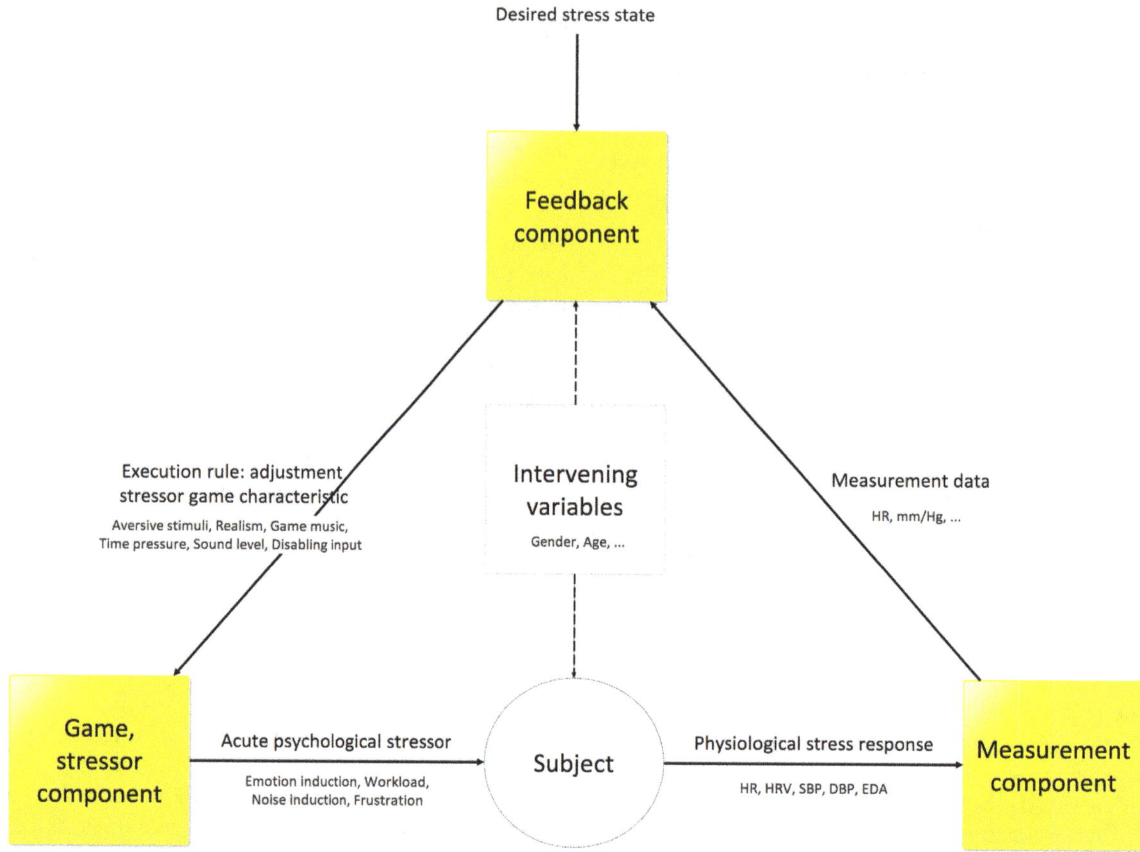

FIGURE 3 | Overview of application.

based on the current stress state, that is expected to result in the alteration of the stress state toward the desired stress state.

Instructions provided to subjects can be altered to fit the needs of the respective paradigm being used. Two general instructions that need to be given in any paradigm are that (1) the subject should perform to the best of their abilities, i.e., find as many notes as possible (monetary incentive could be employed here), and (2) the subject should remain as still as possible in order to ensure valid physiological meaurements. Important to note here is that due to the first instruction, GASICA is expected to also present a certain amount of social-evaluative threat, as the subject feels that they are evaluated on how well they are performing.

Most of the properties of GASICA can be altered by the therapist or researcher using it, as indicated in relevant sections in this manuscript. In this manner we aim to present a generic application that can be used in a multitude of paradigms. Some of the most important alterations include:

- Which elements of a paradigm, such as a baseline measurement, a fitting condition and a manipulation condition are presented, and in which order.
- Determining the used rules and corresponding stressor characteristics.
- Which characteristics are presented during the fitting condition, in which order, and how many times.
- Whether the manipulation condition utilizes a predetermined sequence of stressor characteristic adjustments or utilizes the feedback model fitted during the fitting condition.
- If a task or therapy element will be presented during the manipulation condition and how this is alternated with the characteristic adjustments.
- How long the baseline measurement will be.
- Which stress response types are measured and used to determine the stress state, and the corresponding weights.

Implementation

In **Figure 4** the complete architecture of GASICA is given, containing the implementations of the different components and the implemented connections between the components. The stressor game environment (VBS2) and the feedback model (Python) are run together on one pc, the *stimulus pc*, and the stress response measurement software (Caretaker and Acqknowledge) is run on another pc, the *acquisition pc*. This distinction is made because the software on the different pc's has different requirements: the stressor game environment requires more graphical power, whereas the measurement software mostly requires large memory and fast writing to the hard disk. By separating the components, we can utilize pc hardware that is better suited for different software, and prevent interference between the software packages. Furthermore, an additional module, the *Connection and sync*

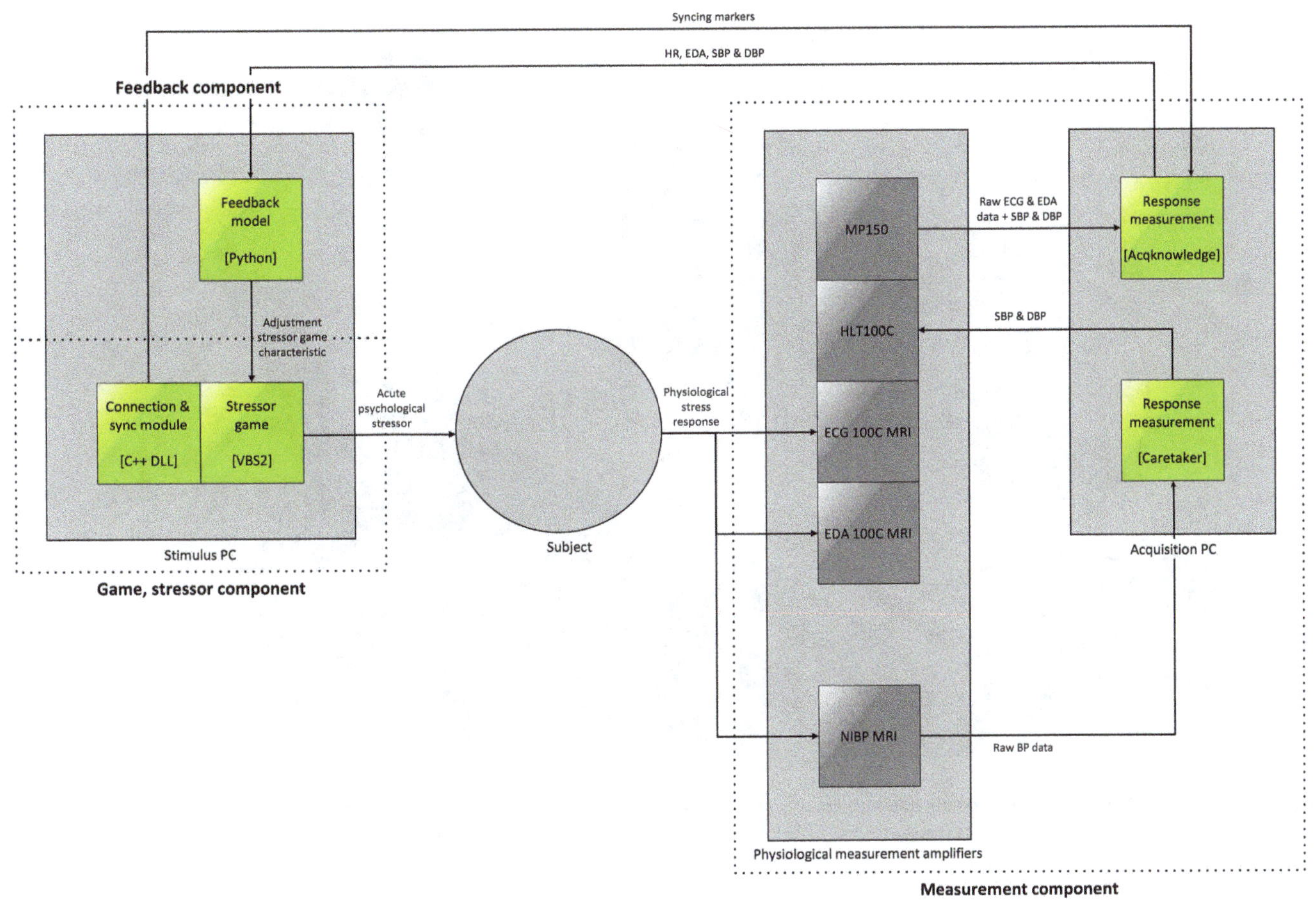

FIGURE 4 | GASICA architecture. Gray elements represent hardware such as computers and amplifiers, green elements represent software, with the software environment or language indicated between brackets. The main components from **Figure 3** are indicated with dotted lines.

module, is developed as a dynamic link library (DLL) in C++ and is utilized as a plugin in VBS2, allowing to connect additional measurement equipment to GASICA using either the parallel or the serial port. Additionally, this module serves to synchronize the measurements in the measurement component with events in the stressor game or in any additional tasks that are used in different paradigms.

Furthermore, the therapist or researcher can determine several properties of GASICA as described above. In order to facilitate this adjustment, all properties can be set through a single configuration file. Even more, all software components are coded as modular open-source code and will made available in due time on gasica.com. This allows therapist or researchers to change any element of the application that could not be altered using the configuration file, for example the way the stress state is determined, or the game design. In **Figure 5** a picture of GASICA in use is included, with the different components from **Figure 4** encircled.

DISCUSSION

We have presented GASICA, an application aimed at controlling the internal stress state in various therapy and research paradigms by online and continuous monitoring of the stress state through (neuro)physiological signals. Here we discuss the strengths and limitations of the application, and the future directions.

STRENGTHS

Through the fulfillment of the requirements of the different components, GASICA is an application that presents several strengths:

(1) Multidimensional
The application allows to present different stressor forms, such as workload, emotion induction, and frustration. This allows to investigate the effects of these specific stressor forms, in isolation or in combination, in different paradigms.
(2) Ecological valid
The stressor forms presented and the instantiations of the stressor game characteristics that present these forms allow for the presentation of ecological valid stressors. This allows for the execution of paradigms that produce results with more generalizable power to real-world situations.
(3) Controllable
The application allows to both control the stressor form and stressor intensity that is presented, aiming to result in the control of the stress state of the subject. If this succeeds,

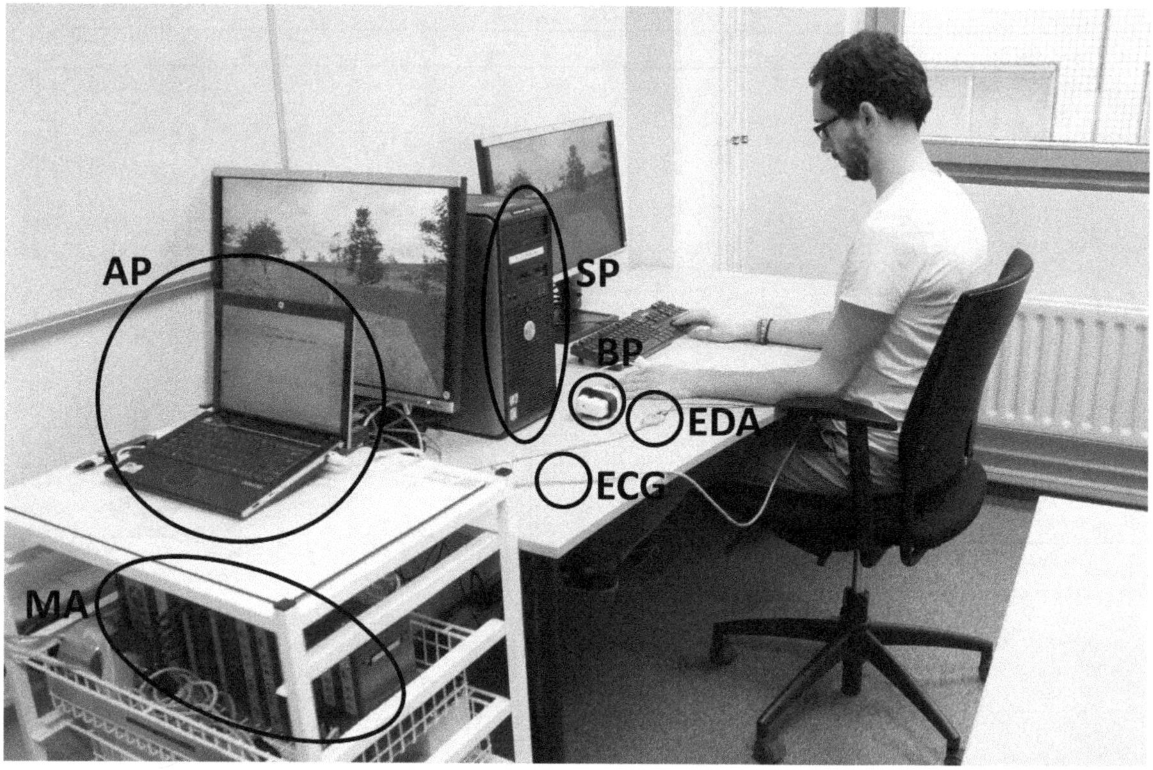

FIGURE 5 | Picture of GASICA in use, with the different components encircled. AP stands for acquisition pc, SP for stimulus pc, BP for blood pressure measurement, EDA for electrodermal activity measurement, ECG for electrocardiography measurement and MA for measurement amplifiers.

it opens many possibilities. For example, it allows to use GASICA to keep the stress state of the subject within desirable bounds given a specific paradigm, for example in therapies such as exposure therapy. Another example is to use the application to keep the stress state of a subject on a certain level for the duration of the paradigm, relevant, for example, in cases where the stress state is an intervening variable on the dependent variable in research.

(4) Generic

The application is generic in several respects. First, the configuration file allows to adjust any of the properties of GASICA, such as the adding of tasks to the application (the task itself can be constructed using the high-level programming language of VBS2), or the possibility to exclude or include stressor game characteristics and alter existing ones, allowing to present the stressor forms that are required in the respective paradigm. Second, the narrative and 3d world can be adjusted (the environment ensures easy import of existing 3d worlds and objects). Third, a wide range of physiological measurements can be used by adding Biopac amplifiers through a simple plug-and-play interface. After the new amplifier is added, the complete GASICA application automatically detects this new signal and utilizes it for control of the stress state. Additionally, measurement equipment from other vendors can be added through the connection and sync module. These properties allow adjustment of the application to make it suitable for different therapy and research paradigms. Furthermore, the entire application will be provided as modular open-source software on gasica.com, in order to allow any adjustments that are not feasible through the configuration file. This generic nature also allows GASICA to be used in additional ways. Examples could be to add neural activity measurement devices and make the measurements from these devices available to the subject, hereby effectively using GASICA as a neurofeedback application. Other examples could be in the entertainment field, where GASICA can be used to optimize the user experience, or for training purposes, aimed at the training of functioning in stressful jobs, such as in the military, aviation, or firefighting.

LIMITATIONS

Several limitations can be anticipated with this application. First, it is to be expected that the rules fitted during the fitting condition capture a relation between stressor and response that is context-dependent, for example dependent of the elapsed time the stressor has been presented. As such, these relations are prone to change during the course of the experiment or therapy. At this moment, the application does not control for this. We aim to investigate these effects during the upcoming validation study and determine possible solutions, such as using *adaptive rules* in the feedback model, i.e., rules that adjust to changing relations between stressors and responses.

Second, currently only a few intervening variables are controlled for in the application. In the upcoming validation study we will analyse the effect of several intervening variables, such as elapsed time of the current paradigm, and include these in the feedback model.

Third, the application utilizes linear regression models to model the relation between continuously instantiated stressor game characteristics and stress response type sizes. However, it is not certain whether this relation is linear. We will use the data from future research to assess what kind of model best fits these relations.

STRESS INDUCTION

One of the important questions regarding the use of GASICA is whether it induces stress, or that the found responses are due to other concepts, most prominently, arousal. As stated in the treatment of these concepts in the introduction, we concur with the distinction proposed by Day and Walker (2007). We feel that according to this distinction GASICA should be considered as a stressor, as GASICA presents many stimuli that have been found to be aversive stimuli, entailing both qualitative appraisal in terms of aversiveness, and meeting the requirement that aversive challenges must be utilized.

Given that it is pivotal to establish with the highest possible certainty that the responses to GASICA are indeed representing stress, we have planned a follow-up validation study to this Technology Report. In this study a large study population is used, containing a control group to control for other factors of the digital stressor game that can contribute to physiological responses, such as motor activity. Furthermore, additional measurements are included, such as additional subjective measurements and cortisol measurements. As cortisol is an important and widely used biomarker for stress that could not be used as an online measurement in the measurement component, we will use it as an offline measurement in this study to gain more insight in the effects of GASICA on stress.

ACKNOWLEDGMENTS

We would like to thank our reviewers for their invaluable and insightful feedback, providing us with new angles to view our application from. This project is part of the research program *Treatment of cognitive disorders based on functional brain imaging*, funded by the Netherlands Initiative Brain and Cognition, a part of the Organization for Scientific Research (NWO) under grant number 056-14-014.

REFERENCES

Adams, E. (2010). *Fundamentals of Game Design, 2nd Edn.* Berkeley: New Riders.

Barlett, C. P., and Rodeheffer, C. (2009). Effects of realism on extended violent and nonviolent video game play on aggressive thoughts, feelings, and physiological arousal. *Aggress. Behav.* 35, 213–224. doi: 10.1002/ab.20279

Bradley, M. M., and Lang, P. J. (1999). *International affective digitized sounds (IADS): stimuli, instruction manual and affective ratings.* Tech. Rep. B-2. Gainesville, FL: The Center for Research in Psychophysiology, University of Florida.

Carnagey, N. L., Anderson, C. A., and Bushman, B. J. (2007). The effect of video game violence on physiological desensitization to real-life violence. *J. Exp. Soc. Psychol.* 43, 489–496. doi: 10.1016/j.jesp.2006.05.003

Dahlquist, L. M., Herbert, L. J., Weiss, K. E., and Jimeno, M. (2010). Virtual-reality distraction and cold-pressor pain tolerance: does avatar point of view matter? *Cyberpsychol. Behav. Soc. Netw.* 13, 587–591. doi: 10.1089/cyber.2009.0263

Day, T. A., and Walker, F. R. (2007). More appraisal please: a commentary on Pfaff et al. (2007) "Relations between mechanisms of CNS arousal and mechanisms of stress." *Stress* 10, 311–313. doi: 10.1080/10253890701638204

Dedovic, K., Renwick, R., Mahani, N. K., Engert, V., Lupien, S., and Pruessner, J. (2005). The Montreal Imaging Stress Task: using functional imaging to investigate the effects of perceiving and processing psychosocial stress in the human brain. *J. Psychiatry Neurosci.* 30, 319–325.

Dickerson, S. S., and Kemeny, M. E. (2004). Acute stressors and cortisol responses: a theoretical integration and synthesis of laboratory research. *Psychol. Bull.* 130, 355–391. doi: 10.1037/0033-2909.130.3.355

Eerola, T., and Vuoskoski, J. K. (2011). A comparison of the discrete and dimensional models of emotion in music. *Psychol. Music* 39, 18–49. doi: 10.1177/0305735610362821

Fairclough, S. H. (2009). Fundamentals of physiological computing. *Interact. Comput.* 21, 133–145. doi: 10.1016/j.intcom.2008.10.011

Hebert, S., Beland, R., Dionne-Fournelle, O., Crete, M., and Lupien, S. (2005). Physiological stress response to video-game playing: the contribution of built-in music. *Life Sci.* 76, 2371–2380. doi: 10.1016/j.lfs.2004.11.011

Hedges, L. V. (1981). Distribution theory for Glass's estimator of effect size and related estimators. *J. Educ. Behav. Stat.* 6, 107–128. doi: 10.3102/10769986006002107

Ivory, J. D., and Kalyanaraman, S. (2007). The effects of technological advancement and violent content in video games on players? Feelings of presence, involvement, physiological arousal, and aggression. *J. Commun.* 57, 532–555. doi: 10.1111/j.1460-2466.2007.00356.x

Jones, F., and Bright, J. (2001). *Stress. Myth, Theory and Research.* Harlow: Pearson Education Limited.

Kirschbaum, C., Pirke, K. M., and Hellhammer, D. H. (1993). The Trier Social Stress Test a tool for investigating psychobiological stress responses in a laboratory setting. *Neuropsychobiology* 28, 76–81. doi: 10.1159/0001 19004

Lang, P., Ohman, A., and Vaitl, D. (1988). *The International Affective Picture System.* Gainesville, FL: The Center for Research in Psychophysiology, University of Florida.

Lovallo, W. R. (2005). *Stress and Health.* Thousand Oaks, CA: Sage Publications.

McFarland, R. A. (1985). Relationship of skin temperature changes to the emotions accompanying music. *Biofeedback Self Regul.* 10, 255–267. doi: 10.1007/BF00999346

Miller, S. B., Friese, M., and Sita, A. (1995). Parental history of hypertension, sodium loading, and cardiovascular response to stress. *Psychosom Med.* 57, 381–389.

Newport, D. J., and Nemeroff, C. B. (2002). "Stress," in *Encyclopedia of the Human Brain*, Vol. 4, ed V. S. Ramachandran (Elsevier), 449–462.

Nyklicek, I., Thayer, J. F., and van Doornen, L. J. (1997). Cardiorespiratory differentation of musically-induced emotions. *J. Psychophysiol.* 11, 304–321.

Pope, A. T., Bogart, A. H., and Bartolome, D. S. (1995). Biocybernetic system evaluates indices of operator engagement in automated task. *Biol. Psychol.* 40, 187–195.

Reuderink, B., Nijholt, A., and Poel, M. (2009). "Affective pacman: a frustrating game for brain-computer interface experiments," in *INTETAIN*, eds A. Nijholt, D. Reidsma, and H. Hondorp (Amsterdam: ICST), 221–227.

Ritterfeld, U., Cody, M., and Vorderer, P. (eds.). (2009). *Serious Games: Mechanisms and Effects.* New York; London: Routledge.

Selander, J., Bluhm, G., Theorell, T., Pershagen, G., Babisch, W., Seiffert, I., et al. (2009). Saliva cortisol and exposure to aircraft noise in six European countries. *Environ. Health Perspect.* 117, 1713–1717. doi: 10.1289/ehp. 0900933

Simulations, B. I. (2011). *Virtual BattleSpace 2.* Prague, Bohemia Interactive.

Smith, A., Whitney, H., Thomas, M., Perry, K., and Brockman, P. (1997). Effects of Caffeine and Noise on Mood, Performance and cardiovascular functioning. *Hum. Psychopharmacol.* 12, 27–33.

Sokhadze, E. M. (2007). Effects of music on the recovery of autonomic and electrocortical activity after stress induced by aversive visual stimuli. *Appl. Psychophysiol. Biofeedback* 32, 31–50. doi: 10.1007/s10484-007-9033-y

Stegeren, A. H., Wolf, O. T., and Kindt, M. (2008). Salivary alpha amylase and cortisol responses to different stress tasks: impact of sex. *Int. J. Psychophysiol.* 69, 33–40. doi: 10.1016/j.ijpsycho.2008.02.008

Tafalla, R. J. (2007). Gender differences in cardiovascular reactivity and game performance related to sensory modality in violent game play. *J. Appl. Soc. Psychol.* 37, 2008–2023. doi: 10.1111/j.1559-1816.2007.00248.x van der Vijgh, B., Beun, R. J., van Rood, M., and Werkhoven, P. (2015). *Meta-analysis of Digital Game and Study Characteristics eliciting Physiological Stress Responses.*

van Rossum, G. (1995). *Python Tutorial,* Technical Report CS-R9526, Centrum Voor Wiskunde en Informatica (CWI), Amsterdam.

Wahlstrom, J., Hagberg, M., Johnson, P. W., Svensson, J., and Rempel, D. (2002). Influence of time pressure and verbal provocation on physiological and psychological reactions during work with a computer mouse. *Eur. J. Appl. Physiol.* 87, 257–263. doi: 10.1007/s00421-002-0611-7

15

Cognitive state monitoring and the design of adaptive instruction in digital environments: lessons learned from cognitive workload assessment using a passive brain-computer interface approach

Peter Gerjets[1]*, Carina Walter[2], Wolfgang Rosenstiel[2], Martin Bogdan[2,3] and Thorsten O. Zander[4]

[1] *Hypermedia Lab, Knowledge Media Research Center, Tübingen, Germany*
[2] *Department of Computer Engineering, University of Tübingen, Tübingen, Germany*
[3] *Department of Computer Engineering, University of Leipzig, Leipzig, Germany*
[4] *Team PhyPA, Biological Psychology and Neuroergonomics, Technical University Berlin, Berlin, Germany*

Correspondence:
Peter Gerjets, Knowledge Media Research Center, Schleichstrasse 6, Tübingen 72076, Germany
e-mail: p.gerjets@iwm-kmrc.de

According to Cognitive Load Theory (CLT), one of the crucial factors for successful learning is the type and amount of working-memory load (WML) learners experience while studying instructional materials. Optimal learning conditions are characterized by providing challenges for learners without inducing cognitive over- or underload. Thus, presenting instruction in a way that WML is constantly held within an optimal range with regard to learners' working-memory capacity might be a good method to provide these optimal conditions. The current paper elaborates how digital learning environments, which achieve this goal can be developed by combining approaches from Cognitive Psychology, Neuroscience, and Computer Science. One of the biggest obstacles that needs to be overcome is the lack of an unobtrusive method of continuously assessing learners' WML in real-time. We propose to solve this problem by applying passive Brain-Computer Interface (BCI) approaches to realistic learning scenarios in digital environments. In this paper we discuss the methodological and theoretical prospects and pitfalls of this approach based on results from the literature and from our own research. We present a strategy on how several inherent challenges of applying BCIs to WML and learning can be met by refining the psychological constructs behind WML, by exploring their neural signatures, by using these insights for sophisticated task designs, and by optimizing algorithms for analyzing electroencephalography (EEG) data. Based on this strategy we applied machine-learning algorithms for cross-task classifications of different levels of WML to tasks that involve studying realistic instructional materials. We obtained very promising results that yield several recommendations for future work.

Keywords: passive brain-computer interface, EEG, cross-task classification, working-memory load, adaptive learning environments, cognitive load theory

INTRODUCTION: PASSIVE BRAIN-COMPUTER INTERFACES FOR ADAPTIVE DIGITAL ENVIRONMENTS

A Brain-Computer Interface (BCI) is a direct link between a human brain and a technical system. It detects patterns in brain activity (by means of so-called classifiers) and translates them into input commands for the machine. Usually, brain activity is recorded noninvasively through electroencephalography (EEG) and is interpreted by a conventional personal computer using machine learning and signal processing techniques (Blankertz et al., 2002). Machine learning algorithms are used to classify different patterns in the EEG that have to be actively produced by patients, e.g., by imaging movements (Wolpaw et al., 1991; Pfurtscheller et al., 1993; Schalk et al., 2004) or that are elicited in reaction to an attended stimulus. The initial, principal goal of BCI-based applications has been to provide direct communication and control channels for patients who have lost their ability to communicate naturally (Wolpaw et al., 2002). As the reliability and usability of BCI systems have improved over the past decade, their applicability and their appeal for other purposes besides patient support has grown also. Today BCI-approaches are developed for applications beyond assistive technologies addressing general problems of human-computer interaction (Zander et al., 2010). According to such a passive BCI approach (Zander and Kothe, 2011), spontaneously generated brain signals related to current changes in cognitive and affective user states can be deployed to support a given interaction. With passive BCIs, new methods for real-time cognitive state assessments become available that might improve human-computer interaction significantly (for exemplary studies in this emerging field see e.g., Lin et al., 2005; Ramsey et al., 2006; Dyson et al., 2010).

Different forms of passive BCIs have been proposed in recent years, for example for detecting the perception of errors (Zander and Jatzev, 2009; Zander et al., 2010), for detecting cheating (Reissland and Zander, 2010), for detecting specific intentions when fixating an object (Zander et al., 2011a; Protzak et al., 2013), or for detecting the perceived loss of control when using a system (Jatzev et al., 2008; Zander and Jatzev, 2012). Passive BCIs can be considered as an implicit, secondary communication channel enriching the ongoing primary human-computer interaction by providing information about ongoing user states. The opportunity to adapt specialized digital environments to current mental states such as inattention, cognitive or perceptual workload, mental fatigue or aversive emotions might be very helpful for users such as system operators, people interacting in augmented environments, or even surgeons and astronauts (Tonin et al., 2010; De Negueruela et al., 2011).

In this paper we will mainly concentrate on issues related to the detection of users' cognitive workload and the automatic adaptation to it. Workload adaptation is a topic that is not only relevant for specialized digital environments as mentioned before but also for much more ubiquitous and generic settings of everyday life such as adaptive learning environments for educational purposes. As will be outlined in the next section, adapting the complexity of instructional materials to learners' cognitive workload has been the main rationale of many instructional design approaches. In the remainder of this paper we will elaborate on the methodological and theoretical prospects and pitfalls of a passive BCI approach to cognitive workload assessment in instructional contexts by discussing results from the literature and from our own research. Based on these discussions, we will present a strategy on how several inherent challenges of applying BCIs to working-memory load (WML) and learning can be met by refining the psychological constructs behind WML, by exploring their neural signatures, by using these insights for sophisticated task designs, and by optimizing algorithms for analyzing EEG data.

COGNITIVE WORKLOAD AND ADAPTIVE INSTRUCTION: A CHALLENGE FOR INSTRUCTIONAL DESIGN

According to important cognitive theories of instructional design (e.g., Cognitive Load Theory, CLT, Sweller et al., 1998; Cognitive Theory of Multimedia Learning, CTML, Mayer, 2009) the type and amount of cognitive load learners experience while studying instructional materials is one of the crucial factors for successful learning. Optimal learning conditions are characterized by providing challenges for learners without inducing cognitive overload. This general rationale is also prevalent in many classic instructional design theories. For instance, Vygotsky's (1978) well-known "zone of proximal development" describes an ideal instructional situation as intermediate between situations that are "too difficult" and situations that are "too easy." Salomon's (1984) AIME-approach focuses on optimizing learners' "amount of invested mental effort" by manipulating the perceived task demands of learning materials in a way that learners' are stimulated to engage in study activities imposing a high level of cognitive workload. Reigeluth's seminal Elaboration Theory (Reigeluth and Stein, 1983) is based on the idea of presenting the same instructional contents in a sequence of increasingly more complex versions to align the cognitive workload imposed onto learners to their growing level of understanding. Thus, presenting instructional materials in a way that learners' cognitive workload is constantly held within an optimal range is not a new idea but rather seems to be unequivocally advocated by many instructional theories as a guideline to provide optimal learning conditions. The different conceptions, however, of what constitutes the nature of cognitive workload, seem to be less unequivocally.

Workload theories in the human factors area like Wickens' (1984) widely adopted Multiple Resource Model assume that there are numerous information-processing resources (like perception, processing and action applied to items of different modalities and representational codes), each of which could potentially be overloaded in a current task performance, thereby generating a bottleneck. On the contrary, cognitive theories of instructional design like CLT or CTML are much more specific with regard to the information-processing resources they consider as pivotal cognitive bottlenecks for processes of learning and comprehension. According to these theories, the workload imposed onto a structure called working memory is the crucial type of cognitive load. Working memory describes the small amount of information that can be held and manipulated in mind simultaneously for the execution of a current cognitive task (Cowan, 2014). A careful management of cognitive load imposed onto working memory is the main instructional rationale of theories like CLT or CTML. This is in line with the main recommendation derived by working memory researchers (e.g., Cowan, 2014) from their work with regard to improving learning and education: It is of fundamental importance that instructional materials are adjusted to the working-memory capabilities of learners.

The concept of WML in CLT and CTML refers back to the multicomponent working memory model by Baddeley (1986, 2000, 2012), which distinguishes verbal and visual temporal storage components (phonological loop and visuospatial sketchpad) from an attentional control system (the central executive, borrowed from the supervisory attentional system postulated by Norman and Shallice, 1986). CLT and CTML focus almost entirely on the capacity limitations of the storage components of working memory as the bottlenecks for learning, assuming that these components constrain the amount of new information that can be processed simultaneously in order to be integrated into long-term memory. According to this view, if the amount of information a learner has to process at some point in time, exceeds the capacity of these storage components, the entire learning process is hindered. Consequently, the scientific literature on CLT and CTML focuses on identifying instructional manipulations that allow influencing the type and amount of WML during learning in order to not overtax students working memory capacity.

WML during learning is commonly assumed to be the result of an interaction between the external task requirements of the instructional design presented to learners and the complexities of the contents to be learned in relation to learners' knowledge prerequisites (cf. Kalyuga et al., 2003). Identical contents can result in lower WML for more (as compared to less) knowledgeable learners due to the chunking of information enabled by the availability of more complex concepts for representing contents. Beyond the cognitive load imposed by the representational holding of contents (also described as intrinsic or essential cognitive load) there are additional components of cognitive load imposed by task requirements of the instructional design itself (e.g., requirements such as searching and handling information, comparing instructional materials, or drawing elaborative inferences). Depending on whether these additional processes required by the instructional design are helpful or hindering for deeper learning they are described as germane or extraneous processes (Sweller et al., 1998; Gerjets and Scheiter, 2003; Gerjets and Hesse, 2004; Cierniak et al., 2009b). This distinction, however, between "positive" (germane) and "negative" (extraneous) components of cognitive load has been subject to severe critique in recent years (cf. Gerjets et al., 2009; De Jong, 2010).

Frameworks like CLT and CTML have elaborated ample advice on how to adapt contents and instructional designs to students' limited working-memory resources. One important caveat in this field, however, consists in the fact that it is not possible to provide a general advice for all types of learners independent of their level of prior knowledge. Due to the interaction between content complexities and learner's knowledge prerequisites, one and the same instructional material can impose different levels of workload onto different learners. There are even "expertise reversal effects" showing that one instructional material *A* as compared to another instructional material *B* imposes higher WML for novice learners, whereas the reverse is true for more advanced learners (Kalyuga et al., 2003). For instance, a so-called integrated graphic that presents pictorial elements in close spatial proximity to corresponding verbal explanations (e.g., labels) imposes a lower level of WML onto novice learners than a non-integrated graphic that provides verbal explanations apart from their pictorial counterparts (e.g., as a figure caption). It is assumed that integrated graphics support novices in searching for verbal explanations of pictorial elements. Interestingly, the inverse pattern has been shown for more advanced learners (e.g., Cierniak et al., 2009a). Advanced learners suffer from higher WML when learning with integrated graphics as compared to non-integrated graphics. This is due to the fact that at some point during learning verbal explanations of pictorial elements become redundant for learners as they are acquainted with these elements. Subsequently, learners might tend to even suffer from integrated graphics with regard to WML because they are forced to process verbal information in working memory that is unnecessary for them to understand the graphics. Consequently, from the viewpoint of instructional-design theories WML is a highly volatile learner characteristic, potentially consisting of different cognitive load components that change during learning not only due to learners' increasing level of knowledge but also due to the changing instructional materials and task requirements presented to learners at each point in time.

Accordingly, an ultimate instructional goal would probably be a moment-to-moment assessment of WML leading to an immediate online adaptation of instructional materials in case of learners getting overwhelmed (or underchallenged) with regard to their currently available working-memory capacity. A natural technological solution to achieve this goal would consist in constructing an adaptive learning environment that—other than traditional intelligent tutor systems (ITS) based on model-tracing (e.g., Corbett, 2001) or based on natural language analysis (e.g., Graesser and McNamara, 2010)—does not aim to diagnose learners' developing knowledge structures directly, but more generically concentrates on the continuous detection of different levels of WML and the online-adaptation to it. Probably, the biggest obstacle to achieve such a technological goal is the lack of appropriate measurement procedures allowing for a continuous and non-obtrusive online tracking of WML. Current measurement methods mostly rely either on subjective workload ratings (Hart and Staveland, 1988; Paas et al., 2003) or on dual-task procedures (Brünken et al., 2003; DeLeeuw and Mayer, 2008; Cierniak et al., 2009b), both of which are likely to disrupt and annoy learners while studying—without allowing for a fine-grained temporal modeling of WML. Despite these drawbacks, first provisional attempts to construct workload-adaptive learning environments based on subjective rating scales yielded promising results, even though adaptation was not instantaneous, as WML could not be assessed continuously (Mihalca et al., 2011). Additionally, the learning process had of course to be interrupted frequently in this study to obtain workload ratings from learners.

Less obtrusive measures of WML that are better integrated into the learning process, such as performance measures obtained on assessment items embedded into the instructional materials are unfortunately not sufficiently specific for cognitive load monitoring, as they do not reveal whether the successful or unsuccessful solution of an assessment item was achieved with a high or low level of working-memory investment. Or as Cowan (2014) puts it: "One potential pitfall to watch for is that, while some students will want to press slightly beyond their zone of comfort and will learn well, others will want an easy time, and may choose to learn less than they would be capable of learning," Thus, the investments of working-memory resources during learning and the success or failure with regard to assessments of learning outcomes are clearly dissociable. Beyond this disadvantage, even repeated assessments during learning will not lead to a continuous measurement and might even frustrate learners in case of high failure rates.

In sum, measures like task performance, rating scales, or dual tasks do not allow for a continuous and non-obtrusive measurement of WML and this fact provides a fundamental problem for workload-adaptive instructional environments. One option that has been advocated to overcome this problem is to identify suitable physiological indicators of WML. For instance, it has been proposed to use physiological measures like pupil dilation or skin conductivity for a continuous WML assessment. However, up to now these measures mostly turned out to be not very reliable and specific indicators of WML (Brünken et al., 2003; Paas et al., 2003). A novel methodological avenue for solving this problem in instructional research might be to obtain more direct physiological measures of neural activity to derive sufficiently specific indicators of WML during learning. This approach can capitalize on a tradition of using EEG parameters as workload indicators in human factors research as well as in neuroscience research (e.g., Gevins and Smith, 2003). In instructional scenarios this approach has been applied very rarely and in a tentative fashion (e.g., Gerlic and Jausovec, 1999; Antonenko and Niederhauser, 2010; Antonenko et al., 2010). In this paper we will follow this line of research by trying to explore the potential of a passive BCI approach for designing workload-adaptive learning technologies based on EEG signals. In the near future, such BCIs may be applied in combination with low cost headset-like EEG sensors using dry electrodes (as they are currently beginning to reach the market, cf., Zander et al., 2011b) to help learners in instructional environments to keep their cognitive workload constantly within an optimal range. Beyond preventing cognitive overload, such BCIs may also help to immediately detect and fix a lack of challenge when learning materials are too simple in relation to a specific learner's prerequisites in terms of prior knowledge or working memory capacity. This approach resembles ITS that have already been developed for other types of learner states (e.g., affective states like boredom or engagement), following the same rationale of using sensor-based measures to control adaptive learning environments (for an overview see Calvo and D'Mello, 2010).

PROMISES AND DRAWBACKS OF EEG-BASED MEASUREMENT OF WML DURING LEARNING: THE ISSUE OF PERCEPTUAL-MOTOR CONFOUNDS

The currently best-studied EEG correlates of WML that would be suitable for a continuous online assessment of learner states are variations in the oscillatory power of the theta and alpha band activity (for a review see Klimesch, 1999). An increase in WML has repeatedly been shown to lead to an increase in theta band activity over frontal-midline electrodes (event-related synchronization, theta ERS; e.g., Gevins et al., 1997; Jensen and Tesche, 2002; Missonnier et al., 2006; Krause et al., 2010; Sauseng et al., 2010) and a decrease in alpha band power over parietal-occipital electrodes (event-related desynchronization, alpha ERD; e.g., Gevins et al., 1997; Stipacek et al., 2003; Krause et al., 2010).

In line with these findings, it has recently been proposed by Antonenko et al. (2010) to use oscillatory power for the measurement of WML in instructional research. To substantiate this idea, the authors discuss two studies that obtained continuous EEG measures to indicate WML during learning with hypermedia (Antonenko and Niederhauser, 2010) and multimedia (Gerlic and Jausovec, 1999). However, in our view both of these studies are subject to one of the main pitfalls that have to be resolved before neural workload measures can find a useful application in the context of a passive BCI to improve learning: In both studies it remains very unclear due to the complex learning materials used for experimentation whether the observed EEG differences between more and less demanding learning materials really go back to differences in WML alone or whether they might be mostly results of some behavioral correlates of workload or of some other perceptual or motor differences between the experimental conditions.

For instance, Gerlic and Jausovec (1999) found that learning about planets from spoken text combined with music and pictorial information (high WML) as compared to learning from written text alone (low WML) yielded alpha ERDs in temporal and occipital electrodes whereas in the text only condition alpha ERDs in frontal and central electrodes occurred. Here, potential differences in WML between the experimental conditions are massively confounded with perceptual differences of the experimental materials. The same criticism applies to the second study cited by Antonenko et al. (2010). This study (Antonenko and Niederhauser, 2010) revealed differences in alpha and theta frequencies when reading hypertext with vs. without link previews, hypothetically indicating a lower level of WML in conditions with link previews. However, conditions with link previews differed also perceptually (pop-up windows showed up) and with regard to motor activity (mouseover was needed for activating previews) from the conditions without previews. Again, these perceptual-motor confounds seem to prevent a clear attribution of the EEG differences found between experimental conditions to levels of WML. In our view, these problems of perceptual-motor confounds seem inevitable when using standard EEG power analyses for comparing different realistic learning materials (instead of comparing more controlled experimental tasks without perceptual-motor confounds).

What implications do these studies have with regard to the prospects of developing workload-adaptive instructional environments based on a passive-BCI approach? First it has to be noted that the standard EEG power analyses used in these experimental studies require a statistically averaging of data across several subjects and trials to identify significant EEG differences between instructional conditions. When it comes to adaptive learning environments, however, single-subject single-trial analyses are necessary to derive a continuous classification of learners' level of WML from EEG data allowing instantaneous reactions to different levels of WML. This requires very different approaches to online data analysis. Second, even if it is possible to classify realistic instructional conditions (inducing different levels of WML) online based on suitable methods to analyze EEG power differences, the question needs to be addressed, whether this classification is really based on differences in WML or on some of the perceptual-motor confounds of the different instructional conditions. In the latter case, it can unfortunately not be expected that the classification method used for the current task will yield transfer to novel instructional situations unless these situations have similar perceptual-motor confounds of different levels of WML. Beyond this problem that a classification based on perceptual-motor confounds is quite uninteresting from a practical perspective, it is also quite uninformative with regard to the theoretical issue of whether we can adapt instructional environments to cognitive workload because the classification method might not be specific enough to address workload only and hence might not really keep track of learners WML. We addressed both caveats (demonstration of single-subject single-trial analyses; avoiding perceptual-motor confounds in classifier training) in two of our own studies that will be reviewed in this paper.

STUDY 1: REALISTIC INSTRUCTIONAL MATERIALS IMPOSING DIFFERENT LEVELS OF WML: DO SINGLE-SUBJECT SINGLE-TRIAL EEG DATA ALLOW FOR A CLASSIFICATION OF THESE LEVELS?

The first caveat that we addressed in a study by Walter et al. (2011) is whether EEG power differences between learners studying two types of realistic instructional materials (inducing different levels of WML) are sufficiently strong and reliable to enable a good classification result when analyzed with BCI methods. The problem of analyzing single-subject single-trial data online is pivotal for the passive BCI approach and requires completely different methods for analyzing oscillatory EEG data than those used by Antonenko and Niederhauser (2010). These methods are based on machine learning algorithms as they have been developed by research on traditional BCIs for patients. In our study, we used realistic materials similar to Gerlic and Jausovec (1999) or Antonenko and Niederhauser (2010) to investigate classification accuracies, being aware, of course, that using realistic instructional materials will inevitably result in the abovementioned confound issues.

The study by Walter et al. (2011) used a within-subject design to manipulate WML. Ten learners (12–14 years) were asked to study two different types of instructional materials involving processes of learning and comprehension at different levels of WML. In a high WML study window, learners had to study graphical representations and explanations of mathematical angle theorems in order to understand the theorems. In a low WML study window, learners had to study a different kind of graphical representations, namely comic strips, in order to understand the stories depicted. Both materials involved complex graphical displays, however, the comic strips where quite easy to understand for learners whereas the angle theorems where quite hard for them to grasp. The two types of materials where presented to learners in an alternating sequence to avoid confounding WML with presentation time. This type of sequencing was chosen to improve experimental control and internal validity. It has to be noted, however, that it is not very representative with regard to realistic instructional situations. Under realistic conditions, there is usually an increase in the objective complexity of learning materials over time, which is, however, not always associated with an increase of learners' level of WML due to learner's improved knowledge prerequisites over time (see Section Cognitive workload and adaptive instruction: A challenge for instructional design for details).

The experimental procedure comprised three parts. First, subjects had to solve a pre-test to assure they had no prior knowledge on angular geometry before participating in the study. A second part consisted of three learning episodes, 11 min each. In each episode subjects were asked to study five angle-theorems as well as five comic strips (in alternating sequence). Each theorem and each comic strip was presented for a 45 s time interval that we define as *study window*. Subsequent to each study window, subjects were requested to answer a question with regard to the interpretation of the theorem or comic strip (four multiple-choice options presented for 10 s). Finally, subjects had to rate their subjective level of cognitive load during the study window on a 7-point Likert scale presented for another 10 s. Overall, subjects were presented with 15 study windows on angle theorems and 15 study windows on comic strips in the second part of the experiment, always alternating between these two types of materials. In a third part of the experiment, first, learning outcome measures were obtained by asking students to solve angle problems. We used a German version of the Carnegie Learning geometry tutor for this task (Schwonke et al., 2007). Finally, a post-test comprising the same items as the pretest was administered in order to allow for direct pre-post comparisons.

During the two types of study windows (angle theorems vs. comic strips), EEG data was collected and features with regard to different characteristics in the EEG frequency bands were extracted. Due to the low number of 30 study windows (15 for each type of instructional material), all artifact free study windows were segmented into smaller epochs of 15 s for each subject and each study window. Accordingly, 45 epochs per subject resulted for each type of instructional material (3 epochs per study window × 5 study windows per learning episode × 3 learning episodes for each type of instructional material), which were used for classification. This segmentation was possible because no significant variation was detected in the signal over a full study window. Concerning the feature selection, we focused on frontal and parietal electrodes with regard to the spectral power within the alpha (8–13 Hz) and theta (4–7 Hz) frequency band. For spectral analysis, an autoregressive model was calculated using the Burg-Algorithm. As there were no theta differences between learning materials, only alpha power values were used as features to classify comic epochs (studying easy materials inducing low levels of WML) vs. theorem epochs (studying difficult materials inducing high levels of WML). As students were not required to take any overt motor action during learning, prima facie no obvious motor confounds of the two types of study windows are to be expected. The results show that during epochs with high levels of WML, a desynchronization of alpha band activity could be observed in parietal (and occipital) brain areas as compared to epochs with low levels of WML. These differences could be successfully classified on a single-subject single-trial basis by using a support vector machine (SVM) with radial basis function (RBF)-Kernel (Lotte et al., 2007). A 10-fold cross validation was conducted to verify the accuracy of the trained SVM. The mean classification accuracy for all 10 learners was 76%. For seven out of the ten learners, an accuracy of 80% or higher could be achieved for detecting epochs with high vs. low levels of WML.

Thus, our results show that it is indeed possible to classify whether learners study realistic instructional materials inducing low vs. high levels of WML with a substantial accuracy based on single-subject single-trial EEG data. However, although our results seem to be practically relevant and methodologically interesting, we would consider them to be subject to the same conceptual critique that we raised when discussing the studies by Gerlic and Jausovec (1999) or Antonenko and Niederhauser (2010) with regard to perceptual-motor confounds. For instance, the angle theorems and the comic strips might differ with regard to certain perceptual characteristics, potentially leading to differences in processing beyond imposing different levels of workload onto working memory (e.g., different eye-movements or different types of semantic processing). Thus, even if there have been no obvious motor confounds of task difficulty in this study (because students were not required to take any overt motor action during learning), there nevertheless might have been perceptual and as a consequence subtle motor confounds because more difficult tasks might have resulted in different eye-movements that could have been picked up by a classifier. Accordingly, our second caveat remains: Even if an EEG-based classification is possible for realistic tasks imposing different levels of WML, this classification might still not be very helpful theoretically because it remains unclear whether a workload classifier trained on realistic tasks really represents a measure of WML or of something else.

ARE THERE SUCCESSFUL CLASSIFICATIONS OF LEVELS OF WML BASED ON OSCILLATORY EEG DATA? A CRITICAL REFLECTION ON RECENT STUDIES AND SOME SUGGESTIONS FOR IMPROVEMENT

Having a closer look at the tasks used for the classification of WML from EEG data in studies outside the field of learning and instruction reveals that problems of perceptual-motor confounds seem to be quite common, shading doubt onto the usefulness of these results as examples for the successful classification of WML. Interestingly, these problems even occur in most studies that use simple and low-level working-memory tasks for classification.

For instance, Heger et al. (2010) compared a resting state situation to a situation where subjects were conducting workload-imposing tasks like flanker tasks (where they have to press keys in reaction to the orientation of the middle arrow of a display of five arrows like: > > < > >) or switching tasks (where they have to press keys to decide whether a number is greater vs. lower than five or whether a number is odd vs. even depending on the dashed or solid framing of the number). Heger et al. (2010) classified the neural signature of the resting state situation vs. the workload-imposing situations with an accuracy of over 90% [using Artificial Neural Networks (ANNs)]. Additionally, they applied the classifier trained on these manipulations to realistic computer-based tasks of low vs. high WML (reading vs. typing) by using a so-called cross-task classification approach (for details with regard to this approach see below). The authors claim that the classifier application to the computer-based tasks was quite successful, although no quantitative results of this cross-task classification are reported. These results seem to be quite impressive at first sight, however, there are severe perceptual-motor confounds in this study that render a clear theoretical interpretation of the findings impossible: Obviously, a striking difference between the two classes used for training and for cross-task classification was whether motor activity was involved or not (key pressing vs. resting and typing vs. reading). Thus, motor activity was strongly confounded with the manipulation of WML. As the representation of motor activity in the EEG itself has a strong alpha component and there are strong oscillatory electromyographic effects (EMG) on the beta and gamma band activity in addition (which were actually used for classification by the authors) this study may mainly demonstrate a classification of motor vs. no-motor activity rather than of high vs. low levels of WML.

A study by Berka et al. (2004) who claim to classify different levels of workload in motor tasks as well as in cognitive tasks might be subject to a more sophisticated motor confound. They used EEG data to distinguish four classes of "vigilance" and report that increasing workload leads to a classification into the high vigilance class for all types of tasks. However, as their classifier mainly relies on alpha band power (which is also subject to ERD during motor activity) in combination with behavioral measures (fast eye blinks), it remains quite unclear whether the classifier is sensitive for increased workload, increased motor activity and eye movements, or both.

Similar arguments apply to the work of Chaouachi et al. (2011) who used digit span tasks (requiring subjects to retain sequences of digits of different length) and a logic task (requiring subjects to induce rules of different difficulties describing sequences of numbers like 2 - 4 - 6) for training and classification (by means of Gaussian Process Regression). The NASA-TLX rating scale (Hart and Staveland, 1988) was used to obtain subjective data on experienced cognitive workload. Their results yielded over 90% accuracy with regard to the prediction which tasks were subjectively rated as simple, intermediate or difficult. Though initially impressive, again the difficulty levels of the tasks used were systematically confounded with the amount of motor activities required. Thus, the results cannot unambiguously be interpreted as a classification of WML. For instance in the easiest condition of the digit span tasks subjects were prompted 20 times to enter the last three digits presented resulting in a pattern of 20 bursts of three key presses in the experimental block. In the most difficult condition of the digit span task they were prompted four times to enter the last eight digits presented resulting in a pattern of four bursts of eight key presses in the experimental block. Thus, not only does the easy block contain 60 key presses and the difficult block 32 key presses but also the temporal distribution was very different. Moreover, a baseline measurement that was used as a standard for the EEG power data from the different experimental blocks was obtained only once at the beginning of the experiment. In combination with the fact that all tasks were presented in an easy to difficult order, the study seems also to confound task difficulty and time delay since baseline measurement, which might be exploited by the classifier. Therefore, systematic drifts of EEG features over time could also be responsible for good classification results.

Another study that reported good within-task classification results for three types of working-memory tasks (two levels of WML each) is the study by Baldwin and Penaranda (2012). They used a reading span task, a visuospatial n-back task, and a Sternberg task for inducing different levels of WML. The reading span task requires simultaneous processing (deciding whether a sentence is correct or not) and storage (memorizing a letter presented at the end of each sentence) for a variable number of sentences (three or four in the low WML condition and six or seven in the high WML condition). The visuospatial n-back task required remembering and comparing the previous locations of a moving square with its current location. In the low WML condition the current location has to be compared with the location one trial before (1-back). In the high WML condition it has to be compared with the location three trials before (3-back). Thus, the task requires updating a list of one vs. three locations in working memory for each trial. Nine different locations were used for presentation and the probability that the current location was identical to the criterion location presented *n* trials before (i.e., positive match) was set to 50%. Subjects received a feedback (answer correct or not) after each trial. The Sternberg task requires deciding whether a number was or was not present in a list of numbers presented before. In the low WML condition the list length was one, two, or three. In the high WML condition the list length was four, five, or six. The six blocks of tasks (two difficulty levels of each of the three tasks) were presented in a randomized order. Each experimental block was presented for 5 min to subjects. For the subsequent EEG analysis each block was segmented into 60 non-overlapping windows of 5 s each (motor responses required to complete the tasks were not excluced from the analysis). The classifiers used to distinguish the levels of WML relied on 50 features, namely the EEG power of five frequency bands (delta, theta, alpha, beta, and gamma) obtained in 10 EEG channels (three frontal, three central, three parietal, and one occipital). ANNs were applied to classify the two levels of WML for all three tasks. The within-task classification, using 50% of the data from the to-be-classified task as training data and 50% for classifier application, resulted in high classification accuracies (approximately 80% on average). As in the studies reported before, however, these results might easily go back to some perceptual-motor confounds as the different experimental conditions (levels of WML) differed strongly with regard to the amount of motor activity contained in the EEG signal used for classification. For instance, in the reading span task the memorized letters had to be typed into an on-screen keyboard every three or four letters in the low WML condition and every seven or eight letters in the high WML condition. Thus, in the easy condition the number of 5-s windows that contain motor signals from typing should approximately be twice as large as in the difficult condition. The same is true for the Sternberg task. In the easy condition, a motor reaction is required after a sequence of one to three numbers, whereas in the difficult condition, a motor reaction is only required after a sequence of four to six numbers. Again, windows containing motor signals should be twice as frequent in the easy condition than in the difficult condition. The effects of these confounds might be severe as some of the EEG frequency bands used for classification (e.g., alpha or gamma) strongly react to motor responses. The n-back task used by the authors seems to have no obvious motor confounds with regard to the number of reactions required, however, the task might suffer from a subtle perceptual confound: The 1-back is a quite easy task with an error rate of approximately 10% whereas the 3-back is a rather difficult task with an error rate of approximately 30% (chance level was set to 50%). As subjects received a feedback (response correct or not) after each trial, the number of 5-s windows containing the cognitive processing of error feedback was three times higher in the difficult condition than in the easy condition. Assuming that error feedback leads to strong neural responses in the EEG (Falkenstein et al., 1991; Spüler et al., 2012a) it cannot be ruled out that this perceptual confound due to feedback presentation has contributed to the strong classification results. Moreover, as the visuospatial n-back requires subjects to memorize one vs. three locations on the screen, it cannot be ruled out that subjects in the difficult condition displayed much more eye-movements during rehearsal than subjects in the easy condition. As the authors do not report to have removed artifacts due to eye movements from the EEG data, this difference might also have contributed to good classification results.

Based on the abovementioned studies, it has to be noted that even if there are no obvious motoric confounds of task difficulty in workload classification studies—as it is, for instance, the case in the n-back task used by Baldwin and Penaranda (2012) or in our own study reported above (Walter et al., 2011)—it is nevertheless possible that perceptual confounds are present as more difficult tasks might result in different visual displays (e.g., more error feedback or more complex graphics) leading to differences in processing that are unrelated to the concept of WML (e.g., eye movements or error detection). Thus, in order to reliably classify WML, which is a precondition for our goal of developing workload-adaptive instructional environments, it is important to train EEG classifiers on tasks that are highly controlled for perceptual and motoric confounds, which probably cannot be fulfilled by the realistic instructional tasks that we eventually intend to classify in instructional environments.

With regard to the issue of avoiding perceptual-motor confounds of WML, the most convincing classification study we found in the literature was conducted by Brouwer et al. (2012), who used a sophisticated approach to workload classification based on a letter n-back task. They implemented three levels of WML (0-back, 1-back, and 2-back), whereby in the easiest condition (0-back) no updating was required as participants only had to compare whether a presented letter was identical to a previously defined target letter. Tasks were presented in blocks consisting of 48 trials of the same level of difficulty (2.5 s per trial, 2 min per block). Overall, 24 blocks were presented in a pseudorandom order (eight blocks of each difficulty level). The first six blocks of each difficulty level were used for classifier training, the remaining two blocks for classifier testing. Similar to the n-back task used by Baldwin and Penaranda (2012) no obvious perceptual-motor confounds were committed. Additionally, compared to the visuospatial n-back task used by Baldwin and Penaranda (2012) there were probably no differences between difficulty levels with regard to eye-movements for the letter n-back task. Moreover, Brouwer et al. (2012) controlled for potential effects of the differential distributions of error feedback received by participants for the three difficulty levels. In order to run the EEG analysis, each block was segmented into non-overlapping windows of different length depending on the analysis (ranging from 2.5 to 120 s per window, which allows to test for the relation between temporal window size and classification accuracy). Motor responses required to complete the tasks and other artifacts like eye blinks were not excluced from the analysis. Different types of classifiers were tested with regard to their ability to detect levels of WML. The classifier that was based on oscillarory power relied on three frequency bands (theta, alpha, and beta) obtained in seven EEG channels (frontal, central, and parietal). A SVM was applied to these features to classify different levels of WML. The results showed that the classification accuracy strongly depended on the temporal window size used for the classification (ranging from 2.5 to 120 s) as well as on the difficulty levels that have to be distinguished. The best classification results (approximately 85% correct on average) were obtained for distinguishing complete blocks of 0-back and 2-back task (i.e., decision after 48 trials or 120 s). However, as the 0-back task involves no updating process at all but relies a comparison of a current stimulus with a predefined target, it might not really be considered a working-memory task (as compared to the 1-back or 2-back task). Distinguishing the latter two (thereby involving a serious detection of the level of WML) yielded classification results of approximately 75% on average (again based on a window size of 48 trials or 120 s). However, the classification accuracy rapidly diminished when the time interval after which the decision had to be made decreased. For instance, for the distinction between 0-back und 2-back tasks the accuracy level was reduced from approximately 85% on average for a window size of 120 s (i.e., one block) to approximately 65% for a window size of 2.5 s (i.e., one trial). Unfortunately, the authors do not report on the accuracy of the more interesting distinction between 1-back and 2-back task for small window sizes but based on the abovementioned results it can be expected to be rather small. Thus, the overall classification results in this study seem to be sound and encouraging—but they are not overwhelming with regard to the prospects of yielding a fast real-time classification of WML as it is needed for developing workload-adaptive instructional environments. We assume that one reason for the moderate classification accuracy for short windows of analysis might be the fact that the motor responses required to complete the tasks as well as other artifacts like eye blinks were not excluced from the analysis in the study of Brouwer et al. (2012). As these artifacts are known to cause strong EEG signals, they can be expected to increase the overall noise level of the data, thereby potentially drowning out the weaker signals resulting from the different levels of WML implemented in the study. Accordingly, it might be a better option to define windows of analysis in a way that a time interval from at least approximately 125 ms before any keypress to approximately 125 ms after any keypress is excluded from the analysis to filter out the strongest motor signals for the sake of data quality. This is probably most important during classifier training. Using such a procedure during classifier application would be anyway quite difficult to implement in a realistic online scenario.

To conclude, several studies have recently been conducted to classify different levels of WML based on oscillatory EEG data. Although many authors report results that are quite impressive at first sight, a closer look usually reveals severe issues with regard to perceptual-motor confounds of the workload manipulations chosen. These confounds render it rather difficult to unequivocally attribute classification accuracies to levels of WML alone. Moreover, as the study of Brouwer et al. (2012) demonstrated, even if motor signals are not confounded with levels of WML, they might nevertheless create high levels of noise in the EEG data that can complicate the effective detection of the more subtle signals resulting from cognitive states. This is particularly the case when time intervals that contain strong motor signals are not excluded from the EEG analysis, which is true for all studies reviewed in this section. However, this type of temporal filtering will probably not suffice to counteract the problem of perceptual-motor artifacts in general. A better option with regard to this issue would probably be the development of more sophisticated methods for the analysis of oscillatory EEG data based on Independent Component Analysis (ICA, Makeig et al., 1996). ICA aims at reconstructing independent sources of neural activity inside the brain from the EEG data observed at surface electrodes. Once ICA-based methods become sufficiently sophisticated to rule out that classifiers strongly rely on the contribution of perceptual and motor sources, confounds like the ones observed in the abovementioned studies might become less severe (see Zander et al., submitted, for an example of how this type of methodological approach might look like). However, until these more advanced methodologies based on ICAs are available for practical application, we would strongly recommend avoiding perceptual-motor confounds when training classifiers for the detection of different levels of WML.

Thus, the rationale that we would advocate with regard to our instructional goal in this paper comprises three parts: First, we would suggest to avoid realistic instructional tasks of different WML for classifier training because these tasks will be necessarily confounded with regard to their perceptual and motor requirements. Second, we would encourage using very well designed tasks from working memory research without perceptual-motor confounds for sound classifier training. And third, in order to render these working-memory tasks relevant with regard to our practical goal, methods of cross-task classification are indicated for the later application of the classifier training to instructional target tasks. However, as the studies reviewed in this section might have sufficiently demonstrated, avoiding perceptual-motor confounds that can be erroneously picked up by classifiers remains a challenge even when using low-level working-memory tasks for classifier training. In the next section we will argue that overcoming this challenge is an important prerequisite for the successful application of cross-task classification methods.

HOW TO ALLOW FOR CLASSIFIER TRANSFER? THE CASE FOR CROSS-TASK CLASSIFICATION

The method of cross-task classification for detecting WML is based on the use of EEG data recorded during solving simple and short, but theoretically well-defined working-memory tasks that induce differences in WML without inducing other substantial differences (particularly with regard to perceptual or motor processing). These tasks are used for classifier training. After the levels of WML induced by these tasks have been calibrated, the classifiers then can be applied to target tasks, for instance, more complex instructional tasks. For cross-task classification (other than for within-task classification) all trials of the training data can be used to calibrate the classifier. Subsequently, each trial of the test data serves as new and independent input data to test the separability of the target classes according to the pretrained classifier model. However, it requires quite sophisticated passive BCI methods to train classifiers on working-memory tasks and to apply these classifiers to more complex learning materials for the detection of different levels of WML by means of cross-task-classification. The main challenges of this approach are (1) identifying or designing appropriate training tasks without confounds for different levels of WML, (2) identifying EEG features related to WML, and (3) developing machine learning algorithms enabling cross-task classification of these features (Schölkopf and Smola, 2002; Lal et al., 2004; Besserve et al., 2007; Brugger et al., 2008). Achieving high classification accuracies requires a good generalizability of the classifier as well as suitable working-memory tasks for classifier training that induce the same type and level of WML than the instructional target tasks.

With regard to our instructional goal, defining a successful classifier for cross-task classification would not only solve the core problem of perceptual-motor confounds when training classifiers with realistic tasks but would also address three other important challenges of detecting levels of WML during complex learning. First, collecting data for classifier training during complex learning tasks is very time consuming for learners, as a sufficiently high number of training trials are needed to calibrate a reliable classifier. Second, realistic learning tasks are not as reproducible as performance tasks because they inherently induce learning effects. Thus, using a set of similar learning tasks of identical complexity does not imply that these tasks will induce the same amount of WML onto learners if administered in a sequence. Rather, the first learning tasks in the sequence might yield much higher levels of workload than the last learning tasks in the sequence due to learners' knowledge gains (cf. the discussion of expertise-reversal effects in Section Cognitive workload and adaptive instruction: A challenge for instructional design). Third, a classifier trained on complex tasks usually remains quite opaque with regard to what characteristics of learners' mental state the classifier actually has picked up. Simple and theoretically well-defined working-memory tasks without perceptual-motor confounds, on the contrary, will be conceptually much more revealing. Thus, an appropriate cross-task classification approach might not only serve to overcome important methodological and practical problems of classifier transfer but might also solve theoretical problems. Up to now, there are only a few studies on applying cross-task classification procedures to workload detection and as can be seen from these studies, defining training tasks for cross-task classification is in no way trivial if perceptual-motor confounds are to be avoided. In the previous section, we already discussed the study by Heger et al. (2010) who used ANNs for cross-task classification but had strong motor confounds in the training tasks (resting state vs. flanker tasks or switching tasks) as well as in in the target tasks (reading vs. typing). Accordingly, the strong cross-task classification results in this study presumably demonstrated the cross-task classification of motor activity vs. no-motor activity but not a cross-task classification of levels of WML.

Gevins et al. (1998) also used ANNs trained on EEG data obtained during solving two types of simple working-memory tasks (verbal and spatial n-back). They were able to successfully discriminate between three levels of WML for each of these tasks. Additionally, they used cross-task classification to distinguish between low and high difficulty levels across the two tasks and reported classification performances above 85%. Although these results are promising at first sight, it has to be noted that subjects basically had to solve the same task (n-back) in a verbal and a spatial version. Using two versions of the same task for cross-task classification is prima facie much simpler than our goal of using rather diverse tasks like a working-memory task and a complex learning task. In our current context, we are obviously more interested in cross-task classification across diverse tasks than in cross-classifying different versions of the same task.

Another study that uses cross-task classification to distinguish different levels of WML across diverse working-memory tasks is the study of Baldwin and Penaranda (2012) that has already been discussed in the previous section. The authors achieved good with-task classification results for three different working-memory tasks. These results might, however, easily go back to some perceptual-motor confounds as described above. For cross-task classification, ANNs were trained on one (or a set of two) of these tasks and tested on a different task, which was not included in the training set. In this analysis, only very poor classification accuracies could be achieved. Actually, according to the authors, the accuracies for each individual subject were near chance level for all possible combinations of tasks used for cross-task classification. From our perspective, these disappointing cross-task classification results could go back to the same perceptual-motor confounds we pointed out earlier as potential explanations of the good within-task classification results: If classifiers can pick up strong perceptual-motor signals that incidentally distinguish between different versions of individual tasks (high vs. low WML), a good accuracy for within-task classification can be expected although this classification does not rely on levels of WML. Unfortunately, if different tasks have different patterns of those distinct perceptual-motor signals, training classifiers on one of these tasks will not yield transfer to the other tasks. Alternatively, the authors themselves assume that the three different tasks they used in their study might induce highly dissimilar features in the EEG signal because they rely on separate types of working memory processes related to different neural structures. In our view, this explanation addresses an important additional issue and strongly points to an urgent need for a better theoretical underpinning of passive BCI approaches to WML with regard to relevant working memory processes, their taxonomy, and their neural basis. In our view, a better theoretical understanding of different working memory processes is not only important for designing suitable sets of training tasks for cross-task classification but also for choosing appropriate strategies for data analysis as will be pointed out in the next section. Thus, for achieving our instructional goal of designing passive BCIs for cognitive load estimation during learning we tried to establish a strong link to state of the art research on working-memory processes.

HOW IS WORKING MEMORY WORKING? THE NEED FOR THEORY ON WORKING MEMORY PROCESSES

When referring back to the multicomponent working memory model by Baddeley (1986, 2000, 2012), which is the basis of most instructional approaches to cognitive load, sets of tasks like those chosen by Baldwin and Penaranda (2012) indeed seem to be quite disparate with regard to the process components involved. Baddeley's model distinguishes different temporal storage components for handling diverse representational codes as well as a central attentional control system for implementing executive functions. The tasks employed by Baldwin and Penaranda (2012) differed on the one hand in their requirements with regard to processing diverse representational codes like letters, numbers, sentences, and spatial locations. On the other hand, they also differed with regard to the attentional control processes involved like updating and matching a set of items (n-back), interleaving sentence processing with maintaining a list of items (reading span) or maintaining a list of items in the presence of distracting stimuli (Sternberg task). Thus, when considering the different working-memory components postulated by Baddeley, these tasks seem to be quite disparate. Accordingly, a strong cross-task classification performance between them might not be expected to occur. In other words, if three tasks are used for cross-task classification, but each task requires different working-memory processes with regard to storage as well as with regard to attentional control, then no strong classifier transfer between these tasks should be hypothesized unless the different processes involved in the tasks are characterized by an identical or very similar neural basis. Taking this line of reasoning very seriously, we propose that a first step for defining a theoretically sound set of training tasks for cross-task classification should be an exact definition of the cognitive processes that need to be picked up by a classifier. From our perspective, this step is crucial to allow for an appropriate classifier transfer with regard to a later target context. Thus, for our current purposes of connecting working-memory tasks and learning tasks by means of cross-task classification it will be necessary to decide first, which of the different working-memory processes we want to track. Accordingly, we have to clarify which working-memory processes are pivotal when it comes to the role of WML for learning.

Instructional theories like CLT and CTML unequivocally focus almost entirely on processing requirements with regard to the storing of specific representational codes in working memory. Thus, they would consider the capacity limitations of the storage components of working memory to be the main bottlenecks for learning, assuming that these components constrain the amount of new information that can be processed simultaneously in order to be integrated into long-term memory. According to these theories, the entire learning process is hindered when the amount of information a learner has to process exceeds the capacity of these storage components. Using this theoretical account as a basis for an approach to cross-task classification would probably imply to define different classifiers for different storage components in order to measure the WML with regard to one specific storage component. Consequently, each classifier would be trained on a set of working-memory tasks using only one representational code and therefore imposing WML only with regard to one specific storage component. Interestingly, however, recent research on the relation between working memory and instruction suggests a quite different theoretical perspective. Many studies in instructional contexts have shown that the individual capacity of the storage components of working memory (as measured, for instance, by simple span tasks) neither predicts comprehension and learning outcomes in the short run (e.g., in studies on multimedia learning, see Schüler et al., 2011 for an overview) nor in the long run (e.g., in studies on school achievement, cf. Hoard et al., 2008; Alloway and Alloway, 2010; Kornmann et al., submitted). Instead, the central executive functions of working memory (that is, the attentional control processes that are usually required to accomplish more comprehensive working-memory tasks; cf. Daneman and Carpenter, 1980; Engle, 2002) seem to be highly predictive for successful learning and comprehension. These findings render only little support for the basic assumption of current instructional theories that capacity limitations of the storage components of working memory are pivotal for learning and comprehension. Rather, they provide evidence for an alternative idea, namely that the requirements imposed onto attentional control processes in working memory might be the crucial constraints for learners that need to be handled by providing workload-adaptive instructional environments.

Working out this idea in further detail first raises the issue of defining more precisely the nature of attentional control processes in working memory. Baddeley's working-memory theory might be a good conceptual starting point in this respect because it already postulates a central attentional control system for implementing different executive functions. Baddeley has modeled this central executive after the supervisory attentional system postulated by Norman and Shallice (1986). According to Norman and Shallice, many cognitive and overt responses are elicited quite automatically and based on activations of well-learned schemata in long-term memory. However, in order to cope with situations that cannot be handled by schema-based processes alone without resulting in errors, they postulate a supervisory attentional system that actively steps in to inhibit automatic responses and to select more appropriate ones. According to this view, the main role of attention control or executive functions in working memory might be to replace automatically activated information by more suitable information in order to avoid inappropriate processing (for a similar recent account of working memory see Oberauer, 2009). This general idea of attentional control is well in line with a latent variable analysis of executive functions conducted by Miyake et al. (2000). In this study the authors measured individual task performances in a set of simple tasks—each loading on one single executive function—as well as in a set of complex executive tasks. This procedure allows analyzing the contributions of each executive function to the individual performances in the complex task. Confirmatory factor analysis indicated that there are three target executive functions that are clearly separable although they are also correlated with one another. According to this analysis, attention control can be decomposed into the three basic executive functions inhibition, shifting, and updating, all of which aim at replacing currently active working-memory contents. The authors summarize their results by claiming that it is important to recognize both the unity and diversity of executive functions, implying that there is one overarching common factor representing the overall control of attention in addition to three specific factors representing the three executive functions.

Coming back to our instructional context, the ideas of Norman and Shallice (1986) and Miyake et al. (2000) might suggest a distinction between (1) those instructional situations that allow for a schema-based processing and therefore require little attentional control and (2) those situations that highly depend on executive processes (e.g., for selecting relevant information and *inhibiting* irrelevant information, for *updating* and organizing memory contents or for *shifting* between different task demands). Interestingly, and in line with this reasoning, most instructional design principles elaborated by CLT and CTML indeed address issues of helping learners to focus on relevant and to ignore irrelevant information, to update and organize memory contents and to shift attention between different task demands (cf. Mayer, 2009). Therefore, these design principles fit nicely into the view that the amount of controlled attention required by a learning task is pivotal to define relevant WML in instructional contexts. Moreover, a focus on requirements with regard to controlled attention (instead of storage requirements) would also be well aligned to core assumptions of many recent working memory theories (e.g., Barrouillet et al., 2004; Engle and Kane, 2004; Cowan,

2005, 2014; Unsworth and Engle, 2007; Oberauer, 2009). These theories agree that attentional control demands rather than temporary storage demands constitute the core of WML. According to this perspective, the limited ability to control attention constitutes the essence of human working memory limitations and also explains individual differences in working memory capacity (Engle and Kane, 2004; Unsworth and Engle, 2007). Using this theoretical account as a basis for cross-task classification would first of all imply a very different approach to the selection of training tasks compared to the approach of focusing on the limitations of different storage components of working memory. In particular, in order to define a theoretically sound set of training tasks for cross-task classification, we would either need a training set that allows a classifier to pick up the overarching common factor representing the general control of attention or we would have to define three training sets that more specifically address the three executive functions identified by Miyake et al. (2000).

An important consequence of these theoretical insights from the cognitive psychology of working-memory in the context of designing passive BCIs for cognitive load estimation would probably be that we need to better specify the neural basis of the general control of attention in working memory as well as the neural signatures of the three target executive functions that constitute controlled attention. This is important mainly because it may help to inform feature selection for analyzing sets of training tasks for different aspects of WML. Based on functional magnetic resonance imaging (fMRI) techniques, it has been shown that working-memory tasks typically involve an interaction of the dorsolateral prefrontal cortex and the intraparietal sulcus, which are also described as anterior and posterior attentional systems in controlled attention tasks (Curtis and D'Esposito, 2003; Klingberg, 2009). This is well in line with known relations between WML and frontal and parietal changes in oscillatory power (Gevins et al., 1997; Jensen and Tesche, 2002; Stipacek et al., 2003; Missonnier et al., 2006; Krause et al., 2010; Sauseng et al., 2010). It has to be noted, however, that due to volume conduction EEG signals obtained in frontal and parietal electrodes do not necessarily indicate that the sources of these signals also originate from frontal or parietal areas of the cortex. Therefore, fMRI data and EEG data resulting from the same cortical processes do not necessarily need to map with regard to the localization of activated voxels in the cortex and the localization of electrodes on the surface of the skull that are responsive to these processes. Nevertheless, fMRI data are highly useful in our context in order to characterize the homogeneity or heterogeneity of brain areas involved in the different working-memory functions we are interested in. Neuroimaging studies (cf. Nee et al., 2012 for a recent review of 37 studies, Smith and Jonides, 1999; Sylvester et al., 2003) as well as some recent EEG studies (Chapman et al., 2007; Kiss et al., 2007; Hanslmayr et al., 2008; Sörqvist and Sætrevik, 2010; Nigbur et al., 2011) suggest, for example, that beyond the general fronto-parietal pattern of activation characteristic for WML, different frontal areas are involved in different working-memory functions. Detailed fMRI studies show, for instance, that the dorsolateral prefrontal cortex (Broca area 9 and 46) is typically activated when holding spatial information, monitoring and manipulating information in working memory, using strategies to facilitate memory, or verifying representations that have been retrieved from long-term memory (Goldman-Rakic, 1994; Owen, 1997; Dobbins et al., 2002; Bor et al., 2004; for an overview see Owen et al., 2005). Closely related areas in the mid-ventrolateral prefrontal cortex (Broca area 45 and 47) are activated during the selection, comparison and evaluation of stimuli held in short-term and long-term memory as well as during the holding of non-spatial information in working memory and the elaborated encoding of information into episodic memory (Goldman-Rakic, 1994; Petrides, 1994; Henson et al., 1999). Compared to the frontal cortex, the posterior areas of the brain that are crucial for working memory—including the parietal cortex—are mainly responsible for the maintenance of information in working memory. Thus, these areas have also been described as a "buffer for perceptual attributes" (Callicott et al., 1999). In line with this characterization, the involvement of different representational codes in working-memory tasks might lead to subtle differences with regard to the activation of these parietal areas. For instance, Knops et al. (2006) demonstrated in an fMRI study that two types of n-back tasks (identity match: "stimulus is the same/not the same as *n* trials before" and comparison: "stimulus is smaller/larger than *n* trials before") with numerical vs. verbal materials activated slightly dissimilar areas in the intraparietal sulcus. Besides prefrontal and parietal areas, also the anterior cingulate cortex (ACC) shows an increased activation during working-memory tasks. Activity in this brain region is often related to increased effort, error detection, and attention (Callicott et al., 1999). Moreover, the brain regions crucial for working memory are not operating in isolation from each other, but are communicating. For instance, a study by Honey et al. (2002) has shown that the connectivity of fronto-parietal brain networks increases when working memory is involved.

What are the implications of these findings from the neuroscience literature on working memory and executive functions with regard to potential approaches to the cross-task classification of WML? First, in line with the functional evidence from cognitive psychology (e.g., Miyake et al., 2000) the neural basis of working memory also seems to be characterized by unity (e.g., fronto-parietal network activation) as well as diversity (e.g., differential involvement of specific brain areas). There seem to be networks that are involved in all working-memory tasks whereas other networks are only involved in specific working-memory tasks. Second, we take this pattern as evidence that it might make sense to look out for a quite broad neural signature indicating the load onto a generic common factor representing the overall control of attention (cf. Klingberg, 2009). Third, although there is evidence that particular areas are involved when it comes to specific working-memory functions (e.g., certain executive functions or functions related to particular representational codes), it might be difficult to distinguish these different functions by means of their neural signatures in the EEG signal. Differences in the areas involved are quite subtle so that detecting these specific signatures might require a further development of more sophisticated methods for the analysis of oscillatory EEG data based on ICAs (Makeig et al., 1996), also including the activity of networks (Mullen et al., 2010). These future methods might allow for better defining (source-based) features, which might enable classifiers to pick up these rather subtle differences with regard to the activated brain areas. In line with this evidence, in our own attempts to classify EEG data from working-memory tasks, we will first try to identify an overarching factor of controlled attention involved in WML. This factor is assumed to represent the unity of executive functions according to the analysis of Miyake et al. (2000) and is considered to be based on the same neural basis (i.e., fronto-parietal networks, Klingberg, 2009) for different learning materials, independent, for instance, from the representational codes involved (e.g., numerical or verbal) or from the specific executive functions required (e.g., inhibition, shifting, updating). After having specified more precisely the nature of the working-memory processes we want our classifier to pick up—based on the cognitive as well as on the neuroscientific working-memory literature—we can now continue to develop a theoretically sound set of training tasks for these processes.

Defining a classifier (based on fronto-parietal patterns of activation in EEG data) that allows extracting the amount of controlled attention required by a task (independent from specific representational codes or executive functions involved) presupposes at least a set of two different working-memory tasks for classifier training, each without perceptual-motor confounds, and both differing substantially with regard to the representational codes and executive functions they involve (to ensure that the classifier will not extract these specific features). An ideal set of working memory-tasks for classifier training in our instructional setting would consist of two working-memory tasks that are both known to be highly correlated with achievements in learning tasks (potentially indicating that the executive functions involved in these tasks are relevant for learning). At the same time they should not be highly correlated with each other (potentially indicating that these tasks do not involve the same combination of executive functions). Actually, a combination of an n-back task with a complex span task—as used in the study of Baldwin and Penaranda (2012)—fulfills these constraints. Both tasks are standard paradigms in working-memory research that predict learning outcomes very well (Daneman and Carpenter, 1980; Engle, 2002; Kornmann et al., submitted) but correlate only weakly with each other (Kane et al., 2007; Redick and Lindsey, 2013), indicating that different executive processes might be involved in task performance. For instance, a reading span task requires *shifting* between a rather complex semantic processing task and a rather simple additive *updating* of a set of items. Contrarily, the n-back task requires a complex *updating* of a set of items involving a replacement (*inhibition*) of previous set members and a reordering of the sequence of set members as well as a *shifting* between these updating task demands and a simple identity-matching task. In the light of this analysis it is quite astonishing that the promising combination of an n-back task and a complex span tasks in the study of Baldwin and Penaranda (2012) yielded no positive cross-task classification result with regard to the Sternberg task. One reason for this finding might be of course that there were differential perceptual-motor confounds of the three tasks in that study (as already mentioned above). Another reason, however, might be that the Sternberg task used in the study does not really represent a working-memory task in the sense that it involves executive demands like *updating*, *shifting*, or *inhibition* (in addition to maintaining a set of items): Subjects had to maintain a sequentially presented list of items for 2 s and after this phase they had to decide whether a certain probe was present in the set or not. Subsequently, a new list was presented. Thus, this task does not involve maintaining a memory set and working on this set or on other items in an interleaved fashion. Therefore, the Sternberg task resembles much more a short-term memory task than a working-memory task. In line with this reasoning, Corbin and Marquer (2013) argue that the Sternberg task can be considered a working-memory task only under very specific conditions, for instance, when additional experimental constraints are imposed on subjects that increase the processing load. Thus, in terms of neural signatures, the Sternberg task may mainly rely on neural networks not involved in executive control whereas the n-back task and the complex span task may rely on neural networks required for executive control, but may differ with regard to the specific mixture of executive functions required for task performance, which explains their rather weak correlation on a behavioral level. In essence, as our overview of the working-memory literature on the behavioral and the neural level reveals, it will not be sufficient to just select a random working-memory task or a random combination of working-memory tasks for successful classifier training when cross-task classification is intended. Rather, a strong link to state of the art research in the cognitive psychology and cognitive neuroscience of working-memory processes is necessary to select appropriate sets of working-memory tasks that are characterized by overlapping task demands with regard to the target construct (controlled attention) and differential mixtures of specific executive functions so that the resulting classifier is not constraint to a specific mixture of these functions.

WHAT HAVE WE LEARNED SO FAR? A SUMMARY IN FIVE LESSONS

As a summary on how the different issues raised in this paper might be overcome in order to achieve the instructional goal of designing passive BCIs for cognitive load estimation during learning we compiled the following list of five lessons learned. These lessons do not only result from research on cognitive load in instructional design (Section Cognitive workload and adaptive instruction: A challenge for instructional design) and from studies on EEG measures of workload during instruction (Section Promises and drawbacks of EEG-based measurement of WML during learning: The issue of perceptual-motor confounds), but also from our own initial studies (Section Study 1: Realistic instructional materials imposing different levels of WML: Do single-subject single-trial EEG data allow for a classification? And what is being classified?), from studies on workload classification (Section Are there successful classifications of levels of WML based on oscillatory EEG data? A critical reflection on recent studies and some suggestions for improvement) and on cross-task classification (Section How to allow for classifier transfer? The case for cross-task classification) as well as from the behavioral and neurocognitive working-memory literature (Section How is working memory working? The need for theory on working memory processes). It should become clear from this list that many details of how to choose tasks for classifier training and how to analyze the EEG data resulting from these tasks might be of crucial importance, even though these details might appear quite oversophisticated at first sight. In order to demonstrate the importance of these lessons we applied them meticulously in designing a follow-up study (Walter et al., submitted) that resulted in a successful cross-task-classification of WML. This study will be summarized in the next section.

LESSON 1 – THE ROLE OF TASK ORDER IN THE CONTEXT OF LEARNING

A randomized task order is usually a good choice for classifier calibration and testing to avoid any confounds of the classes to be detected with the time of presentation. However, when it comes to learning tasks, randomization is hard to implement. WML is a highly volatile learner characteristic that changes during learning not only due to ubiquitous increases in the complexity of instructional materials and task requirements over time (objective complexity) but also due to learners' increasing levels of knowledge (degree of expertise, cf. Section Cognitive workload and adaptive instruction: A challenge for instructional design). Based on these changes, task order plays a different role for learning tasks than for performance tasks where a randomized task order can typically be implemented without hesitation. For learning tasks, randomization is usually not appropriate. In most cases, certain materials will be too complex to be understood at an early phase of instruction while they might be quite easy at a later point in time. This is due to the fact that an increase in expertise over time (i.e., learning) allows handling more complex contents than before without the need to activate a larger number of knowledge structures in working memory (due to the chunking of information into more complex concepts, cf. Section Cognitive workload and adaptive instruction: A challenge for instructional design). Accordingly, two materials with identical objective complexity might impose very different levels of WML at different points in time during learning due to learners' knowledge gains. As a consequence, it is not advisable to present too complex learning tasks at the beginning of an instructional sequence and too simple learning tasks at the end of an instructional sequence. Otherwise, no learning might occur at all because the learning tasks are either much too simple or much too complex in relation to learners' current knowledge prerequisites. This inherent dynamic of WML in the context of learning tasks due to the ongoing acquisition of knowledge implies that it makes no sense to present learning tasks in a randomized task order, as one would typically do with performance tasks: Realistic learning tasks differ exactly from performance tasks with regard to the fact that they cannot be presented in an arbitrary order without jeopardizing their character as learning tasks. This specific characteristic, however, has serious implications for classifier testing and training when designing passive BCIs for cognitive load estimation during learning: Most important, when instructional materials need to be presented in a fixed simple to complex sequence in any realistic learning context, it is inevitable that testing a classifier on such a fixed sequence of learning materials is subject to a confound of objective levels of task complexity and presentation time. From our perspective, it is necessary to take the potentially negative effects of such a confound due to fixed task order explicitly into account (e.g., the effect that a classifier might pick up slow drifts in the EEG signal over time as useful information about task complexity due to the correlation of both factors). We advocate two measures to counteract these potentially negative effects. First, with regard to feature selection for classifier definition, we suggest to use %ERD/ERS ratios (Pfurtscheller and Lopes da Silva, 2005) instead of simple power values to explicitly cancel out slow changes in the EEG signal over time. The %ERD/ERS ratios are calculated by using a baseline signal for comparison that immediately follows or precedes the target window of analysis. Second, for parity reasons we recommend to use the same simple to complex sequence not only for classifier testing on learning tasks but also for classifier training on working-memory tasks (by presenting the working-memory tasks needed to train the classifier in a similar fixed order. When applying %ERD/ERS ratios to both task sequences (classifier training and testing), the baseline as well as the window of analysis will both be subject to potential drifts in the EEG signal over time for all sequences. Accordingly, these drifts cannot be erroneously picked up by a classifier.

LESSON 2 – CLASSES BASED ON SUBJECTIVE RATINGS OF WML

The inherent dynamic of WML due to learning explained in Lesson 1 also has a second implication beyond task order, namely that it might not be useful to define classes of learning tasks for classifier training and testing based on their objective task complexity. Rather, the definition of these classes needs to take into account that the same learning tasks could elicit different levels of WML depending on learners' current degree of expertise as well as on their individual working-memory capacity (cf. Section Cognitive workload and adaptive instruction: A challenge for instructional design). For instance, in a block of 40 learning tasks of similar objective complexity, the first 20 tasks might impose rather high levels of WML onto learners due to their novelty, whereas the last 20 tasks might impose lower levels of WML onto learners due to schema formation (chunking). Accordingly, in line with instructional theories (cf. Section Cognitive workload and adaptive instruction: A challenge for instructional design) we propose that classes based on subjective ratings of WML may be more appropriate for classifier training and classifier testing than classes based on objective task complexity, at least when the target construct for classification is the WML actually experienced by learners (which is the case in the context of adaptive instructional environments). For illustration, consider the example of learning how to solve two-digit addition tasks in the octal numeral system (base-8 number system, e.g., 23 + 77 = 122). This task will be quite demanding with regard to working-memory resources when encountered for the first times. However, with increasing practice, it will become rather easy, comparable to two-digit addition tasks in the decimal numeral system that we are all acquainted with (e.g., 23 + 77 = 100). Thus, the WML actually experienced by learners when solving two-digit addition tasks in the octal numeral system will change to a large extent over time, whereas the objective task complexity remains constant. This example should make clear that the classes that we need to detect in instructional contexts are subjective levels of WML and not objective levels of task complexity.

LESSON 3 – AVOIDING PERCEPTUAL-MOTOR CONFOUNDS

The windows used for analyzing EEG data during classifier training should not contain perceptual-motor confounds that could be erroneously picked up by the classifier. This implies that classifier training cannot be conducted on realistic learning tasks but need to be restricted to more controlled experimental working-memory tasks. Additionally, methods like ICA and connectivity analyses need to be further developed to better rule out motor artifacts in the future (cf. Section Promises and drawbacks of EEG-based measurement of WML during learning and instruction: The issue of perceptual-motor confounds, Study 1: Realistic instructional materials imposing different levels of WML: Do single-subject single-trial EEG data allow for a classification of these levels?, Are there successful classifications of levels of WML based on oscillatory EEG data? A critical reflection on recent studies and some suggestions for improvement, How to allow for classifier transfer? The case for cross-task classification). These methods might eventually allow excluding those components or networks from the set of features for classifier training, which clearly reflect perceptual or motor processing.

LESSON 4 – COMBINING WORKING-MEMORY TASKS

The working memory-tasks used for classifier training should not be confined to a single type of task. Instead combinations of at least two working-memory tasks should be used (preventing the classifier from picking up task-specific features). All working-memory tasks used should be predictive for achievements in learning tasks (potentially indicating that the executive functions involved in these tasks are relevant for learning). At the same time, the tasks should differ with regard to the specific executive functions they require (updating, shifting, inhibition) and with regard to the representational codes (numbers, letters, words etc.) they involve in order to train a generic classifier sensible to general changes in the requirements on controlled attention irrespective of specific executive functions or representational codes. This can be ensured by selecting working-memory tasks that only have a weak correlation with each other (potentially indicating that these tasks do not involve the same combination of executive functions). Additionally, it might be wise to avoid visual-spatial working-memory tasks for classifier training because these tasks might afford rehearsal strategies that produces different pattern of eye-movements for different levels of WML (cf. Section How is working memory working? The need for theory on working memory processes).

LESSON 5 – DIFFICULTY LEVEL OF WORKING-MEMORY TASKS

One should be prepared that the level of WML induced by controlled experimental working-memory tasks used for classifier training could differ from the level of WML induced by realistic learning tasks used for classifier testing. This is a natural implication of the fact that different task are used for classifier training than for classifier testing (cf. Section How to allow for classifier transfer? The case for cross-task classification). Thus, a calibration procedure for cross-task classification might be needed that allows for a scaling to adjust a trained classifier to new testing materials.

STUDY 2: CROSS-TASK CLASSIFICATION OF BASIC WORKING-MEMORY TASKS AND REALISTIC INSTRUCTIONAL TASKS

Based on the five lessons outlined in the previous section, we extended the design of our Study 1 (outlined in Section Study 1: Realistic instructional materials imposing different levels of WML: Do single-subject single-trial EEG data allow for a classification of these levels?, for details see Walter et al., 2011) in several ways (Walter et al., 2013a; Walter et al., submitted). The goal of Study 2 was to develop efficient classification methods to differentiate levels of WML based on cross-task classification. We trained a SVM on two well-controlled working-memory tasks (reading span, numerical n-back), assuming theoretically that they would induce similar types of WML (and accordingly similar types of neural processing) as the two realistic learning tasks we used subsequently for classifier testing (algebra problems). By taking into account the lessons summarized in the previous section, we were able to achieve promising results for cross-tasks classification. 21 subjects participated in the study, however, due to technical problems during data collection, five subjects had to be discarded from the analysis. For the majority of the remaining 16 subjects the cross-task classification reached a significant classifier performance ($p < 0.05$, permutation test), with classifier accuracies up to 95% for the best subjects. The classifier was able to distinguish the subjectively easier vs. harder set of algebra problems with a mean classification accuracy of 73%. In the following we will outline the methodological strategies that we used to overcome the inherent challenges of using cross-task classification for cognitive workload assessment in the context of learning.

TASK DESIGN

Training tasks

According to the considerations in Section How is working memory working? The need for theory on working memory processes, it will not be sufficient to just select a random working-memory task or a random combination of working-memory tasks to train an efficient classifier for cross-task classification. Rather, it will be necessary to select appropriate sets of working-memory tasks overlapping in task demands with regard to our target construct (controlled attention demands due to WML) and differing with regard to specific executive functions (see Lesson 4). As described above, the n-back task in combination with the reading-span task fulfills these requirements. Thus, we decided to use this combination of tasks in Study 2. Both tasks predict achievements in learning tasks very well but correlate only weakly with each other, which might be due to their different profiles with regard to executive functions. A reading span task requires *shifting* between a semantic processing task and a simple additive *updating* of a set of items. The n-back task, on the contrary, requires an *updating* of a set of items together with a replacement (*inhibition*) of previous set members interleaved with an identity-matching task. In addition to these differences, we designed the tasks to cover various representational codes (see Lesson 4). In the n-back task, single-digit numbers had to be memorized (except the number seven, which is the only two-syllable number), whereas the reading span task was based on memorizing letters (from the set B, F, H, J, L, M, Q, R, X) and on verifying sentences. By these design decisions we tried to prevent the classifier from picking up task-specific features. We implemented three levels of task difficulty for each task in a within-subject block design (i.e., 1-back, 2-back, 3-back and readings spans with 2, 4, 6 letters/sentences). We ensured that subjects received identical visual displays in all levels of task difficulty to avoid perceptual confounds (see Lesson 3).

Testing tasks

For classifier testing, two different types of algebra word problems were designed (subtraction problems and fraction problems). For both types of tasks, again three levels of task difficulty were implemented that strongly differed with regard to the level of WML they would induce. To avoid perceptual confounds of task difficulty (see Lesson 3), all word problems contained exactly four numerical pieces of information at each level of task difficulty (either numbers or fractions). Additionally, the word problems were matched for number of words. Thus, we ruled out that more difficult word problems resulted in more numerical of text information or more complex visual displays leading to differences in processing, which may show up in the EEG (see Section Are there successful classifications of levels of WML based on oscillatory EEG data? A critical reflection on recent studies and some suggestions for improvement).

In order to solve the subtraction problems, a variable x had to be calculated by selecting and integrating appropriate numbers. For the first level of task difficulty, subjects merely had to select one out of the four numbers ($x = a$). The second level required them to subtract two relevant numbers ($x = a - b$). The third level, finally, asked for the difference between two differences, thus involving all four given numbers ($x = (a - b) - (c - d)$). This manipulation of task difficult was based on the taxonomy by Schnotz et al. (2010) and can be assumed to induce strong differences in WML.

The fraction problems required subjects to select and instantiate algebraic expressions containing fractions and multiplications in order to determine the value of a variable x. For the first level of task difficulty, the appropriate expression contained one fraction ($x = c \cdot a/b$). For the second difficulty level the expression contained the same fraction two times ($x = c \cdot a/b + d \cdot a/b$). The third level contained two different fractions ($x = c \cdot a/b + d \cdot e/f$). This manipulation of task difficult was based on the taxonomy by Scheiter et al. (2010) and can be assumed to induce strong differences in WML.

In all four tasks, subjects had to react with key presses to provide their answers. They could react either with "yes" or "no" in the working-memory tasks (identity matching in the n-back task and sentence verification in the reading-span task) or with one out of four multiple choice options in the learning tasks used for classifier testing). The motor reaction was exactly the same for both working-memory tasks and both learning tasks. Furthermore, there were no differences in the motor reaction between different levels of tasks difficulty. No feedback was given to subjects in order to avoid confounding task difficulty and ratio of negative feedback (cf. Section Are there successful classifications of levels of WML based on oscillatory EEG data? A critical reflection on recent studies and some suggestions for improvement).

For modeling a realistic learning scenario (cf. Lesson 1), the mathematical word problems were presented in a simple to complex sequence for each learner (within-subject block design). Accordingly, a randomized task order for classifier testing could not be implemented. For parity reasons, we used the same simple to complex sequence for each working-memory task to generate the data used for classifier training. To rule out potential negative effects of such a fixed task order (e.g., slow drifts in the EEG signal that can inform the classifier) we calculated %ERD/ERS ratios using a baseline for comparison that immediately follows or precedes the window of analysis, thus counteracting the potential confound of time and level of WML (for details see below).

DETAILS OF EEG MEASUREMENT

With regard to the windows used for analyzing EEG data, we ensured that they did not contain any motor events or perceptual confounds that could be picked up by a classifier. The windows of analysis always ended at least 125 ms before any keypress to exclude EEG signals based on motor planning (Grabner and De Smedt, 2011). Furthermore, a time interval of 125 ms after any keypress was excluded from the analysis to avoid potential motor artifacts (see Lesson 3). Although these decisions with regard to the EEG analysis as well as with regard to the tasks designs already yielded highly controlled tasks without perceptual-motor confounds, we additionally reduced eye-movement artifacts by optimizing the data pre-processing step (Walter et al., submitted). We applied the artifact-reduction method described by Schlögl et al. (2007).

To counteract the potential confound of time and level of task difficulty, we calculated %ERD/ERS ratios based on power values using two time intervals for each task, one interval that strongly imposes the task-specific WML (activation interval, I_a) and one interval that imposes only a low level of WML (resting interval, I_r). Defining these intervals requires a theoretically based understanding of the working-memory processes involved in the tasks (cf. Section How is working memory working? The need for theory on working memory processes). We ensured that each trial of a task included both intervals to avoid systematic evects of drifts in the EEG signal (see Lesson 1).

In the n-back task, every 2000 ms a new digit was presented for identity matching. Subjects could react by pressing "yes" or "no" anytime. For I_a we used the time interval from stimulus onset until 125 ms before keypress (in this interval identity matching and updating/replacement is required). For I_r we used the time interval from 125 ms after keypress until the next stimulus appeared (in this interval mainly storage is required).

In the reading-span task, a list of sentences was presented for verification (e.g., oranges are blue). After each sentence, subjects could react by pressing "yes" or "no" anytime. After keypress a fixation cross was presented for 500 ms before a letter (that had to be remembered for later recollection) was presented for 1000 ms. For I_a we used the time interval in which the letter was presented (in this interval a shifting between the semantic processing task and an updating of the set of letters to be remembered is required). For I_r we used the time interval from 125 ms after keypress (sentence verification) until the next letter to remember appears (in this interval mainly storage is required).

In both learning tasks, a series of word problems was presented to subjects. First, subjects read a page with facts as long as they wanted. After keypress a problem statement appeared that had to be solved. Subjects could react by pressing a next-button anytime and could then select one out of four multiple-choice options to provide their solution. Subsequently, a fixation cross was presented for 500 ms. For I_a we used the time interval from the onset of the problem statement until 125 ms before keypress for selecting the problem solution (in this interval the necessary facts had to be remembered and inferences had to be drawn for problem solution). For I_r we used the time interval from 125 ms after keypress (i.e., after providing the problem solution) until the next page of facts appeared (in this interval no cognitive processing was required).

DATA ANALYSIS AND RESULTS

Concerning the feature selection, we focused on frontal and parietal electrodes with regard to the spectral power within the theta (4–7 Hz) and alpha (8–13 Hz) frequency band (see Section Promises and drawbacks of EEG-based measurement of WML during learning: The issue of perceptual-motor confounds and Study 1: Realistic instructional materials imposing different levels of WML: Do single-subject single-trial EEG data allow for a classification of these levels?). For spectral analysis, an autoregressive model was calculated with the Burg-Algorithm. The %ERD /ERS values for the 10 postulated frequencies (4, 5, 6, 7, 8, 9, 10, 11, 12, and 13 Hz) were calculated with regard to 10 electrodes (F3, Fz, F4, FC1, FC2, CP1, CP2, P3, Pz, P4) resulting in 10 features for each of the 10 electrodes. For the sake of consistency, these features were used across all subjects and tasks.

Cognitive-load ratings were obtained after each block of working-memory tasks and after each learning task by means of a 7-point Likert scale. These ratings were used for defining task classes (according to subjective levels of WML, see Lesson 3) and for adjusting the complexity levels of the different tasks (see Lesson 5). Since the tasks (n-back task, reading-span task, and subsequent learning tasks used for classifier testing) differed substantially with regard to the subjective level of WML they induced for each of their three difficulty levels, a calibration procedure was applied (see Lesson 5). We selected two out of the three difficulty levels for each task based on subjects' error rates and cognitive-load ratings. For instance, we removed the first level of task difficulty of the subtraction problems from the analysis because it turned out that these tasks were much simpler than the other tasks. The procedure of selecting two out of three difficulty levels for analysis allows us to calibrate difficulty levels across different tasks. For the remaining differences in the difficulty levels across the four tasks, the scaling method of the EEG power values was improved by scaling the data over trials and by adjusting the range of the diverse datasets: First, our training data were z-score normalized resulting in a centered, scaled version of the input-data. Subsequently, we calculated the means and standard deviations of the power values of the training-set. Finally, the testing data were normalized with regard to these means and standard deviations calculated from the training data.

In order to define classes for the training and testing of classifier we analyzed the relation between the objective complexity levels of the four tasks and the subjective cognitive-load ratings. In line with our expectations (see Lesson 1) and with instructional theory (see Section Cognitive workload and adaptive instruction: A challenge for instructional design), it turned out that due to learning the levels of subjectively experienced cognitive load decreased over time within each level of objective task difficulty. As a consequence, we used subjective cognitive-load ratings for defining classes. For this purpose, we calculated the mean value of the subjectively experienced WML for all working-memory tasks solved by a subject as a personal cut-off point to define two classes (low vs. high level of WML according to cognitive-load ratings) for all four tasks (i.e., we defined the two classes for both types of word problems according to the same subjective cut-off point). Using this procedure requires to adjust the objective complexity levels of the tasks for classifier training and testing according to the calibration procedure described in the last paragraph to ensure that the number of trials in both classes is sufficiently balanced for each individual task (i.e., it is necessary to select appropriate complexity levels of all tasks so that all tasks have a similar range of WML as measured by the subjective cognitive-load ratings).

For cross-task classification, we used a SVM with RBF-Kernel that was trained on the combination of the two working-memory tasks and applied to the two realistic learning tasks. As a result, the two levels of WML of the learning tasks could be successfully classified on a single-subject single-trial basis. On average a classification accuracy of 73% could be achieved for the 16 subjects. The classification results were significant for 22 out of the 32 classifications conducted (for each of the 16 subjects two classifications were conducted for the two learning tasks). It has to be noted, though, that these results are based on classification decisions after each trial of the learning tasks. Taking the results of Brouwer et al. (2012) into account, much higher accuracies could be expected when classification decisions would be based on more than one trial of a task.

In conclusion, the methodological strategies that we used to implement the lessons learned so far yielded quite promising results. Our decisions with regard to how to design and analyze Study 2 allowed for a successful cross-task classification of WML when solving complex learning tasks. Thus, the most important precondition for the goal of developing workload-adaptive instructional environments based on passive BCIs, namely the availability of a continuous and non-intrusive assessment of WML during solving realistic learning tasks, seems to be satisfied.

DISCUSSION

In this paper, we discussed and applied several lessons learned on how to implement passive BCI methods to assess WML during learning. A study based on these lessons (Study 2) yielded very promising results for a cross-task classification of WML when solving complex learning tasks (see Section Study 2: Cross-task classification of basic working-memory tasks and realistic instructional tasks). In the remainder of this paper we will discuss the prospects for further improving cross-task classification results and for applying our methods outside the lab in realistic environments, for instance by expanding the feature space used for workload assessment in real-world studies.

FUTURE PROSPECTS FOR IMPROVING CROSS-TASK CLASSIFICATION RESULTS

To improve cross-task classification accuracies even further, a couple of additional methods could be applied to the tasks we used in our studies. One issue that might be addressed by these methods is the fact that, due to learners' knowledge gains over time, the learning tasks needed to be presented in a fixed simple to complex order, which results in a confound of presentation time and objective levels of task complexity. Due to non-stationarities in EEG signals over time, a classifier might pick up slow drifts in the feature space as useful information about task complexity due to the correlation of both factors. Although we tried to diminish this effect by analyzing %ERS/ERD ratios, in future studies, additional methods for covariate shift adaptation might help to further alleviate these drifts and to improve classification accuracies (Satti et al., 2010; Spüler et al., 2012b). Another approach would be to present all tasks in a randomized order of difficulty levels to evaluate the influence of non-stationarities on the cross-task classification results. It should be clear from Lesson 1, however, that this manipulation is not very plausible as a modeling of a realistic learning situation (which is our target scenario) but should only be used to clarify the role of non-stationarities for methodological reasons.

Another interesting option that arises from the task design of Study 2 is to explicitly include very high levels of WML in the analysis that intentionally result in a "cognitive overload." Chanel et al. (2008) found that an excessive increase in WML might lead to disengagement that is detectable by a reversed EEG pattern (i.e., theta-desynchronization and alpha-synchronization), which corresponds to the neural signature of low WML. In our own study we found that absolute difficulty levels varied substantially across different types of tasks. We used the calibration procedure described above to remove difficulty levels, which turned out to be too easy (e.g., arithmetic level 1) or too difficult (e.g., algebra level 3) for learners in terms of error rates and subjective ratings of cognitive load. Interestingly, however, exploratory analyses of these excluded conditions indeed revealed in line with Chanel et al. (2008) the similarity of the neural signatures of conditions with very low levels of WML and very high levels of WML (in the sense of cognitive overload), thereby potentially indicating task disengagement (Walter et al., 2013b). This pattern might be exploited in future studies to better define a zone of optimal workload during learning (high but not too high) and to assess this zone by applying passive BCI methods. Cross-task classification might benefit from this approach because tasks that induce cognitive overload will be better excluded from the high WML class.

ASSESSING WORKLOAD OUTSIDE THE LAB IN REAL-WORLD ENVIRONMENTS

Although we applied our approach of assessing different levels of WML to realistic instructional materials (algebra word problems), the laboratory tasks used for data collection were nevertheless highly controlled with regard to temporal parameters and perceptual-motor confounds. However, if we consider our target scenario of applying passive BCIs in realistic learning scenarios the question remains, whether the methods we developed can be applied successfully outside the lab in real-world environments, where several parameters are expected to differ from the lab. Of course, it is highly interesting in the first step to evoke WML by using well-controlled laboratory tasks as laboratory tasks and designs allow for high control over most of the relevant factors and provide a clear structure that can be aligned to cognitive theories of WML. On the other hand, using well-controlled laboratory tasks moves the whole study further away from realistic settings. It is likely, that the brain works differently in real world scenarios, where tasks appear to be more relevant for the person involved. McDowell et al. (2013) discuss this hypothesis postulating that the activity of the brain increases with the relevance of the tasks it is involved in. Hence, it is of great importance that theoretical and methodological approaches developed in laboratory studies are validated in real world environments. Fortunately, first steps into this direction (e.g., Zander et al., submitted) provide evidence that today's state of the art theories explain at least partially what brain activity is related to realistic workload in real-world environments.

One of the most important issues with regard to real-world studies will be the occurrence of perceptual-motor confounds that have been extensively discussed in this paper. In realistic environments we would clearly expect workload-related behavioral activity, such as specific changes in the pattern of behavior. Due to volume conduction such behavioral activity will be added to the EEG signal through muscularly, ocularly, or translatorly induced effects. Generally, these changes in the potential recorded at EEG electrodes will be bigger in amplitude than those resulting from cortical activity. Hence, it is likely that BCI classifiers might strongly rely on this behavioral information. Thus, in uncontrolled realistic application scenarios it might be quite unclear whether a single-trial detection system used for classification is based on brain activity or on perceptual-motor confounds. This mirrors the methodological problems of many of the studies discussed in this paper.

As a consequence, it is important to better investigate, which signals a BCI classifier picks up when moving out of the controlled laboratory environments. As the EEG is a complex mixture of different signals, complex methodologies have to be applied to identify sources contributing to it. Recent research revealed that methods like ICA (Makeig et al., 1996) are powerful tools for solving this problem. Independent sources of signals can be identified by their temporal, spectral, and spatial properties. From this information the type of process might be inferred that underlies a specific aspect of the overall signal. For instance, data resulting from artifacts might be better discriminated from cortical activity, and cortical activity might be divided into different processes that can be related to specific cognitive and affective states. ICA can even be used to reveal the connectivity of different cortical structures. Such network activity likely carries relevant information about workload, which is not only based on the activation of specific brain areas but also on the information transfer between different areas (e.g., the fronto-parietal networks implementing controlled attention). Different statistical approaches might be utilized in the future to investigate network activity in the EEG. A description of an open-source toolbox including the most commonly used methods can be found in Mullen et al. (2010).

To conclude, we consider passive BCIs to be powerful tools for improving adaptive learning environments in the future, provided that they are properly validated, first, by combining controlled experimental studies and complex real-world studies and, second, by investigating independent components, network activities and classification properties. Moreover, our passive BCI approach might also be transferred to many other aspects of Human-Computer Interaction, using cognitive state monitoring for introducing fundamentally new types of input, like implicit interaction (see Zander et al., 2014).

ACKNOWLEDGMENTS

This research was funded by the Leibniz ScienceCampus Tübingen "Informational Environments." Carina Walter was a doctoral student of the LEAD Graduate School [GSC1028], funded by the Excellence Initiative of the German federal and state governments.

REFERENCES

Alloway, T., and Alloway, R. G. (2010). Investigating the predictive roles of working memory and IQ in academic attainment. *J. Exp. Child Psychol.* 106, 20–29. doi: 10.1016/j.jecp.2009.11.003

Antonenko, P. D., and Niederhauser, D. S. (2010). The influence of leads on cognitive load and learning in a hypertext environment. *Comput. Human Behav.* 38, 1–38. doi: 10.1016/j.chb.2009.10.014

Antonenko, P., Paas, F., Grabner, R., and Gog, T. (2010). Using electroencephalography to measure cognitive load. *Educ. Psychol. Rev.* 22, 425–438. doi: 10.1007/s10648-010-9130-y

Baddeley, A. (1986). *Working Memory.* Oxford: Clarendon Press.

Baddeley, A. (2000). The episodic buffer: a new component of working memory? *Trends Cogn. Sci.* 4, 417–423. doi: 10.1016/S1364-6613(00)01538-2

Baddeley, A. (2012). Working memory: theories, models, and controversies. *Annu. Rev. Psychol.* 63, 1–29. doi: 10.1146/annurev-psych-120710-100422

Baldwin, C. J., and Penaranda, B. N. (2012). Adaptive training using an artificial neural network and EEG metrics for within- and cross-task workload classification. *Neuroimage* 59, 48–56. doi: 10.1016/j.neuroimage.2011.07.047

Barrouillet, P., Bernardin, S., and Camos, V. (2004). Time constraints and resource sharing in adults' working memory spans. *J. Exp. Psychol. Gen.* 133, 83–100. doi: 10.1037/0096-3445.133.1.83

Berka, C., Levendowski, D., and Cvetinovic, M. (2004). Real-time analysis of EEG indexes of alertness, cognition and memory acquired with a wireless EEG headset. *Int. J. Hum. Comp. Interact.* 17, 151–170. doi: 10.1207/s15327590ijhc1702_3

Besserve, M., Jerbi, K., Laurent, F., Baillet, S., Martinerie, J., and Garnero, L. (2007). Classification methods for ongoing EEG and MEG signals. *Biol. Res.* 40, 415–437. doi: 10.4067/S0716-97602007000500005

Blankertz, B., Curio, G., and Müller, K. R. (2002). "Classifying single trial EEG: towards brain computer interfacing," in *Advances in Neural Information Processing Systems (NIPS 01) 14* (Vancouver), 157–164.

Bor, D., Cumming, N., Scott, C. E. M., and Owen, A. M. (2004). Prefrontal cortical involvement in encoding strategies, independent of stimulus modality. *Eur. J. Neurosci.* 19, 3365–3370. doi: 10.1111/j.1460-9568.2004.03438.x

Brouwer, A. M., Hogervorst, M. A., van Erp, J. B. F., Heffelaar, T., Zimmerman, P. H., and Oostenveld, R. (2012). Estimating workload using EEG spectral power and ERPs in the n-back task. *J. Neural Eng.* 9, 1–14. doi: 10.1088/1741-2560/9/4/045008

Brugger, D., Rosenstiel, W., and Bogdan, M. (2008). Automatic cluster detection in Kohonen's SOM. *IEEE Trans. Neural Netw.* 19, 442–459. doi: 10.1109/TNN.2007.909556

Brünken, R., Plass, J. L., and Leutner, D. (2003). Direct measurement of cognitive load in multimedia learning. *Educ. Psychol.* 38, 53–61. doi: 10.1207/S15326985EP3801_7

Callicott, J. H., Mattay, V. S., Bertolino, A., Finn, K., Coppola, R., Frank, J. A., et al. (1999). Physiological characteristics of capacity constraints in working memory as revealed by functional MRI. *Cereb. Cortex* 9, 20–26. doi: 10.1093/cercor/9.1.20

Calvo, R., and D'Mello, S. (2010). Affect detection: an interdisciplinary review of models, methods, and their applications. *IEEE Trans. Affect. Comput.* 1, 18–37. doi: 10.1109/T-AFFC.2010.1

Chanel, G., Rebetez, C., Bétrancourt, M., and Pun, T. (2008). "Boredom, engagement and anxiety as indicators for adaptation to difficulty in games," in *Proceedings of the 12th International Conference on Entertainment and Media in Ubiquitous Era - MindTrek '08* (Tampere), 13–17. doi: 10.1145/1457199.1457203

Chaouachi, M., Jraidi, I., and Frasson, C. (2011). "Modeling mental workload using EEG features for intelligent systems," in *Proceedings of UMAP* 2011 (Girona), 50–61. doi: 10.1007/978-3-642-22362-4_5

Chapman, R. M., Nowlis, G. H., McCrary, J. W., Chapman, J. A., Sandoval, T. C., Guillily, M. D., et al. (2007). Brain event-related potentials: diagnosing early-stage Alzheimer's disease. *Neurobiol. Aging* 28, 194–201. doi: 10.1016/j.neurobiolaging.2005.12.008

Cierniak, G., Scheiter, K., and Gerjets, P. (2009a). "Expertise reversal in multimedia learning: subjective load ratings and viewing behavior as cognitive process indicators," in *Proceedings of the 31st Annual Conference of the Cognitive Science Society,* eds N. A. Taatgen and H. van Rijn (Austin, TX: Cognitive Science Society), 1906–1911.

Cierniak, G., Scheiter, K., and Gerjets, P. (2009b). Explaining the split-attention effect: is the reduction of extraneous cognitive load accompanied by an increase in germane cognitive load? *Comput. Human Behav.* 25, 315–324. doi: 10.1016/j.chb.2008.12.020

Corbett, A. (2001). "Cognitive computer tutors: solving the two-sigma problem," in *Proceedings of the Eighth International Conference on User Modeling*, ed M. G. Bauer (Berlin: Springer), 137–147.

Corbin, L., and Marquer, J. (2013). Is Sternberg's memory scanning task really a short-term memory task? *Swiss J. Psychol.* 72, 181–196. doi: 10.1024/1421-0185/a000112

Cowan, N. (2005). *Working-Memory-Capacity.* Hove: Psychology Press. doi: 10.4324/9780203342398

Cowan, N. (2014). Working memory underpins cognitive development, learning, and education. *Educ. Psychol. Rev.* 26, 197–223. doi: 10.1007/s10648-013-9246-y

Curtis, C. E., and D'Esposito, M. (2003). Persistent activity in the prefrontal cortex during workload. *Trends Cogn. Sci.* 7, 415–423. doi: 10.1016/S1364-6613(03)00197-9

Daneman, M., and Carpenter, P. A. (1980). Individual differences in working memory and reading. *J. Verb. Learn. Verb. Behav.* 19, 450–466. doi: 10.1016/S0022-5371(80)90312-6

De Jong, T. (2010). Cognitive load theory, educational research, and instructional design: some food for thought. *Instr. Sci.* 38, 105–134. doi: 10.1007/s11251-009-9110-0

DeLeeuw, K. E., and Mayer, R. E. (2008). A comparison of three measures of cognitive load: evidence for separable measures of intrinsic, extraneous, and germane load. *J. Educ. Psychol.* 100, 223–234. doi: 10.1037/0022-0663.100.1.223

De Negueruela, C., Broschart, M., Menon, C., and Millán, J. D. (2011). Brain-computer interfaces for space applications. *Pers. Ubiquitous Comput.* 15, 527–537. doi: 10.1007/s00779-010-0322-8

Dobbins, I. G., Foley, H., Schacter, D. L., and Wagner, A. D. (2002). Executive control during episodic retrieval: multiple prefrontal processes subserve source memory. *Neuron* 35, 989–996. doi: 10.1016/S0896-6273(02)00858-9

Dyson, M., Sepulveda, F., and Gan, J. Q. (2010). Localisation of cognitive tasks used in EEG-based BCIs. *Clin. Neurophysiol.* 121, 1481–1493. doi: 10.1016/j.clinph.2010.03.011

Engle, R. (2002). Working memory capacity as executive attention. *Curr. Dir. Psychol. Sci.* 11, 19–23. doi: 10.1111/1467-8721.00160

Engle, R. W., and Kane, M. J. (2004). "Executive attention, working memory capacity, and a two-factor theory of cognitive control," in *The Psychology of Learning and Motivation*, ed H. Ross (New York, NY: Elsevier), 145–199.

Falkenstein, M., Hohnsbein, J., Hoormann, J. B., and Blanke, L. (1991). Effects of crossmodal divided attention on late ERP components. II. Error processing in choice reaction tasks. *Electroencephalogr. Clin. Neurophysiol.* 78, 447–455. doi: 10.1016/0013-4694(91)90062-9

Gerjets, P., and Hesse, F. W. (2004). When are powerful learning environments effective? The role of learning activities and of students' conceptions of educational technology. *Int. J. Educ. Res.* 41, 445–465. doi: 10.1016/j.ijer.2005.08.011

Gerjets, P., and Scheiter, K. (2003). Goal configurations and processing strategies as moderators between instructional design and cognitive load: evidence from hypertext-based instruction. *Educ. Psychol.* 38, 33–41. doi: 10.1207/S15326985EP3801_5

Gerjets, P., Scheiter, K., and Cierniak, G. (2009). The scientific value of cognitive load theory: a research agenda based on the structuralist view of theories. *Educ. Psychol. Rev.* 21, 43–54. doi: 10.1007/s10648-008-9096-1

Gerlic, I., and Jausovec, N. (1999). Multimedia: differences in cognitive processes observed with EEG. *J. Tech. Res. Dev.* 47, 5–14. doi: 10.1007/BF02299630

Gevins, A., and Smith, M. (2003). Neurophysiological measures of cognitive workload during human-computer interaction. *Theor. Issues Ergon. Sci.* 4, 113–131. doi: 10.1080/14639220210159717

Gevins, A., Smith, M. E., Leong, H., McEvoy, L., Whitfield, S., Du, R., et al. (1998). Monitoring working memory load during computer-based tasks with EEG pattern recognition methods. *Hum. Factors* 40, 79–91. doi: 10.1518/001872098779480578

Gevins, A., Smith, M. E., McEvoy, C. L., and Yu, D. (1997). High-resolution EEG mapping of cortical activation related to working memory: effects of task difficulty, type of processing, and practice. *Cereb. Cortex* 7, 374–385. doi: 10.1093/cercor/7.4.374

Goldman-Rakic, P. S. (1994). Working memory dysfunction in schizophrenia. *J. Neuropsychiatr. Clin. Neurosci.* 6, 348–357.

Grabner, R., and De Smedt, B. (2011). Neurophysiological evidence for the validity of verbal strategy reports in mental arithmetic. *Biol. Psychol.* 87, 128–136. doi: 10.1016/j.biopsycho.2011.02.019

Graesser, A. C., and McNamara, D. S. (2010). Self-regulated learning in learning environments with pedagogical agents that interact in natural language. *Educ. Psychol.* 45, 234–244. doi: 10.1080/00461520.2010.515933

Hanslmayr, S., Pastoetter, B., Baeuml, K.-H., Gruber, S., Wimber, M., and Klimesch, W. (2008). The electrophysiological dynamics of interference during the Stroop task. *J. Cogn. Neurosci.* 20, 215–225. doi: 10.1162/jocn.2008.20020

Hart, S. G., and Staveland, L. E. (1988). "Development of NASA-TLX (Task Load Index): results of empirical and theoretical research," in *Human Mental Workload*, eds P. A. Hancock and N. Meshkati (Amsterdam: North Holland Press), 139–183.

Heger, D., Putze, F., and Schultz, T. (2010). "Online workload recognition from EEG data during cognitive tests and human-machine interaction," in *Lecture Notes in Artificial Intelligence:* Vol. 6359. *KI 2010: Advances in Artificial Intelligence*, eds T. Dillmann, J. Beyerer, U. Hanebeck, and T. Schultz (Heidelberg: Springer), 410–417.

Henson, R. N., Shallice, T., and Dolan, R. J. (1999). Right prefrontal cortex and episodic memory retrieval: a functional MRI test of the monitoring hypothesis. *Brain* 122, 1367–1381. doi: 10.1093/brain/122.7.1367

Hoard, M. K., Geary, D. C., Byrd-Craven, J., and Nugent, L. (2008). Mathematical cognition in intellectually precocious first graders. *Dev. Neuropsychol.* 33, 251–276. doi: 10.1080/87565640801982338

Honey, G. D., Fu, C. H., Kim, J., Brammer, M. J., Croudace, T. J., Suckling, J., et al. (2002). Effects of verbal working memory load on corticocortical connectivity modeled by path analysis of functional magnetic resonance imaging data. *Neuroimage* 17, 573–582. doi: 10.1006/nimg.2002.1193

Jatzev, S., Zander, T. O., Filippis, M. D., Kothe, C., Welke, S., and Rötting, M. (2008). "Examining causes for nonstationarities: the loss of controllability is a factor which induces nonstationarities," in *Proceedings of the 4th International BCI Workshop & Training Course* (Graz: Verlag der Technischen Universität Graz), 138–143.

Jensen, O., and Tesche, C. D. (2002). Frontal theta activity in humans increases with memory load in a working memory task. *Eur. J. Neurosci.* 15, 1395–1399. doi: 10.1046/j.1460-9568.2002.01975.x

Kalyuga, S., Ayres, P., Chandler, P., and Sweller, J. (2003). The expertise reversal effect. *Educ. Psychol.* 38, 23–31. doi: 10.1207/S15326985EP3801_4

Kane, M. J., Conway, A. R., Miura, T. K., and Colflesh, G. J. (2007). Working memory, attention control, and the n-back task: a question of construct validity. *J. Exp. Psychol. Learn. Mem. Cogn.* 33, 615–622. doi: 10.1037/0278-7393.33.3.615

Kiss, I., Watter, S., Heisz, J. J., and Shedden, J. M. (2007). Control processes in verbal working memory: an event-related potential study. *Brain Res.* 1172, 67–81. doi: 10.1016/j.brainres.2007.06.083

Klimesch, W. (1999). EEG alpha and theta oscillations reflect cognitive and memory performance: a review and analysis. *Brain Res. Rev.* 29, 69–195. doi: 10.1016/S0165-0173(98)00056-3

Klingberg, T. (2009). *The overflowing brain.* New York, NY: Oxford University Press.

Knops, A., Nuerk, H.-C., Fimm, B., Vohn, R., and Willmes, K. (2006). A special role for numbers in working memory? An fMRI study. *Neuroimage* 29, 1–14. doi: 10.1016/j.neuroimage.2005.07.009

Krause, C. M., Pesonen, M., and Haemaelaeinen, H. (2010). Brain oscillatory 4-30 Hz electroencephalogram responses in adolescents during a visual memory task. *Neuroreport* 21, 767–771. doi: 10.1097/WNR.0b013e32833bfcbb

Lal, T., Hinterberger, T., Widman, G., Schröder, M., Hill, J., Rosenstiel, W., et al. (2004). "Methods towards invasive human brain computer interfaces. Advances in neural information processing systems," in *Proceedings NIPS 17* (Vancouver), 737–744.

Lin, C.-T., Wu, R.-C., Liang, S.-F., Chao, W.-H., and Jung, T.-P. (2005). EEG-based drowsiness estimation for safety driving using independent component analysis. *IEEE Trans. Circuits Syst. I Reg. Papers* 52, 2726–2738. doi: 10.1109/TCSI.2005.857555

Lotte, F., Congedo, M., Lécuyer, A., Lamarche, F., and Arnaldi, B. (2007). A review of classification algorithms for EEG-based brain-computer interfaces. *J. Neural Eng.* 4, R1. doi: 10.1088/1741-2560/4/2/R01

Makeig, S., Bell, A., Jung, T., and Sejnowski, T. (1996). Independent component analysis of electroencephalographic data. *Adv. Neural Inf. Process. Syst.* 8, 145–151.

Mayer, R. E. (2009). *Multimedia Learning 2nd Edn.* New York, NY: Cambridge University Press. doi: 10.1017/CBO9780511811678

McDowell, K., Chin-Teng, L., Oie, K. S., Tzyy-Ping, J., Gordon, S., Whitaker, K. W., et al. (2013). Real-world neuroimaging technologies. *Access IEEE* 1, 131–149. doi: 10.1109/ACCESS.2013.2260791

Mihalca, L., Salden, R. J. C. M., Corbalan, G., Paas, F., and Miclea, M. (2011). Effectiveness of cognitive-load based adaptive instruction in genetics education. *Comput. Human Behav.* 27, 82–88. doi: 10.1016/j.chb.2010.05.027

Missonnier, P., Deiber, M., Gold, G., Millet, P., Gex-Fabry, P. M., Fazio-Costa, L., et al. (2006). Frontal theta event-related synchronization: comparison of directed attention and working memory load effects. *J. Neural Transm.* 113, 1477–1486. doi: 10.1007/s00702-005-0443-9

Miyake, A., Friedman, N. P., Emerson, M. J., Witzki, A. H., and Howerter, A. (2000). The unity and diversity of executive functions and their contributions to complex 'frontal lobe' tasks: a latent variable analysis. *Cogn. Psychol.* 41, 49–100. doi: 10.1006/cogp.1999.0734

Mullen, T., Delorme, A., Kothe, C., and Makeig, S. (2010). An electrophysiological information flow toolbox for EEGLAB. *Biol. Cybern.* 83, 35–45.

Nee, D. E., Brown, J. W., Askren, M. K., Berman, M. G., Demiralp, E., Krawitz, A., et al. (2012). A meta-analysis of executive components of working memory. *Cereb. Cortex* 23, 264–282. doi: 10.1093/cercor/bhs007

Nigbur, R., Ivanova, G., and Stürmer, B. (2011). Theta power as a marker for cognitive interference. *Clin. Neurophysiol.* 122, 2185–2194. doi: 10.1016/j.clinph.2011.03.030

Norman, D. A., and Shallice, T. (1986). "Attention to action: willed and automatic control of behavior," in *Consciousness and Self-Regulation:* Vol. 4. *Advances in Research and Theory,* eds R. Davidson, G. E. Schwartz, and D. Shapiro (New York, NY: Plenum Press), 2–18.

Oberauer, K. (2009). Design for a working memory. *Psychol. Learn. Motiv.* 51, 45–100. doi: 10.1016/S0079-7421(09)51002-X

Owen, A. M. (1997). The functional organization of working memory processes within human lateral frontal cortex: the contribution of functional neuroimaging. *Eur. J. Neurosci.* 9, 1329–1339. doi: 10.1111/j.1460-9568.1997.tb01487.x

Owen, A. M., McMillan, K. M., Laird, A. R., and Bullmore, E. (2005). N-back working memory paradigm: a meta-analysis of normative functional neuroimaging studies. *Hum. Brain Mapp.* 25, 46–59. doi: 10.1002/hbm.20131

Paas, F., Tuovinen, J. E., Tabbers, H., and Van Gerven, P. (2003). Cognitive load measurement as a means to advance cognitive load theory. *Educ. Psychol.* 38, 63–71. doi: 10.1207/S15326985EP3801_8

Petrides, M. (1994). Frontal lobes and behaviour. *Curr. Opin. Neurobiol.* 4, 207–211. doi: 10.1016/0959-4388(94)90074-4

Pfurtscheller, G., Flotzinger, D., and Kalcher, J. (1993). Brain-computer interface: a new communication device for handicapped persons. *J. Microcomput. Appl.* 16, 293–299. doi: 10.1006/jmca.1993.1030

Pfurtscheller, G., and Lopes da Silva, F. H. (2005). "Event-related desynchronization (ERD) and event-related synchronization (ERS)," in *Electroencephalography: Basic Principles, Clinical Applications and Related Field,* eds E. Niedermeyer and F. H. Lopes da Silva (Philadelphia, PA: Lippincott, Williams and Wilkins), 1003–1016.

Protzak, J., Ihme, K., and Zander, T. O. (2013). "A passive brain-computer interface for supporting gaze-based human-machine interaction," in *Universal Access in Human-Computer Interaction. Design Methods, Tools, and Interaction Techniques for eInclusion*, eds C. Stephanidis and M. Antona (Berlin: Springer), 662–671.

Ramsey, N. F., van de Heuvel, M. P., Kho, K. H., and Leijten, F. S. (2006). Towards human BCI applications based on cognitive brain systems: an investigation of neural signals recorded from the dorsolateral prefrontal cortex. *IEEE Trans. Neural Syst. Rehabil. Eng.* 14, 214–217. doi: 10.1109/TNSRE.2006.875582

Redick, T. S., and Lindsey, D. R. (2013). Complex span and n-back measures of working memory: a meta-analysis. *Psychon. Bull. Rev.* 20, 1102–1113. doi: 10.3758/s13423-013-0453-9

Reigeluth, C. M., and Stein, F. S. (1983). "The elaboration theory of instruction," in *Instructional-Design Theories and Models: An Overview of their Current Status,* ed C. M. Reigeluth (Hillsdale, NJ: Erlbaum Associates), 335–381.

Reissland, J., and Zander, T. O. (2010). "Automated detection of bluffing in a game - revealing a complex covert user state with a passive BCI," in *Human Factors: A System View of Human, Technology and Organisation*, eds D. de Waard, A. Axelsson, M. Berglund, B. Peters, and C. Weikert (Maastricht, NL: Shaker Publishing), 435–443.

Salomon, G. (1984). Television is "easy" and print is "tough": the differential investment of mental effort in learning as a function of perception and attribution. *J. Educ. Psychol.* 76, 647–658. doi: 10.1037/0022-0663.76.4.647

Satti, A., Guan, C., Coyle, D., and Prasad, G. (2010). "A covariate shift minimisation method to alleviate non-stationarity effects for an adaptive brain-computer interface," in *Proceedings of the 20th International Conference on Pattern Recognition (ICPR),* ed J. E. Guerrero (Los Alamitos, CA: IEEE Computer Society), 105–108.

Sauseng, P., Griesmayr, B., Freunberger, R., and Klimesch, W. (2010). Control mechanisms in working memory: a possible function of EEG theta oscillations. *Neurosci. Biobehav. Rev.* 34, 1015–1022. doi: 10.1016/j.neubiorev.2009.12.006

Schalk, G., McFarland, D. J., Hinterberger, T., Birbaumer, N., and Wolpaw, J. R. (2004). BCI2000: a general-purpose brain-computer interface (BCI) system. *IEEE Trans. Biomed. Eng.* 51, 1034–1043. doi: 10.1109/TBME.2004.827072

Scheiter, K., Gerjets, P., and Schuh, J. (2010). The acquisition of problem-solving skills in mathematics: how animations can aid understanding of structural problem features and solution procedures. *Instr. Sci.* 38, 487–502. doi: 10.1007/s11251-009-9114-9

Schlögl, A., Keinrath, C., Zimmermann, D., Scherer, R., Leeb, R., and Pfurtscheller, G. (2007). A fully automated correction method of EOG artifacts in EEG recordings. *Clin. Neurophysiol.* 118, 98–104. doi: 10.1016/j.clinph.2006.09.003

Schnotz, W., Horz, H., McElvany, N., Schroeder, S., Ullrich, M., Baumert, J., et al. (2010). "Das BITE-Projekt: Integrative Verarbeitung von Bildern und Texten in der Sekundarstufe I," in *Kompetenzmodellierung: Zwischenbilanz des DFG-Schwerpunktprogramms und Perspektiven des Forschungsansatzes (Zeitschrift für Pädagogik: Beiheft No. 56),* eds E. Klieme, D. Leutner, and M. Kenk (Weinheim: Beltz), 143–153.

Schölkopf, B., and Smola, A. (2002). *Learning with Kernels: Support Vector Machines, Regularization, Optimization and Beyond.* Cambridge, MA: MIT Press.

Schüler, A., Scheiter, K., and van Genuchten, E. (2011). The role of working memory in multimedia instruction: is working memory working during learning from text and pictures? *Educ. Psychol. Rev.* 23, 389–411. doi: 10.1007/s10648-011-9168-5

Schwonke, R., Wittwer, J., Aleven, V., Salden, R., Krieg, C., and Renkl, A. (2007). "Can tutored problem solving benefit from faded worked-out examples?" in *Proceedings of the 2nd European Cognitive Science Conference*, eds S. Vosniadou, D. Kayser, and A. Protopapas (New York, NY: Erlbaum), 59–64.

Smith, E. E., and Jonides, J. (1999). Storage and executive processes in the frontal lobes. *Science* 283, 1657–1661. doi: 10.1126/science.283.5408.1657

Sörqvist, P., and Sætrevik, B. (2010). The neural basis of updating: distinguishing substitution processes from other concurrent processes. *Scand. J. Psychol.* 51, 357–362. doi: 10.1111/j.1467-9450.2010.00817.x

Spüler, M., Bensch, M., Kleih, S., Rosenstiel, W., Bogdan, M., and Kübler, A. (2012a). Online use of error-related potentials in healthy users and people with severe motor impairment increases performance of a P300-BCI. *Clin. Neurophysiol.* 123, 1328–1337. doi: 10.1016/j.clinph.2011.11.082

Spüler, M., Rosenstiel, W., and Bogdan, M. (2012b). Principal component based covariate shift adaption to reduce non-stationarity in a MEG-based brain-computer interface. *EURASIP J. Adv. Signal Process.* 2012:129. doi: 10.1186/1687-6180-2012-129

Stipacek, A., Grabner, R. H., Neuper, C., Fink, A., and Neubauer, A. C. (2003). Sensitivity of human EEG alpha band desynchronization to different working memory components and increasing levels of memory load. *Neurosci. Lett.* 353, 193–196. doi: 10.1016/j.neulet.2003.09.044

Sweller, J., van Merriënboer, J. J., and Paas, F. F. (1998). Cognitive architecture and instructional design. *Educ. Psychol. Rev.* 10, 251–296. doi: 10.1023/A:1022193728205

Sylvester, C. Y., Wager, T. D., Lacey, S. C., Hernandez, L., Nichols, T. E., Smith, E. E., et al. (2003). Switching attention and resolving interference: fMRI measures of executive functions. *Neuropsychologia* 41, 357–370. doi: 10.1016/S0028-3932(02)00167-7

Tonin, L., Leeb, R., Tavella, M., Perdikis, S., and del Millan, J. R. (2010). "The role of shared-control in BCI-based telepresence," in *Proceedings of the 2010 IEEE International Conference on Systems Man and Cybernetics (SMC)*, ed O. Kaynak (Red Hook, NY: Curran Associates), 1462–1466.

Unsworth, N., and Engle, R. W. (2007). The nature of individual differences in working memory capacity: active maintenance in primary memory and controlled search from secondary memory. *Psychol. Rev.* 114, 104–132. doi: 10.1037/0033-295X.114.1.104

Vygotsky, L. (1978). *Mind in Society: the Development of Higher Psychological Processes.* Cambridge, MA: Harvard University Press.

Walter, C., Cierniak, G., Gerjets, P., Rosenstiel, W., and Bogdan, M. (2011). "Classifying mental states with machine learning algorithms using alpha activity decline," in *Proceedings of the 19th European Symposium on Artificial Neuronal Networks,* (Brugge: ESANN), 405–410.

Walter, C., Schmidt, S., Rosenstiel, W., Bogdan, M., and Gerjets, P. (2013b). "Alpha- and theta frequencies as indicators for optimal cognitive load during learning," in *Paper Presented at the 6th International Cognitive Load Theory Conference* (Toulouse).

Walter, C., Schmidt, S., Rosenstiel, W., Gerjets, P., and Bogdan, M. (2013a). "Using cross-task classification for classifying workload levels in complex learning tasks," in *Proceedings of the 5th IEEE Humaine Association Conference on Affective Computing and Intelligent Interaction (ACII 2013)*, eds T. Pun, C. Pelachaud, and N. Sebe (Los Alamitos, CA: IEEE Computer Society), 876–881. doi: 10.1109/ACII.2013.164

Wickens, C. D. (1984). "Processing resources in attention," in *Varieties of Attention,* eds R. Parasuraman and D. R. Davies (New York, NY: Academic Press), 63–102.

Wolpaw, J., Birbaumer, N., McFarland, D., Pfurtscheller, G., and Vaughan, T. (2002). Brain-computer interfaces for communication and control. *Clin. Neurophysiol.* 113, 767–791. doi: 10.1016/S1388-2457(02)00057-3

Wolpaw, J. R., McFarland, D. J., Neat, G. W., and Forneris, C. A. (1991). An EEG-based brain-computer interface for cursor control. *Electroencephalogr. Clin. Neurophysiol.* 78, 252–259. doi: 10.1016/0013-4694(91)90040-B

Zander, T., and Jatzev, S. (2009). "Detecting affective covert user states with passive brain-computer interfaces," in *Proceedings of the 3rd International Conference on Affective Computing and Intelligent Interaction (ACII 2009)*, eds J. Cohn, A. Nijholt, and M. Pantic (Los Alamitos, CA: IEEE Computer Society), 1–9.

Zander, T., Lehne, M., Ihme, K., Jatzev, S., Correia, J., Kothe, C., et al. (2011b). A dry EEG-system for scientific reasearch and brain-computer interfaces. *Front. Neurosci.* 5, 1–10. doi: 10.3389/fnins.2011.00053

Zander, T. O., Brönstrup, J., Lorenz, R., and Krol, L. R. (2014). "Towards BCI-based implicit control in human–computer interaction," in *Advances in Physiological Computing,* eds S. H. Fairclough and K. Gilleade (London: Springer), 67–90. doi: 10.1007/978-1-4471-6392-3_4

Zander, T. O., Gaertner, M., Kothe, C., and Vilimek, R. (2011a). Combining eye gaze input with a brain-computer interface for touchless human-computer interaction. *Int. J. Hum. Comput. Interact.* 27, 38–51. doi: 10.1080/10447318.2011.535752

Zander, T. O., and Jatzev, S. (2012). Context-aware brain-computer interfaces: exploring the information space of user, technical system and environment. *J. Neural Eng.* 9:016003. doi: 10.1088/1741-2560/9/1/016003

Zander, T. O., and Kothe, C. (2011). Towards passive brain-computer interfaces: applying brain-computer interface technology to human-machine systems in general. *J. Neural Eng.* 8:025005. doi: 10.1088/1741-2560/8/2/025005

Zander, T. O., Kothe, C., Jatzev, S., and Gaertner, M. (2010). "Enhancing human computer interaction with input from active and passive brain-computer interfaces," in *Brain-Computer Interfaces: Applying our Minds to Human-Computer Interaction,* eds D. Tan and A. Nijholt (London: Springer), 24–29.

16

Hybrid fNIRS-EEG based classification of auditory and visual perception processes

Felix Putze[1]*, Sebastian Hesslinger[1], Chun-Yu Tse[2,3], YunYing Huang[4], Christian Herff[1], Cuntai Guan[5] and Tanja Schultz[1]

[1] *Cognitive Systems Lab, Institute of Anthropomatics and Robotics, Karlsruhe Institute of Technology, Karlsruhe, Germany*
[2] *Department of Psychology, Center for Cognition and Brain Studies, The Chinese University of Hong Kong, Hong Kong, China*
[3] *Temasek Laboratories, National University of Singapore, Singapore, Singapore*
[4] *Nuffield Department of Clinical Neurosciences, John Radcliffe Hospital, Oxford, UK*
[5] *Institute for Infocomm Research (I2R), A*STAR, Singapore, Singapore*

Correspondence:
Felix Putze, Cognitive Systems Lab, Institute of Anthropomatics and Robotics, Karlsruhe Institute of Technology, Adenauerring 4, Karlsruhe 76131, Germany
e-mail: felix.putze@kit.edu

For multimodal Human-Computer Interaction (HCI), it is very useful to identify the modalities on which the user is currently processing information. This would enable a system to select complementary output modalities to reduce the user's workload. In this paper, we develop a hybrid Brain-Computer Interface (BCI) which uses Electroencephalography (EEG) and functional Near Infrared Spectroscopy (fNIRS) to discriminate and detect visual and auditory stimulus processing. We describe the experimental setup we used for collection of our data corpus with 12 subjects. On this data, we performed cross-validation evaluation, of which we report accuracy for different classification conditions. The results show that the subject-dependent systems achieved a classification accuracy of 97.8% for discriminating visual and auditory perception processes from each other and a classification accuracy of up to 94.8% for detecting modality-specific processes independently of other cognitive activity. The same classification conditions could also be discriminated in a subject-independent fashion with accuracy of up to 94.6 and 86.7%, respectively. We also look at the contributions of the two signal types and show that the fusion of classifiers using different features significantly increases accuracy.

Keywords: brain-computer interface, EEG, fNIRS, visual and auditory perception

1. INTRODUCTION

For the last decade, multimodal user interfaces have become omnipresent in the field of human-computer interaction and in commercially available devices (Turk, 2014). Multimodality refers to the possibility to operate a system using multiple input modalities but also to the ability of a system to present information using different output modalities. For example, a system may present information on a screen using text, images and videos or it may present the same information acoustically by using speech synthesis and sounds. However, such a system has to select an output modality for each given situation. One important aspect it should consider when making this decision is the user's workload level which can negatively influence task performance and user satisfaction, if too high. The output modality of the system which imposes the smaller workload on the user does not only depend on the actions of the system itself, but also on concurrently executed cognitive tasks. Especially in dynamic and mobile application scenarios, users of a system are frequently exposed to external stimuli from other devices, people or their general environment.

According to the multiple resource theory of Wickens (2008), the impact of a dual task on the workload level depends on the type of cognitive resources which are required by both tasks. If the overlap is large, the limited resources have to be shared between both tasks and overall workload will increase compared to a pair of tasks with less overlap, even if the total individual task load is identical. For example, Yang et al. (2012) showed a study in which they combine a primary driving task with additional auditory and visual task of three difficulty levels. They showed that the difference in the performance level of the driving task depends on the modality of the secondary task: According to their results, secondary visual tasks had a stronger impact on the driving than secondary auditory tasks, even if individual workload of the auditory tasks was slightly higher than of the visual tasks. For Human-Computer Interaction (HCI), this implies that when the interaction strategy of the system must must select from different output channels by which it can transfer information to the user, its behavior should take into account the cognitive processes which are already ongoing. It is possible to model the resource demands of cognitive tasks induced by the system itself (see for example Cao et al., 2009). For example, we know that presenting information using speech synthesis requires auditory perceptual resources while presenting information using a graphical display will require visual perceptual resources. However, doing the same for independent parallel tasks is impossible in an open-world scenario where the number of potential distractions is virtually unlimited. Therefore, we have to employ sensors to infer which cognitive resources are occupied.

To some degree, perceptual load can be estimated from context information gathered using sensors like microphones or cameras. However, if, for example, the user wears earmuffs or head phones, acoustic sensors cannot reliably relate acoustic scene events to processes of auditory perception. Therefore, we need a more direct method to estimate those mental states. A Brain-Computer Interface (BCI) is a "system that measures central activity and converts it into artificial output that replaces, restores, enhances supplements, or improves natural central nervous system output" (Wolpaw and Wolpaw, 2012). BCIs can therefore help to detect or discriminate perceptual processes for different modalities directly from measures of brain activity and are therefore strong candidates to reliably discriminate and detect modality-specific perceptual processes. As BCIs have many additional uses for active interface control or for passive user monitoring, they may be already in place for other tasks and would not require any additional equipment.

Our system combines two different signal types [Electroencephalography (EEG) and functional Near Infrared Spectroscopy (fNIRS)] to exploit their complementary nature and to investigate their individual potential for classifying modality-specific perceptual processes: EEG is the traditional signal for BCIs, recording electrical cortical activity using electrodes. fNIRS on the other hand captures the hemodynamic response by exploiting the fact that oxygenated and de-oxygenated blood absorb different proportions of light of different wavelengths in the near-infrared spectrum. fNIRS captures different correlates of brain activity than EEG: While EEG measures an electrical process, fNIRS measures metabolic response to cognitive activity. This fact makes it plausible that a fusion of both signal types can give a more robust estimation of a person's cognitive state.

BCIs based on EEG have been actively researched since the 1970s, for example in computer control for locked-in patients (e.g., Wolpaw et al., 1991; Sitaram et al., 2007). BCIs based on fNIRS have become increasingly popular since the middle of last decade (Sitaram et al., 2007). The term hybrid BCI generally describes a combination of several individual BCI systems (or the combination of a BCI with another interface) (Pfurtscheller et al., 2010). A sequential hybrid BCI employs two BCIs one after another. One application of a sequential BCI is to have the first system act as a "brain switch" to trigger the second system. A sequential hybrid BCI usually resorts to different types of brain activity measured by a single signal type (e.g., correcting mistakes of a P300 speller by detecting error potentials, Spüler et al., 2012). In contrast, a simultaneous hybrid BCI system usually combines entirely different types of brain signals to improve the robustness of the joint system. The first simultaneous hybrid BCI that is based on synchronous measures of fNIRS and EEG was proposed by Fazli et al. (2012) for classification of motor imagery and motor execution recordings. The authors reported an improvement in recognition accuracy by combining both signal types.

Zander and Kothe (2011) defined Passive BCI as follows: "a passive BCI is one that derives its outputs from arbitrary brain activity arising without the purpose of voluntary control, for enriching a humanmachine interaction with implicit information on the actual user state." A number of such systems exist to classify the user's workload level, for example presented by Heger et al. (2010) or Kothe and Makeig (2011). Those systems used different EEG feature extraction techniques that are usually related to the frequency power distribution to classify low and high workload conditions. Other researchers derived features from Event Related Potentials (ERPs) in time domain (Allison and Polich, 2008; Brouwer et al., 2012) or used Common Spatial Patterns (Dijksterhuis et al., 2013) to discriminate workload levels. Workload level is typically assessed from subjective questionnaires or task difficulty. Sassaroli et al. (2008) placed fNIRS optodes on the forehead to measure concentration changes of oxyhemoglobin and deoxyhemoglobin in the prefrontal cortex during memory tasks and discriminated between three different levels of workload in three subjects. Similarly, Bunce et al. (2011) discriminate different workload levels for a complex Warship Commander Task, for which task difficulty was manipulated to create different levels of workload. They recorded fNIRS from 16 optodes at the dorsolateral prefrontal cortex and saw significant differences in oxygenation between low and high workload conditions. They also observed a difference in signal response to different difficulty settings for expert and novice users, which was mirrored by the behavioral data. Herff et al. (2014) showed that it is possible to classify different levels of n-back difficulty corresponding to different levels of mental workload on a single trials for prefrontal fNIRS signals with an accuracy of up to 78%. Hirshfield et al. (2009) combined EEG and fNIRS data for workload estimation in a counting task and saw better results for fNIRS in comparison to frequency based EEG-features. The authors reported surprisingly low accuracy for their EEG-based classifier and suspected problems with coverage of relevant sites and montage-specific artifacts. In contrast, Coffey et al. (2012) presented results from a similar study but showed worse results for the fNIRS features. From the available literature, it is hard to judge the relative discriminative power of the different signal types. On the one hand, Coffey et al. (2012) and Hirshfield et al. (2009) cover only a small aspect of general passive BCI research as they both concentrate on the classification of workload and use similar fNIRS montages. On the other hand, the experiments are too different to expect identical results (different cognitive tasks, different features, etc.). Therefore, there is too little data available for a final call on the synergistic potential between both modalities and their applicability to specific classification tasks. This paper contributes to an answer of this question by investigating a very different fNIRS montage, by including different types of EEG features to ensure adequate classification accuracy and by looking at a more specific aspect of cognitive activity, namely processing of different input modalities.

All the systems mentioned above modeled workload as a monolithic construct and did not classify the resource types which contributed to a given overall workload level. While there exist user studies, e.g., Heger et al. (2011), which show that it is possible to improve human-computer interaction using this construct, many use cases—like the mentioned selection between auditory and visual output modalities—require a more fine grained model of mental workload, like the already mentioned multiple resource theory (Wickens, 2008). Neural evidence from a study by Keitel et al. (2012) of subjects switching between bimodal and unimodal processing also indicated that cognitive resources for visual and auditory processing should be modeled separately. Most basic visual processing takes place in the visual cortex of the human brain, located in the occipital lobe, while auditory stimuli are processed in the auditory cortex located in the temporal lobes. This clear localization of important modality-specific areas in the cortex accessible for non-invasive sensors hints at the feasibility of separating both types of processing modes.

In this paper, we investigate how reliably a hybrid BCI using synchronous EEG and functional fNIRS signals can perform such classification tasks. We describe an experimental setup in which natural visual and auditory stimuli are presented in isolation and in parallel to the subject of which both EEG and fNIRS data is recorded. On a corpus of 12 recorded sessions, we train BCIs using features from one or both signal types to differentiate and detect the different perceptual modalities. This paper contributes a number of substantial findings to the field of passive BCIs for HCI: We trained and evaluated classifiers which can either discriminate between predominantly visual and predominantly auditory perceptual activity or which were able to detect visual and auditory activity independently of each other. The latter is ecologically important as many real-life tasks demand both visual and auditory resources. We showed that both types of classifiers achieved a very high accuracy both in a subject-dependent and subject-independent setup. We investigated the potential of combining different feature types derived from different signals to achieve a more robust and accurate recognition result. Finally, we look at the evaluation of the system on continuous data.

2. MATERIALS AND METHODS

2.1. PARTICIPANTS

Twelve healthy young adults (6 male, 6 female), age between 21 and 30 years (mean age 23.6, *SD* 2.6 years) without any known history of neurological disorders participated in this study. All of them have normal or corrected-to-normal visual acuity, normal auditory acuity, and were paid for their participation. The experimental protocol was approved by the local ethical committee of National University of Singapore, and performed in accordance with the policy of the Declaration of Helsinki. Written informed consent was obtained from all subjects and the nature of the study was fully explained prior to the start of the study. All subjects had previous experience with BCI operation or EEG/fNIRS recordings.

2.2. EXPERIMENTAL PROCEDURE

Subjects were seated in a sound-attenuated room with a distance of approximately one meter from a widescreen monitor (24″ BenQ XL2420T LED Monitor, 120 Hz, 1920 × 1080), which was equipped with two loudspeakers on both sides (DELL AX210 Stereo Speaker). During the experiment, subjects were presented with movie and audio clips, i.e., silent movies (no sound; `VIS`), audiobooks (no video; `AUD`), and movies with both video and audio (`MIX`). We have chosen natural, complex stimuli in contrast to more controlled, artificially generated stimuli to keep subjects engaged with the materials and to achieve a realistic setup.

Besides any stimulus material, the screen always showed a fixation cross. Subjects were given the task to look at the cross at all times to avoid an accumulation of artifacts. When there was no video shown, e.g., during audio clips and during rest periods, the screen pictured the fixation cross on a dark gray background. In addition to the auditory, visual and audiovisual trials, there were `IDLE` trials. During `IDLE`, we showed a dark gray screen with a fixation cross in the same way as during the rest period between different stimuli. Therefore, subjects were not be able to distinguish this condition from the rest period. In contrast to the rest periods, `IDLE` trials did not follow immediately after a segment of stimulus processing and can therefore be assumed to be free of fading cognitive activity. `IDLE` trials were assumed to not contain any systematic processing of stimuli. While subjects received other visual or auditory stimulations from the environment during `IDLE` trials, those stimulations were not task relevant and of lesser intensity compared to the prepared stimuli. In contrast to `AUD`, `VIS`, and `MIX` trials, there was no additional resting period after `IDLE` trials.

The entire recording, which had a total duration of nearly 1 h, consisted of five blocks. **Figure 1** gives an overview of the block design. The first block consisted of three continuous clips (60 s audio, 60 s video, 60 s audio and video with a break of 20 s between each of them. This block had a fixed duration of 3 min 40 s. The remaining four blocks had random durations of approximately 13 min each. The blocks 2–5 followed a design with random stimulus durations of 12.5 ± 2.5 s (uniformly distributed) and rest periods of 20 ± 5 s (uniformly distributed). The stimulus order of different modalities was randomized within each block. However, there was no two consecutive stimuli of the same modality. **Figure 2** shows an example of four consecutive trials in the experiment. Counted over all blocks, there were 30 trials of each category `AUD`, `VIS`, `MIX`, and `IDLE`.

The stimuli of one modality in one block formed a coherent story. During the experiment, subjects were instructed to memorize as much of these stories (`AUD`/`VIS`/`MIX` story) as possible. In order to ensure that subjects paid attention to the task, they filled out a set of multiple choice questions (one for each story) after each block. This included questions on contents, e.g., "what happens after…?", as well as general questions,

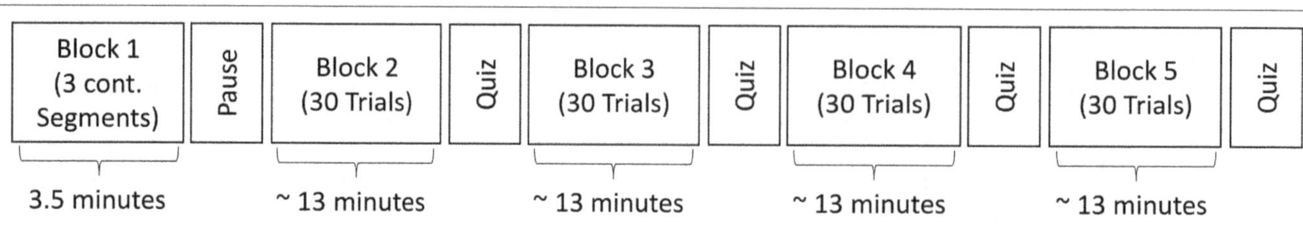

FIGURE 1 | Block design of the experimental setup.

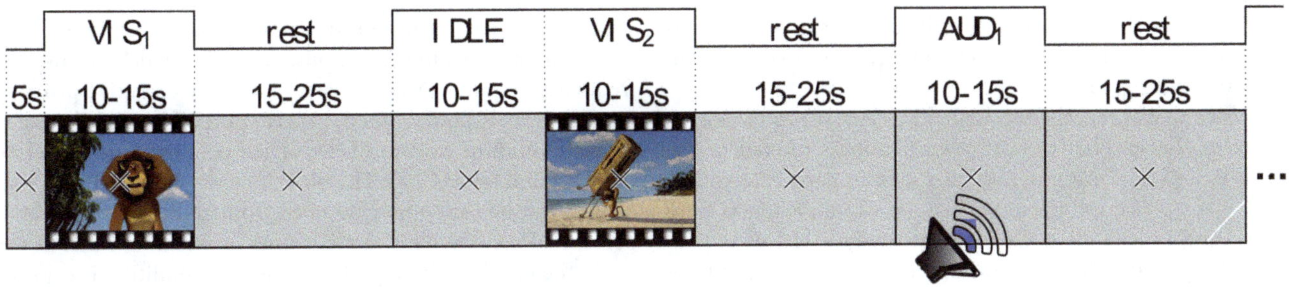

FIGURE 2 | Example of four consecutive trials with all perceptual modalities.

such as "how many different voices appeared?" or "what was the color of ...?". According to their answers, all subjects paid attention throughout the entire experiment. In the auditory condition, subjects achieved an averaged correct answer rate of 85%, whereas in the visual condition there is a correct answer rate of 82%.

2.3. DATA ACQUISITION

For fNIRS recording, a frequency-domain oximeter (Imagent, ISS, Inc., Champaign, IL, USA) was employed. Frequency-modulated near-infrared light from laser diodes (690 nm or 830 nm, 110 MHz) was conducted to the participants head with 64 optical source fibers (32 for each wavelength), pairwise co-localized in light source bundles. A rigid custom-made head-mount system (montage) was used to hold the source and detector fibers to cover three different areas on the head: one for the visual cortex and one on each side of the temporal cortex. The multi-distance approach as described in Wolf et al. (2003); Joseph et al. (2006) was applied in order to create overlapping light channels. **Figure 3** shows the arrangement of sources and detectors in three probes (one at the occipital cortex and two at the temporal lobe). For each probe, two columns of detectors were placed between two rows of sources each to the left and the right, at source-detector distances of 1.7–2.5 cm. See **Figure 3A** for the placement of the probes and **Figure 3B** for the arrangement of the sources and detectors. After separating source-detector pairs of different probes into three distinct areas, there were a total of 60 channels on the visual probe and 55 channels on each auditory probe. Thus, there was a total number of $n_c = 170$ channels. The sampling frequency used was 19.5 Hz.

EEG was simultaneously recorded with an asalab ANT neuro amplifier and digitized with a sampling rate of 256 Hz. The custom-made head-mount system, used for the optical fibers, also enabled us to place the following 12 Ag/AgCl electrodes according to the standard 10–20 system: Fz, Cz, Pz, Oz, O1, O2, FT7, FT8, TP7, TP8, M1, M2. Both M1, and M2 were used as reference.

After the montage was positioned, the locations of fNIRS optrodes, EEG electrodes, as well as the nasion, pre-auricular points and 123 random scalp coordinates were digitized with Visor (ANT BV) and ASA 4.5 3D digitizer. Using each subject's structural MRI, these digitized points were then coregistered, following Whalen et al. (2008), in order to have all subjects' data in a common space.

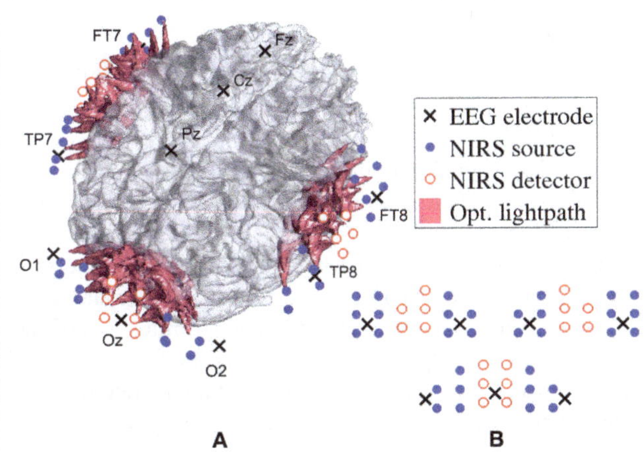

FIGURE 3 | Locations of EEG electrodes, fNIRS optrodes, and their corresponding optical lightpath. The arrangement of fNIRS sources and detectors is shown projected on the brain in **(A)** and as unwrapped schematic in **(B)** for the two auditory probes (top left and right) and the visual probe (bottom).

2.4. PREPROCESSING

The preprocessing of both fNIRS and EEG data were performed offline. Optical data included an AC, a DC, and a phase component; however, only the AC intensities were used in this study. Data from each AC channel were normalized by dividing it by its mean, pulse-corrected following Gratton and Corballis (1995), median filtered with a filter length of 8 s, and downsampled from 19.5 to 1 Hz. The downsampled optical density changes ΔOD_c were converted to changes in concentration of oxyhemoglobin (HbO) and deoxyhemoglobin (HbR) using the modified Beer-Lambert law (MBLL) (Sassaroli and Fantini, 2004).

The parameters for differential path-length factor and wavelength-dependent extinction coefficient within this study were based on standard parameters in the HOMER2 package, which was used for conversion process (Huppert et al., 2009). Values of molar extinction coefficients were taken from http://omlc.ogi.edu/spectra/hemoglobin/[1]. Finally, common average referencing (CAR) was applied to the converted data

[1]compiled by Scott Prahl using data from: W. B. Gratzer, Med. Res. Council Labs, Holly Hill, London, and N. Kollias, Wellman Laboratories, Harvard Medical School, Boston.

in order to reduce noise and artifacts that are common in all channels (Ang et al., 2012). Thereby, the mean of all channels is substracted from each individual channel c. It is performed on both ΔHbO and ΔHbR.

EEG data were preprocessed with EEGLAB 2013a (Delorme and Makeig, 2004). First the data was bandpass filtered in the range of 0.5–48 Hz using a FIR filter of standard filter order of 6 ($= \frac{3}{\text{low cutoff}} \cdot$ sampling rate). Then, non-brain artifacts were rejected using Independent Component Analysis (ICA) as proposed by Jung et al. (2000). In this process, all 10 channels were converted to 10 independent components. One component of each subject was rejected based on prefrontal eye blink artifacts. Finally, the prestimulus mean of 100 ms was substracted from all stimulus-locked data epochs.

2.5. GRAND AVERAGES

In the following, we calculate Grand Averages of both fNIRS and EEG signals (in time domain and frequency domain) for the different types of stimuli. This is done to investigate the general sensitivity of the signals to differences in modality and to motivate the feasibility of different feature types which we define later for classification.

Figure 4 shows the averaged haemodynamic response function (HRF) for selected channels of all 12 subjects for labels `AUD` (blue), `VIS` (red), and `IDLE` (black). The stimulus locked data trials (blocks 2–5) are epoched by extracting the first 10 s of each stimulus, and a 2 s prestimulus baseline was substracted from each channel. There was a clear peak in the HRF in response to a `VIS` stimulus on channels from the occipital cortex (channels 141 and 311 in the figure) and a return to baseline after the stimulus is over after 12.5 s. This effect is absent for an `AUD` stimulus. Conversely, the channels from the auditory cortex (channels 30 and 133 in the figure) react much stronger to a `AUD` than to a `VIS` stimulus.

Figure 5 shows the first second of ERP waveforms of conditions `AUD` (blue), `VIS` (red), and `IDLE` (black), averaged across all 12 subjects. It shows distinctive pattern for auditory and visual stimuli when comparing electrodes at the visual cortex with electrodes at more frontal positions. It is also widely known that frequency responses can be used to identify cognitive processes. **Figure 6** shows power spectral density on a logarithmic scale at a frontal midline position (Fz), at the ocipital cortex (Oz) and the temporal lobe (FT7). The plots indicate that especially visual activity can be easily discriminated from auditory activity an no perceptual activity. This fact becomes especially evident at electrode site Oz. The alpha peak for the `AUD` condition is expected, but unusually pronounced. We attribute this to the fact that the `VIS` stimuli are richer compared to the `AUD` stimuli as they often contain multiple parallel points of interest and visual attractors at once. The difference between `VIS` and `AUD` trials does also not only involve perceptual processes but also other aspects of cognition, as they differ in content, processing codes and other parameters. On the one hand, this is a situation specific to the scenario we employed. On the other hand, we argue that this difference between visual and auditory information processing pertains for most natural conditions. We will investigate this issue by looking at the discriminability of `AUD` and `IDLE` conditions and also at the influence of alpha power on overall performance.

2.6. CLASSIFICATION

In this study, we first aimed to classify auditory against visual perception processes. Second, we wanted to detect auditory or visual processes, i.e., we classify modality-specific activity vs. no activity. Third, we wanted to detect a certain perception process in presence of other perception processes.

To demonstrate the expected benefits of combining the fNIRS and EEG signals, we first explored two individual classifiers for each signal domain, before we examined their combination by estimating a meta classifier. The two individual fNIRS classifiers were based on the evoked deflection from baseline HbO (`HbO` classifier) and HbR (`HbR` classifier). The EEG classifiers were

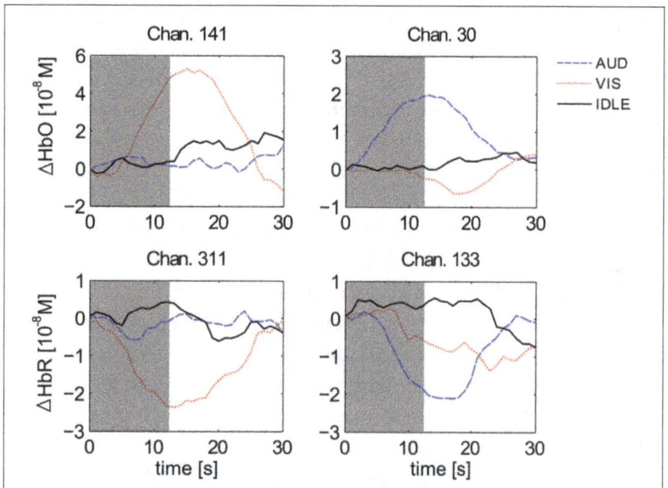

FIGURE 4 | Grand averaged HRFs of HbO (top) and HbR (bottom) for visual (left) and auditory (right) channels. Depicted are averages for the classes `AUD` (blue), `VIS` (red), and `IDLE` (black). The area shaded in gray marks the average duration of a stimulus presentation.

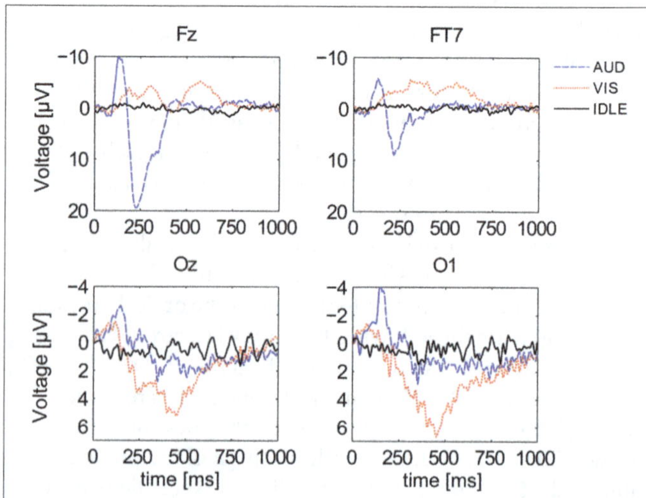

FIGURE 5 | Grand averaged ERPs of all 3 conditions at 4 different channel locations. Depicted are averages for the classes `AUD` (blue), `VIS` (red), and `IDLE` (black).

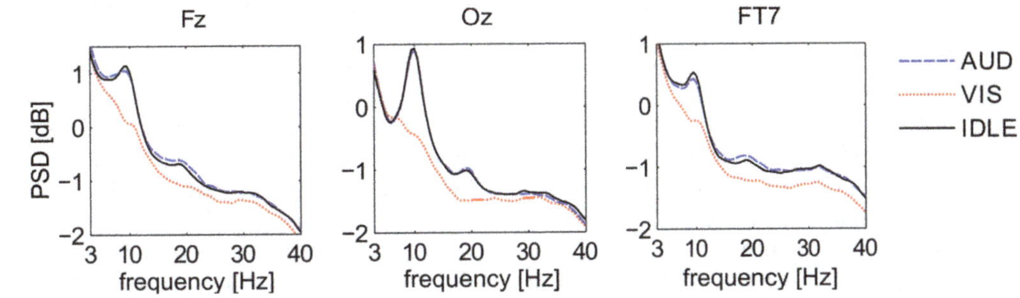

FIGURE 6 | Power Spectral Density of three EEG signals at Fz, Oz, FT7 for three different conditions. Depicted are averages for the classes AUD (blue), VIS (red), and IDLE (black).

based on induced band power changes (POW classifier) and the downsampled ERP waveform (ERP classifier).

2.6.1. fNIRS features

Assuming an idealized haemodynamic stimulus response, i.e., a rise in HbO (HbO features) and a decrease in HbR (HbR features), stimulus-locked fNIRS features were extracted by taking the mean of the first few samples (i.e., $t_{opt} - \frac{w}{2}, \ldots, t_{opt}$) substracted from the mean of the follwing samples (i.e., $t_{opt}, \ldots, t_{opt} + \frac{w}{2}$) in all channels c of each trial, similar to Leamy et al. (2011). Equation 1 illustrates how the feature was calculated.

$$f_c^{\mathrm{HbO}} = \frac{2}{w}\left(\sum_{t_{opt}}^{t_{opt}+\frac{w}{2}} \Delta\overline{[\mathrm{HbO}]}_c(t) - \sum_{t_{opt}-\frac{w}{2}}^{t_{opt}} \Delta\overline{[\mathrm{HbO}]}_c(t)\right)$$

$$f_c^{\mathrm{HbR}} = \frac{2}{w}\left(\sum_{t_{opt}}^{t_{opt}+\frac{w}{2}} \Delta\overline{[\mathrm{HbR}]}_c(t) - \sum_{t_{opt}-\frac{w}{2}}^{t_{opt}} \Delta\overline{[\mathrm{HbR}]}_c(t)\right) \quad (1)$$

2.6.2. EEG features

For POW, the entire 10 s of all 10 channels were transformed to the spectral domain using Welch's method, and every other frequency component in the range of 3–40 Hz was concatenated to a 38-dimensional feature vector per channel. ERP features were always based on the first second (onset) of each trial. First, the ERP waveform underlied a median filter ($k_{med} = 5 \approx 0.02$s), followed by a moving average filter ($k_{avg} = 13 \approx 0.05$s). A final downsampling of the resulting waveform ($k_{down} = k_{avg}$) produced a 20-dimensional feature vector for each channel.

In the end, all features, i.e., HbO, HbR, POW, and ERP, were standardized to zero mean and unit standard deviation (z-normalization).

Four individual classifiers were trained based upon these four different feature types. Each classifier yielded a probability distribution across (the two) classes. Using those individual class probability values, we further evaluated a META classifier, based on decision fusion: The META classifier was based on the weighted sum $p^{\mathrm{meta}} = \sum_m w_m \cdot p_m$ of the class probability values p_m of each of the four individual classifiers (m = HbO, HbR, POW, and ERP) with weight w_m. The class with higher p^{meta}, i.e., the maximum likelihood class, was then selected as the result of the META classifier.

The weights w_m were estimated based on the classification accuracy on evaluation data (i.e., labeled data which is not part of the training data but available when building the classifier). Specifically, those classification accuracies that were higher than baseline (pure chance, i.e., 0.5 for the balanced binary classification conditions) were linearly scaled to the interval [0, 1], while those that were below baseline were weighted with 0, and thus, not incorporated. Afterwards, the weight vector $\overline{w} = [w_{\mathrm{HbO}}, w_{\mathrm{HbR}}, w_{\mathrm{POW}}, w_{\mathrm{ERP}}]^T$ was divided by its 1-norm in order to sum all of its elements to 1.

For the first three classifiers (HbO, HbR, and POW) a regularized linear discriminant analysis (LDA) classifier was employed (implemented following, Schlogl and Brunner, 2008 with a shrinkage factor of 0.5, as determined on evaluation data), while a soft-margin linear support vector machine (SVM) was used for the ERP classifier (using the LibSVM implementation by Chang and Lin, 2011 with default parameters). This was done because we expected the first three feature sets to be normally distributed (i.e., LDA is optimal), while we expected the more complex and variable temporal patterns of an ERP to require a more robust classification scheme. Note that this design choice was validated by evaluating both types of classifiers for all types of features on a representative subset of the data corpus. This ensured that in the reported results we used the classifier which leads to the optimal classification accuracy for every feature set.

For evaluation of the proposed hybrid BCI, we define a number of binary classification tasks. We call each different classification task a *condition*. Classification was performed for each modality and feature type separately as well as for the combined META classifier. In the subject-dependent case, we applied leave-one-trial-out cross-validation (resulting in 60 folds for 60 trials per subject). To estimate parameters of feature extraction and classification (t_{opt} and w from Equation 1 for each fold, fusion weights w_m), we performed another nested 10-fold cross-validation (i.e., in each fold, we have 53 trials for training and 6 trials (5 trials in the last fold) for evaluation) for the train set of each fold. The averaged accuracy in the inner cross-validation is used for parameter selection in the outer cross-validation. This procedure avoided overfitting of the parameters to the training data. In the subject-independent case, we performed leave-one-subject-out cross-validation, resulting in a training set of 660 trials and a test set of 60 trials per fold.

To evaluate those classifiers for the discrimination and detection of modality-specific processing, we define a number of binary classification conditions. **Table 1** lists all defined classification conditions with the corresponding classes. All classification conditions are evaluated in a cross-validation scheme as described above. For each condition, we investigate both a subject-dependent classifier and a subject-independent classifier setup. As evaluation metric, we look at classification accuracy. Furthermore, we compare the performance of the individual classifiers (which only use one type of feature) with the META classifier and analyze the contribution of the two types of signals (EEG and fNIRS) to the different classification conditions. Additionally, we analyze the generalizability of the different detectors for modality-specific activity (lines 1–3 in **Table 1**) by evaluating the classifiers on trials with and without other independent perceptual and cognitive activity. Finally, we look at the classification performance on continuous data. For this purpose, we evaluate a subset of the classification conditions on windows extracted from continuous recordings without alignment to a stimulus onset.

3. RESULTS

Table 2 summarizes the recognition accuracy for all different conditions for the subject-dependent evaluation. The first entry is a discriminative task in which the classifier learns to separate visual and auditory perceptual activity. We see that for all four individual classifiers, a reliable classification is possible, albeit EEG-based features perform much better (HbO: 79.4% vs. POW: 93.6%). The fusion of all four classifiers, META, yields the best performance, significantly better (paired, one-sided t-test, $\alpha = 0.05$ with Bonferroni-Holm correction for multiple comparisons) than the best individual classifier by a difference 4.2% absolute. This is in line with the results of the meta analysis by D'Mello and Kory (2012), who found modest, but consistent improvements by combining different modalities for the classification of inner states. **Figure 7** shows a detailed breakdown of recognition results across all subjects for the example of AUD vs. VIS. We see that for every subject, recognition performance for every feature type was above the trivial classification accuracy of 50% and the performance of META was above 80% for all subjects.

In the next step, we evaluated subject-independent classification on the same conditions. The results are presented in **Table 3**. Averaged across all conditions, classification accuracy degrades by 6.5% compared to the subject-dependent results, resulting from higher variance caused by individual differences. Still, we managed to achieve robust results for all conditions, i.e., subject-independent discrimination visual and auditory processes is feasible. We therefore decided to report subsequent analyses for the subject-independent systems as those are much preferable from an HCI perspective.

The AUD vs. VIS condition denotes a discriminination task, i.e., it classifies a given stimulus as either auditory or visual. However, for an HCI application, those two processing modes are not mutually exclusive as auditory and visual perception can occur in parallel and can also be both absent in idle situations. We therefore need to define conditions which train a detector for specific perceptual activity, independently of the presence or absence of the other modality. Our first approach toward such a detector for auditory or visual perceptual activity is to define the AUD vs. IDLE and the VIS vs. IDLE conditions. A classifier trained on these conditions should be able to identify neural activity induced by the specific perceptual modality. In **Tables 2, 3**, we see that those conditions can be classified with high accuracy of 95.6% and 96.4% (subject-dependent), respectively. To test whether this neural activity can still be detected in the presence of other perceptual processes, we evaluate the classifiers trained on those conditions also on MIX trials. We would expect a perfect classifier to classify each of those MIX trials as VIS for the visual detector and AUD for the auditory detector. The top two rows of **Table 4** summarize the results and show that the classifier still correctly detects the modality it is trained for in most cases.

A problem of those conditions is that it is not clear that a detector trained on them has actually detected specific visual or auditory activities. Instead, it may be the case that it has detected general cognitive activity which was present in both the AUD and VIS trials, but not in the IDLE trials. To analyze this possibility, we evaluated the classifier of the AUD vs. IDLE condition on VIS trials (and accordingly for VIS vs. IDLE evaluated on AUD). We present the results in the bottom two rows of **Table 4**. Both classifiers were very inconsistent in their results and

Table 1 | Binary classification conditions for evaluation.

Condition	Class 1	Class 2
AUD vs. VIS	AUD	VIS
AUD vs. IDLE	AUD	IDLE
VIS vs. IDLE	VIS	IDLE
allAUD vs. nonAUD	AUD, MIX	VIS, IDLE
allVIS vs. nonVIS	VIS, MIX	AUD, IDLE

For each condition, we list the class labels which define the corresponding classes.

Table 2 | Stimulus-locked classification accuracies (in %) for *subject-dependent* classification.

	HbO	HbR	POW	ERP	META	p
AUD vs. VIS	79.4 (2.5)	74.3 (3.3)	93.6 (1.6)	93.3 (1.6)	**97.8*** (0.7)	0.006
AUD vs. IDLE	80.0 (2.7)	74.7 (3.1)	71.9 (3.0)	91.4 (1.7)	**95.6*** (1.6)	0.028
VIS vs. IDLE	83.8 (2.7)	78.1 (3.3)	90.7 (1.7)	81.9 (2.8)	**96.4*** (0.9)	0.002
allAUD vs. nonAUD	67.2 (3.1)	62.8 (3.3)	69.7 (2.0)	85.9 (1.7)	**89.0*** (1.5)	0.003
allVIS vs. nonVIS	68.5 (2.9)	64.7 (2.9)	91.5 (1.9)	81.9 (1.9)	**94.8*** (1.3)	0.019
Average	75.8	70.9	83.5	86.9	94.7	–

An asterisk in the META column indicates a significant improvement ($\alpha = 0.05$) over the best corresponding individual feature type. Given in parantheses are standard errors of the mean. The last column indicates the p value of the statistical comparison of META and the best single-feature classifier. Highest classification accuracy for each condition is given in bold font.

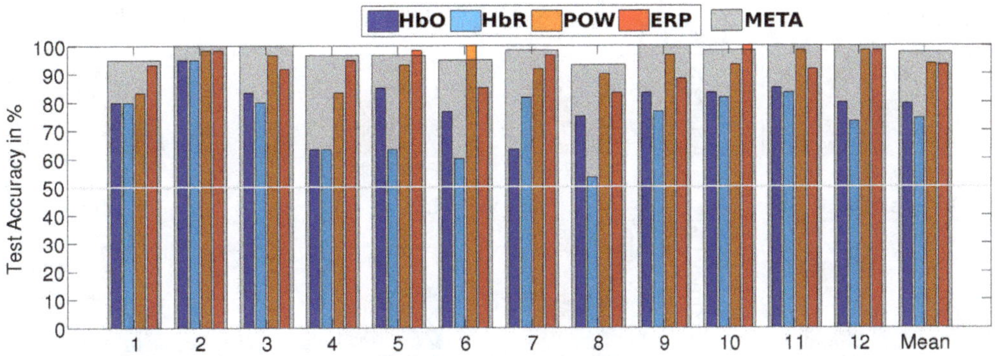

FIGURE 7 | Stimulus-locked recognition rates of AUD vs. VIS for subject-dependent, as well as for subject-independent classification. Recognition rates of the META classifier are indicated by a gray overlay on top of the individual classifiers' bars.

Table 3 | Stimulus-locked classification accuracies (in %) for *subject-independent* classification.

	HbO	HbR	POW	ERP	META	*p*
AUD vs. VIS	70.3 (2.2)	65.7 (2.2)	84.3 (2.2)	90.4 (1.3)	**94.6*** (1.3)	0.02
AUD vs. IDLE	64.0 (1.9)	61.9 (1.6)	66.1 (1.4)	84.2 (2.1)	**86.9*** (2.0)	0.002
VIS vs. IDLE	72.2 (2.8)	69.0 (4.0)	82.5 (2.9)	75.3 (2.6)	**89.9*** (1.8)	0.01
allAUD vs. nonAUD	60.6 (2.0)	58.8 (1.4)	41.7 (7.2)	**85.6** (2.1)	84.7 (1.3)	0.85
allVIS vs. nonVIS	62.7 (2.6)	62.0 (2.6)	84.2 (1.9)	73.1 (2.8)	**86.7*** (1.4)	0.003
Average	66.0	63.5	71.8	81.7	88.6	–

An asterisk in the META column indicates a significant improvement ($\alpha = 0.05$) over the best corresponding individual feature type. Given in parantheses are standard errors of the mean. The last column indicates the p value of the statistical comparison of META and the best single-feature classifier. Highest classification accuracy for each condition is given in bold font.

Table 4 | Subject-independent classification accuracy of classifiers (in %) for AUD vs. IDLE and VIS vs. IDLE, evaluated on different trials from outside the respective training set.

Trained on...	Evaluated on...	HbO	HbR	POW	ERP	META
AUD vs. IDLE	MIX	67.1	63.6	47.5	88.6	88.4
VIS vs. IDLE	MIX	69.3	68.4	69.0	84.7	77.6
AUD vs. IDLE	VIS	66.3	66.7	52.6	48.8	48.5
VIS vs. IDLE	AUD	59.5	61.4	49.3	50.5	48.2

"detected" modality-specific activity in nearly half of the trials, which actually did not contain such activity.

To train a classifier which is more sensitive for the modality-specific neural characteristics, we needed to include non-IDLE trials in the training data as negative examples. For this purpose, we defined the condition allAUD vs. nonAUD, where the allAUD class was defined as allAUD = {AUD, MIX} and the nonAD was defined as nonAUD = {IDLE, VIS}. Now, allAUD

Table 5 | Subject independent correct classification rate (in %) and confusion matrix for the allAUD vs. nonAUD and the allVIS vs. nonVIS conditions, broken down by original labels.

	AUD	VIS	IDLE	MIX
allAUD	328	53	54	278
nonAUD	32	307	306	82
% correct	91.1	85.3	85.0	77.2
allVIS	65	339	64	318
nonVIS	295	21	296	42
% correct	81.9	84.2	82.2	88.3

contains all data with auditory processing, while nonAUD contained all data without, but potentially with other perceptual activity. The condition allVIS vs. nonVIS was defined analogously. **Tables 2, 3** document that a detector trained on these conditions was able to achieve a high classification accuracy. This result shows that the new detectors did not only learn to separate general activity from a resting state (as did the detectors defined earlier). If that would have been the case, we would have seen a classification accuracy of 75% or less: For example, if we make this assumption in the allVIS vs. nonVIS condition, we would expect 100% accuracy for the VIS, MIX and IDLE trials, and 0% accuracy for the AUD trials, which would be incorrectly classified as they contain general activity but none which is specific to visual processing. This baseline of 75% is outperformed by our classifiers for detection. This result indicates that we were indeed able to detect specific perceptual activity, even in the presence of other perceptual processes. For additional evidence, we look at how often the original labels (AUD, VIS, IDLE, MIX) were classified correctly in the two new detection setups by the META classifier. The results are summarized in **Table 5** as a confusion matrix. We see that all classes are correctly classified in more than 75% of all cases, indicating that we detected the modality-specific characteristics in contrast to general cognitive activity.

The results we presented in **Tables 2, 3** indicate that fusion was useful to achieve a high recognition accuracy. Still, there was a remarkable difference between the results achieved by the

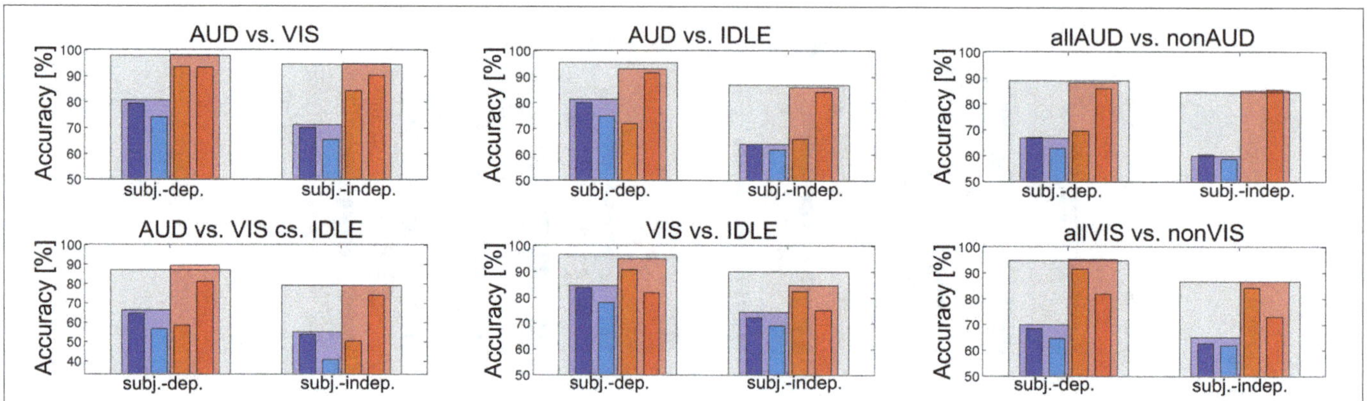

FIGURE 8 | fNIRS-META (red) vs. EEG-META (blue) evaluated for both subject-dependent and subject-independent classification for different conditions.

classifiers using fNIRS features and by classifiers using EEG features. This was true across all investigated conditions and for both subject dependent and subject independent classification. We suspect that the advantage of the META classifier was mostly due to the combination of the two EEG based classifiers. In **Figure 8**, we investigated this question by comparing two fusion classifiers EEG-META and fNIRS-META which combined only the two fNIRS features or the two EEG features, respectively. The results show that for the majority of the conditions, the EEG-META classifier performed as good as or even better than the overall META classifier. However, the fNIRS features contributed significantly to the classification accuracy for both conditions AUD vs. IDLE and VIS vs. IDLE ($p = 0.003$ and $p = 0.01$, respectively for the difference of EEG-META and META in the subject-dependent case).

To exclude that the difference was due to the specific fNIRS feature under-performing in this evaluation, we repeated the analysis with other established fNIRS features (average amplitude, value of largest amplitude increase or decrease). The analysis showed that we could not achieve improvements by exchanging fNIRS feature calculation compared to the original feature. We conclude that the difference in accuracy was not caused by decisions during feature extraction. Overall, we see that fNIRS-based features were outperformed by the combination of EEG based features for the most investigated conditions but that it could still contribute to a high classification accuracy in some of the cases.

There are however some caveats to the dominance of EEG features. First, the ERP classifier is the only one of the four feature types which is fundamentally dependent on temporal alignment to the stimulus onset and therefore not suited for many applications of continuous classification. While the employed fNIRS features also use information on the stimulus onset (as they essentially characterize the slope of the signal), only the ERP features rely on specific oscillatory properties in a range of milliseconds (compare **Figures 5** and **4**), which cannot be extracted reliably without a stimulus locking. Second, concerning the POW classifier, we see in **Figure 6** a large difference in alpha power between VIS and AUD. As both types of trials induce cognitive activity, we did not expect the AUD trials to exhibit alpha power (i.e., idling rhythm) nearly at an IDLE level. We cannot completely rule out that this effect is caused at least in parts by the experimental design (e.g., because visual stimuli and auditory stimuli differed in complexity) or subject selection (e.g., all subjects were familiar with similar recording setups and therefore easily relaxed). Therefore, we need to verify that the discrimination ability of the POW classifier does not solely depend on differences in alpha power. For that purpose, we repeated the evaluation of AUD vs. VIS with different sets of band pass filters, of which some excluded the alpha band completely. Results are summarized in **Figure 9**. We see that as expected, feature sets including the alpha band performed best. Accuracy dropped by a maximum of 9.4% relative when removing the alpha band (for the subject dependent evaluation from 1–40 Hz to 13–40 Hz). This indicates the upper frequency bands still contain useful discriminating information.

The previous analysis showed that different features contributed to different degrees to the classification result. Therefore, we were interested in studying which features were stable predictors of the ground truth labels on a single trial basis. The successful person-independent classification was already an indication that such stable, generalizable features exist. To investigate which features contributed to the detection of different modalities, we calculated the correlation of each feature with the ground truth labels for the conditions VIS vs. IDLE and AUD vs. IDLE.

For the POW features, we ranked the electrode by their highest absolute correlation across the whole frequency range for each subject. To see which features predicted the ground truth well across all subjects, we averaged those ranks. The resulting average rankings are presented in the first two columns of **Table 6**. We note that for the VIS vs. IDLE condition, electodes at the occipital cortex were most strongly correlated to the ground truth. In contrast, for the AUD vs. IDLE condition, those electrodes can be found at the bottom of the ranking. For this condition, the highest ranking electrodes were at the central-midline (it was expected that electrodes above the auditory cortex would not contribute strongly to the AUD vs. IDLE condition as activity in the auditory cortex cannot be captured well by EEG). The low *SD* also indicates that the derived rankings are stable across subjects. We can therefore conclude that the POW features were generalizable and neurologically plausible.

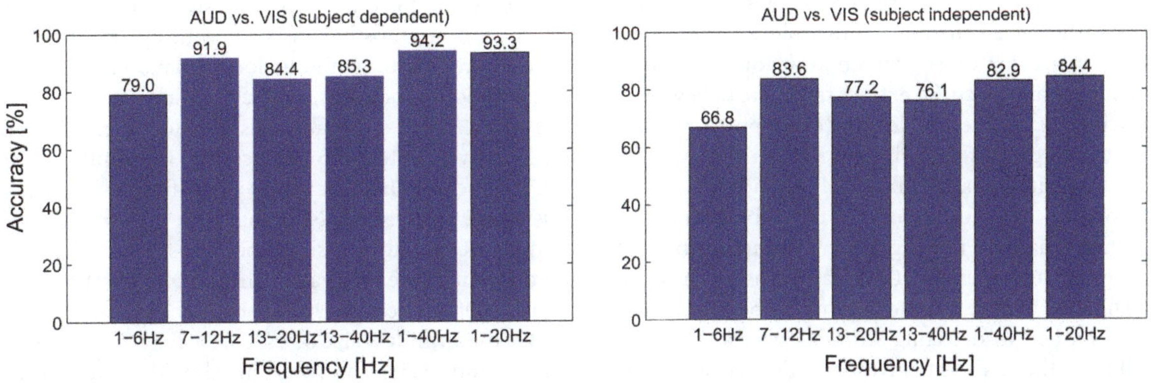

FIGURE 9 | Classification accuracy for different filter boundaries for the POW feature set, evaluated for both subject-dependent (left half) and subject-independent (right half) classification for different conditions.

Table 6 | Average rankings of electrode positions derived from correlation of POW and ERP features to ground truth labels.

Rank	VIS vs. IDLE	AUD vs. IDLE	VIS vs. IDLE	AUD vs. IDLE
1	Oz (2.5)	Pz (2.3)	O1 (2.6)	Cz (3.0)
2	O2 (2.2)	Cz (2.4)	O2 (2.9)	Fz (1.4)
3	Pz (2.2)	Fz (1.7)	Oz (3.1)	Pz (3.0)
4	TP8 (3.2)	TP8 (2.3)	TP8 (3.0)	TP7 (2.7)
5	TP7 (2.8)	TP7 (1.9)	Fz (2.2)	FT8 (2.7)
6	Fz (3.4)	FT7 (3.0)	TP7 (2.9)	TP8 (2.3)
7	O1 (1.5)	O2 (2.8)	Pz (3.1)	FT7 (2.4)
8	Cz (2.2)	FT8 (3.0)	Cz (2.3)	O1 (0.8)
9	FT8 (3.6)	O1 (3.3)	FT7 (2.6)	Oz (1.6)
10	FT7 (2.4)	Oz (2.6)	FT8 (3.0)	O2 (2.1)

Table 7 | Resulting *p*-values for Friedman tests to investigate whether the calculated average feature rankings are statistically significant.

Feature	Condition	Ranking by ...	*p*-value
ERP	AUD vs. IDLE	Electrodes	$< 10^{-5}$
ERP	AUD vs. IDLE	Time windows	$< 10^{-10}$
ERP	VIS vs. IDLE	Electrodes	0.12
ERP	VIS vs. IDLE	Time windows	$< 10^{-10}$
POW	AUD vs. IDLE	Electrodes	$< 10^{-3}$
POW	AUD vs. IDLE	Frequency bands	$< 10^{-10}$
POW	VIS vs. IDLE	Electrodes	$< 10^{-2}$
POW	VIS vs. IDLE	Frequency bands	$< 10^{-10}$

We then ranked the frequency band features by their highest absolute correlation across the whole electrode set for each subject and average those ranks across subjects. We observed the highest average ranks at 9.5 Hz and at 18.5 Hz. Especially for the first peak in the alpha band, we observed a low *SD* of 6.2, which indicates that those features were stable across subjects.

For the ERP features, we repeated this analysis (with time windows in place of frequency bands). The two rightmost columns of **Table 6** show a similar picture as for the POW features regarding the contribution of individual electrodes: Features from electrodes at the occipital cortex were highly discriminative in the VIS vs. IDLE condition, features from central-midline electrodes carried most information in the AUD vs. IDLE condition. Regarding time windows, we observe the best rank for the window starting at 312 ms, which corresponds well to the expected P300 component following a stimulus onset. With a *SD* of 2.9, this feature was also ranked highly across all subjects.

To investigate the reliability of the derived rankings, we conducted Friedman tests on the rankings of all participants. Those showed that all investigated rankings (with one exception) yielded a significant difference in average ranks of the items. The resulting *p*-values are given in **Table 7**. This indicates that the rankings actually represent a reliable, person-independent ordering of features.

The analysis for fNIRS features differed from the EEG feature analysis because of the signal characteristics. For example, the fNIRS channels were spatially very close to each other and highly correlated. Therefore, we did not look at features from single fNIRS channels. Instead, we differentiated between the different probes. For the VIS vs. IDLE condition, the channel which yielded the highest absolute correlation was located above the visual cortex for 75% of all subjects (averaged across both HbO and HbR). For the AUD vs. IDLE condition, the channel with the highest absolute correlation was located above the auditory cortex for 91.6% of all subjects. This indicates that the fNIRS signals also yielded neurologically plausible features which generalized well across subjects. When comparing HbO and HbR features, the HbO features were correlated slightly higher to the ground truth (19.6% higher maximum correlation) than the HbR features, which corresponds to their higher classification accuracy.

The classification setups which we investigated up to this point are all defined on trials which are locked at the onset of a stimulus. The detection of onsets of perceptual activity is an important use case for HCI applications: The onset of a perceptual activity often marks a natural transition point to react to a change of user state. On the other hand, there are use cases where the detection of ongoing perceptual activity is relevant. To investigate how the implemented classifiers perform on continuous stimulus presentation, we evaluated classification and detection on the three continuous segments (60 s of each AUD, VIS, MIX) which were recorded in the first block for each subject. As data is sparse for those segments, we only regard the subject-independent approach. To extract trials, the data was segmented into windows of a certain length (overlapping by 50%). We evaluated the impact of the window size on the classification accuracy: For window sizes of 1, 2, 4, 8, and 16 s, we end up with 120, 60, 30, 15, and 8 windows per subject and class, respectively. Those trials are not aligned to a stimulus onset. We used the same procedure to extract POW features as for the onset-locked case. The ERP feature was the basis of the best non-fusion classifier but is limited to detecting stimulus onsets. Therefore, we excluded it from the analysis to investigate the performance of the remaining classifiers. For both feature types based on fNIRS, we modified the feature extraction to calculate the mean of the window, normalized by the mean of the already elapsed data. The other aspects of the classifier were left unchanged.

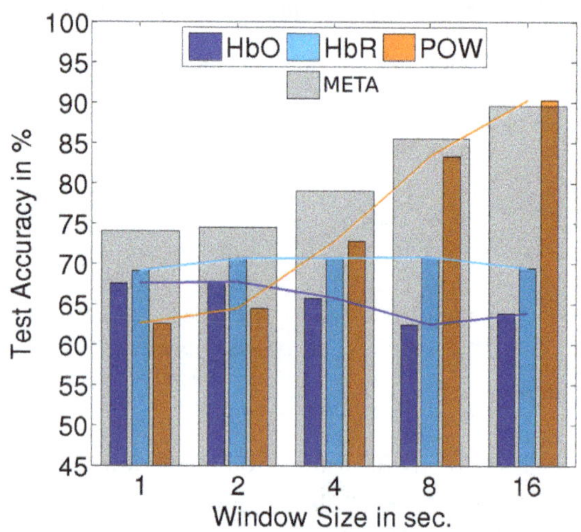

FIGURE 10 | Accuracy for subject-independent classification of AUD vs. VIS on continuous data. Results are in dependency of window size.

Figures 10, 11 summarize the results of continuous evaluation. The results are mostly consistent with our expectations and the previous results on stimulus-locked data. For all three regarded classification conditions, we achieve an accuracy of more than 75% for META, i.e., reliable classification does not solely depend on low-level bottom-up processes at the stimulus onset. Up to the threshold of 16 s, there was a benefit of using larger windows for feature calculation. Note that with growing window size, the number of trials for classification drops, which also has an impact on the confidence interval for the random baseline (Mueller-Putz et al., 2008). The upper limit of the 1% confidence interval is 52.4% for a window size of 1 s, 53.4% for 2 s, 54.9% for 4 s, 56.9% for 8 s, and 59.5% for 16 s. This should be kept in mind when interpreting the results, especially for larger window sizes. The EEG feature yields a better classification accuracy than the two fNIRS-based classifiers in two of the three cases. For the allAUD vs. nonAUD situation however, the POW classifier does not exceed the random baseline and only the two fNIRS based classifiers can achieve satisfactory results. Therefore, we see that when ERP features are missing in the continuous case, the fNIRS features can substantially contribute to classification accuracy in the case of allAUD vs. nonAUD.

4. DISCUSSION

The results from the previous section indicate that both the discrimination and detection of modality-specific perceptual processes in the brain is feasible both in a subject-dependent as well as a subject-independent setup with high recognition accuracy. We see that the fusion of multiple features from different signal types led to improvement in recognition accuracy significantly. However, in general fNIRS-based features were outperformed by features based on the EEG signal. In the future, we will look closer into other reasons for this gap and potential remedies for it. One difference between fNIRS and EEG signals is the lack of advanced artifact removal techniques for fNIRS that have been applied with some success in other research on fNIRS BCIs (Molavi and Dumont, 2012). Another difference is that the coverage of fNIRS optodes was limited mainly to the sensory areas, but our

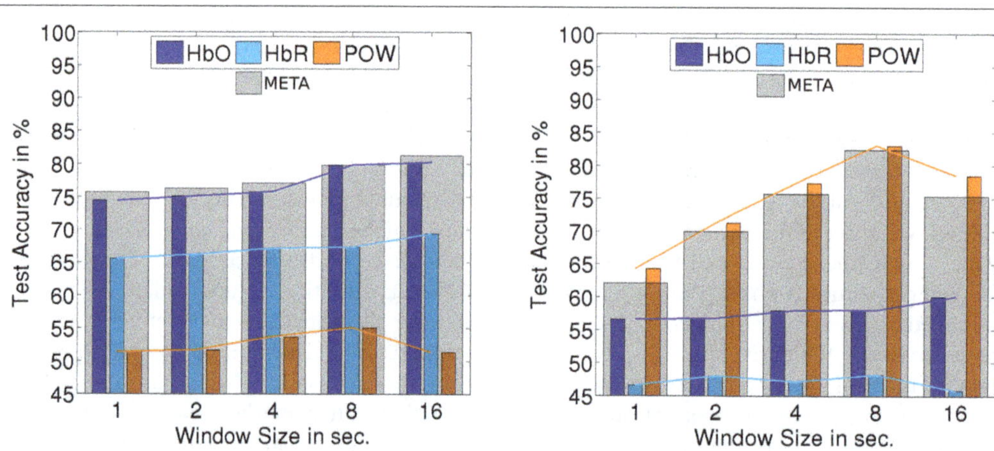

FIGURE 11 | Accuracy for subject-independent classification of allAUD vs. nonAUD (left) and allVIS vs. nonVIS (right) on continuous data. Results are in dependency of window size.

EEG measures may include robust effects generated from other brain regions, such as the frontal-parietal network. Activities in these regions may be reflecting higher cognitive processes triggered by the different modalities, other than purely perceptual ones. It may be worthwhile to extend the fNIRS setup to include those regions as well. Still, we already saw that fNIRS features can contribute significantly to certain classification tasks. While evaluation on stimulus-locked data allows a very controlled evaluation process and is supported by the very high accuracy we can achieve, this condition is not very realistic for most HCI applications. In many cases, stimuli will continue over longer periods of time. Features like the ERP feature explicitly model the onset of a perceptual process but will not provide useful information for ongoing processes. In future work, we will investigate such continuous classification on the longer, continuous data segments of the recorded corpus.

Following the general guidelines of Fairclough (2009), one limitation in validity of the present study is the fact that there may be other confounding variables that can explain the differences in the observed neurological responses to the stimuli of different modalities. Subjects were following the same task for all types of stimuli; still, factors like different memory load or increased need for attention management due to multiple parallel stimuli for visual trials may contribute to the separability of the classes. We address this partially by identifying the expected effects, for example in **Figure 4** comparing fNIRS signals from visual and auditory cortex. Also the fact that detection of both visual and auditory processing worked on MIX trials shows that the learned patterns were not only present in the dedicated data segments but were to some extend generalizable. Still, we require additional experiments with different tasks and other conditions to reveal whether it is possible to train a fully generalizable detector and discriminator for perceptual processes. Finally, we also have to look into a more granular model with a higher sensitivity than the presented dichotomic characterization of perceptual workload.

The evaluation was performed in a laboratory setting but with natural and complex stimulus material. The results indicate that such a system is robust enough to use it for the improvement an HCI system in a realistic scenario. We saw that both EEG and fNIRS contributed to a high classification accuracy; in most cases, the results for the EEG-based classifiers were more accurate than for the fNIRS based ones. Whether the additional effort which is required to apply and evaluate a hybrid BCI (compared to a BCI with only one signal type) depends on the specific application. When only one specific classification condition is relevant (e.g., to detect processing of visual stimuli), there is always a single optimal signal type which is sufficient to achieve robust classification. The benefit of a hybrid system is that it can potentially cover multiple different situations for which no generally superior signal type exists. Another aspect for the applicability of the presented system for BCI is the response latency, which also depends on the choice of employed features. The ERP features react very rapidly to but are limited to situations, in which a stimulus onset is present. Such short response latency (less than 1 s) may be useful when an HCI system needs to immediately switch communication channels or interrupt communication to avoid perceptual overload of the user (for example, when the user unexpectedly engages in a secondary task besides communicating with the HCI system). In such situations, the limitation to onsets is also not problematic. On the other hand, if the system needs to assume that the user is already engaged in a secondary task when it starts to observe him or her (i.e., to determine the initial communication channel at the beginning of a session), it is not sufficient anymore to only respond to stimulus onsets. For those cases, it may be worthwhile to accept the latency required by the fNIRS features and also the POW feature for a classification of continuous perceptual activity.

We conclude that we demonstrated the first passive hybrid BCI for the discrimination and detection of perceptual activity. We showed that robust classification is possible both in a subject-dependent and a subject-independent fashion. While the EEG features outperformed the fNIRS features for most parts of the evaluation, the fusion of multiple signals and features was beneficial and increased the versatility of the BCI.

ACKNOWLEDGMENTS

This work was supported by the IGEL (Informatik-GrEnzenLos) scholarship of the KIT. We are also thankful to Prof. Trevor Penney of the National University of Singapore for providing access to the fNIRS system used in this project as well as the staff and students from Temasek Lab at NUS (Kian Wong, Tania Kong, Xiao Qin Cheng, and Xiaowei Zhou) for their intensive support throughout the entire data collection. We acknowledge support by Deutsche Forschungsgemeinschaft and Open Access Publishing Fund of Karlsruhe Institute of Technology.

REFERENCES

Allison, B. Z., and Polich, J. (2008). Workload assessment of computer gaming using a single-stimulus event-related potential paradigm. *Biol. Psychol.* 77, 277–283. doi: 10.1016/j.biopsycho.2007.10.014

Ang, K. K., Yu, J., and Guan, C. (2012). "Extracting effective features from high density nirs-based BCI for assessing numerical cognition," in *Acoustics, Speech and Signal Processing (ICASSP), 2012 IEEE International Conference on* (Kyoto: IEEE), 2233–2236.

Brouwer, A.-M., Hogervorst, M. A., van Erp, J. B. F., Heffelaar, T., Zimmerman, P. H., and Oostenveld, R. (2012). Estimating workload using EEG spectral power and ERPs in the n-back task. *J. Neural Eng.* 9:045008. doi: 10.1088/1741-2560/9/4/045008

Bunce, S. C., Izzetoglu, K., Ayaz, H., Shewokis, P., Izzetoglu, M., Pourrezaei, K., et al. (2011). "Implementation of fNIRS for monitoring levels of expertise and mental workload," in *Foundations of Augmented Cognition. Directing the Future of Adaptive Systems, Number 6780 in Lecture Notes in Computer Science*, eds D. D. Schmorrow and C. M. Fidopiastis (Berlin, Heidelberg: Springer), 13–22.

Cao, Y., Theune, M., and Nijholt, A. (2009). "Modality effects on cognitive load and performance in high-load information presentation," in *Proceedings of the 14th International Conference on Intelligent User Interfaces, IUI '09* (New York, NY: ACM), 335–344.

Chang, C.-C., and Lin, C.-J. (2011). LIBSVM: a library for support vector machines. *ACM Trans. Intell. Syst. Technol.* 2, 27:1–27:27. doi: 10.1145/1961189.1961199

Coffey, E. B. J., Brouwer, A.-M., and Erp, J. B. F. v. (2012). Measuring workload using a combination of electroencephalography and near infrared spectroscopy. *Proc. Hum. Fact. Ergonom. Soc. Ann. Meeting* 56, 1822–1826. doi: 10.1177/1071181312561367

Delorme, A., and Makeig, S. (2004). EEGLAB: an open source toolbox for analysis of single-trial eeg dynamics including independent component analysis. *J. Neurosci. Methods* 134, 9–21. doi: 10.1016/j.jneumeth.2003.10.009

Dijksterhuis, C., Waard, D. d., and Mulder, B. L. J. M. (2013). Classifying visuomotor workload in a driving simulator using subject specific spatial brain patterns. *Front. Neurosci.* 7:149. doi: 10.3389/fnins.2013.00149

D'Mello, S., and Kory, J. (2012). "Consistent but modest: a meta-analysis on unimodal and multimodal affect detection accuracies from 30 studies," in *Proceedings of the 14th ACM International Conference on Multimodal Interaction* (Santa Monica, CA: ACM), 31–38.

Fairclough, S. H. (2009). Fundamentals of physiological computing. *Inter. Comput.* 21, 133–145. doi: 10.1016/j.intcom.2008.10.011

Fazli, S., Mehnert, J., Steinbrink, J., Curio, G., Villringer, A., Müller, K.-R., et al. (2012). Enhanced performance by a hybrid NIRS–EEG brain computer interface. *Neuroimage* 59, 519–529. doi: 10.1016/j.neuroimage.2011.07.084

Gratton, G., and Corballis, P. M. (1995). Removing the heart from the brain: compensation for the pulse artifact in the photon migration signal. *Psychophysiology* 32, 292–299. doi: 10.1111/j.1469-8986.1995.tb02958.x

Heger, D., Putze, F., and Schultz, T. (2010). "Online workload recognition from eeg data during cognitive tests and human-machine interaction," in *KI 2010: Advances in Artificial Intelligence* (Karlsruhe: Springer), 410–417.

Heger, D., Putze, F., and Schultz, T. (2011). An EEG adaptive information system for an empathic robot. *Int. J. Soc. Robot.* 3, 415–425. doi: 10.1007/s12369-011-0107-x

Herff, C., Heger, D., Fortmann, O., Hennrich, J., Putze, F., and Schultz, T. (2014). Mental workload during n-back taskquantified in the prefrontal cortex using fNIRS. *Front. Hum. Neurosci.* 7:935. doi: 10.3389/fnhum.2013.00935

Hirshfield, L. M., Chauncey, K., Gulotta, R., Girouard, A., Solovey, E. T., Jacob, R. J. K., et al. (2009). "Combining electroencephalograph and functional near infrared spectroscopy to explore users mental workload," in *Foundations of Augmented Cognition. Neuroergonomics and Operational Neuroscience, Number 5638 in Lecture Notes in Computer Science*, eds D. D. Schmorrow, I. V. Estabrooke, and M. Grootjen (Berlin, Heidelberg: Springer), 239–247.

Huppert, T. J., Diamond, S. G., Franceschini, M. A., and Boas, D. A. (2009). Homer: a review of time-series analysis methods for near-infrared spectroscopy of the brain. *Appl. Opt.* 48, D280–D298. doi: 10.1364/AO.48.00D280

Joseph, D. K., Huppert, T. J., Franceschini, M. A., and Boas, D. A. (2006). Diffuse optical tomography system to image brain activation with improved spatial resolution and validation with functional magnetic resonance imaging. *Appl. Opt.* 45, 8142–8151. doi: 10.1364/AO.45.008142

Jung, T.-P., Makeig, S., Westerfield, M., Townsend, J., Courchesne, E., and Sejnowski, T. J. (2000). Removal of eye activity artifacts from visual event-related potentials in normal and clinical subjects. *Clin. Neurophysiol.* 111, 1745–1758. doi: 10.1016/S1388-2457(00)00386-2

Keitel, C., Maess, B., Schröger, E., and Müller, M. M. (2012). Early visual and auditory processing rely on modality-specific attentional resources. *Neuroimage* 70, 240–249. doi: 10.1016/j.neuroimage.2012.12.046

Kothe, C. A., and Makeig, S. (2011). "Estimation of task workload from eeg data: new and current tools and perspectives," in *Engineering in Medicine and Biology Society, EMBC, 2011 Annual International Conference of the IEEE* (Boston, MA: IEEE), 6547–6551.

Leamy, D. J., Collins, R., and Ward, T. E. (2011). "Combining fNIRS and EEG to improve motor cortex activity classification during an imagined movement-based task," in *Foundations of Augmented Cognition. Directing the Future of Adaptive Systems* (Orlando, FL: Springer), 177–185. doi: 10.1007/978-3-642-21852-1-22

Molavi, B., and Dumont, G. A. (2012). Wavelet-based motion artifact removal for functional near-infrared spectroscopy. *Physiol. Meas.* 33, 259–270. doi: 10.1088/0967-3334/33/2/259

Mueller-Putz, G., Scherer, R., Brunner, C., Leeb, R., and Pfurtscheller, G. (2008). Better than random: a closer look on BCI results. *Int. J. Bioelectromagn.* 10, 52–55.

Pfurtscheller, G., Allison, B. Z., Brunner, C., Bauernfeind, G., Solis-Escalante, T., Scherer, R., et al. (2010). The hybrid BCI. *Front. Neurosci.* 4:30. doi: 10.3389/fnpro.2010.00003

Sassaroli, A., and Fantini, S. (2004). Comment on the modified BeerLambert law for scattering media. *Phys. Med. Biol.* 49, N255. doi: 10.1088/0031-9155/49/14/N07

Sassaroli, A., Zheng, F., Hirshfield, L. M., Girouard, A., Solovey, E. T., Jacob, R. J. K., et al. (2008). Discrimination of mental workload levels in human subjecs with functional near–infrared spectroscopy. *J. Innov. Opt. Health Sci.* 01, 227–237. doi: 10.1142/S1793545808000224

Schlogl, A., and Brunner, C. (2008). Biosig: a free and open source software library for bci research. *Computer* 41, 44–50. doi: 10.1109/MC.2008.407

Sitaram, R., Zhang, H., Guan, C., Thulasidas, M., Hoshi, Y., Ishikawa, A., et al. (2007). Temporal classification of multichannel near-infrared spectroscopy signals of motor imagery for developing a brain–computer interface. *Neuroimage* 34, 1416–1427. doi: 10.1016/j.neuroimage.2006.11.005

Spüler, M., Bensch, M., Kleih, S., Rosenstiel, W., Bogdan, M., and Kübler, A. (2012). Online use of error-related potentials in healthy users and people with severe motor impairment increases performance of a p300-BCI. *Clin. Neurophysiol.* 123, 1328–1337. doi: 10.1016/j.clinph.2011.11.082

Turk, M. (2014). Multimodal interaction: a review. *Patt. Recogn. Lett.* 36, 189–195. doi: 10.1016/j.patrec.2013.07.003

Whalen, C., Maclin, E. L., Fabiani, M., and Gratton, G. (2008). Validation of a method for coregistering scalp recording locations with 3d structural mr images. *Hum. Brain Mapp.* 29, 1288–1301. doi: 10.1002/hbm.20465

Wickens, C. D. (2008). Multiple resources and mental workload. *Hum. Factors* 50, 449–455. doi: 10.1518/001872008X288394

Wolf, M., Wolf, U., Choi, J. H., Toronov, V., Adelina Paunescu, L., Michalos, A., et al. (2003). Fast cerebral functional signal in the 100-ms range detected in the visual cortex by frequency-domain near-infrared spectrophotometry. *Psychophysiology* 40, 521–528. doi: 10.1111/1469-8986.00054

Wolpaw, J. R., McFarland, D. J., Neat, G. W., and Forneris, C. A. (1991). An eeg-based brain-computer interface for cursor control. *Electroencephalogr. Clin. Neurophysiol.* 78, 252–259. doi: 10.1016/0013-4694(91)90040-B

Wolpaw, J. R., and Wolpaw, E. W. (2012). *Brain-Computer Interfaces: Principles and Practice.* Oxford; New York: Oxford University Press.

Yang, Y., Reimer, B., Mehler, B., Wong, A., and McDonald, M. (2012). "Exploring differences in the impact of auditory and visual demands on driver behavior," in *Proceedings of the 4th International Conference on Automotive User Interfaces and Interactive Vehicular Applications, AutomotiveUI '12* (New York, NY: ACM), 173–177.

Zander, T. O., and Kothe, C. (2011). Towards passive brain–computer interfaces: applying brain–computer interface technology to human–machine systems in general. *J. Neural Eng.* 8:025005. doi: 10.1088/1741-2560/8/2/025005

Permissions

All chapters in this book were first published by Frontiers; hereby published with permission under the Creative Commons Attribution License or equivalent. Every chapter published in this book has been scrutinized by our experts. Their significance has been extensively debated. The topics covered herein carry significant findings which will fuel the growth of the discipline. They may even be implemented as practical applications or may be referred to as a beginning point for another development.

The contributors of this book come from diverse backgrounds, making this book a truly international effort. This book will bring forth new frontiers with its revolutionizing research information and detailed analysis of the nascent developments around the world.

We would like to thank all the contributing authors for lending their expertise to make the book truly unique. They have played a crucial role in the development of this book. Without their invaluable contributions this book wouldn't have been possible. They have made vital efforts to compile up to date information on the varied aspects of this subject to make this book a valuable addition to the collection of many professionals and students.

This book was conceptualized with the vision of imparting up-to-date information and advanced data in this field. To ensure the same, a matchless editorial board was set up. Every individual on the board went through rigorous rounds of assessment to prove their worth. After which they invested a large part of their time researching and compiling the most relevant data for our readers.

The editorial board has been involved in producing this book since its inception. They have spent rigorous hours researching and exploring the diverse topics which have resulted in the successful publishing of this book. They have passed on their knowledge of decades through this book. To expedite this challenging task, the publisher supported the team at every step. A small team of assistant editors was also appointed to further simplify the editing procedure and attain best results for the readers.

Apart from the editorial board, the designing team has also invested a significant amount of their time inunderstanding the subject and creating the most relevant covers. They scrutinized every image to scout for the most suitable representation of the subject and create an appropriate cover for the book.

The publishing team has been an ardent support to the editorial, designing and production team. Their endless efforts to recruit the best for this project, has resulted in the accomplishment of this book. They are a veteran in the field of academics and their pool of knowledge is as vast as their experience in printing. Their expertise and guidance has proved useful at every step. Their uncompromising quality standards have made this book an exceptional effort. Their encouragement from time to time has been an inspiration for everyone.

The publisher and the editorial board hope that this book will prove to be a valuable piece of knowledge for researchers, students, practitioners and scholars across the globe.

List of Contributors

Alberto Betella, Riccardo Zucca, Ryszard Cetnarski, Xerxes D. Arsiwalla and Pedro Omedas
Synthetic, Perceptive, Emotive and Cognitive Systems group (SPECS), Universitat Pompeu Fabra, Barcelona, Spain

Alberto Greco, Antonio Lanatà, Alessandro Tognetti and Danilo De Rossi
Research Centre "E. Piaggio", University of Pisa, Pisa, Italy
Information Engineering Department, University of Pisa, Pisa, Italy

Daniele Mazzei
Research Centre "E. Piaggio", University of Pisa, Pisa, Italy

Paul F. M. J. Verschure
Synthetic, Perceptive, Emotive and Cognitive Systems group (SPECS), Universitat Pompeu Fabra, Barcelona, Spain
ICREA, Institució Catalana de Recerca i Estudis Avançats, Barcelona, Spain

Maarten A. Hogervorst
TNO Human Factors, Netherlands Organisation for Applied Scientific Research, Soesterberg, Netherlands
TNO, Perceptual and Cognitive Systems, Soesterberg, Netherlands

Ricardo Chavarriaga, Aleksander Sobolewski and José del R. Millán
Defitech Chair in Non-Invasive Brain-Machine Interface, Center for Neuroprosthetics, School of Engineering, Ecole Polytechnique Fédérale de Lausanne, Lausanne, Switzerland

Chris Dijksterhuis, Dick de Waard, Ben L. J. M. Mulder and Ritske de Jong
Department of Psychology, University of Groningen, Groningen, Netherlands

Tzyy-Ping Jung
Swartz Center for Computational Neuroscience, Institute for Neural Computation, University of California, San Diego, La Jolla, CA, USA
Department of Bioengineering, Jacobs School of Engineering, University of California San Diego, La Jolla, CA, USA
Center for Advanced Neurological Engineering, Institute of Engineering in Medicine, University of California, San Diego, La Jolla, CA, USA

Karel A. Brookhuis
Department of Psychology, University of Groningen, Groningen, Netherlands
Department of Infrastructure Systems and Services, Delft University of Technology, Delft, Netherlands

Yu-Te Wang
Department of Computer Science and Engineering, Jacobs School of Engineering, University of California San Diego, La Jolla, CA, USA
Swartz Center for Computational Neuroscience, Institute for Neural Computation, University of California San Diego, La Jolla, CA, USA

Kuan-Chih Huang, Teng-Yi Huang and Chin-Teng Lin
Department of Electrical Engineering, National Chiao-Tung University, Hsinchu, Taiwan

Chun-Shu Wei
Swartz Center for Computational Neuroscience, Institute for Neural Computation, University of California San Diego, La Jolla, CA, USA
Department of Bioengineering, Jacobs School of Engineering, University of California San Diego, La Jolla, CA, USA

Chung-Kuan Cheng
Department of Computer Science and Engineering, Jacobs School of Engineering, University of California San Diego, La Jolla, CA, USA
Center for Advanced Neurological Engineering, Institute of Engineering in Medicine, University of California San Diego, La Jolla, CA, USA

Chih-Sheng Huang and Chin-Teng Lin
Brain Research Center, National Chiao-Tung University, Hsinchu, Taiwan
Institute of Electrical Control Engineering, National Chiao-Tung University, Hsinchu, Taiwan

Chun-Ling Lin
Brain Research Center, National Chiao-Tung University, Hsinchu, Taiwan
Department of Electrical Engineering, Ming Chi University of Technology, New Taipei City, Taiwan

Li-Wei Ko
Brain Research Center, National Chiao-Tung University, Hsinchu, Taiwan
Institute of Bioinformatics and Systems Biology, National Chiao-Tung University, Hsinchu, Taiwan
Department of Biological Science and Technology, National Chiao-Tung University, Hsinchu, Taiwan

Shen-Yi Liu and Tung-Ping Su
Brain Research Center, National Chiao-Tung University, Hsinchu, Taiwan
Department of Psychiatry, Taipei Veterans General Hospital, Taipei, Taiwan

Lawrence A. Farwell
Brain Fingerprinting Laboratories, Inc./Brain Fingerprinting, LLC, Seattle, WA, USA

Drew C. Richardson
Federal Bureau of Investigation, FBI Laboratory, Quantico, VA, USA

Graham M. Richardson
Department of Cell and Developmental Biology, Vanderbilt University, Nashville, TN, USA

John J. Furedy
Department of Psychology, University of Toronto, Toronto, ON, Canada

Jaime A. Pineda
Department of Cognitive Science, University of California, San Diego, La Jolla, CA, USA
Neurosciences Group, University of California, San Diego, La Jolla, CA, USA

Mark Grichanik, Vanessa Williams, Michelle Trieu and Hailey Chang
Department of Cognitive Science, University of California, San Diego, La Jolla, CA, USA

Christian Keysers
Netherlands Institute for Neuroscience, KNAW, Amsterdam, Netherlands
Department of Neuroscience, University Medical Center Groningen, University of Groningen, Netherlands

Christian Mühl
Institut National de Recherche en Informatique et en Automatique, Bordeaux Sud-Ouest, Talence, France

Camille Jeunet
Institut National de Recherche en Informatique et en Automatique, Bordeaux Sud-Ouest, Talence, France
Laboratoire Handicap et Système Nerveux, University of Bordeaux, Bordeaux, France

Fabien Lotte
Institut National de Recherche en Informatique et en Automatique, Bordeaux Sud-Ouest, Talence, France
Laboratoire Bordelais de Recherche en Informatique (LaBRI), Talence, France

Yi-Hsuan Yang
Music and Audio Computing Lab, Research Center for IT Innovation, Academia Sinica, Taipei, Taiwan

Yuan-Pin Lin
Swartz Center for Computational Neuroscience, Institute for Neural Computation, University of California, San Diego, La Jolla, CA, USA
Center for Advanced Neurological Engineering, Institute of Engineering in Medicine, University of California, San Diego, La Jolla, CA, USA

Koji Kashihara
Information Solution, Institute of Technology and Science, The University of Tokushima, Tokushima, Japan

Megan Strait and Matthias Scheutz
Human-Robot Interaction Laboratory, Department of Computer Science, Tufts University, Medford, MA, USA

Anne-Marie Brouwer
TNO Human Factors, Netherlands Organisation for Applied Scientific Research, Soesterberg, Netherlands
TNO, Perceptual and Cognitive Systems, Soesterberg, Netherlands
Perceptual and Cognitive Systems, Netherlands Organisation for Applied Scientific Research TNO, Soesterberg, Netherlands

Thorsten O. Zander
Team PhyPA, Biological Psychology and Neuroergonomics, Technical University Berlin, Berlin, Germany

Jan B. F. van Erp
Perceptual and Cognitive Systems, Netherlands Organisation for Applied Scientific Research TNO, Soesterberg, Netherlands
Human Media Interaction, Twente University, Enschede, Netherlands
TNO Human Factors, Netherlands Organisation for Applied Scientific Research, Soesterberg, Netherlands

Johannes E. Korteling
Training Performance Innovations, Netherlands Organisation for Applied Scientific Research TNO, Soesterberg, Netherlands

Adelbert W. Bronkhorst
Perceptual and Cognitive Systems, Netherlands Organisation for Applied Scientific Research TNO, Soesterberg, Netherlands
Cognitive Psychology, VU University, Amsterdam, Netherlands

Benny van der Vijgh and Maarten van Rood
Buys Ballot Laboratory, Department of Information and Computing Sciences, Utrecht University, Utrecht, Netherlands
Department of Neurology and Neurosurgery, University Medical Center Utrecht, Utrecht, Netherlands

Robbert J. Beun and Peter Werkhoven
Buys Ballot Laboratory, Department of Information and Computing Sciences, Utrecht University, Utrecht, Netherlands

Peter Gerjets
Hypermedia Lab, Knowledge Media Research Center, Tübingen, Germany

Carina Walter and Wolfgang Rosenstiel
Department of Computer Engineering, University of Tübingen, Tübingen, Germany

Martin Bogdan
Department of Computer Engineering, University of Tübingen, Tübingen, Germany
Department of Computer Engineering, University of Leipzig, Leipzig, Germany

Felix Putze, Sebastian Hesslinger, Christian Herff and Tanja Schultz
Cognitive Systems Lab, Institute of Anthropomatics and Robotics, Karlsruhe Institute of Technology, Karlsruhe, Germany

Chun-Yu Tse
Department of Psychology, Center for Cognition and Brain Studies, The Chinese University of Hong Kong, Hong Kong, China
Temasek Laboratories, National University of Singapore, Singapore, Singapore

YunYing Huang
Nuffield Department of Clinical Neurosciences, John Radcliffe Hospital, Oxford, UK

Cuntai Guan
Institute for Infocomm Research (I2R), A*STAR, Singapore, Singapore

Index

www.ingramcontent.com/pod-product-compliance
Lightning Source LLC
LaVergne TN
LVHW082213200926
848484LV00008B/2249